Healthcare Delivery in the Information Age

Series Editor
Nilmini Wickramasinghe
STE 406, Chicago, IL
USA

The healthcare industry is uniquely structured so that the receiver of the services (the patient) often isn't the predominant payer for those services (the insurance company). Healthcare interventions are often complex and typically involve multiple players including providers, payers, patients and regulators. This leads to economic dilemmas such as moral hazard, information asymmetry, and tangential considerations of cost versus quality creating obstacles on the road to delivering efficient and effective healthcare. Relevant data, pertinent information, and germane knowledge play a vital role in relieving these problems and can be most effectively obtained via prudently structured and well designed healthcare technology. Some of the major challenges facing today's healthcare organizations include demographic (longer life expectancy and an aging population), technology (incorporating advances that keep people healthier), and financial (escalating costs technological innovation) problems. In order to realize technology's full potential it is imperative to understand the healthcare-technology paradigm, develop sustainability models for the effective use of technology in a specific context, then successfully design and implement patient-centric technology solutions. Many of the problems with technology are connected to the platform-centric nature of these systems which cannot support seamless transfer of data and information, leading to inferior healthcare delivery. This new series focuses on designing effective and efficient technologically enabled healthcare processes to support the delivery of superior healthcare and provide better access, quality and value. It's main goal will be to identify the barriers and facilitators in moving from idea generation to concept realization and will navigate the key challenges in the field: bringing readers solutions and recommendations while identifying key factors in developing technology-enabled healthcare solutions.

More information about this series at http://www.springer.com/series/8783

Nilmini Wickramasinghe • Indrit Troshani
Joseph Tan
Editors

Contemporary Consumer Health Informatics

Springer

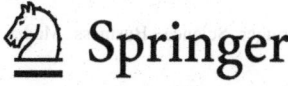

Editors
Nilmini Wickramasinghe
Deakin University and Epworth HealthCare
Victoria
Australia

Joseph Tan
McMaster University
Hamilton
Canada

Indrit Troshani
The University of Adelaide
South Australia
Australia

ISSN 2191-5946 ISSN 2191-5954 (electronic)
Healthcare Delivery in the Information Age
ISBN 978-3-319-79868-4 ISBN 978-3-319-25973-4 (eBook)
DOI 10.1007/978-3-319-25973-4

Springer Cham Heidelberg New York Dordrecht London

Softcover reprint of the hardcover 1st edition 2016

Printed on acid-free paper

Springer International Publishing AG Switzerland is part of Springer Science+Business Media (www.springer.com)

For our families
This series is dedicated to Leo Cussen:
Learned scholar, colleague extraordinaire
and good friend.

Foreword

Healthcare is in a time of crisis with no country able to meet future needs doing things the way they have been done in the past. The combination of increasing age accompanied by a rapid advance in chronic diseases coupled with a declining birthrate points to a shortage of medical professionals' right when they are needed the most. Clearly, new thinking is in order. Fortunately, information technology (IT) is available in various forms and context to help in creating and implementing new ways of thinking to meet the healthcare needs of the future. As such, this is a very important and timely book.

Countries around the world are struggling with aspects of *contemporary consumer health informatics* in making sensible and sustainable use of IT. The authors do an exemplary job in bringing issues to the fore with well developed reasoning and suggestions for solution covered in a series of well thought-out chapters. The area and issues are extremely diverse as the chapters bring to notice. Numerous disciplines are involved, not always in agreement. The relevant stakeholders cover the gamut from individual citizens to the World Health Organization. To address this wide range of issues and stakeholders is not easy and the authors have done an exemplary job.

Ultimately, quality of life is a global goal which can be brought about by improving healthcare. IT plays a crucial role as an enabler in effectively and efficiently implementing healthcare solutions. In this sense, informatics is pivotal in bridging IT with prospective healthcare implementation, that is, getting systems used and useful for those intended. However, all is not without problems. As with any new way of thinking, disruptions to the traditional way of doing things need to be taken into consideration and sensitively dealt with. Many stakeholders are likely not even aware of the entrenched nature of doing things that is in contradiction with healthcare innovation.

Education is a critical success factor in attaining the objectives noted in the chapters. With appropriate education, enhanced healthcare can be achieved and made sustainable in a cost-effective fashion through the intelligent application of IT and associated systems. Contemporary Consumer Health Informatics is a step in that direction with expectations of use in a variety of educational settings. As such, this book can be seminal in assisting in the kind of changes in thinking that are critical to a bright healthcare future.

Doug Vogel
Association for Information Systems Fellow and Past President
eHealth Research Institute Director
School of Management
Harbin Institute of Technology, China

Preface

Over the past decade, the traditional doctor–patient relationship has been shifting to a more consultative scenario as the patient/consumer increasingly takes on a more active role in understanding, managing and making decisions about his/her health. Further, as many areas across the globe continue to face shortages of medical professionals, there is a shift towards helping those needing care to somehow help themselves. IT sits at the centre of these shifts. Increasingly, consumers rely on IT-enabled applications to access health information, resources and tools. This phenomenon has been called consumer health informatics (CHI).

CHI has become a key branch of medical informatics and incorporates key concepts and constructs from various disciplines including: nursing informatics, public health, information systems, psychology, health promotion, health education, library science and communication science to name a few. Critical to CHI is a patient-centric focus. CHI uses technology to support and analyse health consumers' needs for information, support health-related decision-making and provide resources supporting self-care. CHI systems run a wide gamut from personal health records, health-related websites, smartphone and IPad apps, monitoring devices and social networking for healthcare purposes. Research in this growing area strives to study, recommend and implement methods for making information accessible to consumers. Research and practice also seek to model and integrate consumers' preferences in the design and development of health technologies, which may be either independent or interconnected to clinical systems.

The introduction of IT into healthcare delivery and especially e-health solutions are representative of disruptive technologies that are challenging key traditional relationships in healthcare such as the: provider–patient, payer–patient, provider–healthcare organisation and patient–policy maker. CHI takes a socio-technical perspective and delves deep into the underlying people, process and technology perspectives and thereby helps us fully understand the impacts of the tools, techniques, technologies and tactics of today's information age on healthcare delivery. Without such an in depth and detailed assessment of all the implications of information communication technologies (ICT) on the web of healthcare players it is not possible for healthcare delivery to address the current challenges of escalating costs, changing population demographics and impacts of key disease such as chronic diseases and still provide a healthcare value proposition of excellence. Such an assessment, must also recognise that healthcare, to a great extent, is a function of local culture, norms and practices, which presents both a challenge and opportunity for CHI to facilitate the realisation of value-driven healthcare delivery for all healthcare systems. Therefore, there is a need to know (and, thereby a need for a point of entry resource) for those engaged in health information systems research and practice to develop, at minimum, a foundational understanding of CHI. This book tries at least in part to fill this void.

Contemporaneous with the growth of CHI in practice and research, we are also witnessing, unsurprisingly, a growth in courses and degrees, which are beginning to be offered in this domain, some of which are funded by national health informatics efforts. These courses vary in breadth and depth of coverage but one unifying challenge at present is the lack of a comprehensive learning resource that attempts to capture all the key aspects, challenges, barriers and facilitators to facilitate a fuller and appropriate understanding of this important unique field. Once more, we hope this publication will meet this need too. Thus, we believe not only is such a book timely, it is and will be a key resource for both practitioner and student as well as academic, consultant and general public as we all try to grapple, manage and thrive with this new and evolving area of CHI.

The book consists of 25 chapters that cover many different perspectives of CHI. For instance, many chapters focus on mobile technology solutions for diabetes management, weight and fitness considerations, for example, chapters by Hamper, Kouliev et al, Wickramasinghe and Goldberg. While other considerations regarding mobile solutions are explored by Edirisinghe et al., Sako et al., Kou and Wickramasinghe and Dos et al. Other technologies that are significant in the CHI domain include web technologies, e-health and social media. These are central in the respective discussions contained in the chapters by Gururajan et al., Blooma et al., Troshani and Wickramasinghe, Kordzadeh and Hadyan et al. Finally, recognising that consumers of health informatics are varied and divergent several chapters examine specific contexts and solutions such as nursing, for example, Wickramasinghe et al or oncology, for example, Wickramasinghe et al. or they look at critical issues to ensure such solutions will be successful including Ramprasad and Syn, Bozan, Alotaibi and Alkhattabi, Han-Lin et al. and Mogimi and Wickramasinghe. Taken together these chapters provide a comprehensive view of many of the critical issues in CHI and also serve to highlight the breadth of this nascent field.

We are only just witnessing the impacts of CHI and in the next decades this field will grow and expand and hopefully provide superior healthcare to all. We hope our readers will enjoy this compilation of chapters we have provided and find it informative, interesting and inspire them to explore this field further.

The Editors
Nilmini Wickramasinghe
Indrit Troshani
Joseph Tan

References

Esenbach, G. (2000). Consumer health informatics. *British Medical Journal, 320*(7251):1713–1716

Hersey, J. C., Matheson, J., Lohr, K. N. (1997). Consumer health informatics and patient decision-making. Rockville: Agency for Health Care Policy and Research (AHCPR research report No 98-N001.)

Greenes, R. A., Shortliffe, E. H. (1990). Medical informatics. An emerging academic discipline and institutional priority. *Journal of the American Medical Association, 263*:1114–1120.

Shortliffe, E. H., Perrault, L. (1990). Medical informatics: Computer applications in health care. Reading: Addison-Wesley.

Van Bemmel, J. H., Musen, M. A. (1997). Handbook of medical informatics. Heidelberg: Springer.

Coulter, A. (1999). Paternalism or partnership? Patients have grown up—and there's no going back. *British Medical Journal, 319:*719–720.

Eysenbach, G., Sa, E. R., Diepgen, T. L. (1999). Shopping around the Internet today and tomorrow: Towards the millennium of cybermedicine. *British Medical Journal, 319.* Full version: www.bmj.com/cgi/content/full/319/7220/1294. Accessed 31 May 2000.

Smith, R. (1997). The future of healthcare systems. *British Medical Journal, 314:*1495–1496.

Ferguson, T. (1997). Health online and the empowered medical consumer. *Joint Committee Journal on Quality Improvement, 23:*251–257.

Acknowledgements

This book would not have been possible without the assistance, cooperation and support of many people: the contributors, reviewers, our respective institutions, our colleagues, students, families, friends and staff at Springer. We thank you all and appreciate all your efforts in helping us make this book come to be.

Contents

About the Editors

Prof. Nilmini Wickramasinghe (Ph.D.; M.B.A.; Grad.Dip.Mgt.St.; B.Sc. Amus.A, piano; Amus.A, violin) has a well-recognised research record in the field of healthcare and IT/IS. Her expertise is in the strategic application and management of technology for effecting superior healthcare solutions. She currently is the professor director of Health Informatics Management at Epworth HealthCare and a professor at Deakin University.

Dr. Indrit Troshani is a Senior Lecturer in Information Systems at the University of Adelaide Business School. He holds a PhD from Edith Cowan University (Western Australia) and an MSc (Sunderland, UK). His research interests include adoption and diffusion of network innovations and mobile services in healthcare and financial services industry. His work has been published in several journals including Information Technology & People, Electronic Markets, Journal of Computer Information Systems, Journal of Engineering and Technology Management and Industrial Management & Data Systems.

Prof. Joseph Tan specialises in innovative design, implementation and diffusion of advancing e-technology to improve health services delivery system efficiencies and effectiveness. Professor Tan's research interests cut across multiple disciplines, with emphasis on the application of strategic e-business and e-health models to improve health systems operational efficiencies, individual or group decision effectiveness and community health behaviours. He teaches health IT project management and special topics in e-Health.

Chapter 1
Reliability of Qualitative Data Using Text Analysis: A Queensland Health Case Study

Raj Gururajan, Kevin Clark, Susan Moller, Prema Sankaran, Abdul Hafeez Baig, Nilmini Wickramasinghe and Rashmi Gururajan

Background

Analytics is the process of developing insights or recommendations for actions from historical data (Sharda et al. 2013). Analytics represents a combination of management sciences, computer technology and statistical techniques to identify and solve real-life issues. While there are many views to analytics, in the health domain, there are four major components discussed: descriptive, prescriptive, diagnostic and predictive analytics (Banerjee et al. 2013). Descriptive analytics investigates what has happened and explores issues related to past events. Diagnostics analytics explores why an event has occurred and provides possible causes for such an occurrence. Prescriptive analytics provides reasons as to what should be done about what has happened or about an event occurrence. Predictive analytics discusses matters that are likely to happen.

The modern view of these four components of analytics may differ across interest groups, but these appear to be followed in many health organisations. While quantitative data has been used to anchor these views in the past, in recent years, especially

R. Gururajan (✉) · K. Clark · S. Moller · P. Sankaran · A. Hafeez Baig
60 Baker Ave, Kew East 3102, Australia
e-mail: gururaja@usq.edu.au

K. Clark
e-mail: Kevin.Clark@health.qld.gov.au

P. Sankaran
e-mail: premsank@gmail.com

A. Hafeez Baig
e-mail: abdulhb@usq.edu.au

N. Wickramasinghe
Deakin University and Epworth HealthCare, 60 Baker Ave, Kew East 3102, Australia
e-mail: n.wickramasinghe@deakin.edu.au

R. Gururajan
Medical Student, Monash University, Melbourne, Australia

N. Wickramasinghe et al. (eds.), *Contemporary Consumer Health Informatics*,
Healthcare Delivery in the Information Age, DOI 10.1007/978-3-319-25973-4_1

in public health agencies, qualitative data may be used to complement quantitative data in decision-making processes. There appear to be two main reasons for the notion that qualitative data is also essential in major decision-making processes. The first reason is the involvement of many stakeholders commenting on various service quality provisions using social media, as well as internal data gathering forums. The second reason is that there is a general notion that the quantitative data collection process is quite restrictive and may not capture all aspects of stakeholder views.

While the involvement of many stakeholders is encouraging, there is also a dangerous possibility that the data could be diluted because of varying views, especially in unstructured forms of data collection. Therefore, assuring reliability and validity is essential. While many techniques, such as the reliability analysis, are available in quantitative data, researchers normally use 'saturation' as a reliability surrogate in qualitative data. We used analytics to provide reliability and validity in qualitative data analysis.

Health Text Analytics

Text analytics refers to deriving high-quality information from text, usually using methods that involve structuring of input text. For example, an unstructured data source can be made available to an application for analyses, and a set of arbitrary patterns based on keywords can be developed, resulting in an output. This process is called text analytics and typically involves tasks such as text categorisation, text clustering and concept extraction. While these processes have been followed in many text analyses, the major difference between text analysis and text analytics is the opportunity to unearth insights and extract value out of information. Unearthing insights requires a comprehensive understanding of the context, stakeholders, their emotional aspects, the problem or issue on hand and the ability to articulate these as part of the analysis leading to text analytics.

In this study, we applied text analytics to a set of interviews conducted in a public service agency in Queensland, Australia. The interviews were conducted in many wards with varying functionalities and mainly explored a technology implementation.

The scope of the study is restricted to Queensland Health (QH) and the implementation of a radically new technology called the 'Patient Journey Board' (PJB). The PJB is a touch-screen technology where patient data are consolidated so that carers such as doctors, nurses and allied health professionals can see the data in an unambiguous manner. Data entries are updated on a progressive basis following patient assessment to maintain accuracy and currency.

Methodology

As stated earlier, the scope of this chapter is restricted to qualitative data only. Data was collected from staff in QH wards involved in client care and focused on their behavioural patterns of acceptance and usage of technologies, as well as their opinion on the usage of these technologies. The participants were recruited specifically for this purpose. The recruitment and scheduling aspects were managed by QH through their regular processes.

The qualitative method employed in this study included semi-structured in-depth interviews to gain a sufficient understanding on the topic from QH professionals in their work settings. The aim of these interviews was to identify any unknown factors that may affect the adoption of technology.

In order to extract opinions about technology in specific domains such as QH, the selection of sample is crucial. It is important that the opinions expressed by QH professionals should be unbiased and pertaining to technology only—rather than the effects of technology on current workflows, especially within the scope of this study. The samples for this project consisted of four sets of people from QH. The first set comprised the senior managers who have oversight of strategic operations. The second set is ward managers who have oversight of tactical aspects. The third set is ward professionals who have oversight on operational aspects. The last set of samples included others and was comprised of people who did not fall under the first three categories.

While information systems research identifies a range of sampling techniques such as random and clustering, the sampling technique used for this study may be classified as 'purposive' sampling. The study was conducted with QH to meet their immediate needs. As the assessment is 'real', extreme care is needed to be exercised to preserve the integrity of QH values and standards. This warranted high levels of experience in conducting the assessment and professional knowledge about the assessment aspects. In order to assure completeness in assessments, this approach of 'purposive sampling' was followed in this study.

The instruments of this research consisted of two broad categories of questions. The first category related to the adoption and use of technology. The second category consisted of 'influencing' variables. The influencing variables are those that have an influence on the technology adoption but beyond the technology itself. For example, these variables can be organisational or procedural issues. Open-ended questions were included in the instrument to obtain unbiased and non-leading information. Prior to administering the questions, a complete peer review and a pilot study were conducted in order to ascertain the validity of the instrument.

Qualitative Data Analysis

The qualitative data analysis consisted of two phases. The first phase involved generating a set of initial analytics to determine the direction of extracting evidence, and the second phase involved providing reliability and validity.

In terms of initial analytics, the data was analysed in three different ways. The first set of analytics involved a word frequency cloud using the interview transcripts. The purpose of this analytic process was to assure that we explored relevant and appropriate themes, and the word cloud provided assurance through a keyword search. The second set of analytics was undertaken to develop a pictorial representation of the interview data, representing major themes explored. The interconnection between key themes and the links between the themes provided visual assurance that relevant and appropriate themes were considered in the interviews. The third set of analytics involved exploring the occurrences of keywords in terms of frequency distribution. This provided a pseudo statistical validity.

Word Frequency Cloud The word frequency cloud is a technique in NVivo that documents the most frequently appearing words in a transcript. For the purpose of this study, the number of most frequent words was fixed at 100, and the transcripts of all interviews were run en bloc.

The procedure basically analyses words based on their occurrence, their distance and their context and develops a frequency table of occurrence and percentage. Once this was established, words that did not appear more than a certain arbitrarily chosen number in the overall context were assumed to be less significant in the overall context of the study and removed from the word-frequency-run procedure. This procedure was repeated many times to remove any words that did not make sense or add value to the analysis (e.g. words like 'yes', 'I', etc.). Figure 1.1 is a screenshot of the 'word cloud' to provide an initial viewpoint for further in-depth qualitative analysis.

Using NVivo, researchers generated a word frequency map to assure that keywords were addressed in the interviews. The word frequency cloud shown in Fig. 1.1 indicates keywords extracted from interview transcripts and provides an initial direction for further study.

The word cloud demonstrates that many key concepts were included. For example, patient, board, ward, good, information, etc., were the words used by interviewees and represented the gamut of topics discussed. The topics were discussed with the interviewer (in this case, the researcher), and it provided another level of reliability to ensure that each participant had the same opportunity to discuss these terms. The proximity and the size of the words represent the importance and connection between keywords (Fig. 1.1).

The word cloud and word frequency table (Fig. 1.1) provided an initial path for further analysis as the cloud indicated that keywords were captured in the interview process, thus indicating 'reliability'. Furthermore, the research team conducted over 60 interviews, and the themes were found to be saturated around the twelfth interview, indicating that the qualitative process employed in this study was reliable and appropriate. In fact, after the sixth interview, most of the technology-related issues were saturated in the interview process, thus indicating a very high level of reliability.

Pictorial Representation of Interconnections While the word cloud provides keywords and their relationships, it does not represent the major themes. In order to generate major themes, the research team used Leximancer, a text analytics application. The interview transcripts were submitted to this application, and the parameters were set for 1000 iterations so that major themes and their relationships could be understood. Figure 1.2 is a pictorial representation of what was accomplished.

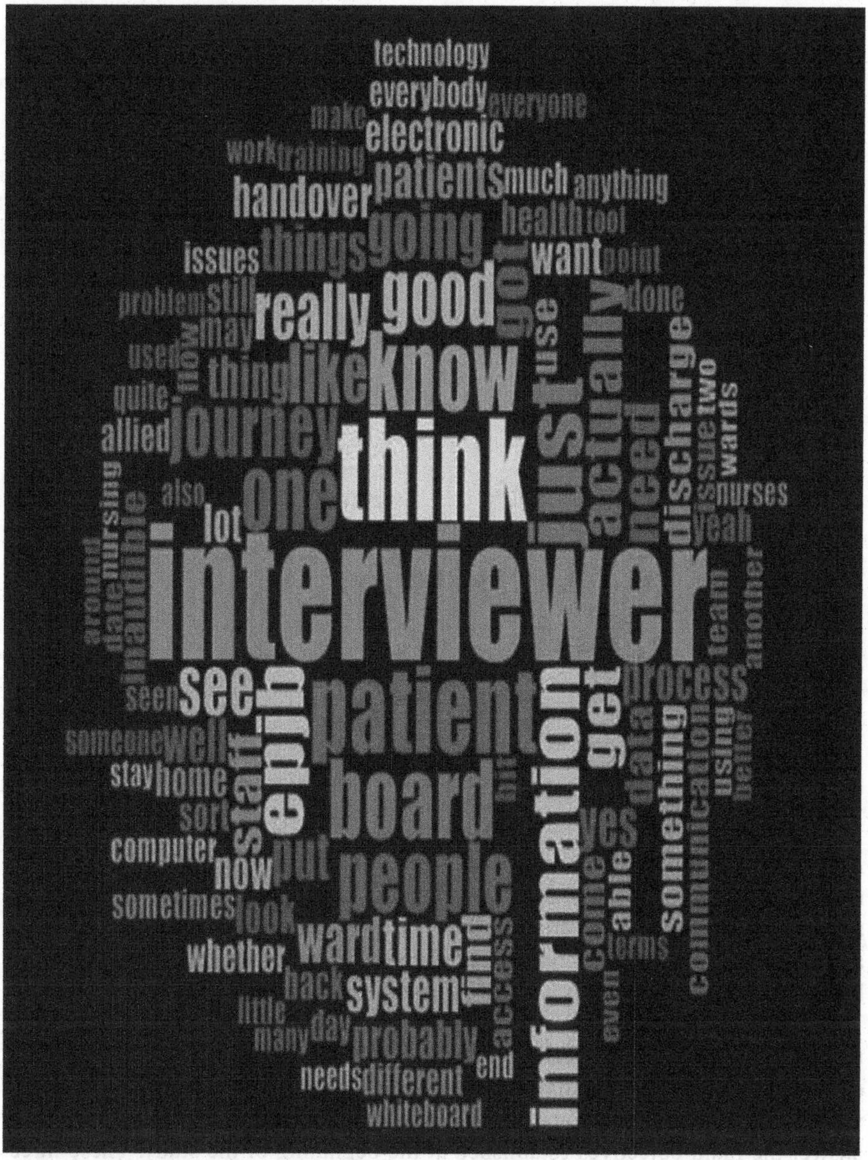

Fig. 1.1 Summary of visual aspects

From Fig. 1.2, the analytics application returned three major themes—patients, nurses and people. The three circles are overlapping with almost the same perimeter thickness, indicating the equal importance of these three themes. Main issues within the themes are shown as 'text' labels, for example 'time' in the nurse circle indicates an issue among nurses. Similarly, labels like satisfaction, allied, care, etc., indicate the range of subthemes among the main theme discussed. The lines between these subthemes indicate relationships between the themes.

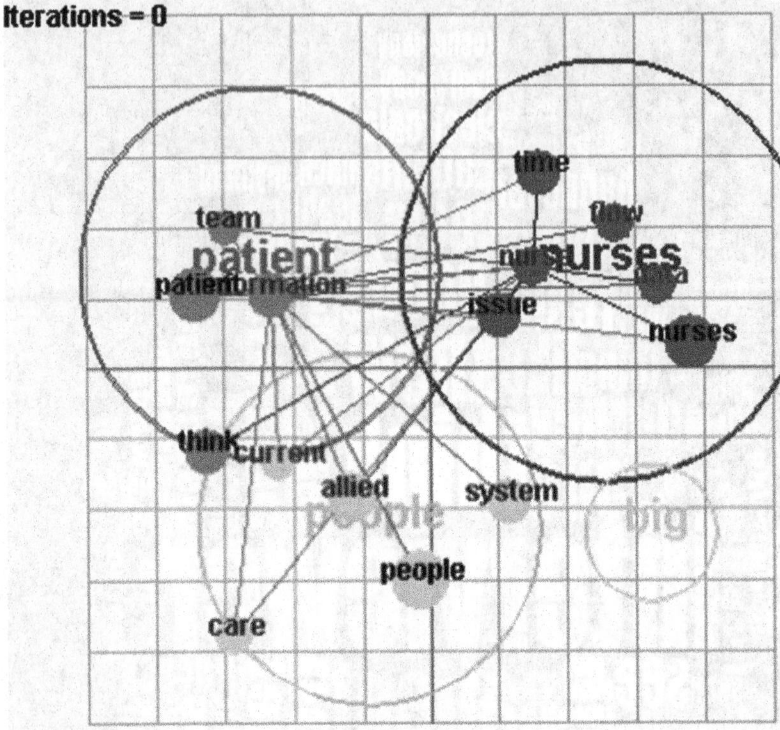

Fig. 1.2 Summary of the analytics application returned three major themes

Keyword Occurrence The keyword occurrence is a technique used in this study to understand how many times a keyword features during the interview as a way of assessing the importance of the keyword. NVivo produced a frequency distribution and allocated a weight to each keyword so that the strength of each keyword could be assessed. The following is a list of keywords extracted (Table 1.1):

EPJB electronic patient journey boardThe above analytics provided a glimpse of the total picture and highlighted trends to be explored in more detail. The purpose of conducting these three initial steps was to ensure that the research was exploring what it intended to explore and that interviews were conducted in a way so as to answer the main objectives established at the beginning of the study. These three analytics provided adequate reliability and confidence to further explore the text data (Fig. 1.3).

The research team conducted manual analyses based on the word query facility within the software application to explore main themes. At this stage, interview transcripts were split into pre-technology implementation and post-technology implementation. The following two sections provide a summary of interview comments on the main issues identified during the text analysis process (Fig. 1.4).

Table 1.1 Summary of key-words occurrence

Word	Count	Weighted percentage (%)
Interviewer	367	2.05
Think	267	1.49
Patient	220	1.23
Just	202	1.13
Board	193	1.08
Know	193	1.08
One	174	0.97
EPJB	172	0.96
Information	172	0.96
People	166	0.93
Good	144	0.80
Journey	137	0.76
Like	133	0.74
Get	131	0.73
Actually	130	0.73
See	129	0.72
Got	123	0.69
Going	122	0.68
Really	121	0.68
Need	111	0.62
Staff	103	0.58
Put	100	0.56
Time	100	0.56
Ward	94	0.52
Things	91	0.51
Yes	91	0.51
Find	86	0.48
Thing	83	0.46
Patients	82	0.46
System	82	0.46
Process	81	0.45
Well	79	0.44
Data	78	0.44
Discharge	78	0.44
Handover	74	0.41
Want	73	0.41
Use	72	0.40
Lot	71	0.40
Now	71	0.40
Look	70	0.39

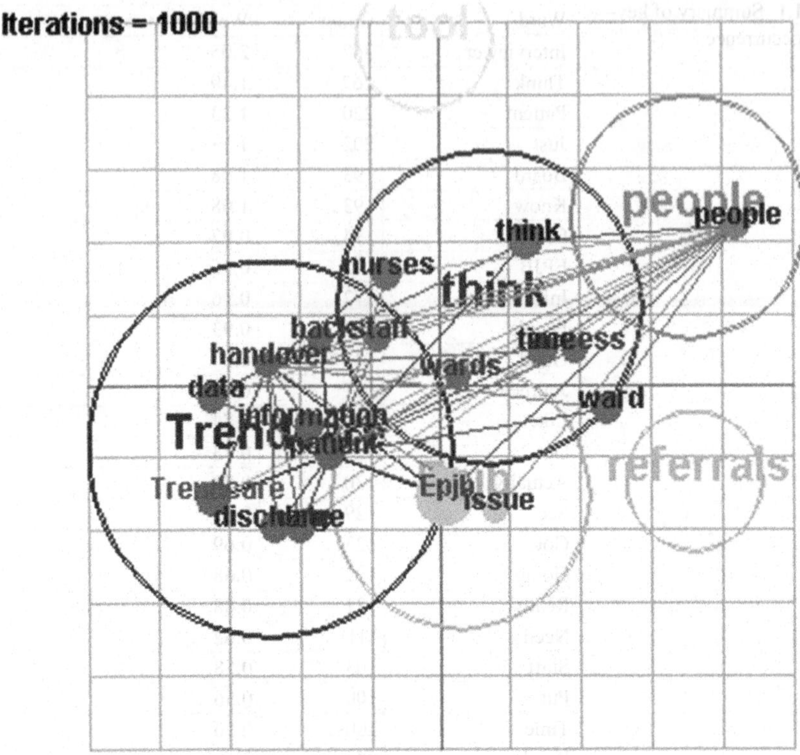

Fig. 1.3 Summary of post-analysis themes

The research team also conducted a tree map to verify reliability of the themes in a pictorial manner.

Tree Map The next stage in the data analysis process was generating a tree map. The purpose of the tree map was to ascertain that the themes that were extracted adequately met the objectives and were represented by the keywords. In generating the tree map, the visual provision indicates the weight of the keywords as shown by the size of the rectangle allocated to the keywords.

In the word frequency table (Table 1.1), prominent words depicting this study appear on the left side of the diagram. As shown, these words, while indicating frequency and relative importance, also indicate the main theme of the study. This was further confirmed with a cluster analysis as shown in Fig. 1.5.

Results of the Analytics

Ease of Use Well we used to have the electronic patient journey board (EPJB) as a whiteboard and that just replaced it, and it is much easier. They only have to—they're probably not putting in so much as it's pulling other information from other

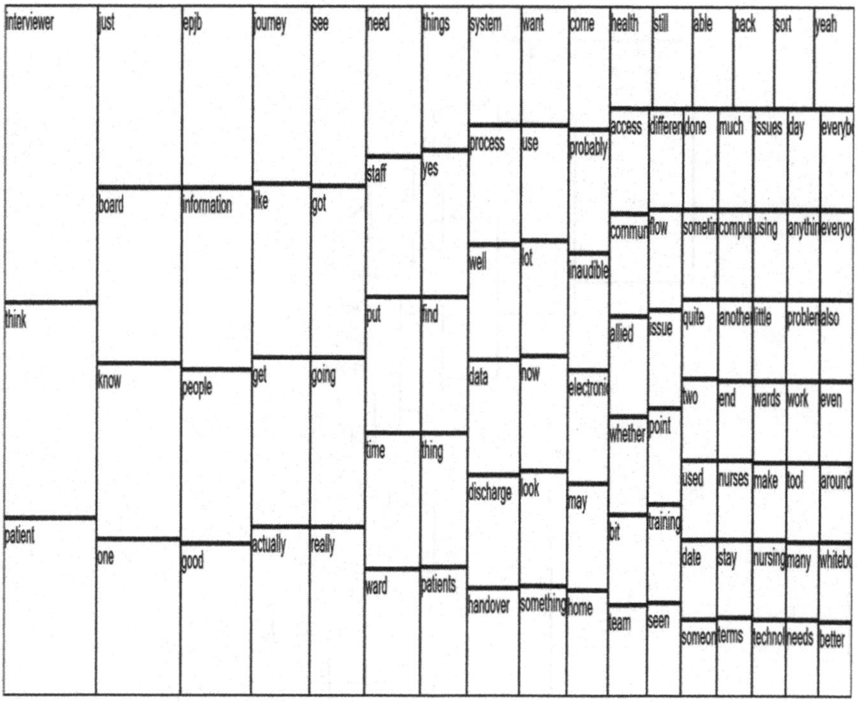

Fig. 1.4 Summary of post-analysis themes

places, they're not having to put in as much as they did before. They seem to be … I haven't heard any complaints, there's nobody whingeing or griping you know. It's just having the time for them to do it and the EPJB just makes it convenient because it's done on that main screen. It's done with six types of a key, the dates in; it's easy enough when they're handing over like I said to do it as they're speaking. I usually sit there in there of a morning and do it. They might say she's not going home Wednesday now she's been extended till next Friday so then you just enter that date and there's just more consistency with it and if that's what they want us to do as they hounded us for that to put in length of discharges or stays or whatever.

Time Savings Yes, because what we did to reduce time was basically instead of each nurse handing over, we've gone to just handing over the whole ward. The oncoming TL is to have the EPJB up and click on the next name as they're speaking and then they're to go out of that handover and then they sight their patients. The TLs liked it from the TL handover sheet it showed them who the physios were already on, stuff like that.

Uptake I'd probably say 70–80 %. I think they really like it, put it this way they wouldn't like to go back to the old way of writing it up on the board.

Currency of Information Before we had the EPJB we never had to enter discharge dates. We used to get in trouble for it and we would try to and you'd go in there

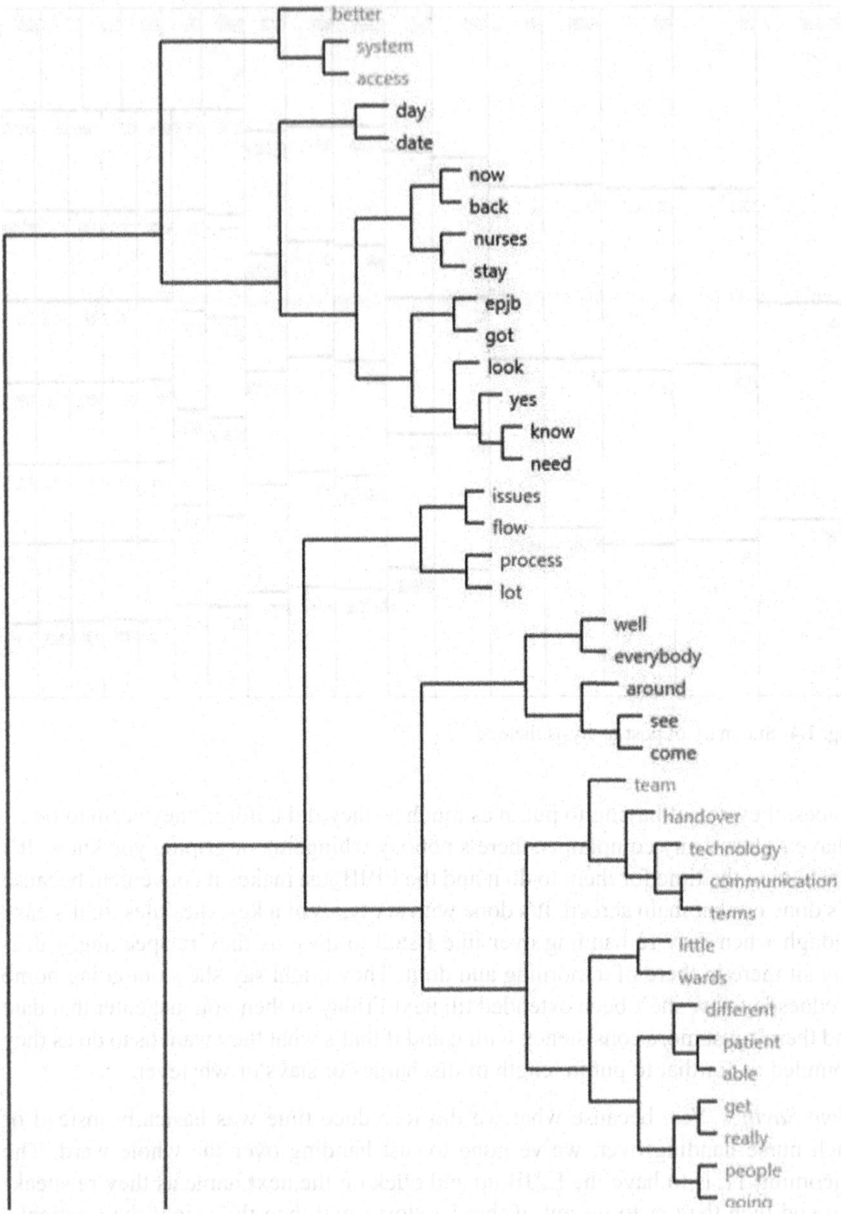

Fig. 1.5 Summary of post-analysis themes

and it's locked by another user and it would be just be good if Trend could pull that information from the EPJB.

Old White Board Versus EPJB Well how are they going to do it to if we're to go back to the old white board it's just so messy and so untidy and a lot of the time wasn't getting updated but this way they have to update it because it's a handover sheet do you know what I mean? It's the patient's journey basically.

Training Needs No it doesn't take long for them to learn because everything's there. You've just got to tick things and you've got your drop down's like if someone's had a fall if it's high medium or low and there's forms to fill out which we teach them what to do. It all goes in the UR notes, everything's there. It's not like we have to write too much and that's a good thing. If we don't have to write then the nurses will do it. We've basically got train the trainer now. Enough of our staff can train the new ones

Positive Impact The EPJB has made a huge difference to the impact on our length of stays and a huge impact on giving the staff a lot more knowledge as to where we're at with our patients. They know where we're up to with our patient care—they know that the physio's seen them, they don't have to go to the UR chart and flick through and say 'Oh, I think a physio's seen them' whereas now we can look at the EPJB—'physio's seen them' we know that for sure

Access Yes that's right because out on the ward they've got their computers and they can do exactly what they want and then it comes to me on here so I know who's gone home and who's going home tomorrow. So bed management—so if name says 'we need some beds' she can sit on there and look. I don't have to get out of my chair to go and run and find the nurses and say 'hey, what's going on out here?' It's good having a comments section down here.

Attitude I feel they're coming to like it the more they use it, the more they realise it is a good system so I'd mark it probably another 8.

From the analytics and manual analysis of available data, we extracted the table of key factors (Table 1.2):

Table 1.2 Summary of comfort of the technology adoption

Implementation factors	Rate of change
Easy to use	Yes
Saves time	Yes—handovers
Good uptake	Staff like it
Satisfactory	Yes
Training required	Minimal
Positive impact	Yes
Communications	Improved
Access to computers	Satisfactory
Attitude: Rating—8/10	High level of acceptance

Table 1.2 highlights that users confirmed the technology as being easy to use, reduces time and improves communications. When these three factors are viewed in unison, it is possible to assert that the first objective is accomplished.

Similarly, it is clear that users were satisfied with the technology, and the text data indicates a high level of acceptance. Therefore, it is possible to assert that the second objective has been accomplished.

From the interviews, users were not able to assert regarding the level of quality of services. While there were positive references to this effect, the research did not generate sufficient data to assert this objective.

Conclusions

The text analytics process was useful in establishing the reliability of data as well as for understanding the direction to be taken in conducting qualitative analysis of open-ended semi-structured interviews used to gather interview data. Due to the type of data being collected, it was difficult to collect data in a strictly unified way due to the volume and variation in user-functional aspects.

The research team used various techniques such as word cloud, frequency map and intelligence iterative analysis to guide the data analysis process. Further, text analytics helped the research team to verify whether the interviews were conducted properly and whether the interview data would adequately address the range of themes the research sought to explore.

With this initial direction established, NVivo was used to create themes and nodes and create other structures for analysing and categorising the data. These structures helped identifying the strength of the themes and exploring their inter-relationships. The research team did not expand further upon this aspect of analysis as it is adequately addressed with standard qualitative analysis. This chapter discusses and reports on the three analytic processes that were the focus of this particular research in assuring reliability of data collected.

Bibliography

Banerjee, A., Bandyopadhyay, T., & Acharya, P. (2013). Data analytics: Hyped up aspirations or true potential? *Vikalpa, 38*(4), 1–11.

Brown, S. A., & Venkatesh, V. (2005). Model of adoption of technology in the household: A baseline model test and extension incorporating household life cycle. *MIS Quarterly, 29*(4), 399–426.

Childers, T. L., Carr, C. L., Peck, J., & Carson, S. (2001). Hedonic and utilitarian motivations for online retail shopping behavior. *Journal of Retailing, 77*(4), 511–535.

Finkelstein, S., Speedie, S., Zhou, X., Pothouff, S., & Ratner, E. (2011). Perception, satisfaction and utilisation of the VALUE home telehealth service. *Journal of Telemedicine and Telecare, 17*(6), 288–292.

Kim, S. S., & Malhotra, N. K. (2005). A longitudinal model of continued is use: An integrative view of four mechanisms underlying post-adoption phenomena. *Management Science, 51*(5), 741–755.

Kim, S. S., Malhotra, N. K., & Narasimhan, S. (2005). Two competing perspectives on automatic use: A theoretical and empirical comparison. *Information Systems Research, 16*(4), 418–432.

Kim, H. W., Chan, H. C., & Gupta, S. (2007). Value-based adoption of mobile internet: An empirical investigation. *Decision Support Systems, 43*(1), 111–126.

Limayem, M., & Hirt, S. G. (2003). Force of habit and information systems usage: Theory and initial validation. *Journal of the AIS, 4*(1), 65–97.

Limayem, M., Hirt, S. G., & Cheung, C. M. K. (2007). How habit limits the predictive power of intentions: The case of IS continuance. *MIS Quarterly, 31*(4), 705–737.

Metzger, L. (2011). Telehealth in home healthcare. PhD Thesis—Marywood University.

Remenyi, D., Williams, B., Money, A., & Swartz, E. (1998). *Doing research in business and management.* London: Sage.

Sharda, R., Adomako Asamoah, D., & Ponna, N. (2013). Research and pedagogy in business analytics: Opportunities and illustrative examples. *Journal of Computing & Information Technology, 21*(3), 171–183. doi:10.2498/cit.1002194.

van der Heijden, H. (2004). User acceptance of hedonic information systems. *MIS Quarterly, 28*(4), 695–704.

Prof. Raj Gururajan has an experience of 25 years in research and teaching in the information systems domain. Much of his research focuses in the area of health informatics. He has over 200 publications. Currently, Raj is a professor at the University of Southern Queensland (USQ).

Kevin Clark is a nurse unit manager who has 4 years of experience in applying lean thinking to healthcare-specific people and process redesign, cultural change, quality and safety related to the patient experience. Furthermore, he has experience and detailed knowledge of the current state and national healthcare systems' challenges and opportunities through my work on the Queensland Clinical Senate Executive and the Queensland Clinical Education and Training Council.

Susan Moller is the principle project officer of 'Electronic Patient Journey Boards' at Queensland Health. She has experience as a nurse unit manager and held positions at St Vincent's Private Hospital, Perninsula Maternal & Neonatal Service.

Prema Sankaran has an experience of 14 years in teaching in the finance domain and 6 years of research experience from industry. She has both academic and commercial publications. Currently, Prema is a Professor and Dean at Thiagarajar School of Management (TSM), Madurai, India.

Dr. Abdul Hafeez Baig is a senior lecturer in information systems at the USQ. Much of his research focuses in the area of health informatics.

Prof. Nilmini Wickramasinghe (PhD; MBA; GradDipMgtSt; BSc. Amus.A (piano); Amus.A (violin)) has a well-recognised research record in the field of health care and IT/IS. Her expertise is in the strategic application and management of technology for effecting superior health care solutions. Currently, she is the professor and director of health informatics management at Epworth HealthCare and professor at Deakin University.

Rashmi Gururajan is a final-year medical student at Monash University in Melbourne, Australia. She has a keen interest in chronic disease, particularly diabetes research. To date, she has been awarded three research scholarships in order to investigate diabetes in an Indigenous population, and the reasons for readmission to hospital with diabetic complications. Rashmi will complete her medical studies in December 2016 and hopes to continue her house officership in Melbourne.

Chapter 2
Exercise, Diet Counselling, and Management for the Adults with Diabetes Mellitus: An Indian Case Study

Dharnini Pathy, Raj Gururajan, Abdul Hafeez-Baig, Nilmini Wickramasinghe and Rashmi Gururajan

Introduction

The two major clinical forms of diabetes mellitus are insulin-dependent diabetes mellitus (IDDM or type 1) and non-insulin-dependent diabetes mellitus (NIDDM or type 2) as classified by WHO (1999). In type 2 diabetes mellitus, there is a progressive inadequacy of insulin production. The inadequacy seems to stem from a failure of the pancreas to be able to compensate adequately for the progressive decline in sensitivity to insulin in the target tissues. Insulin sensitivity decreases as the body fat content increases, and excessive weight gain is the most important trigger for the onset of type 2 diabetes in those who are genetically susceptible to it. A high-fat, low-fibre diet and inactivity are other lifestyle characteristics that decrease insulin sensitivity, predisposing individuals to this type of diabetes (Webb 2002).

With the forces of globalization and industrialization proceeding at an increasing rate, the prevalence of diabetes is predicted to increase dramatically over the next few decades. The resulting burden of complication and premature mortality will continue to present itself as a major and growing public health problem for most countries (Diabetes Atlas 2003).

The UN resolution on diabetes has been to eradicate the global epidemic of this chronic disease. Diabetes causes about 5 % of all deaths globally each year. About 80 % of people with diabetes are in low- and middle-income countries, and they are

R. Gururajan (✉) · D. Pathy · A. Hafeez-Baig
60 Baker Ave, Kew East, VIC 3102, Australia
e-mail: Raj.Gururajam@usq.edu.au

A. Hafeez-Baig
e-mail: abdulhb@usq.edu.au

N. Wickramasinghe
Deakin University and Epworth HealthCare, 60 Baker Ave, Kew East 3102, Australia
e-mail: n.wickramasinghe@deakin.edu.au

R. Gururajan
Medical Student, Monash University, Melbourne, Australia

N. Wickramasinghe et al. (eds.), *Contemporary Consumer Health Informatics*, Healthcare Delivery in the Information Age, DOI 10.1007/978-3-319-25973-4_2

in the age range of 45–64 years. Without urgent action, deaths due to diabetes are likely to increase by more than 50 % in the next 10 years (Abegunde et al. 2007).

In type 2 diabetes mellitus, as the disease progresses, abnormal catabolism of protein and fat becomes part of the picture, since carbohydrates are not utilized in a normal fashion for the production of energy. Eventually, fat metabolism gets deranged with abnormal accumulation of end products (Heinz 1959). Both acute and chronic complications develop in subjects with type 2 diabetes mellitus over a period of time. Diabetes can first become manifest with either the symptomatic hyperglycaemia or a medical emergency which can be caused by severe hyperglycaemia, ketoacidosis, or severe hyperlipidaemia. Most symptoms of diabetes are related to hyperglycaemia or accumulation of glucose in various tissues (Whitney and Rolfes 2002).

Metabolic, genetic, and other factors affect major diabetic complications such as retinopathy, nephropathy, and neuropathy. Retinopathy is early background lesions in capillaries of the eye usually resulting from microaneurysms (Williams and Anderson 1989). It is estimated that more than 2.5 million people worldwide are affected by diabetic retinopathy, the leading cause of blindness (Sadikot 2008). Diabetic nephropathy develops gradually through several stages related to clinical and tissue findings. Nephropathy is the most common cause of kidney failure, which is responsible for huge dialysis costs; about 10–20 % of those affected die of renal failure (Williams and Anderson 1989). In India, it has been estimated that one out of every three to four patients undergoing dialysis or renal transplants has kidney problems resulting from diabetes (Sadikot 2008).

Neuropathy is the development of nerve damage and diminished transmission of nerve impulses that affect muscle function and sensory perception in various parts of the body. Later, the person loses sensation in the hands and feet. Injuries to these areas may go unnoticed, and infections can progress rapidly. With loss of circulation and nerve function, undetected injury and infection may lead to gangrene, necessitating amputation of the limbs (Williams and Anderson 1989). People with diabetes are 15–40 times more likely to require limb amputations compared to the general population. In most countries, diabetes is the second biggest cause of lower limb amputations, after accidents (Sadikot 2008).

There is no doubt that diabetes with its complications and related diseases, such as high blood pressure, lipid abnormalities, and obesity, especially visceral obesity, has led to a significant increase in the number of people with the early onset of cardiovascular disease (CVD), and death has reached pandemic proportions. In fact, diabetes is a global killer, rivaling human immunodeficiency virus/acquired immune deficiency syndrome (HIV/AIDS) in its deadly reach and causing some 3.8 million deaths a year (Sadikot 2008).

The short-term complications include cell distension and toxicity due to accumulation of polyols. Blurred vision can be caused due to accumulation of sorbitol and fructose. Polyol accumulation can alter the function of peripheral nerves. The structures of blood vessels and nerves become damaged leading to loss of circulation and nerve function. Infections are likely to occur due to poor circulation coupled with glucose-rich blood and urine (Whitney and Rolfes 2002).

Diet has been the mainstay of treatment in the management of diabetes mellitus for many centuries. The discovery and introduction of insulin and oral hypoglycaemic agents led to the laxity of the rigid regulations. However, the importance of diet as the first line of treatment has been realized and reinstated in present times. Dietary strategies for nutritional management of individuals with diabetes should be focused on the dietary factors that have the greatest impact on the regulation of carbohydrate and lipoprotein metabolism. Dietary strategies should be developed to gain long-term patient compliance (Brown 1990). Although the optimal dietary composition is not well established, the benefits of modest caloric restriction, use of high-fibre diets, are well recognized. Recent clinical interventions with modest caloric restriction and increased physical activity have shown that the onset of diabetes can be significantly delayed and possibly prevented with modest weight loss (Mooradian 2003).

Attempts to manage diabetes mellitus were made by Egyptians in 3500 B.C. In India, as early as 2500 years ago, Sushrutha and Charaka had realized the importance of dietary regulation for the treatment of type 2 diabetes mellitus. Measures were adopted to correct obesity in diabetics. The use of sugar, jaggery, molasses, wines, ghee, butter, and meat was prohibited (Krall 1962).

Aretaeus, the Greek physician, in second century A.D., advised diabetics to have milk, cereals, starch, autumn fruits, and sweet wines. Dodson in the eighteenth century noted that the sweet taste in urine was actually due to the presence of sugar. He also advocated a diet rich in all nutrients, especially carbohydrate to compensate for the loss in the urine (Krall 1962).

Beginning with Rollo (1797) up to 1923, when insulin was introduced, the dietary treatment was largely based on the following principles: a reduction or elimination of carbohydrate and, if necessary, reduction of total energy intake. With the exception of a few who followed the low-carbohydrate diet based on green leafy vegetables (Mc Cance and Lawrence 1929), the treatment by and large had shifted to a moderate high-carbohydrate diet with restricted calories (Robinwitch 1930). Himsworth (1942) noted a striking correlation between mortality and fat consumption. A fall in the diabetic mortality during World War I was attributed to a reduction in fat and increase in carbohydrate intake. This trend is noticed even today with the urban populations eating a diet higher in fat calories and an increase in the incidence of type 2 diabetes mellitus.

The shift to a high-protein diet was noticed in the early 1950s. Protein-rich diet from plant, animal, or mixed protein sources were found to be equally effective in the control of blood sugar levels (Conway 1953; Coleman 1953; Bryant 1953).

The importance of the carbohydrate component of the diet was realized in the early 1960s. The changing trends in the diabetic diet during the twentieth century have been reviewed by Ajgaonkar (1964). Major dietary manipulations have centred around carbohydrates and fat. The span of almost 50 years, from 1917 to 1960, registered a gradual and steady increase in the carbohydrate component, and this was accompanied by a parallel decline in the fat component.

Need for the Study Several studies have reported an alarming increase in the incidence of type 2 diabetes mellitus even in young Indians (Ramachandran 2005; Mohan et al. 2007; Abegunde et al. 2007). The search is on for an effective treatment with diet counselling and exercise which can reduce the plasma glucose values and reduce the microvascular and macrovascular complications related to the disease.

Dietary changes are important. Unlike trying out one single food or a group of foods as supplements to improve the disease, the current study has tried to change the dietary aspects of the subject. Periodic intensive counselling on diet was given to improve the diet, to manage the disease, and to achieve the goals of reducing fasting and postprandial plasma glucose levels in subjects with diabetes mellitus. A prescribed exercise regimen was also given along with diet counselling to manage the disease and evaluate the combined effect of diet with exercise.

Evidence-based studies have been carried out in the West, but in India there is incomplete evidence related to diet and diabetes and hence an urgent need to come out with evidence-based studies. Increasingly, evidence suggests that the normalization of blood glucose and lipid profiles is valid. In line with other moves towards evidence-based medicine, increasing efforts have been made to standardize the diet composition for subjects with diabetes mellitus. It is important to recognize that all dietary recommendations will change over time as new data become available. It is essential to exercise judgement while assessing the evidence and to take responsibility for recommending changes.

Review of Literature

Diabetes mellitus has been defined as a genetically and clinically heterogeneous group of disorders, all of which show glucose intolerance. It is characterized by a partial or total lack of functioning insulin and alterations in carbohydrate, protein, and fat metabolism. The insulin defect maybe due to a failure in the formation, liberation, or action of insulin (Robinson and Lawler 1982). It was known in antiquity and remains today a health problem which causes coronary artery disease, blindness, renal failure, and amputations (Crabbe 1987). Diabetes is one of the most common chronic illnesses to afflict man worldwide.

Classification of Diabetes Mellitus

Increasing evidence indicates differences between insulin-dependent and non-insulin-dependent diabetes, and epidemiological studies have provided newer clinical and pathogenetic information (Williams and Anderson 1989).

Type 1 Diabetes Mellitus Type 1 was formerly classified as juvenile-onset diabetes mellitus. It indicates the processes of beta-cell destruction that may ultimately lead to diabetes mellitus in which "insulin is required for survival" to prevent the development of ketoacidosis, coma, and death (WHO 1999). It occurs between 1 and 40 years of age and includes 10–20% of all diabetes cases. These subjects secrete little, if any, insulin and thus become insulin dependent, requiring both insulin injections and a carefully controlled diet. This type of diabetes occurs suddenly, exhibiting many of the symptoms classic to diabetes and can be difficult to control

(Townsend and Roth 2000). Subjects require lifelong dependence on insulin injections for survival. Though it usually occurs in children and adolescents, it can also occur during adulthood.

Type 2 Diabetes Mellitus Type 2 diabetes mellitus was previously called as adult-onset diabetes and usually occurs after the age of 40. Its onset is gradual as the amount of insulin produced each day gradually diminishes (Williams 1993). It is not uncommon for the subject to have no symptoms and to be totally ignorant of his or her condition until it is discovered accidentally during a routine urine or blood test or after a heart attack or a stroke. This is the most common form of diabetes and is characterized by disorders of insulin action and insulin secretion. The specific reasons for development of these abnormalities are not yet known (WHO 1999).

Malnutrition-Related Diabetes Mellitus Malnutrition-related diabetes mellitus (MRDM) is mainly seen in some tropical countries such as India, and it occurs in young people between 15 and 30 years of age. Generally, people with this type of diabetes mellitus are lean and undernourished. The pancreas fails to produce adequate insulin, and as a result, people with this type of diabetes require insulin. In contrast to type 1, these subjects generally do not develop ketoacidosis when insulin injections are discontinued (WHO 1999).

Impaired Glucose Tolerance Subjects in whom the fasting level is lower than that required for the diagnosis of diabetes mellitus but in whom the values obtained during the glucose tolerance tests lie between normal and diabetic values are considered to be glucose intolerant. People with impaired glucose tolerance (IGT) are at a greater risk of developing type 2 diabetes mellitus and hence have been given a separate category.

Gestational Diabetes Gestational diabetes mellitus can occur between the 16th and 28th week of pregnancy. It is a carbohydrate intolerance resulting in hyperglycaemia of variable severity with onset or first recognition during pregnancy (WHO 1999). Usually, gestational diabetes disappears after the infant is born. However, diabetes mellitus can develop 5–10 years after the pregnancy (Townsend and Roth 2000).

Potentially Modifiable or Reversible Risk Factors The potentially modifiable risk factors are those which can be modified and helped in preventing or postponing the disease. They are classified into minor and major modifiable risk factors.

Minor Modifiable Risk Factors The minor modifiable risk factors include obesity, physical inactivity, alcohol consumption, stress, and dietary factors.

Obesity A positive association between overweight and obesity and type 2 diabetes mellitus has been well established (Seshiah 1989). Although Asian Indians generally have lower body mass index (BMI) than many other races, the association of BMI with glucose intolerance is as strong as in any other population. In the past two decades, the rates of obesity have tripled in developing countries that have been adopting a Western lifestyle involving decreased physical activity and overconsumption of energy-dense foods (Hussain et al. 2007).

Physical Inactivity In type 2 diabetes mellitus, exercise can enhance peripheral glucose uptake by muscle and apparent increased insulin sensitivity (Bogardus et al. 1984). Regular physical activity appears to blunt the rise in blood glucose following carbohydrate ingestion and may increase insulin sensitivity for 2 or 3 days afterwards (Wheeler et al. 1987). Evidence supports the hypothesis that sedentary habits and low cardiorespiratory fitness are responsible for the progression from normal glucose metabolism to type 2 diabetes mellitus and that they are independent predictors of cardiovascular events and premature mortality in individuals diagnosed with diabetes mellitus (Boule et al. 2001). Regular physical activity can retard the progression from one stage to another, and it may even reverse the process.

Alcohol Consumption There are varied results regarding the relation of alcohol consumption and type 2 diabetes mellitus. Few studies have supported the view that moderate alcohol consumption decreases risk of type 2 diabetes mellitus (Holbrook et al. 1990; Tsumara et al. 1999; Beulens et al. 2005). Wheeler et al. (2004) reported that in people with diabetes, moderate alcohol consumption does not acutely affect glycaemic control and is associated with a decrease in coronary heart disease and a reduced risk of mortality. On the other hand, binge drinking and high alcohol consumption increased the risk of type 2 diabetes mellitus (Carlsson et al. 2003). Hence, no conclusive reports exist on alcohol and type 2 diabetes mellitus.

Stress Stress results when something causes the body to behave as if it were under attack. Sources of stress can be physical, such as injury or illness, or they can be mental, such as problems in marriage, home, job, health, or finances (Webster 2003). In people with diabetes, stress can alter blood glucose levels in two ways. First, people under stress may not take good care of themselves. They may drink more alcohol or exercise less. They may forget, or not have time, to check their glucose levels or plan good meals. Secondly, stress hormones may also alter blood glucose levels directly (Krall and Beaser 1989). Stress blocks the body from releasing insulin in people with type 2 diabetes, so cutting stress may be more helpful for these people (Seshiah 1989). The pervasive impact of depression on quality of life and its potential negative effect on diabetes management warrant recognition and treatment of the effective disorder in diabetic individuals (Gavard et al. 1993). Controlling stress with relaxation therapy seems to help for some people.

Major Modifiable Risk Factors

Major modifiable risk factors are hyperglycaemia, hypertension, microalbuminuria, and smoking.

Hyperglycaemia and Impaired Glucose Tolerance IGT and/or impaired fasting glucose (IFG) is intermediate between normoglycaemia and diabetes and represent risk categories for the future development of diabetes, as about one third of the IGT subjects develop type 2 diabetes mellitus (Khatib 2006; Ramachandran 2003). Several studies (Gerich 1998; Pratley and Weyer 2002; Irons et al. 2004) have indicated that IGT precedes diabetes. Hence, IGT has acquired great importance as a point of intervention in recent times in type 2 diabetes mellitus (Mohan et al. 2007).

Hypertension Hypertension occurs about twice as frequently in people with diabetes than in the general population (Garcia et al. 1974). Hypertension and diabetes together considerably accelerate the development of coronary artery disease along with other macrovascular and microvascular complications (Singh et al. 1998). Age, sex, obesity, renal disease, and duration of diabetes may influence the association between diabetes and hypertension. Hypertension-related factors may act synergistically with arterial wall abnormalities, cellular dysfunction, lipo protein abnormalities, and platelet derangements to accelerate atherosclerosis (Anderson and Giel 1994). The association of coronary artery disease and hypertension with diabetes is greater in urban than in rural subjects (Singh et al. 1998). The risk classification of blood pressure levels is given in Table 2.1.

Microalbuminuria The term microalbuminuria indicates an albumin excretion rate (AER) greater than the range of normal values. By convention, microalbuminuria indicates an AER of 30–300 mg/24 h. Microalbuminuria predicts renal failure in subjects with type 1 and premature cardiovascular mortality in subjects with type 2 diabetes mellitus. Studies have shown an increased cardiovascular mortality in type 2 diabetes mellitus subjects with microalbuminuria (Jarret et al. 1984; Mogensen 1984; Schmitz and Vaeth 1988). As possible explanation for this association, several changes in CVD factors have been documented in microalbuminuric diabetic subjects including high levels of blood pressure, triglycerides (TGs), and fibrinogen (Mattock et al. 1988; Jensen et al. 1988; James and Pearson 1993). According to Dinneen and Gerstein (1997), microalbuminuria is a strong predictor of cardiovascular mortality and cardiovascular morbidity in subjects with type 2 diabetes mellitus.

As many as 7 % of patients with type 2 diabetes mellitus may already have microalbuminuria at the time they are diagnosed with diabetes (Gross et al. 2005). In UK Prospective Diabetes Study (UKPDS), the incidence of microalbuminuria was 2 % per year in patients with type 2 diabetes mellitus, and the 10-year prevalence after diagnosis was 25 % (Adler et al. 2003; Gross et al. 2005).

Smoking Cigarette smoking is not only one of the most potent risk factors for atherosclerosis in humans but also the factor that if reduced or eliminated, clearly results in a reduction of risk (National Heart, Lung and Blood Institute 1971). There are consistent results showing enhanced risk for micro- and macrovascular disease,

Table 2.1 Risk classification of blood pressure. (Source: Chobanian et al. (2003))

Classification	Blood pressure values (mmHg)	
	Systolic	Diastolic
Normal	< 120	< 80
Prehypertensive	120–139	80–89
Stage I hypertension	140–159	90–99
Stage II hypertension	=160	1=100

as well as premature mortality from the combination of smoking and diabetes. Advocacy for tobacco control through public policy initiatives is also an appropriate and potentially effective way to reduce the burden of excess morbidity and mortality that tobacco use confers on those with diabetes (American Diabetes Association 2004). Morton et al. (2008) suggested that smoking cessation programmes should target diabetic subjects to more effectively prevent complications and promote successful management of diabetes.

Complications of Type 2 Diabetes Mellitus

Degenerative complications are the cause of most diabetes morbidity and mortality. People with chronic diabetes mellitus have increased risk of developing complicating problems that reflect the tissue damaging effect over a period of time (Williams and Anderson 1989).

Microvascular Complications

Glucose metabolism changes in tissues where glucose transport into the cell does not depend on insulin. When the extracellular glucose level is high, cellular glucose concentration rises and glucose is converted to sorbitol and fructose by polyol pathway. Sorbitol and fructose cannot leave the cell, and they promote osmotic accumulation of water with subsequent swelling and cellular dysfunction especially in the lens of the eye (Mahan and Arlin 1992). The microvascular complications occurring in type 2 diabetes mellitus are retinopathy, neuropathy, and nephropathy.

Retinopathy About 10 % of persons with type 1 diabetes mellitus who develop retinal malformations (vitreous haemorrhage, retinal detachment, *cotton-wool* spots) in eye will eventually become blind. Older persons with type 2 diabetes mellitus can develop blindness from macular oedema with surrounding microaneurysms and hard exudates, even in the absence of proliferating retinal malformations (Williams and Anderson 1989).

Diabetic retinopathy is generally classified as either background or proliferative. Background retinopathy includes such features as small haemorrhages in the middle layers of the retina. Retinal oedema may require intervention because it is sometimes associated with visual deterioration. Proliferative retinopathy is characterized by the formation of new blood vessels on the surface of the retina and can lead to vitreous haemorrhage. Laser photocoagulation can often prevent proliferative retinopathy from progressing to blindness; therefore, close surveillance for the existence or progression of retinopathy in patients with diabetes is crucial (Watkins 2003).

Neuropathy Diabetic neuropathy is recognized by the American Diabetes Association (ADA) as “the presence of symptoms and/or signs of peripheral nerve dysfunction in people with diabetes after the exclusion of other causes". As with other microvascular complications, risk of developing diabetic neuropathy is proportional to both the magnitude and duration of hyperglycaemia, and some individuals may possess genetic attributes that affect their predisposition to developing such complications. Persons with diminished transmission of nerve impulses that affect the muscle function and sensory perception is due to abnormality in metabolism of sorbitol and myoinositol (Boulton et al. 2005, 2004). Foot problems can easily occur from decreased function of both nerves and blood circulation to and from the feet (Levin 1991).

Nephropathy Prolonged hyperglycaemia brings about thickening of basement membrane of the glomerulus and causes irreversible damage to the glomeruli (Mc Lester and Darby 1952). The earliest clinical sign of diabetic renal disease is proteinuria, and it is the initial indicator of diabetic nephropathy. The process of microscopic capillary lesions and hyalinization of both afferent and efferent glomerular arterioles, characteristic of Kimmelstiel–Wilson disease, maybe present (Myers et al. 1995).

Macrovascular Complications

These develop at an earlier age and are the major cause of death in subjects with type 2 diabetes mellitus. A common consequence of peripheral vascular disease is reduced circulation, coldness in the extremities, and fatigue. Some of the degenerative complications of diabetes mellitus are coronary artery disease, cerebrovascular disease, peripheral vascular disease (gangrene), and hypertension (Mahan and Arlin 1992). The macrovascular complications leading to different kinds of CVD have been discussed below:

Atherosclerosis Atherosclerosis is the most common complication of diabetes and is the most leading cause of death in diabetics (Marks and Krall 1971), accounting for more than half of all diabetic mortality (Laing et al. 2003; Paterson et al. 2007). Diabetes is associated with a three- or fourfold increase in risk of CVD (Coulston 1994). The increased mortality from CVD in the absence of major risk factors such as cigarette smoking, hypertension, and serum cholesterol concentration is seen more in diabetics than nondiabetics (Betteridge 1994).

Serum Lipid Abnormalities The lipid profile is significantly altered in diabetic subjects as compared to nondiabetics (Udawat et al. 2001). Hypercholesterolemia and other lipid and lipoprotein abnormalities are collectively referred to as diabetic dyslipidemia, and they contribute to vascular risk (Betteridge 1994). The major concern is the high percentage of low-density lipoprotein (LDL) and dyslipidemia in majority of the diabetic subjects (Roy 1987).

The National Cholesterol Education Programme (NCEP) has defined the categories of CVD risk according to levels of lipids as shown in Table 2.2.

Passmore and Eastwood (1986) defines serum lipid abnormality as increased levels of TGs or cholesterol or both in the serum; however, it involves other physical and biochemical changes in the plasma such as turbidity, viscosity, and other changes in lipoproteins. Diabetes mellitus is an important disorder which profoundly affects the lipid metabolism in acute and chronic ways. Abnormalities of plasma lipids in diabetes have long attracted attention due to association between hyperlipidaemia and atherosclerosis (Manzato et al. 1993). The aggressive change of lifestyle modifications can reduce or delay the need for medical intervention. Appropriate lifestyle and medical interventions will reduce the occurrence of CVD and allow people with diabetes to live healthier and longer lives (Buse et al. 2007).

Hypercholesterolemia It is known to be a potent risk factor which occurs more commonly in diabetics than in the general population (New et al. 1963). There is an increase in TG-rich lipoproteins attributed to overproduction of very low-density lipoprotein (VLDL) and poor peripheral clearance of VLDL consequent to lesser expression of Apo B100 receptors on endothelial cell surface (Jackson et al. 1992).

Dyslipidemia The cluster of lipid abnormalities associated with type 2 diabetes mellitus is defined by increase in TG and small, dense LDL concentrations, and decrease in HDL cholesterol (HDL-C) is characterized as dyslipidemia associated with type 2 diabetes mellitus (Krauss and Siri 2004). Hypertriglyceridemia is known to be highly prevalent in the untreated diabetic subjects usually accompanied by a decrease in HDL-C. Hypertriglyceridemia associated with diabetes improves during therapy with insulin (Brunzell et al. 1985). Hypertriglyceridemia in diabetics has been reported to be associated with increased VLDL synthesis and impaired VLDL and chylomicron catabolism (Dunn 1982).

Low HDL level occurs in both type 1 and type 2 diabetes mellitus subjects (Rabkin et al. 1983). HDL-C level increases during therapy with insulin and with weight loss. This increase in HDL-C is associated with lowering of VLDL cholesterol levels and replacement of TGs with cholesterol on the core of HDL-C (Brunzell et al. 1985).

The lipid profile in patients with type 2 diabetes mellitus is characterized by elevated TGs, low levels of HDL-C, and small, dense LDL cholesterol (LDL-C)

Table 2.2 Classification of lipid levels. (Source: NCEP Guidelines (2001))

Serum lipids(mg/dL)	Desirable	Boderline high	High	Very high	
Total cholestrol	< 200	200–239	=240		
Serum TGs	<150	150–199	200–499	=500	
	Optimal	Near optimal/ above optimal	Borderline high	High	Very high
LDL-C	<100	100–129	130–159	160–189	=190
	High	Low			
HDL-C	>60	<40			

HDL high-density lipoprotein, *LDL low-density lipoprotein, LDL-C* LDL cholesterol, *HDL-C* HDL cholesterol, *TG* triglyceride

particles and is believed to be a key factor in promoting atherosclerosis in these patients. In all persons with diabetes mellitus, current treatment guidelines recommend reduction of LDL-C to less than 100 mg/dL, regardless of baseline lipid levels. Lowering LDL-C to less than 70 mg/dL may provide even greater benefits, particularly in very-high-risk subjects with type 2 diabetes mellitus and coronary heart disease (Falko et al. 2005; Gadi and Samaha 2007).

Diet Counselling and Type 2 Diabetes Mellitus

Diet counselling is an ongoing process in which a health professional, usually a registered dietitian, assesses the dietary pattern and intake of the individuals. The diet counsellor identifies areas where change is needed, provides information, educational materials, support, and follow-up to help the individual make and maintain the needed dietary changes.

Information elicited using a food frequency questionnaire provides a more accurate picture of a person's typical eating patterns (Kaufman 1964). The diet counsellor finds out how often the client consumes certain foods from different food groups, number of servings of dairy products, fruits, vegetables, grains and cereals, meats, or fats he or she consumes in a typical day, week, or month.

Twenty-four-hour dietary recall method is a listing of all the foods and beverages a person had consumed within the previous 24-h period. The diet counsellor may ask a person to recall the first thing he or she ate or drank the previous morning. The counsellor then records the estimated amounts of all the food and beverages the person consumed the rest of the day. The 24-h food recall can be used to provide an estimate of energy and nutrient intake. However, people tend to over- or underestimate intake of certain foods and hence may not accurately represent typical food intake (Robinson et al. 1986).

Daily food records are also useful in assessing food intake. An individual keeps a written record of the amounts of all food and beverages consumed over a given period of time. The diet counsellor can then use the food records to analyse actual energy and nutrient intake. Three-day food records kept over two weekdays and one weekend day are often used (Kaufman 1964).

The initial interview and dietary assessment provide the basis for identifying behaviours that need to be changed. Sometimes a person already has a good idea of what dietary changes are needed but may require help making the changes. The diet counsellor bridges this and helps educate a person on the health effects of different dietary choices. The diet counsellor and client work together, to identify areas where change is needed and prioritize changes.

Making dietary change is a gradual process. An individual may start with one or two easier dietary changes the first few weeks and gradually make additional or more difficult changes over several weeks or months (Robinson et al. 1986). In making dietary changes, each individual's situation and background must be carefully considered. Factors that affect food decisions include an individual's ethnic and religious background, group affiliation, socioeconomic status, and world view. Timing of meals and calorie content of the foods to use at each meal has to be considered (Joshi 2002).

Family members are encouraged to attend diet counselling sessions with the client, especially if they share responsibility for food selection and preparation. Although the individual must make food choices and take responsibility for dietary changes, having the support and understanding of family makes success more likely.

The challenge for the client lies not in making the initial dietary changes but in maintaining them over the long term. Diet counselling is an ongoing process that can take months or years. In follow-up sessions, the individual and the diet counsellor analyse food records together and sort out problematic behaviours that are especially difficult to change. Diet counselling involves teaching to interpret labels, to prepare variety of foods for meals, and providing sources for information on foods. Follow-up counselling also allows the opportunity to re-evaluate goals and strategies for achieving those goals (Robinson et al. 1986).

Diet counselling is an important primary intervention which should provide the basis for choosing the appropriate diet to the subject with diabetes. The major problem to be faced is the quantification of the advice. It is necessary that when counselling is imparted in terms of food, the relative proportions of different foods within the dietary mixture should be specified.

Nutrition and diet counselling has positive outcomes. Therefore, key counselling points should be introduced or reinforced in subject settings, in conjunction with multiple-session protocols (Schiller et al. 1998). Counselling on nutrition can result in marked increases in reported fruit and vegetable consumption in an ethnically mixed group of people (Steptoe et al. 2003).

The first report of the Finnish Diabetes Prevention Study (Lindstrom et al. 2003) demonstrated that lifestyle counselling could reduce subjects' weights. Lifestyle counselling has a direct role in reducing the risk for incidence of diabetes (Tuomilehto et al. 2001). Lifestyle counselling among subjects with IGT can improve the attainment of diet, weight, and exercise goals, even after active counselling is finished.

Research Methods

The present study was carried out to assess the effect of periodic intensive counselling on diet alone and counselling on diet and exercise on the body weight, BMI, plasma glucose, glycosylated haemoglobin (HbA1c), serum lipid profile, and blood pressure levels of adults with type 2 diabetes mellitus. The above parameters were also assessed for another group of subjects who served as the control and who were given only one-time counselling on diet and exercise.

Design of the Study This study was an experimental study with a pretest, posttest design with a control group. The study was designed to assess the effect of periodic intensive counselling on diet and periodic intensive counselling on diet and exercise on the anthropometric measurements, plasma glucose, HbA1c, serum lipid profile, and blood pressure levels of adult subjects with type 2 diabetes mellitus.

Selection of the Sample One hundred and fifty adult subjects with type 2 diabetes mellitus who fulfilled the inclusion criteria were selected for the study. These subjects were from Dr. V. Seshiah Diabetes mellitus Care and Research Institute, Chennai, a private referral centre in Tamil Nadu. Fifty subjects were assigned to one of the following three groups:

Group I: Subjects who were willing to attend only one counselling session on diet and exercise
Group II: Subjects who were willing to attend counselling only on diet with periodic follow-up
Group III: Subjects who were willing to attend counselling for both diet and exercise with periodic follow-up

Criteria for Selection of the Subjects The subjects were selected for the study according to the following inclusion and exclusion criteria.

Inclusion Criteria Following inclusion criteria was used to select the population of this research study:

1. Adults with type 2 diabetes mellitus diagnosed within the last one and a half years and on oral hypoglycaemic drugs
2. Subjects in the age group of 40–60 years belonging to both sexes
3. Willingness of the subjects to participate in the study

Exclusion Criteria Following exclusion criteria were used to select the population of this research study:

1. Subjects who are on insulin for management of diabetes mellitus
2. Subjects who are suffering from any other major health complications
3. Subjects pregnant at the time of the study

Experimental Procedure At the beginning of the study, the baseline data were collected for the subjects belonging to all the three groups. Intervention was given for the experimental groups for a period of 180 days, and periodical assessment was also carried out.

Group I—Subjects willing to attend only one counselling on diet and exercise. This group received the diet advice and exercise regimen prescribed by the dietitians at the centre.

Group II—Subjects who were willing to attend counselling only on diet with periodic follow-up. A detailed diet history of the subjects was taken, and then an individualized diet prescription was given to each one of the subjects, taking into consideration the energy requirement, likes and dislikes of the subject, allergies if any, and the pattern of the diet followed by the family. The individual diet prescription was given based on the following guidelines.

The ratio of the break-up of calories for carbohydrates:protein:fat was 60:20:20, respectively.

- The ratio of cereal to vegetable exchange was maintained as 1:2 at lunch and dinner.
- Simple sugars were reduced in the diet.
- Saturated fats were reduced in the diet.
- Mid-morning and mid-afternoon fat-rich snacks were replaced by protein-rich foods such as sprouts or sundal.
- Two fruit exchanges were included in the diet.
- Oil consumption was prescribed as half a kilogram per month per person.

Group III—Subjects who were willing to attend counselling on both diet and exercise with periodic follow-up. A detailed diet history of the subjects was taken, and then an individualized diet was prescribed as per the guidelines enumerated, in the subjects of Group II. Every subject was advised a brisk walk at a moderate pace for at least 45 min, for 5–6 days a week.

Results and Discussion

The present study was designed to determine the effect of periodical intensive counselling on diet, and counselling on diet and exercise on the anthropometric measurements, plasma glucose, HbA1c levels, serum lipid profile and blood pressure levels of subjects with type 2 diabetes mellitus. The effectiveness of diet counselling and diet counselling with exercise was compared with subjects who received only one-time counselling on diet and exercise. There were three groups each comprising 50 subjects. The study was carried out for a period of 180 days. The dropouts were found to be 10, 14, and 8 % in Groups I, II, and III, respectively. The total dropout was found to be 10.7 %.

The data collected were processed, tabulated and subjected to descriptive analysis. The anthropometric measurements, plasma glucose, HbA1c levels, serum lipid parameters, and blood pressure levels were subjected to inferential statistical analysis.

Gender and Age Distribution Distribution of subjects according to gender and the mean age shows that the mean age range of the subjects was 50.4–51.9 years. The mean age of the subjects in Group I (51.9 ± 5.3 years) was slightly higher than that found in Groups II and III, whereas the mean age of the subjects in Group II was almost equal to that of Group III subjects.

Occupation of the Subjects The type of physical activity has been classified based on the occupation of the people and is presented in Table 2.3.

Subjects were classified according to their type of activity based on their occupation. Percentage distribution of the subjects classified on the basis of their type of activity is presented in Table 2.4.

Majority of the subjects in all the three groups were found to be involved in sedentary type of activity. Around 2 % of the subjects in Groups I and II were found to be involved in moderate type of activity. In Group III, 8.7 % of the subjects were found to be involved in moderate type of activity. None of the subjects were involved in heavy type of activity.

Income of the Subjects The income of the subjects was categorized as very low income (less than ₹ 2101), low income (₹ 2101–4500), middle income (₹ 4501–7500), and high income (above ₹ 7500) as per the classification given by the Housing and Urban Development Corporation (HUDCO 2003).

Clinical Symptoms of Type 2 Diabetes Mellitus The percentage distribution of subjects based on the presence of symptoms of type 2 diabetes mellitus is shown, and it can be inferred that 47.8 % of subjects in Group III did not show any symptoms of type 2 diabetes mellitus. Whereas 58.1 % in Group II and 55.6 % in Group I did not show any symptoms. The clinical symptoms are precursors to the complications of type 2 diabetes mellitus. Maintaining near-normal blood parameters helps to postpone the complications associated with type 2 diabetes mellitus. This can be achieved by taking steps to follow the right diet with a regular exercise regimen. Nocturia, vision impairment and weight lòss were not seen in any of the subjects chosen for the study. Around 2.2 % of the subjects in Group I showed symptoms of polyuria. Polyphagia and tiredness were experienced by 6.7 % of the subjects in Group I. In Group II, 4.7 % of the subjects experienced polyphagia, 11.6 % experienced giddiness, and 14 % experienced tiredness. In Group III, 6.5 % experienced polyphagia, 13 % experienced giddiness, and 10.9 % experienced tiredness. About 9–13 % of the subjects in all the groups experienced a combination of two symptoms (HUDCO 2003).

Table 2.3 Classification of activities based on occupation. (Source: Gopalan et al. (2004))

Activities	Occupation	
	Male	Female
Sedentary	Teacher, tailor, barber, executive, shoemaker, priest, peon, postman, retired personnel	Teacher, tailor, executive, house wife, nurse
Moderate	Fisherman, potter, goldsmith, carpenter, mason, rickshaw puller, electrician, industrial labourer, cooli, weaver, driver	Servant maid, cooli, weaver, beedi-maker, agricultural labourer
Heavy	Stonecutter, blacksmith, woodcutter, mine worker	Stonecutter

Table 2.4 Percentage distribution of subjects based on their type of activity

Group	Sedentary		Moderate	
	Number	Percent	Number	Percent
Group I	44	97.8	1	2.2
Group II	42	97.7	1	2.3
Group III	42	91.3	4	8.7

Dietary Pattern of the Subjects Majority of the subjects in Group I (93.3%), Group II (88.4%), and Group III (91.3%) had three square meals a day. Majority of the subjects in all the three groups were nonvegetarians (72–79%) and the others were lacto-vegetarians.

The frequency of consumption of foods, by the subjects belonging to all the three groups on Day 1 and Day 180 of the study period, is presented in Tables 2.6, 2.7, and 2.8. Results showed that majority of the subjects in Group I (86.7%) and Group II (97.7%) and all the subjects in the Group III were consuming rice daily, in all the meals initially. There was a slight increase in the percentage of subjects eating rice daily in Group I and Group II at the end of the study period. Wheat, rava, and vermicelli were consumed two to three times a week by majority of the subjects.

Pulses are the major contributors of protein in the diet for Indians. The most frequently (91.1%) consumed pulse, consumed about two to three times a week, by Group I was red gram dhal. This was followed by whole Bengal gram or channa. At the end of the study, consumption of green gram dhal was found to be increased. In Group II (95.4%), the most frequently consumed pulse was green gram dhal, followed by red gram dhal. At the end of the study, there was an increase in the consumption of green gram (whole), dry peas, and Bengal gram dhal. In Group III, green gram dhal was frequently (93.5%) consumed two to three times a week, followed by red gram dhal. At the end of the study, there was an increased consumption of whole pulses such as green gram and peas. Bengal gram dhal was also used frequently.

Amaranth gangeticus, a green leafy vegetable, was found to be consumed on a daily basis by 47–61% of the subjects belonging to all the groups at the beginning of the study, and an increase in the consumption was noticed at the end of the study in Groups II and III. Majority (53–74%) of the subjects consumed green leafy vegetables such as cabbage, drumstick leaves, and arai keerai two to three times a week. Such a summary of frequency of consumption of food by the subjects in Group I can be seen in Appendix 1.

The consumption of green leafy vegetables, two to three times a week, had increased in Groups II and III at the end of the study.

Roots and tubers such as potato, carrot, beetroot, radish, and yam were consumed two to three times a week by majority of the subjects. Consumption of carrot and beetroot had increased for subjects in Group II at the end of the study. Onion was consumed by 78–91% of the subjects daily at the start of the study.

Among the list of other vegetables, tomato was consumed daily by majority of the subjects in all the three groups. Drumstick was used by 74–86% of the subjects at the beginning of the study. It is a commonly available vegetable used along with brinjal to make a vegetable side dish. French beans, ladies finger, brinjal, and field beans were used two to three times a week by majority of the subjects. Plantain stem, which is rich in fibre, was consumed by about 50% of the subjects at the beginning of the study.

Gourds such as ash gourd, ridge gourd, and snake gourd were frequently used by 10–22% of the subjects in all the groups at the start of the study. At the end of the study, the consumption of gourds had gone up in subjects of Groups II and III. Bitter gourd was used by majority (56–78 %) of the subjects, two to three times a week.

Regarding the intake of flesh foods, fish was consumed by 45–55 % of the subjects belonging to all the three groups, two to three times a week at the beginning of the study whereas the majority of the subjects were not consuming seafoods such as crabs and prawns. Chicken was consumed by 47–60 % of the subjects belonging to all the three groups, at the beginning of the study. Mutton was consumed once a week by 20–29 % of the subjects, at the start of the study. The consumption of mutton had reduced to 11–14 % in the subjects of Groups II and III as against an increase to 31 % in Group I at the end of the study. Organ meats such as liver, pork, and also beef were consumed by only 2 % of the subjects. These foods are rich in saturated fats and are preferably restricted in the diet of subjects with diabetes mellitus. Egg was consumed more than once a week, by 38–56 % of the subjects, at the beginning of the study. A similar pattern was noticed in egg consumption at the end of the study in all the subjects.

Regarding consumption of nuts, groundnuts were consumed by 26–33 % of the subjects, two to four times a week, at the beginning of the study. At the end of the study, groundnut consumption had gone up by 7 % in subjects of Group II and 10 % in subjects of Group III.

Coconut, which is high in saturated fats, was included in the diet two to three times a week, by 56–69 % of the subjects belonging to all the three groups at the beginning of the study. Similar pattern was noted at the end of the study.

Among fruits, apple was the most commonly consumed fruit in all the groups. Banana and guava were the next commonly consumed fruits in all the groups. Other fruits such as papaya and watermelon were consumed two to three times a week.

Milk, which is a good source of protein, was consumed daily or in the form of curd or buttermilk by all the subjects. All the subjects used sunflower oil, which is high in polyunsaturated fatty acids (PUFAs), for cooking purposes. Apart from sunflower oil, other sources of fat were also used in the diet. About 30 % of the subjects used ghee in their diet. Gingelly oil was used by 45.5 % of the subjects. Gingelly oil is high in both monounsaturated (MUFA) and PUFAs . Groundnut oil, which is rich in MUFA, was used by 19.4 % of the subjects.

Diet has long been regarded as the key element in the treatment of diabetes. Incidence of diabetes is reduced during famine condition, and obesity increases the risk for diabetes. All nutritional factors, either excess fat or carbohydrate, which contribute to higher intake of calories and enhance body weight, have been etiologically associated with diabetes.

Indians predominantly use a plant-based diet. In India, people who consume nonvegetarian foods use it only once or twice a week. It is usually restricted to Wednesdays and Sundays. On Tuesdays, Fridays, and Saturdays, usually nonvegetarian foods are not consumed. During some of the auspicious days, people traditionally do not consume nonvegetarian foods.

Whole Bengal gram, whole green gram and peas are used for making sundal (a steamed snack item). Red gram dhal is used for making sambhar (dhal stew) and rasam, which are frequently used side dishes. Green gram dhal and whole green gram are used for making side dishes with or without vegetables for chappathi (unleavened bread).

Coriander and mint leaves are used often in the preparation or garnishing of side dishes. Onions and tomatoes are used on a daily basis by majority of the subjects because they are used for various preparations such as fresh salads, pachadis, gravies, and curries. Tomato is also used in other side dishes such as rasam and sambhar. Garlic was also used often in a similar manner for gravies and curries. Consumption of plantain stem was emphasized as a fibre-rich vegetable, which could be used in salads, and as a vegetable side dish. This could have been the reason for the increased usage of plantain stem at the end of the study. A fried snack or bakery item was replaced by sundal (groundnuts or boiled whole pulses) at teatime, as emphasized in the diet counselling sessions.

Chicken was cooked without the skin and was largely prepared in the gravy form. Mutton, which is rich in saturated fats, was restricted in the diet of subjects with type 2 diabetes mellitus as emphasized in the diet counselling sessions. Egg yolk contains myristic acid which is most atherogenic among the saturated fatty acids and is estimated to have four times the effect of other saturated fatty acids (Durrington 1993). The cholesterol content of egg yolk is high, and hence subjects were advised to take egg white.

Energy and Nutrient Intake of the Subjects in Different Groups

1. The mean daily energy and macronutrient intakes of the subjects in Group I, every month for a period of 6 months are studied.

   Data analysis shows that energy intake of subjects in Group I was around 1627±463 calories in the beginning of the study, which had increased to 1700±353 calories by the end of the study. There was a trend towards an increased intake of calories from the beginning to the end of the study. Estimated energy requirements for these subjects based on their body weight were 1600–1800 calories per day. The intake of energy of the subjects was found to be well within the prescribed allowance. With regard to the carbohydrate and protein intake, there was an increase, from the beginning to the end of the study. There was a minimal increase in the intake of fat by the end of the study.
2. The mean daily energy and macronutrient intakes of the subjects in Group II, every month for a period of 6 months are studied.

   Data analysis shows that energy intake of subjects in Group II was 1450±318 calories in the beginning of the study, which had decreased to 1430±297 calories by the end of the study. There was a trend towards a decreased intake of calories from the beginning to the end of the study. Estimated energy requirements for these subjects based on their body weight were 1600–1800 calories. The intake of energy of the subjects was well within the prescribed allowance. With regard to the carbohydrate and protein intake, there has been a decrease from the beginning to the end of the study. There has been an increase in the intake of fat by the end of the study.

3. The mean daily energy and macronutrient intakes of the subjects in Group III, every month for a period of 6 months are studied and analysed.

   The data analysis shows that energy intake of subjects in Group III was around 1600±400 calories in the beginning of the study, which had decreased to 1495±323 calories by the end of the study. There was a trend towards a decreased intake of calories from the beginning to the end of the study. Estimated energy requirements for these subjects based on their body weight were 1700–1800 calories per day. The intake of energy of the subjects was well within the prescribed allowance. With regard to the carbohydrate and protein intakes, there was a decrease from the beginning to the end of the study. There was not much change in the intake of fat by the end of the study.

4. The mean energy and macronutrient intakes of the subjects in Groups I, II, and III on different days of the study period are studied and analysed.

   The data analysis shows that the energy and fat intakes of subjects belonging to all the three groups did not show any significant change between different periods of evaluation. With respect to carbohydrate intake of subjects in Group II, there was a significant reduction at the end of 180 days, whereas in Group III, the reduction was significant both at 90 and 180 days. Though the protein intake of subjects in Groups II and III were found to be reduced at the end of 90 and 180 days, it was statistically significant ($p < 0.05$) only for Group II. Group I showed a nonsignificant increase in protein intake.

5. The comparison of energy and nutrient intakes between Groups I and II is studied and analysed.

   The data analysis shows that the energy intake of Group I subjects was higher at all the three periods of evaluation compared to the intake of Group II subjects. The difference in their energy intake was significant at all the three periods of evaluation. The carbohydrate and protein intakes of subjects of Group I were higher compared to Group II, and the difference was statistically significant at the end of 90 and 180 days. The difference in fat intake was not significant between the groups. Both the groups showed a trend towards a slight increase in fat intake.

6. The comparison of energy and nutrient intakes between Groups I and III is analysed.

   The data analysis shows that the energy and protein intakes of subjects of Group I was higher than that of Group III at all the three periods of evaluation. Carbohydrate intake of Group I was lesser than subjects of Group III at day one of the study, subsequent to which, at the end of 90 and 180 days, the carbohydrate intake of Group I was higher than that of Group III. Significant differences in energy, carbohydrate, and protein intakes were noticed at 180 days of the study period. The difference in carbohydrate intake was significant at 90 days also. The difference in fat intake was not significant at all the three periods of evaluation between Groups I and III.

7. The comparison of energy and nutrient intakes between Groups II and III is analysed.

   The data analysis shows that the intakes of energy, carbohydrate, and protein were higher in subjects of Group III as compared to Group II at all the three periods of evaluation. The intake of fat was higher in Group III as compared to Group II at day one and after 90 days of the study period. The differences in energy and carbohydrate intakes were significant at the beginning of the study between Groups II and III.
8. The percentage of energy provided by each nutrient on different days of the study period in the diet of the subjects is analysed.

   The data analysis shows that in all the three groups, the carbohydrate, protein, and fat intakes were well within the prescribed limits. Recommended intake for carbohydrate is 60–65 %, protein is 15–20 %, and fat is 20–25 % of the day's total kilocalories. The ratio of carbohydrates:protein:fat in the diet of subjects of Group I was 66:14:20, Group II was 64:14:22, and Group III was 64:14:22. The percentage of calories from protein has remained constant in all the three groups. Subjects of Groups II and III were found to maintain a similar pattern of nutrient intake.
9. The percentage of total and types of fat intakes by the subjects in the three groups, at different periods of evaluation, has been presented in table below.

As shown in Table 2.5, in subjects of Group I, the percentage intake of saturated and monounsaturated fats had reduced with an increase in polyunsaturated fats. In Group II, the monounsaturated fats intake had increased compared to the intake of saturated fats. In Group III, there was an increased intake in monounsaturated fats and saturated fats. In Groups I and II, the intake of polyunsaturated fats had increased, but in Group III, there was a slight reduction in the intake of polyunsaturated fats.

The Step 2 diet, designed by the National Heart, Lung, and Blood Association's National Cholesterol Education Programme (NCEP) for prevention of CVD, prescribes total fat of less than 30 % of the calories. The fat intake of the subjects in all the three groups was well within these limits ranging from 20 to 22 % of the total calories. Step 1 diet (NCEP) prescribes saturated fat to be less than 10 % of the calories, and Step 2 diet prescribes less than 7 % of the calories. The saturated fat intake

Table 2.5 Percentage of total fat intake and fatty acid profile

Nutrient	Group I			Group II			Group III		
	Day 1	Day 90	Day 180	Day 1	Day 90	Day 180	Day 1	Day 90	Day 180
Total Fat	19.6	20.0	20.5	19.7	23.0	24.5	20.8	22.9	23.3
SFA	3.7	3.3	3.6	4.2	4.7	4.8	3.4	5.4	5.3
MUFA	6.2	5.7	5.6	5.6	5.9	6.5	5.7	5.9	6.5
PUFA	9.7	11.0	11.3	9.9	12.4	13.2	11.7	11.6	11.5

SFA saturated fatty acid, *MUFA* monounsaturated fatty acid, *PUFA* polyunsaturated fatty acid

of the subjects in all the three groups was well within these limits ranging from 3 to 5 % of the total calories. About 30 % of the subjects (29.9 %) used ghee in their diet. But the amounts used were minimal.

Monounsaturated fats are recommended to be up to 15 % of the calories. The monounsaturated fat intake was ranging from 5.6 to 6.7 % of the calories. Majority of the subjects (72–79 %) were nonvegetarians, but they consumed nonvegetarian foods only twice a week. Fish was consumed only once a week. Gingelly oil, a rich source of MUFA and PUFAs, was used by 45.5 % of the subjects. Groundnut oil, which is rich in MUFA, was used by 19.4 % of the subjects.

Polyunsaturated fats are recommended to be less than 10 % of the total calories. The intake of the subjects has been 10–13 % of the calories. This could have been because of the increased use of polyunsaturated fats in the diet by the subjects.

Nutrition recommendations for type 2 diabetes mellitus emphasize weight reduction and calorie management, considering that energy balance and weight loss strategies are important in the management of the condition (ADA 2007). Monitoring carbohydrate, whether by carbohydrate counting, exchanges, or experience-based estimation, remains a key strategy in achieving glycaemic control (ADA 2007). The subjects of Groups II and III showed a statistically significant reduction in the carbohydrate intake after 180 days which is the first step towards glycaemic management. A dietary pattern that includes carbohydrate from fruits, vegetables, whole grains, legumes, and low-fat milk is encouraged for good health (ADA 2007). The subjects of Groups II and III were advised to include fruits, vegetables, whole grains, and legumes in their diet.

For individuals with diabetes and normal renal function, there is insufficient evidence to suggest that usual protein intake (15–20 % of energy) should be modified (ADA 2007). The subjects were advised to take a normal protein intake of 20 % of the total calories. Milk and milk products, pulses, and flesh foods were included in the diet for enriching the diet with protein products.

The primary goal with respect to dietary fat in individuals with diabetes is to limit saturated fatty acids, trans fatty acids, and cholesterol intakes so as to reduce risk of CVD. Dietary goals for individuals with diabetes are the same as for individuals with pre-existing CVD, since the two groups appear to have equivalent cardiovascular risk. Thus, saturated fatty acids less than 7 % of total energy, minimal intake of trans fatty acids, and cholesterol intake, less than 200 mg daily are recommended (ADA 2007). The subjects were advised to reduce their intake of mutton, egg yolk, butter, and ghee to restrict saturated fats and cholesterol in their diet. They were encouraged to use chicken and fish in their diet.

According to the diet prescribed to the subjects, the proportion of carbohydrates, proteins, and fats was 60:20:20 % of the calories. The actual intake of the subjects has been 65:15:20 for carbohydrate, protein, and fat, respectively, with slight modifications between the groups.

Several treatments, such as glycaemic and blood pressure control to reduce microvascular complications, eye examinations with timely follow-up and laser treatment to prevent vision loss, that can substantially reduce and prevent diabetes-related complications have been established. Prevention of gangrene and related amputations can be done by taking care of foot-related problems. Lipid control and blood pressure control are used to reduce nephropathy and CVD. Diet prescriptions and exercise prescriptions play an important role in the management of the disease. There is no lack of effective therapy or treatment for diabetes mellitus. Successful and effective implementation of these treatments for people with type 2 diabetes mellitus is the real challenge. Numerous barriers to implementation are located at several levels including the societal, health care system and at patient levels (Engelgau et al. 2003). With this perspective, the present study was designed to determine the effect of periodical intensive counselling, on diet and exercise for a period of 6 months, on the anthropometric measurements, plasma glucose measurements and HbA1c, serum lipid parameters, and blood pressure levels of subjects with type 2 diabetes mellitus.

Furthermore, it can also be concluded there was a nonsignificant increase in mean body weight of the subjects in Group I at the end of 90 days and a significant ($p < 0.05$) decrease at the end of 180 days. A nonsignificant increase in BMI values was noticed at the end of 90 days and then a significant decrease at the end of 180 days. Fasting and postprandial plasma glucose showed a nonsignificant increase at the end of 90 days and a nonsignificant decrease at the end of 180 days. There was a decrease in the HbA1c values at the end of the study, but it was not statistically significant. There was a decrease in serum total cholesterol, LDL, and TG levels at the end of the study. HDL levels remained the same, and VLDL showed an increase. A decrease was noticed in total cholestrol:HDL (TC:HDL) and TG:HDL ratios. All these changes were not statistically significant. Systolic blood pressure levels showed a statistically significant decrease at the end of 90 days and a nonsignificant decrease at the end of 180 days. Diastolic blood pressure levels showed a nonsignificant increase at the end of 90 days and a nonsignificant decrease at the end of 180 days.

The mean values of the anthropometric measurements, plasma glucose, HbA1c levels, serum lipid parameters, and blood pressure levels of the subjects in Group II at different periods of evaluation were also analysed. Data analysis showed that there was a statistically significant ($p < 0.05$) decrease in the body weight at the end of 90 days and a nonsignificant decrease at the end of 180 days in subjects of Group II. There was a statistically significant reduction noted in BMI values at the end of 90 days and a nonsignificant decrease at the end of 180 days. Fasting plasma glucose levels showed a statistically significant ($p < 0.05$) decrease at 90 and 180 days as compared to the beginning of the study. The postprandial glucose levels showed a nonsignificant decrease at the end of 90 days and at the end of 180 days. There was a nonsignificant increase in the mean HbA1c values of the subjects in Group II at 180 days.

There was a statistically significant ($p < 0.05$) reduction in serum total cholesterol and serum LDL-C levels at the end of the study as compared to the beginning of the study in Group II subjects. No significant differences were noted in HDL, VLDL levels, and TC:HDL ratio at the end of the study as compared to the beginning of the study. Serum TG levels and TG:HDL ratio showed a nonsignificant increase at the end of 180 days as compared to the beginning of the study. Systolic and diastolic blood pressure levels showed a nonsignificant increase after 90 days and a nonsignificant decrease after 180 days as compared to the beginning of the study.

The mean values of the anthropometric measurements, plasma glucose parameters, HbA1c, serum lipid parameters, and blood pressure levels of the subjects in Group III at different periods were also evaluated. In Group III subjects, there was a statistically significant ($p < 0.05$) decrease in both the body weight and the BMI at the end of 90 days and a nonsignificant decrease at the end of 180 days as compared to the beginning of the study.

Fasting plasma glucose levels showed a statistically significant ($p < 0.05$) decrease at the end of both 90 and 180 days as compared to the beginning of the study. There was a decrease in the postprandial glucose levels at the end of 90 days and a statistically significant ($p < 0.05$) decrease at the end of 180 days. There was a nonsignificant decrease in glycosylated haemoglobin levels at the end of 180 days.

There was a statistically significant ($p < 0.05$) reduction in serum total cholesterol and LDL-C levels at the end of 180 days as compared to the beginning of the study in Group III subjects. There was no significant change in the serum HDL-C and VLDL levels. Serum TG level showed a nonsignificant decrease at the end of 180 days of the study.

There was a statistically significant ($p < 0.05$) decrease in TC:HDL ratio at the end of 180 days. A nonsignificant decrease in TG:HDL ratio was noticed at the end of 180 days. Systolic and diastolic blood pressure levels showed a nonsignificant decrease at the end of both 90 and 180 days as compared to the beginning of the study.

There was no significant correlation noticed between the BMI and serum total cholesterol levels of the subjects in all the three groups at different periods of evaluation. Subjects of Groups II and III did not show any significant correlation between body weight and fasting plasma glucose levels at different periods of evaluation. Subjects of Group I showed a statistically significant correlation ($p < 0.05$) between mean body weight and fasting plasma glucose levels at day one and at the end of 180 days of the study. No significant correlation was found between mean body weight and postprandial plasma glucose levels in the subjects of all the three groups at different periods of evaluation.

The present study was conducted on subjects with type 2 diabetes mellitus to assess the risk factors related to the complications of the disease. There was a general trend noticed towards a reduction in BMI, plasma glucose levels, serum lipid parameters, and blood pressure levels that are the indicators of development of complications such as cardiac disease and nephrological complications. Subjects of Group II and Group III have shown a statistically significant reduction in the BMI. Reduction in body weight and BMI are essential for good glycaemic control and reduction in risk factors for CVD, a trend to be followed by subjects with type 2 diabetes mellitus. The periodical intensive counselling on diet and exercise has helped in managing the body weight and BMI of these subjects. Reduction in body weight and BMI will help in the overall control of the condition.

Plasma glucose levels and HbA1c showed a general trend towards reduction in subjects of Groups II and III. This is an indicator of glycaemic control, which is very important in the management of diabetes and to prevent the complications related to increased lipid levels and cardiac disease. Good glycaemic control also prevents the progression of kidney disease.

Serum lipid parameters such as total cholesterol and LDL-C levels have shown a statistically significant reduction at the end of 180 days in subjects of Groups II and III. These are very encouraging as they are markers to indicate cardiac health. No significant change was observed in HDL-C levels in all the three groups.

Subjects of Group III showed a nonsignificant reduction in both systolic and diastolic blood pressure levels at the end of 90 days and 180 days. Subjects of Group II showed a nonsignificant reduction in blood pressure level at 180 days.

Summary of Findings In brief, findings of this research study can be summarized as follows:

- Sedentary lifestyle, which increases the risk of type 2 diabetes mellitus, was reported by 97.8 % of the subjects in Group I, 97.7 % of the subjects in Group II, and 91.3 % of the subjects in Group III.
- Majority of the subjects in Group I (95.6 %), Group II (100 %), and Group III (97.8 %) belonged to the high-income group.
- Majority of the subjects were non-smokers, but a small percentage of the subjects in Group I (6.7 %), Group II (9.3 %), and Group III (10.9 %) were smokers.
- Majority of the subjects did not consume alcohol, but a small percentage of the subjects in Group I (6.7 %), Group II (9.3 %), and Group III (19.6 %) consumed alcohol at least once a week.
- A large proportion of the subjects did not have any of the classic symptoms of type 2 diabetes mellitus. Subjects of Group I (6.7 %), Group II (4.7 %), and Group III (6.5 %) showed symptoms of polyphagia.
- Giddiness was experienced by subjects in Group I (8.9 %), Group II (11.6 %), and Group III (13 %). Tiredness was experienced by subjects in Group I (9.7 %), Group II (14.0 %), and Group III (10.9 %).
- Majority of the subjects had close relatives who were diabetics, in Group I (57.8 %), Group II (72.1 %), and Group III (76.1 %).
- Among the cereals, rice was consumed more often by all the subjects as compared to other cereals such as ragi, rava, and wheat, which were consumed less frequently at the beginning of the study.
- The subjects in all the three groups consumed pulses such as Bengal gram, red gram, and green gram dhals frequently.
- Flesh foods such as egg, fish, and chicken were commonly consumed by the subjects in all the three groups.
- Milk and buttermilk were frequently consumed by the subjects in all the three groups.
- Apple was the most commonly consumed fruit followed by guava and papaya, as compared to the other fruits in all the three groups.

- Green leafy vegetables, which are rich sources of ß-carotene, Vitamin C, and fibre, were consumed in higher amounts by all the subjects and more frequently by the subjects in Groups II and III.
- Among nuts, groundnut was frequently consumed in moderate amounts by all the subjects.
- Sunflower oil was used by all the subjects. The next commonly used oil was gingelly oil.

Appendixes

Appendix 1

Table 2.6 Frequency of consumption of foods by subjects in Group I

Food stuff	Never		Rarely		2–3 times/week		Daily	
	Day 1	Day 180	Day 1	Day 180	Day 1	Day 180	Day 1	Day 180
Fruits								
Apple	44.40	44.20	4.40	2.20	42.10	42.80	9.10	10.80
Banana	53.30	53.00	8.90	10.70	33.30	32.80	4.50	3.50
Grapes	88.90	91.10	4.40	5.40	6.70	3.50	–	–
Guava	46.70	46.90	11.00	12.50	37.80	36.10	4.50	4.50
Mango	73.30	73.30	2.20	–	17.80	19.30	6.70	7.40
Melon, water	75.60	75.60	4.40	5.60	20.00	18.80	–	–
Orange	64.40	60.40	4.40	8.50	26.60	27.50	4.60	3.60
Papaya	51.10	51.10	15.60	17.20	31.20	29.60	2.10	2.10
Sweet lime	75.60	73.40	–	–	17.80	19.00	6.60	7.60
Milk and milk products								
Curd/buttermilk	–	–	–	–	8.00	2.00	92.00	98.00
Ghee	64.00	64	10.00	12	26.00	24.00	–	–
Milk	–	–	–	–	–	–	100.00	100.00
Sugars								
Honey	97.80	97.80	2.20	2.20	–	–	–	–
Jaggery	80.00	79.00	11.10	15.30	6.70	5.70	2.20	–
Sugar	91.10	90.10	4.40	–	2.20	7.60	2.30	2.30

Table 2.7 Frequency of consumption of foods by subjects in Group II

Food stuff	Never		Rarely		2–3 times/week		Daily	
	Day 1	Day 180	Day 1	Day 180	Day 1	Day 180	Day 1	Day 180
Cereals								
Oats	88.40	75.40	–	–	11.60	24.60	–	–
Rava	27.90	21.00	7.00	10.00	65.10	69.00	–	–
Rice	–	–	–	–	2.30	1.00	97.70	99.00
Vermicelli	44.20	33. 00	7.00	5.00	48.80	62.00	–	–
Wheat	7.00	–	4.70	–	55.90	50.00	32.40	50.00
Pulses and legumes								
Bengal gram dhal	23.30	18.90	18.60	–	53.50	75.50	4.60	5.60
Bengal gram whole	34.90	24.90	13.90	18.90	51.20	54.00	–	2.20
Black gram dhal	4.70	5.00	11.60	–	44.20	55.80	39.50	39.20
Green gram dhal	2.30	2.30	2.30	2.30	95.40	93.10	–	2.30
Green gram whole	27.90	23.00	9.40	6.50	62.70	70.50	–	–
Red gram dhal	41.90	18.20	11.70	10.20	46.40	71.60	–	–
Peas, dry	2.00	2.00	2.30	–	86.40	88.00	9.30	10.00
Soya beans	81.40	77.40	4.60	6.00	11.70	16.60	2.30	–
Leafy vegetables								
Amaranth	44.20	40.00	–	–	–	–	55.80	60.00
Arai keerai	30.20	25.20	2.30	–	60.50	72.80	7.00	2.00
Cabbage	27.90	22.00	11.70	12.20	58.10	65.80	2.30	–
Coriander leaves	14.00	14.00	7.00	4.90	74.50	73.50	4.50	7.60
Drumstick leaves	30.20	25.00	4.60	2.00	65.20	73.00	–	–
Mint leaves	20.90	18.90	7.00	8.10	69.70	70.70	2.40	2.30
Roots and tubers								
Beetroot	62.80	58.00	16.30	14.70	20.90	27.30	–	–
Carrot	32.60	25.60	9.30	7.60	55.80	62.80	2.30	4.00
Colocasia	76.70	74.00	11.70	5.00	11.60	21.00	–	–

Table 2.7 (continued)

Food stuff	Never		Rarely		2–3 times/week		Daily	
	Day 1	Day 180	Day 1	Day 180	Day 1	Day 180	Day 1	Day 180
Garlic	95.30	96.00	–	–	2.30	–	2.40	4.00
Onion	4.70	2.70	–	–	4.60	2.30	90.70	95.00
Potato	60.50	58.00	9.30	6.90	27.90	35.10	2.30	
Radish	30.20	28.00	7.00	10.40	62.80	61.60	–	–
Yam, elephant	62.80	58.00	16.30	17.00	20.90	25.00	–	–
Yam, ordinary	69.50	75.00	9.30	7.00	21.20	18.00	–	–
Other vegetables								
Brinjal	9.30	8.00	2.30	–	86.10	92.00	2.30	–
Cauliflower	100.00	98.00	–	–	–	2.00	–	–
Cho-cho marrow	76.70	73.00	2.30	–	21.00	27.00	–	–
Cucumber	34.90	28.00	16.30	4.60	37.20	55.20	11.60	12.20
Drumstick	7.00	7.00	2.30	2.00	85.90	91.00	4.80	–
Field beans	55.80	57.80	16.30	7.20	27.90	35.00	–	–
French beans	2.30	2.00	4.60	–	90.80	98.00	2.30	–
Gourd others	87.30	86.40	4.70	2.60	8.00	11.00	–	–
Bitter gourd	20.90	15.00	20.90	9.30	55.90	72.50	2.30	3.20
Knol-khol	97.70	95.40	–	–	2.30	4.60	–	–
Ladies finger	7.00	7.00	2.30	–	88.40	93.00	2.30	–
Peas, green	23.30	26.20	11.70	14.50	60.40	59.30	4.60	–
Plantain, green	97.70	97.00	2.30	3.00	–	–	–	–
Plantain stem	27.90	23.00	16.30	18.00	55.80	59.00	–	–
Tomato	2.30	2.30	–	–	–	–	97.70	97.70
Flesh foods								
Chicken	39.50	30.20	14.00	–	46.50	69.80	–	–
Crab	81.30	80.40	9.40	9.40	9.30	10.20	–	–
Egg	41.90	37.20	–	–	55.90	60.50	2.30	2.30

Table 2.7 (continued)

Food stuff	Never		Rarely		2–3 times/week		Daily	
	Day 1	Day 180	Day 1	Day 180	Day 1	Day 180	Day 1	Day 180
Fish	32.60	30.60	9.40	–	55.70	69.40	2.30	–
Liver	100.00	100.00	–	–	–	–	–	–
Mutton	53.50	51.20	16.30	34.80	27.90	14.00	2.30	–
Prawn	72.10	72.10	16.30	20.00	11.60	7.90	–	–
Nuts								
Almond	90.70	85.00	7.00	–	2.30	15.00	–	–
Cashewnut	81.40	74.40	14.00	21.00	4.60	4.60	–	–
Coconut, fresh	18.60	18.00	2.30	–	65.00	68.80	14.10	13.20
Groundnut	53.50	51.70	16.30	10.70	25.60	32.70	4.60	4.90
Fruits								
Apple	25.60	18.60	–	–	72.20	71.50	2.20	9.90
Banana	62.80	60.60	–	–	27.90	29.80	9.30	9.60
Grapes	81.40	70.10	–	–	16.20	29.90	2.40	–
Guava	46.50	37.20	4.70	–	44.10	62.80	4.70	–
Mango	76.70	68.70	–	15.00	23.30	16.30	–	–
Melon, water	65.10	50.00	2.30	–	32.60	50.00	–	–
Orange	60.50	50.00	–	–	27.90	36.10	11.60	13.90
Papaya	55.80	55.00	2.30	2.80	37.30	33.20	4.60	9.00
Sweet lime	69.80	65.10	2.30	–	23.30	25.50	4.70	9.40
Milk and milk products								
Curd/buttermilk	–	–	4.00	5.00	–	–	96.00	95.00
Ghee	–	–	10.00	10.00	20.00	20.00	–	–
Milk	–	–	–	–	–	–	100.00	100
Sugars								
Honey	97.70	97.70	2.30	2.30	–	–	–	–
Jaggery	74.40	73.40	11.70	19.60	11.70	7.00	2.20	–
Sugar	79.10	79.00	4.70	11.00	7.00	10.00	9.20	–

Table 2.8 Frequency of consumption of foods by subjects in Group III

Food stuff	Never		Rarely		2–3 times/week		Daily	
	Day 1	Day 180	Day 1	Day 180	Day 1	Day 180	Day 1	Day 180
Cereals								
Oats	76.10	62.10	–	–	15.20	37.90	8.70	–
Rava	32.60	21.00	6.50	8.20	60.90	70.80	–	–
Rice	–	–	–	–		–	100.00	100.00
Vermicelli	60.90	37.60	13.10	17.00	26.00	45.40	–	–
Wheat	2.20	2.20	4.40	2.20	47.65	47.60	45.75	48.00
Pulses and legumes								
Bengal gram dhal	23.90	11.90	19.60	–	54.30	83.70	2.20	4.40
Bengal gram whole	19.60	16.00	4.30	19.30	73.90	62.50	2.20	2.20
Black gram dhal	4.30	5.00	2.20	–	71.80	59.10	21.70	36.00
Green gram dhal	4.30	–	2.20	–	93.50	97.70	–	2.30
Green gram whole	26.10	20.00	13.00	12.00	58.60	68.00	2.30	–
Red gram dhal	41.30	20.00	13.00	20.40	43.50	59.60	2.20	–
Peas, dry	5.00	5.00	–	–	90.70	95.00	4.30	–
Soya beans	71.70	68.50	10.80	5.00	17.50	26.50	–	–
Leafy vegetables								
Amaranth	37.00	32.00	–	–	2.20	–	60.80	68.00
Arai keerai	17.40	11.40	–	–	73.90	85.60	8.70	3.00
Cabbage	21.70	18.00	6.50	3.00	69.60	79.00	2.20	
Coriander leaves	13.00	13.00	10.80	–	73.90	80.20	2.30	6.80
Drumstick leaves	34.80	28.60	8.70	2.30	56.50	69.10		
Mint leaves	15.20	12.90	10.80	7.70	74.00	77.20	–	2.20

Table 2.8 (continued)

Food stuff	Never		Rarely		2–3 times/week		Daily	
	Day 1	Day 180	Day 1	Day 180	Day 1	Day 180	Day 1	Day 180
Roots and tubers								
Beet root	60.90	57.00	13.10	12.00	26.00	31.00	–	–
Carrot	32.60	25.00	4.40	10.40	58.70	58.60	4.30	6.00
Colocasia	73.90	73.00	15.20	11.00	10.90	16.00	–	–
Garlic	95.70	95.00	–	–	2.20	–	2.10	5.00
Onion	4.30	1.30	–	–	6.50	7.50	89.20	91.20
Potato	58.70	59.40	13.00	7.00	28.30	33.60	–	–
Radish	32.60	27.00	8.70	22.00	58.70	51.00	–	–
Yam, elephant	63.00	57.00	13.00	20.50	24.00	22.50	–	–
Yam, ordinary	84.80	82.00	2.20	4.80	13.00	13.20	–	–
Other vegetables								
Brinjal	19.60	12.60	6.50	–	73.90	87.40	–	–
Cauliflower	97.80	96.80	–	–	2.20	3.20	–	–
Cho-cho marrow	76.10	72.00	4.40	–	19.50	28.00	–	–
Cucumber	34.80	29.00	15.20	4.30	39.00	54.20	11.00	12.50
Drumstick	17.40	15.20	8.70	–	73.90	84.80	–	–
Field beans	39.10	39.10	19.60	16.20	41.30	44.70	–	–
French beans	6.50	5.00	–	–	91.30	95.00	2.20	–
Gourd others	78.00	75.00	4.05	3.25	18.30	21.80	–	–
Bitter gourd	21.70	14.70	15.20	8.90	58.70	72.00	4.40	4.40
Knol-khol	95.70	93.50	–	–	4.30	6.50	–	–
Ladies finger	6.50	6.50	6.50	–	87.00	93.50	–	–
Peas, green	28.30	30.30	8.70	7.40	63.00	62.30	–	–
Plantain, green	97.80	95.60	–	4.40	2.20	–	–	–
Plantain stem	19.60	17.60	26.10	28.40	54.30	54.00		–

Table 2.8 (continued)

Food stuff	Never		Rarely		2–3 times/week		Daily	
	Day 1	Day 180	Day 1	Day 180	Day 1	Day 180	Day 1	Day 180
Tomato	6.50	6.70	–	–	2.20	–	91.30	93.30
Flesh foods								
Chicken	43.50	37.00	6.50	–	50.00	63.00	–	–
Crab	76.00	76.10	10.90	10.90	13.10	13.00	–	–
Egg	47.80	41.30	8.70	5.40	41.30	51.10	2.20	2.20
Fish	43.50	43.50	10.90	–	45.60	56.50	–	–
Liver	65.20	65.20	19.60	19.60	15.20	15.20	–	–
Mutton	63.00	63.00	17.40	26.10	19.60	10.90	–	–
Prawn	100.00	100.00	–	–	–	–	–	–
Nuts								
Almond	82.60	78.30	4.30	–	10.90	21.70	2.20	–
Cashewnut	78.30	74.30	8.60	19.00	13.10	6.70	–	–
Coconut, fresh	34.80	35.70	–	–	58.60	62.00	6.60	2.30
Groundnut	47.80	46.90	19.60	10.00	32.60	43.10	–	–
Fruits								
Apple	34.80	32.60	13.00	–	39.20	59.60	13.00	7.80
Banana	67.40	63.10	4.30	–	17.30	25.90	11.00	11.00
Grapes	80.40	76.10	6.50	–	10.90	23.90	2.20	–
Guava	50.00	43.50	13.00	–	30.40	43.30	6.60	13.20
Mango	80.40	78.20	4.40	7.70	15.20	14.10	–	–
Melon, water	63.00	50.00	8.60	–	28.40	50.00	–	–
Orange	73.90	69.60	4.40	–	12.90	17.30	8.80	13.10
Papaya	46.20	43.60	12.50	3.70	28.10	35.20	13.20	17.50
Sweet lime	76.10	71.70	6.50	–	13.00	19.60	4.40	8.70
Milk and milk products								

Table 2.8 (continued)

Food stuff	Never		Rarely		2–3 times/week		Daily	
	Day 1	Day 180	Day 1	Day 180	Day 1	Day 180	Day 1	Day 180
Curd/buttermilk	–	–	–	–	10.00	8.00	90.00	92.00
Ghee	–	–	13.00	4.40	13.00	19.60	–	–
Milk	–	–	–	–	–	–	100.00	100.00
Sugars								
Honey	95.70	95.70	4.30	4.30	–	–	–	–
Jaggery	84.80	83.30	8.60	12.30	6.60	4.40	–	–
Sugar	93.50	93.50	–	2.20	4.40	4.30	2.10	–

References

Abegunde, D. O., Mathers, C. D., Adam, T., Ortegon, M., & Strong, K. (2007). The burden and costs of chronic diseases in low-income and middle-income countries. *Lancet, 370,* 1929–1938.

Adler, A. I., Stevens, R. J., Manley, S. E., Bilous, R. W., Cull, C. A., Holman, R. R., & UKPDS Group. (2003). Development and progression of nephropathy in type 2 diabetes: The United Kingdom Prospective Diabetes Study (UKPDS 64). *Kidney International, 63,* 225–232.

Ajgaonkar, S. S., & Ajgaonkar, V. S. (1964). Diet for the Diabetic. *Antiseptic, 64,* 209.

American Diabetes Association. (1987). Nutritional recommendations and principles for individuals with diabetes mellitus (1986). *Diabetes Care, 10,* 126.

American Diabetes Association. (2000). Nutritional recommendations and principles for individuals, with diabetes mellitus. *Diabetes Care, 23*(1), S1–S46.

American Diabetes Association. (2002). Standards of medical care for subjects with diabetes mellitus. *Diabetes Care, 25,* S33–S49.

American Diabetes Association. (2003). Evidence-based nutrition principles and recommendations for the treatment and prevention of diabetes and related complications. *Diabetes Care, 26,* S51–S61.

American Diabetes Association. (2004). Smoking and diabetes. *Diabetes Care, 27,* S74–S75.

Anderson, J. W. (1986). Fibre and health an overview. *The American Journal of Gastroenterology, 81,* 892.

Anderson, J. W., & Giel, P. B. (1994). Nutritional management of diabetes mellitus. In M. E. Shills, J. A. Olson, & M. Shike (Eds.), *Modern nutrition in health and disease* (8th ed.). Philadelphia: Lea and Febiger.

Betteridge, D. J. (1994). Diabetic dyslipidemia. *The American journal of medicine, 96*(Suppl. 6A), 25S–31S.

Beulens, J. W. J., Stolk, R. P., van der Schouw Y. T., Grobbee, D. E., Hendriks, H. F. J., & Bots, M. L. (2005). Alcohol consumption and risk of Type 2 diabetes among older women. *Diabetes Care, 28,* 2933–2938.

Bogardus, C., Ravussin, E., Robbins, D. C., Wolfe, R. R., Horton, E. S., & Sims, E. A. (1984). Effects of physical training and diet therapy on carbohydrate metabolism in subjects with glucose intolerance and non-insulin-dependent diabetes mellitus. *Diabetes, 33,* 311–318.

Boule, N. G., Haddad, E., Kenny, G. P., Wells, G. A., & Sigal, R. J. (2001). Exercise and glycemic control in diabetics. *JAMA, 286,* 2941–2942.

Boulton, A. J. M., Malik, R. A., Arezzo, J. C., & Sosenko, J. M. (2004). Diabetic somatic neuropathies. *Diabetes Care, 27,* 1458–1486.

Boulton, A. J. M., Vinik, A. I., Arezzo, J. C., Bril, V., Feldman, E. L., Freeman, R., et al. (2005). Diabetic neuropathies: A statement by the American Diabetes Association. *Diabetes Care, 28,* 956–962.

Brown, M. L. (1990). *Present knowledge in nutrition* (6th ed.). Washington, DC: International Life Sciences Institute Nutrition Foundation.

Brunzell, J. D., Chait, A., & Beirman, E. L. (1985). Plasma lipoprotein in human diabetes mellitus—A prospective study. *Diabetologia, 23,* 24.

Bryant, E. (1953). Effect of protein source on maintaining blood sugar levels after breakfast. *JADA, 29,* 239. (Cited in Coleman MC, Tuttle WW and Daum K (1953)).

Buse, J. B., Ginsberg, H. N., Bakris, G. L., Clark, N. G., Costa, F., Eckel, R., Fonseca, V., Gerstein, H. C., Grundy, S., Nesto, R. W., Pignone, M. P., Plutzky, J. Porte, D., Redberg, R., Stitzel, K. F., & Stone, N. J. (2007). Primary prevention of cardiovascular diseases in people with diabetes mellitus: A scientific statement from the American Heart Association and the American Diabetes Association. *Diabetes Care, 30,* 162–172.

Carlsson, S., Hammar, N., Grill, V., & Kaprio, J. (2003). Alcohol consumption and the incidence of type 2 diabetes. A 20-year follow-up of the Finnish Twin Cohort Study. *Diabetes Care, 26,* 2785–2790.

Coleman, M. C., Tuttle, W. W., & Daum, K. (1953). Effect of protein source on maintaining blood sugar levels after breakfast. *Journal American Dietetic Association, 29,* 239.

Conway. (1953). Effect of protein source on maintaining blood sugar levels after breakfast. *JADA, 29,* 239. (Cited in Coleman MC, Tuttle WW, and Daum K (1953)).

Coulston, A. M. (1994). Nutrition considerations in the control of diabetes mellitus. *Nutrition-Today, 29,* 6–11.

Crabbe. (1987). *Handbook of diabetes nutritional management.* Rockville: Aspen Publishing.

Diabetes Atlas. (2003). *Executive summary* (2nd ed.). International Diabetes Federation.

Dinneen, S. F., & Gerstein, H. C. (1997). The association of microalbuminuria and mortality in non-insulin dependent diabetes mellitus. *Archives of Internal Medicine, 157,* 1413–1418.

Dunn, F. L. (1982). Hyperlipidemia and diabetes. *Medical Clinics North America, 77,* 1347–1360.

Durrington P. N. (1993). Dietary fat and coronary heart diseases. In: Poutter N.

Engelgau, M. M., Venkat Narayan, K. M., Saaddine, J. B., & Vinicor, F. (2003). Addressing the burden of diabetes in the 21st century: BetterCare and primary prevention. *Journal of the American Society of Nephrology, 14,* S88–S91.

Falko, J. M., Moser R. J., Mesis, S. B., & Caulin-Glaser, T. (2005). Cardiovascular disease risk of type 2 diabetes mellitus and metabolic syndrome: Focus on aggressive management of syndrome. Management of Dyslipidemia. *Current Diabetes Reviews, 1,* 127–135.

Gadi, R., & Samaha, F. F. (2007). Dyslipidemia in type 2 diabetes mellitus. *Current Diabetes Reports, 7,* 228–234.

Garcia, M. J., Namara PM, M., Gordon, T., & Kannel, W. B. (1974). Morbidity and mortality in diabetics in the Framingham population. Sixteen year follow-up study. *Diabetes, 23,* 105–111.

Gavard, J. A., Lustman, P. J., & Clouse, R. E. (1993). Prevalence of Depression in adults with diabetes. *Diabetes Care, 16,* 1167–1178.

Gerich, J. E. (1998). The genetic basis of type 2 diabetes mellitus: Impaired insulin secretion versus impaired insulin sensitivity. *Endocrine Reviews, 19,* 491–503.

Gopalan, C., Rama Sashi, B. V., & Balasubramanian, C. (2004). Nutrition value of Indian foods, Revised Edition 2004, NIN ICMR, Hydrabad.

Gross, J. L., de Azevedo M. J., Silveiro, S. P., Canani, L. H., Caramori, M. L., & Zelmanovitz, T. (2005). Diabetic nephropathy: Diagnosis, prevention, and treatment. *Diabetes Care, 28,* 164–176.

Heinz, H. J. (1959). *The Heinz handbook of nutrition.* London: The Blackiston Division McGraw Hill Book Company Inc.

Himsworth, H. P. (1942). *Proceedings of the Royal Society of Medicine, 42,* 323.

Holbrook, T. L., Barrett-Connor, E., & Wingard, D. L. (1990). A prospective population-based study of alcohol use and non-insulin-dependent diabetes mellitus. *American Journal of Epidemiology, 132,* 902–909.

Hussain, A., Vaaler, S., Sayeed, M. A., Mahtab, H., Ali, S. M. K., & Khan, A. K. A. (2007). Type 2 diabetes and impaired fasting blood glucose in rural a population-based study. *European Journal of Public Health, 17,* 291–296.

Irons, B. K., Mazzolini, T. A., & Greene, R. S. (2004). Delaying the onset of type 2 diabetes mellitus in subjects with prediabetes. *Pharmacotherapy, 24,* 362–371.

Jackson, C. A., Yudkin, J. S., & Forrest, R. D. (1992). A comparison of the relationships of the glucose tolerance test and the glycated haemoglobin assay with diabetic vascular disease in the community: The Islington Diabetes Survey. *Diabetes Research and Clinical Practice, 17,* 111–123.

James, W. P. T., & Pearson, D. W. M. (1993). Diabetes. In J. S. Garrow & W. F. T. James (Eds.), *Human nutrition and dietetics* (9th ed.). Edinburgh: Churchill Livingstone.

Jarette, R. J. (1979). *Nutrition and disease.* London: Croom Helm Limited.

Jarret, R. J., Viberti, G. C., Argyropoulos, A., Hill, R. D., Mahmud, V., & Murrels, T. J. (1984). Microalbuminuri a predicts mortality in non insulin dependent diabetes. *DiabeticMed, 1,* 17–19.

Jensen, T., Stender, S., & Deckert, T. (1988). Abnormalities in plasma concentrations of Lipoproteins and fibrinogen in type 1 (insulin-dependent) diabetic subjects with increased urinary albumin excretion. *Diabetologia, 31,* 142–145.

Joshi, S. A. (2002). *Nutrition and dietetics* (2nd ed.). New Delhi: Tata McGraw Hill Publishing Company Ltd.

Kaufman, M. (1964). Diet management and therapy the many dimensions of diet counselling for diabetes. *American Journal of Clinical Nutrition, 15,* 45.

Khatib, O. M. N. (2006). Guidelines for the prevention, management and care of diabetes mellitus. *EMRO Technical Publication Series, 32,* 81.

Krall, L. P. (1962). *Joslin diabetes manual* (by members of the staff of the Joslin, Diabetes Foundation) (11th ed.). Philadelphia: Lea & Febiger.

Krall, L. P., & Beaser, R. S. (1989). *Joslin's diabetic manual* (12th ed.). Philadelphia: Lea and Febiger.

Krauss, R. M., & Siri, P. W. (2004). Dyslipidemia in type 2 diabetes. *Medical Clinics of North America, 88,* 897–909.

Laing, S. P., Swerdlow, A. J., Slater, S. D., Burden, A. C., Morris, A., Waugh, N. R., et al. (2003). Mortality from heart disease in a cohort of 23,000 subjects with insulin-treated diabetes. *Diabetologia, 46,* 760–765.

Levin, M. E. (1991). The diabetic foot: A primer for nephrologists. *Seminars in Dialysis, 4,* 258–264.

Lindstrom, J., Louheranta, A., Mannelin, M., Rastas, M., Salminen, V., Eriksson, J., et al. (2003). The Finnish Diabetes Prevention Study (DPS): Lifestyle intervention and 3-year results on diet and physical activity. *Diabetes Care, 26,* 3230–3236.

Mahan, K. L., & Arlin, M. T. (1992). *Krause's food nutrition and diet therapy* (8th ed.). Philadelphia: W.B. Saunders Co.

Mahan, L. K., & Escott-Stump, S. (1996). *Krause's food nutrition and diet therapy* (9th ed.). Philadelphia: W.B. Saunders Company.

Manzato, E., Bragnetto, L., Zambon, A., Lapolla, A., Zmpon, S., Crepaldi, G., Fedele, D. (1993). Lipoprotein abnormalities in well-treated type II diabetic subjects. *Diabetes Care, 16,* 469–475.

Marks, H. H., & Krall, L. P. (1971). Onset, course prognosis, and mortality in diabetes me Mellitus. In A. Marble, P. White, R. F. Bradley, & L. P. Krall (Eds.), *Joslin's diabetes mellitus* (11th ed., pp. 209–254). Philadelphia: Lea & Febiger.

Mattock, M. B., Keen, H., Viberti, G. C., el-Gohari, M. R., Murrells, T. J., Scott, G. S., et al. (1988). Coronary heart disease and urinary albumin excretion rate in type 2 (non-insulin-dependent) diabetic subjects. *Diabetologia, 31,* 82–87.

Mc Cance, R. A., & Lawrence, R. D. (1929). Nutrition in diabetes. *Nutrition Abstracts and Reviews, 33,* 1–15. (Cited in Stowers JM (1963)).

Mc Lester, J. S., & Darby, W. J. (1952). *Nutrition and diet in health and disease* (6th ed.). Philadelphia: W.B. Saunders Co.

Mogensen, C. E. (1984). Microalbuminuria predicts clinical proteinuria and early mortality in maturity-onset diabetes. *The New England Journal of Medicine, 310,* 356–360.

Mohan, V., Sandeep, S., Deepa, R., Shah, B., & Varghese, C. (2007). Epidemiology of type 2 diabetes, Indian scenario. *The Indian Journal of Medical Research, 125,* 217–230.

Mooradian, A. D. (2003). Cardiovascular disease in type 2 diabetes mellitus. *Archives of Internal Medicine, 163,* 33–40.

Morton, D. J., Garrett, M., Reid, J., & Wingard, D. L. (2008). Current smoking and type 2 diabetes among subjects in selected Indian health service clinics 1998–2003. *American Journal of Public Health, 98,* 560–565.

Myers, B. D., Nelson, R. G., Tan, M., Beck, G. J., Bennett, P. H., Knowler, W. C., et al. (1995). Progression of overt nephropathy in non-insulin-dependent diabetes. *Kidney International, 47,* 1781–1789.

National Cholesterol Education Programme (NCEP) Expert Panel. (2001). *Report of the NCEP on detection evaluation and treatment and high blood cholesterol in adults*. Washington, DC: NIH Publications.

National Heart, Lung and Blood Institute Task Force on Arteriosclerosis. (1971). *Arteriosclerosis* (pp. 72–137). Washington, DC: Department of Health. Education and Welfare Publication (NIH).

New, M. I., Roberts, T. N., Bierman, E. L., & Reader, G. G. (1963). The significance of blood lipid alterations in diabetes mellitus. *Diabetes, 12,* 208.
Passmore, D. S. R., & Eastwood, M. A. (1986). *Human nutrition and dietetics* (8th ed.). Great Britain: English language Book Society.
Paterson, A. D., Rutledge, B. N., Cleary, P. A., Lachin, J. M., & Crow, R. S. (2007). The effect of intensive diabetes treatment on resting heart rate in type 1 diabetes. *Diabetes Care, 30,* 2107–2112.
Pratley, R. E., & Weyer, C. (2002). Progression from IGT to type 2 diabetes mellitus. The central role of impaired early insulin secretion. *Current Diabetes Reports, 2,* 242–248.
Rabkin, S. W., Boyko, E., & Streja, D. A. (1983). Changes in HDL cholesterol after initiation of insulin therapy in NIDDM in relation to changes in body weight. *American Journal of Medicine, 285,* 14.
Ramachandran, A. (2002). Urban India a breeding ground for diabetes. *Diabetes Voice, 47,* 18–20.
Ramachandran, A. (2003). Successful multiple risk factor intervention in type 2 diabetes. *DiabetesVoice, 48,* 44–46.
Ramachandran, A. (2005). Epidemiology of diabetes in India-three decades of research. *The Journal of the Association of Physicians of India, 53,* 34–38.
Robinson, C. H., & Lawler, M. (1982). *Normal and therapeutic nutrition* (16th ed.). USA: Macmillan.
Robinson, C. H., Lawler, M. R., Chenoweth, W. L., & Garwick, A. E. (1986). *Normal and therapeutic nutrition* (7th ed.). USA: Macmillan Publishing Company.
Robinwitch. (1930). Nutrition in Diabetes Nutrition Abstracts and Reviews, 33, 1–15. (Cited in Stowers JM (1963)).
Rollo, J. (1797). Nutrition in Diabetes Nutrition Abstracts and Reviews, 33, 1–15. (Cited in Stowers JM (1963)).
Roy, V. C. M. (1987). The problems of diabetes mellitus in India cited in Workshop manual diet Digestion. Diabetes. Indian Dietetic Association 12–14.
Sadikot, S. M. (2008). Can the United Nations Help Fashion a Global Response to Diabetes? The UN Chronicle.
Schiller, M. R., Miller, M., Moore, C., Davis, E., Dunn, A., Mulligan, K., et al. (1998). Subjects report positive Nutrition Counselling outcomes. *Journal of the American Dietetic Association, 98,* 977–982.
Schmitz, A., & Vaeth, M. (1988). Microalbuminuria: A major risk factor in non-insulin-dependent diabetes. A 10-year follow-up study of 503 subjects. *Diabetic Medicine: A Journal of the British Diabetic Association, 5,* 126–134.
Server P., & Thorn S. (1995). *Cardiovascular diseases: Risk factors and interventures* (1st ed.). Oxford: Radcliffe Medical Press Ltd.
Seshiah, V. (1989). Diabetes mellitus. New Delhi: Jaypee Brothers.
Singh, R. B., Bajaj, S., Niaz, M. A., Rastogi, S. S., & Moshiri, M. (1998). Prevalence of type 2 diabetes mellitus and risk of hypertension and coronary artery disease in rural and urban population with low rates of obesity. *International Journal of Cardiology, 66,* 65–72.
Steptoe, A., Perkins-Porras, L., McKay, C., Rink, E., Hilton, S., & Cappuccio, F. P. (2003). Behavioral counselling to increase consumption of fruit and vegetables in low income adults: Randomised trial. *British Medical Journal, 326,* 855.
Townsend, C. E., & Roth, R. A. (2000). *Nutrition and diet therapy* (7th ed.). New York: Delmar Publishers.
Tsumara, K., Hayashi, T., Suematsu, C., Endo, G., Fujii, S., & Okada, K. (1999). Daily alcohol consumption and the risk of type 2 diabetes in Japanese men, the Osaka Health Survey. *Diabetes Care, 22,* 1432–1437.
Tuomilehto, J., Lindstrom, J., Eriksson, J. G., Valle, T. T., Hamalainen, H., Ilanne-Parikka, P., et al. (2001). Prevention of type 2 diabetes mellitus by changes in lifestyle among subjects with impaired glucose tolerance. *The New England Journal of Medicine, 344,* 1343–1350.
Udawat, H., Goyal, R. K., & Maheshwari, S. (2001). Coronary risk and dyslipidemia in type 2 diabetic subjects. *The Journal of the Association of Physicians of India, 56,* 970–973.

Watkins, P. J. (2003). Retinopathy. *British Medical Journal, 326,* 924–926.
Webb, G. P. (2002). *Nutrition: A health promotion approach* (2nd ed.). USA: Arnold Publishers.
Webster. (2003). *New world medical dictionary* (2nd ed.). USA: Wiley.
Wheeler, M. L., Delahanty, L., & Wylie-Rosett, J. (1987). Diet and exercise in non insulin-dependent diabetes mellitus: Implications for dietitians from the NIH Consensus Development Conference. *Journal of the American Dietetic Association, 87,* 480–485.
Wheeler, M. L., Franz, M. J., & Froehlich, J. C. (2004). Alcohol consumption and type 2 diabetes. *American Diabetes Association, 1,* 7.
Whitney, E. N., & Rolfes, S. R. (2002). *Understanding nutrition* (9th ed.). Belmont: Wadsworth Group a Division of Thomson Learning Inc.
Williams, S. R. (1993). *Nutrition and diet therapy* (7th ed.). St. Louis: Mosby-Year Book Inc.
Williams, S. R., & Anderson, S. L. (1989). *Nutrition and diet therapy* (7th ed.). USA: Mosby-Year Book Inc.
World Health Organization. (1999). Definition diagnosis and classification of diabetes mellitus, Department of Non-communicable Disease Surveillance. Report of a WHO Consultation, Geneva.
World Health Organization. (2003). Diet, Nutrition and prevention of chronic diseases. Report of a Joint WHO/FAO Expert Consultation, Geneva: WHO Technical Report Series 916.
World Health Organization. (2004). Expert consultation. Appropriate body-mass index for Asian populations and its implications for policy and intervention strategies. *Lancet, 363,* 157–163.

Prof. Raj Gururajan has been researching and teaching in the information systems domain for 25 years. He focuses much of his research in the area of health informatics and has over 200 publications. Currently Raj is a professor at University of Southern Queensland (USQ).

Dr. Abdul Hafeez-Baig is a senior lecturer in information systems at USQ. Much of his research is focussed within the health informatics domain.

Prof. Nilmini Wickramasinghe (Ph.D.; M.B.A.; Grad.Dip.Mgt.St.; B.Sc. Amus.A, piano; Amus.A, violin) has a well-recognized research record in the field of healthcare and IT/IS. Her expertise is in the strategic application and management of technology for effecting superior healthcare solutions. She currently is the professor director of Health Informatics Management at Epworth HealthCare and a professor at Deakin University.

Rashmi Gururajan is a final-year medical student at Monash University in Melbourne, Australia. She has a keen interest in chronic disease, particularly diabetes research. To date, she has been awarded three research scholarships in order to investigate diabetes in an Indigenous population, and the reasons for readmission to hospital with diabetic complications. Rashmi will complete her medical studies in December 2016 and hopes to continue her house officership in Melbourne.

Chapter 3
Dementia Monitoring with Artificial Intelligence

Andreas Hamper and Isabella Eigner

Introduction

The demographic trend is fundamentally changing the social structures of most Western countries: An increasing number of older people, an increasingly longer expected lifetime, and a low birth rate force the current health-care system to face major challenges. At the same time, all health-care sectors are in high demand for qualified personnel. The shortages are imminent for doctors, hospitals, and especially health-care providers in elderly care (Bundesagentur für Arbeit 2015). These challenges make it increasingly difficult to ensure good nursing care for people with age-related diseases. An outstanding disease is age-related dementia. In Germany, 1.4 million people currently suffer from dementia. Due to the demographic change, this number will increase to approximately 1.8 million in the year 2030.

According to the German dementia report, the rate of people with dementia today is about 1600 per 100,000 inhabitants. This number is expected to double within the next 30 years (Sütterlin et al. 2011). Therefore, dealing with this disease has an extraordinary social as well as scientific relevance (Fig. 3.1).

Approximately 720,000 people with dementia—and thus the majority of dementia patients—are currently treated in home care. Many institutions participate in this care process, such as ambulatory care services, doctors and social auxiliary institutions as well as support groups for family members. Therefore, dementia management is considered a viable example for multidisciplinary and multi-sectoral disease management. The individual needs of the patients differ in many ways: Depending on the stage of the disease and the daily condition, the need for assistance may be temporary but can also get too intensive and time-consuming to be handled in

A. Hamper (✉) · I. Eigner
University Erlangen-Nuremberg, Institute of Information Systems,
90403 Nuremberg, Germany
e-mail: andreas.hamper@fau.de

I. Eigner
e-mail: isabella.eigner@fau.de

N. Wickramasinghe et al. (eds.), *Contemporary Consumer Health Informatics*,
Healthcare Delivery in the Information Age, DOI 10.1007/978-3-319-25973-4_3

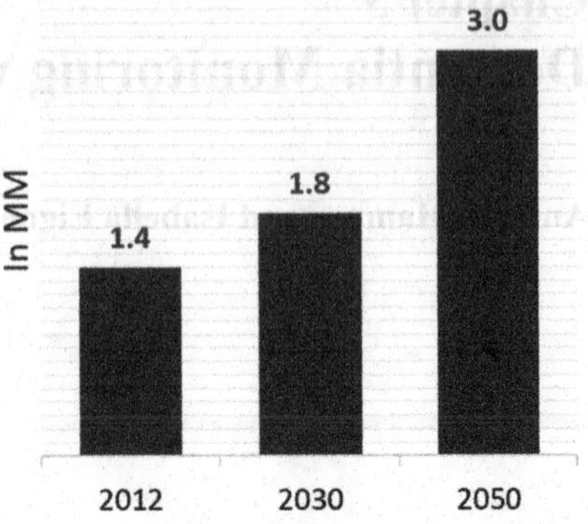

Fig. 3.1 Prognosis of dementia in Germany (rounded; BMFSFJ 2013)

outpatient care (MDS 2008). Practice shows that disease management, the coordination of care professions, and the tailoring of provided services for individual care are less than optimal. Reasons for this are incomplete or delayed information-sharing between stakeholders, heterogeneous sources for disease-related data as well as the lack of individually created supply concepts (BMFSFJ 2007). This results in the need for a simple and automatic collection and storage of disease-related data to optimize available information for all involved professional actors and family members.

The German research project "SAKI," funded by the Federal German Government, addresses the special needs of people with dementia in their home environment. It also focuses on the needs of caregivers and family members. The support system integrates primary care, outpatient care, and informal care provided by family members through a common platform. Critical situations and deviations from normal behavior are recognized automatically by the system and caregivers are informed based on an escalating scale. The project goal is to improve the cooperation of stakeholders in the care process and to increase the patient's and caregivers' sense of security.

Background

Ambient assisted living (AAL) includes concepts, products, and services that follow the goal of raising and securing the quality of life by using information and communication technologies. The main objectives of AAL applications address benefits for single individuals regarding their quality of life, their well-being and security, achieve higher efficiency with limited health-care resources, and support to establish a higher standard of living in societies. The scope of AAL applications for elderly people includes health, safety, security, independence, mobility, and social interaction (Dohr et al. 2010).

As one of the most prominent areas of ambient intelligence, AAL systems provide sensitive, adaptive electronic environments that communicate and interact with people and objects in order to meet various needs. Within this environment, a set of different technologies is needed to gather and process data to detect context-oriented relationships between the user and objects in the home environment. In a first step, various sensors collect data and forward them accordingly to the relevant stakeholders. This data is then either processed by external systems or directly on-site to gather insights on the patient's status. Data can simply be collected from individual sensors or can be combined with other data in a "sensor fusion," which leads to a higher complexity in the structure of the data. Therefore, complex data cannot be merged and processed directly by individual sensors but require powerful microprocessors for post-processing. Finally, the collected data is interpreted by the ambient system using specific algorithmic patterns, which decide on further action, for example, by automatically alarming relatives or caregivers in emergency situations and providing information about the patient's status (Aarts and Wichert 2009).

According to a study conducted by Georgieff (2008), the most relevant areas of application for AAL products are telemedicine, outpatient care, and smart homes. Typical applications in the field of telemedicine or outpatient care include the monitoring of heart rate, blood pressure, and body temperature or the continuous monitoring of patients with chronic conditions such as dementia. Opportunities for ambient systems in smart homes include services in the home environment, such as the detection of present people, recognition of open windows or doors, monitoring of temperatures, automatic gas or smoke detection, and intruder alarm or fall detection (Rosas et al. 2014). Based on these applications, Georgieff categorizes AAL systems into four main areas:

- Health and home care
- Household assistance
- Security and privacy
- Communication and social environment (Georgieff 2008)

The area of *health and home care* includes systems that are used for health care and welfare, the treatment of chronic diseases and the treatment of specific age-related diseases (Becks 2007). Furthermore, assistance systems for medication reminders, exercise programs, and the training of cognitive abilities and motor support in the home environment exist. Applications for *household assistance* deal with issues of supporting the use of technical equipment, for example, providing better ergonomics and additional information, automatic home appliances, touchscreen surfaces, special materials, self-cleaning devices, and interconnected devices, such as heating, lighting, and security systems. To improve *security and privacy* issues in the AAL context, alarm and emergency call systems, access control systems, and motion and presence detectors are available (Becks 2007). With *social integration* as an important factor considering the demographic change, integrated communication networks and social integration and interaction systems, such as support systems for leisure, social, and cultural activities and mobility, can be offered to improve the communication behavior and social interactions of patients (Georgieff 2008).

Classification of AAL Technology

Across the aforementioned AAL areas, a range of different technologies is used to enable applications to collect and process different types of data while integrating patients, caregivers, doctors, and relatives in the ongoing information process. These technologies can be categorized into sensors and sensor networks, video systems, wearables, and assistance and information systems.

Sensors and Sensor Networks

Applications and Approach

The basis for an intelligent home environment (smart home) which supports AAL applications of all kinds is a sensor network that can noninvasively detect different types of activities or interactions with objects. By identifying various kinds of activities, a computer system can control simple mechanisms, such as turning on the lights, but also generate much more complex information about the health and well-being of the resident (De Silva et al. 2012). By analyzing the sensor data using data mining or machine-learning techniques, activity models can be developed. These models serve as a basis for further analysis of the residents' behavior (Chen et al. 2012). Thus, neurodegenerative diseases, such as Alzheimer's, as well as other health problems can already be recognized at an early stage (Tunca et al. 2014). In addition, emergencies can be detected on time by identifying unusual behavior to enable faster reaction in critical situations (Fernandez-Luque et al. 2014). For the monitoring of vital parameters, current approaches already use wearable technologies to gather data and activities of patients. To enable more comfort in everyday life, multi-modal sensors within the home environment of the patient can also be used to detect different activities in a less invasive way. A project conducted by Tunca et al. (2014) uses a variety of sensors to track activities under real-life conditions. Using Zigbee for data transmission, the different sensors are able to communicate and transfer their data to a base station. Further analysis on the data are sent and managed on an additional computer. Other sensor-based systems to monitor activities are developed in the projects "GiraffPlus" (De Silva et al. 2012) and "alert intelligent device (DIA) system" (Fernandez-Luque et al. 2014).

The correct detection of data of different activities is the foundation for the integration of other technologies that support humans in a smart home environment unobtrusively in everyday life (Valero et al. 2013). To support long-term health and well-being, both the physiological and activity data are combined to gather further insights of the patients' status and behavior (Nugent et al. 2013). Received sensor data is processed by software and classified by matching the received data with known patterns to detect activities ("activity labeling"). For the monitoring of elderly persons, it is of particular interest to find correlations between the behavior and the health status of the patient. According to Tunca et al., information about the patients' physical condition can be made by the interpretation of the time, duration, and frequency of certain activities. For example, changes in sleeping times can be an indicator of serious diseases. Furthermore, prolonged execution times of daily activities can be a sign of a decline of cognitive abilities, for example, suggesting reevaluating the severity of dementia (Tunca et al. 2014). In addition, it is also possible to detect trends in overall health development using sensor data over a longer period of time. Based on historical records, the future start time and duration of activities through the use of stochastic prediction models, such as the Hidden Markov Model, can be determined. As a result, in case of abnormal behavior, early measures can be taken (Lotfi et al. 2012).

Technologies and Data

Among others, there are sensors for measuring temperature, humidity, pressure, electromagnetic fields, distance between objects, position and velocity, or smell (Bizer et al. 2006). In general, these sensors can be divided into two groups based on their activity type (Bick et al. 2008). There are passive sensors, such as radio frequency identification (RFID) tags, which draw their energy from the electromagnetic environment of the recipient but usually only have a short range of 20–30 cm. Active sensors or tags, on the other hand, come with their own energy source and a greater range of several meters (Georgieff 2008). In order for the sensors to communicate with each other, AAL environments are divided into three different layers: The lower layer is responsible for the collection of information (sensors, wireless networks), the middle layer ("middleware") supports addressing individual devices such as the interoperability of devices, protocols, and data security, and the upper layer provides value-added services using the collected information (Bick and Kummer 2008). Using common communication standards such as ZigBee, Ant+, Bluetooth, RFID, general packet radio service (GPRS), the Universal Mobile Telecommunications System (UMTS), and long-term evolution (LTE), the different levels can communicate with each other (Fig. 3.2; Mulvenna et al. 2011).

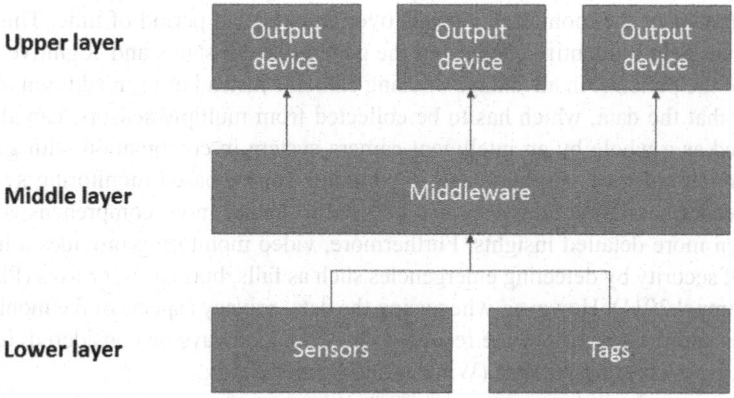

Fig. 3.2 Layered system of ambient environments. (Bick and Kummer 2008)

To detect and distinguish different activities, both sensors and video monitoring systems are common approaches for patient monitoring. Smart homes use a variety of sensors to collect and process the required data. These sensors involve FSR sensors, photocells, digital and sonic rangefinders, contact, temperature and infrared sensors as well as sensors to detect humidity or vibrations.

In a project of Tunca et al. (2014), a total of 27 different activities can be determined by identifying corresponding patterns in the interpretation of sensor data, including eating, washing, reading, internet use, various household activities, using the toilet, shaving, brushing teeth, making phone calls, listening to music, talking, or visiting guests. As the various activities of daily living can be performed in different ways with the same result, sensor data from multiple sources has to be combined to develop a context for daily activities. In addition, false sensor data, which may arise due to noise, lack of activation of sensors, or technical errors (Chen et al. 2012) has to be minimized. As an example, the activity of brushing teeth is described as follows, using various sensors in the bathroom: a contact sensor on the bathroom door, a photocell in the bathroom cabinet, and a digital rangefinder on the tap. When the bathroom door closes after a person has entered the room, the installed contact sensor at the door is activated and sends a signal when the door is closed. The photocell is activated when the door of the bathroom cabinet is opened and the required utensils are taken. If the faucet is used, the installed tap sensor reports a signal to monitor the usage time. Based on these assumptions, specific limits for the proper recognition of an activity are defined for each sensor (Tunca et al. 2014).

Video Systems

Approach and Applications

In addition to recording activities through sensors or sensor networks, it is possible to expand an intelligent monitoring system by using computer vision technologies. Based on cameras, activities as well as physiological data can be recorded. By detecting movements and positions of a person, activity models can be built to observe the behavior of the monitored persons over an extended period of time. This data can again help to identify changes in the general health status and cognitive functions of the patient. An advantage of using cameras instead of or in addition to sensors is that the data, which has to be collected from multiple sensors, can also be captured as a whole by an intelligent camera system in combination with gesture recognition software. An approach to combine camera-based monitoring systems with sensor-based solutions can also be used to gather more comprehensive data for even more detailed insights. Furthermore, video monitoring provides a higher level of security by detecting emergencies such as falls, burglaries, or fires (Planinc and Kampel 2011). However, when using the data, privacy aspects of the monitored persons and the security of the recorded data should always be considered, for example, by encrypting the data (Winkler and Rinner 2014).

Technologies and Data

A video-assisted monitoring system can use traditional red, green, and blue (RGB) cameras. Through multiple cameras with a split field of view, background subtraction techniques, and the subsequent detection of human silhouettes, data can be extracted. Furthermore, by using infrared cameras or depth-based decomposition of images, movements of persons can be registered. Newer red, green, and blue depth (RGB-D) cameras using an additional depth sensor can capture much more accurate data on human activities in comparison to a silhouette-based method. Therefore, more subtle movements and gestures can be recorded. In addition, the posture of a person can be determined based on the matching of skeletal data. To ensure the privacy of the monitored person, there are various possibilities for image editing. Depending on the desired degree of privacy, it is possible to use either a real image, a silhouette with a blurred or pixelated image, a pure silhouette, a three-dimensional (3D) avatar, or ultimately not a person at all in a video sequence (Chaaraoui et al. 2014). An example of an RGB-D camera is the Microsoft "Kinect (1.0)," used in the project "vision@home" to track activities of older people (Chaaraoui et al. 2014).

Another possibility is the use of time-of-flight (TOF) cameras. These cameras can create a 3D image with a geometrically exact mapping of the room. This camera technology has an advantage when dealing with color and lightning issues, such as the same background and clothing color, shadows, changing light conditions, or completely dark environments, as the interpretation of the image is not based on visual but on geometric data (Amoretti et al. 2013). Due to the fact that 3D images composed by pixels are recorded, a certain level of abstraction is available to improve the privacy of the monitored person. An example of an inexpensive TOF camera is Microsoft's "Kinect (2.0)." A monitoring system using this kind of camera to detect activities is developed as part of the European project "PERSONA" (Amoretti et al. 2013). Camera monitoring systems based on TOF can distinguish between static and dynamic activities. Static activities, such as standing or sitting, can be extracted directly from available data. Dynamic activities, such as movements, can only be correctly detected through the interpretation of longer sequences (Amoretti et al. 2013). Due to the high bandwidth the amount of collected data requires (Fleck and Strasser 2008), there are several methods for data reduction. Besides the traditional method to directly send the video or 3D data to a central server to process the data externally, it is also possible to process the signals directly on-site within an intelligent camera network. The resulting algorithm-based decisions can then be forwarded to the external server, requiring fewer bandwidth (Cardinaux et al. 2011).

The detection of falls using computer vision can also be based on fixed cameras or 3D sensors set up in the living environment of the monitored person. In case of an alarm, the image signals of the monitored person can be forwarded as a video stream to supervisors, who can verify the correctness of an alarm (Cucchiara et al. 2007). In a 2D image, the system can recognize a fall by using a rectangular box ("bounding box") or ellipse to map the silhouette of the monitored person and detect sudden changes in the aspect ratios. In a system with multiple cameras, voxels (grid points) can be used in a 3D lattice to detect the position of the person (upright, on the floor or in between). Another approach to gather this kind of information is to detect the position of a person's head and interpret its movement path and speed. However, there are no camera-based systems in place yet that can interpret all types of falls correctly without confusing them with other activities of daily life (Planinc and Kampel 2011). Examples of research projects based on this technology are the "emergency call system through computer vision ("Notrufsystem durch computergestütztes Sehen")" by the Vienna University of Technology (Planinc and Kampel 2011) or "sens@home" by the Fraunhofer Research Institut (Fraunhofer AAL 2009). To protect privacy, images of the video streams can be automatically anonymized by the system (Planinc and Kampel 2011).

Wearables

Applications and Approach

Monitoring

As part of telemedicine, monitoring elderly patients by using wearable sensors is an issue of increasing importance, especially in light of demographic change. The development of smaller sensors provides extended possibilities of using portable sensor systems for remote monitoring of patients. Therefore, wearable sensors with diagnostic or monitoring functions can retrieve physiological or biochemical data about the patient, which can then be forwarded to a doctor, a family member, or an emergency center (Patel et al. 2012). These new technical possibilities are especially advantageous for older people living in rural areas or people who cannot visit a doctor due to physical impairments.

An example of a commercially available system for monitoring of physical health is the "Wearable Wellness System" from the Italian manufacturer Smartex (Smartex 2015). This system consists of a piece of clothing with integrated sensors and a mini-PC as a receiver box for the collection, processing, and storage of data. In addition, Smartex offers software for the configuration of the electronics as well as management and visualization of the resulting data. The portable system is able to collect electrocardiographic signals, as well as respiratory signals through electrodes integrated in the fabric. A built-in accelerometer additionally records body movements (Smartex 2015). In contrast to the Smartex system, the "Body Guardian Remote Monitoring System" developed by Preventice provides the ability to query biometric data in real time. Using a portable sensor plaster attached to the skin of the patient, ECG, heart rate, respiration, activity, and body position can be monitored. The data is received on a smartphone, encrypted, and forwarded to a server where it can be accessed by doctors or hospitals. This way, doctors can monitor their patients' status in real time without having to leave the office or the hospital (Preventice 2015).

Besides vital parameters, changes in sleeping behavior can also reveal important information on a patient's status. Attached directly to a patient's chest, the "Nox-

T3" can record sleeping behavior by monitoring breathing, respiratory rate, heart rate, blood oxygen levels, electromyography (EMG), electrocardiogram (ECG), electroencephalogram (EEG), periodic limb movement (PLM), noise, position, and activity during sleep. The recorded data can then be downloaded from the device and be evaluated for further analysis (nox medical 2015). The large amounts of data, which can be recorded by portable systems for patient monitoring, must be processed accordingly to derive more clinically relevant information. With appropriate signal processing, pattern recognition, and data analysis (Patel et al. 2012), the determined energy expenditure as well as various kinds of activities can be deducted (Kunze 2008).

Fall Detection
With increasing age, the risk of falls steadily increases with multiple risk factors (Vieregge et al. 2008). Several systems are already commercially available for the detection of falls through wearable sensors, for example, the "Fall Detection Technology" developed in the project "Alert 1 Medical Alert System" by Alert 1 (Alert 1 2015), the "Auto Alert" fall sensor from Philips (Philips Lifeline 2015), or the "Vigi'Fall" fall sensor from Vigilio (Vigilio 2015). These sensors can be worn around the neck, on the belt, or on the wrist. For simple sensors, such as the Alert 1, a fall is detected based on acceleration or vibration sensors (Noury et al. 2008). In more recent developments, such as the Vigi'Fall, the wearable sensor also processes the current posture of the person (horizontally or vertically), the duration of immobility, and the position (in bed or out of bed) in addition to the acceleration data. When combined with an in-room infrared sensor, the presence of a person in the room and their position can be detected. In comparison to conventionally worn sensors, the Vigi'Fall has the advantage that it can be adhesively put directly on the body and can therefore discreetly and continuously record accurate data. The recorded data is sent to a receiver box which acts as middleware to process the data from the sensors and interprets it according to a prescribed pattern. In an emergency, the receiver box sets up a telephone connection to a preselected person or service facility (Alert 1 2015); other systems also set up special emergency services (Philips Lifeline 2015; Vigilio 2015).

Technologies and Data

Monitoring
Through integration of sensors in clothing ("e-textile-based systems"), important parameters of the cardiovascular system can be monitored continuously. Sensors can record ECGs based on dry textile electrodes and measure the respiration and blood pressure of a patient (Kunze 2008). In addition to the stationary sensors, piezoelectric sensors, pulse oximeters, phonocardiograms, and accelerometers can also be integrated into portable monitoring systems. These systems are able to record not only quantitative data, such as EMG, ECG, EEG, PLM, blood oxygen levels, respiratory rate, blood pressure, heart rate, or heart sound but also qualitative

data concerning sleeping behavior, body movements, or physical pain. Utilizing ultra-wideband transmission standards such as Bluetooth or Zigbee, sensors can be combined in a so-called Body Area Network (BAN, according to IEEE 802.15.4) to communicate wirelessly with each other. Further signal processing is done by a smartphone, personal digital assistant (PDA), or a mini PC as a receiver box (Radhakrishnan et al. 2014) and if necessary can be forwarded to a hospital or doctor. Using modern smartphones, telemonitoring data can be visualized in a simple way. In contrast to traditional technologies for the detection and visualization of monitoring information, smartphones offer a "ready-to-use" platform, independent from place or time of the user. With the increasing computing power of handheld devices, they can not only be used to display data but also to process it, reducing the amount of required external hardware (Patel et al. 2012).

Fall Detection

To detect falls using wearable sensors, the collection of data is managed as follows: First, activities of daily living must be clearly distinguished from a fall. According to Noury et al. (2008), the critical phase of a fall consists in the sudden movement of the body toward the ground, ending with a vertical shock on the ground. This phase has a duration of approximately 300–500 ms. If afterwards no further movement is registered for a specified amount of time, software interprets the event as a fall and initiates further action. The data sent to the receiver box is primarily relevant for emergency calls, but can also be used to create activity profiles, which can be helpful to detect and prevent emerging physical problems. By interpreting the recorded motions, the occurrence or alteration of chronic diseases can also be recognized by detecting certain behavioral patterns. This can be realized by combining data drawn from fall detection, motion detection, and the detection of unusual movements (Luštrek et al. 2009). It is also important that the privacy of the monitored persons is respected, since in theory every move can be recorded (Noury et al. 2008).

Assistance and Information Systems

Approach and Applications

Elderly people living alone at home often require assistance with daily activities due to increasing age-related problems concerning memory, orientation, and perception. By integrating technologies to aid with these activities, a greater degree of independence can be achieved (Hervás et al. 2013). This results in reduced time, effort, and costs for personal care through family or professional caregivers. In addition, the operation of household appliances with increasingly complex functions can be facilitated by the system. For example, in the "Smart Kitchen" system developed by Blasco et al. (2013), various types of sensors and transmission routes are used to facilitate cooking activities for elderly people.

An additional issue for elderly people living at home alone is medication management. One in ten elderly who are admitted to a hospital are subject to the absence of or false medication (Krähenbühl-Melcher et al. 2007). Therefore, assistance systems such as the "Philips Medication Dispensing Service" (2014) support patients to enable independent medication management by automatically dispensing the right medication at the right time. The data collected by automatic systems for medication can also be helpful for monitoring the progress of the disease and therapy. An increasing number of missed drug intakes can, for example, indicate a worsening of the condition for patients with dementia. By recording the drug-related information, medical or hospital treatments can be performed more precisely and effectively. This can lead to cost savings for health-care systems and an improvement in quality of life for Alzheimer's patients, for example, due to less inpatient treatment.

Technologies and Data

In the example of the Philips medication dispenser, it is possible to deliver up to 60 medicine cups for a maximum of 40 days and up to six times daily to the patient. In addition, the affected person can be reminded when the ingestion of the medication is due. Information and instructions can also be added to the medication plan. Furthermore, there is a possibility to adjust doses of medication depending on the situation; the medication itself is inaccessible to the patient within the device and is only distributed at defined times. If a medication has been skipped, the device can furthermore connect to a family member via phone to make sure that the medication is taken (Philips 2014). In a study by Urzaiz et al. (2013), the basic concept of automatic medication in the context of AAL is further developed with the "LADY medication dispenser" by integrating all stakeholders in the care environment. The following scenario displays the process of an automatic medication dispenser system according to Urzaiz et al. When it's time to take medication, an alarm is activated both visually and by audio. The message "TAKE MEDICINE" appears on the integrated display of the dispenser that provides each medication from individual storage compartments. A sensor detects if the drug is removed from the tray and automatically takes a photo of the patient from a built-in camera. If the medication is not taken from the tray, the alarm will continue to run at predetermined intervals until the medicine is taken or otherwise a message is sent to a caregiver or relative. Using a smartphone app, the caregiver or relative can provide data of prescriptions, levels, and history of medication to and from the dispenser. If a drug is no longer present in sufficient numbers in the dispenser, an automatic order is sent to the pharmacist (Urzaiz et al. 2013).

Another application for in-home assistance developed by Hervás et al. (2011) is based on a smartphone app optimized for elderly people, which utilizes a smartphone camera in combination with QR codes attached to objects of the living environment. By reading the QR code attached to an object, usage information on different devices can be displayed. Thus, it is possible to visualize the functions of the buttons of home appliances, which are currently focused by smartphone camera in a 2D or augmented reality view. This system is generally not intended to collect data about its users but to serve as an assistant and information system. Data is only recorded and retrieved within the residential environment. Through an URL contained in the QR code, recorded data about devices and the living environment can be retrieved from a server and downloaded to the apartment, including a list of parameters with the position and functions of individual objects (Hervás et al. 2011).

A Concept for AI Technology for Dementia Monitoring

While many sensor technologies are available on the market, an AAL solution must focus on the selected use case and the involved stakeholders. This can be the patient himself or other actors involved in the care process. The SAKI project focuses on developing an intelligent monitoring system for people with dementia. While the patient can stay in a familiar home environment, all actors involved in the care process should be supported with relevant information and recommendations, which are based on medical and behavioral data of the patient. The collection of this data takes place via wearable sensors and stationary sensors in the home environment. The analysis of the recorded data is done in real time with the aid of an artificial intelligence (AI) system that acts as a personal assistant in the management of the patient's disease. While numerous sensors and sensor platforms are available on the market, this project aims at combining existing sensors to create user-centered solutions for multiple stakeholders involved in the care process (Fig. 3.3).

Traditional rule-based approaches are limited when it comes to massive amounts of multivariate data as they occur in the context of dementia care. Artificial neural networks (ANNs) offer great advantages over this conventional rule-based approach. The complexity of detecting changes in behavior and habits in the progression of dementia can be tackled by using the context-sensitive application of mathematical algorithms instead of a rigid rule base. Currently, rule-based approaches abstract complex situations to simplified models which are not satisfactory.

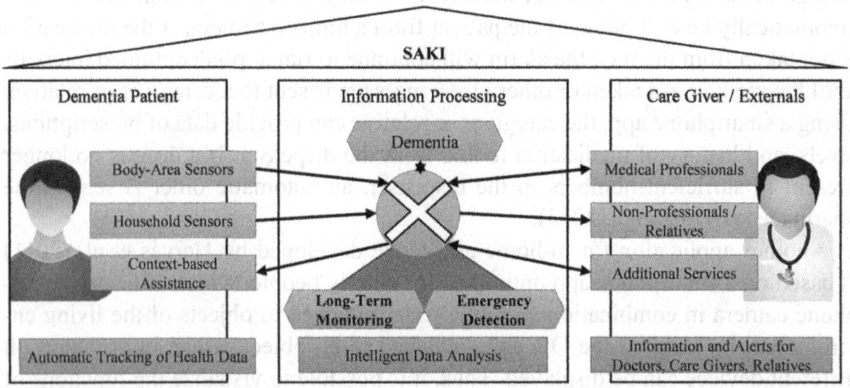

Fig. 3.3 SAKI concept

ANNs are not programmed in a traditional way, but trained on a use-case. This characteristic of machine learning makes the AI approach suitable for this project as typically none or little explicit knowledge is available in the care environment: This technological approach focuses on reducing the enormous amounts of data generated during the 24/7 monitoring from sensors, health indicators, etc. to a small number of usable results (meaningful data reduction).

In the context of this project, self-learning ability means that the system can independently react in defined situations that are learned from initially provided training data. The objective in the training process is to enable the system to handle unknown behavioral patterns and health-related data and provide an interpretation and detection of situations. Symptoms like the degradation of short-term memory, increase of reaction time, and changes in language and motor skills of dementia patients may indicate a progress of the disease and should therefore be automatically detected by the system. Depending on the severity of the (imminent) state, relevant information and proposed instructions are forwarded to the responsible actor in the care process. Necessary data is also added to the care records at the professional caregiver regularly. In this way, quality of care, patient safety, and the sense of security for family members are increased. At the same time, the transparency of the entire care process can be significantly increased. By optimizing resources and reducing the required time for documentation, additional time can be spent on personal interactions with the patient. This leads to a significant improvement in the quality of disease management.

The practical applicability of the use of AI is tested in the specific context of "dementia care at home." Economical, ethical, technological, and user-specific implications play a significant role in this setting.

A major challenge is to provide tailored and suitable information for each participating actor in the care process. Mobile devices like smartphones and tablets are predominant technologies to bundle information from local and external sources. Aggregating care data and providing on-demand information about the patient's status is a main goal in the project. A methodological focus of this project lies on real-life usability: Whereas existing solutions focus on the technological part of dementia monitoring, this project involves the users in the development process by following a user-centered design approach.

Three user groups are focused in the project:

- *Patients*: Dementia patients in early stages who are trying to stay independent and capable of managing their daily life
- *Family members*: Relatives of dementia patients who are involved in the care process or interested in the patient's well-being and safety
- *Professional care providers*: Doctors and ambulant care personnel who need accurate information about the long-term dementia progress

The development of specific sensors is not part of this project. Instead, already established and available AAL sensor solutions build the project's technological base. In addition, widely available electronics like "Activity Tracker" bracelets are included as wearable sensors. Popular examples are the "Nike + FuelBand," "Fitbit

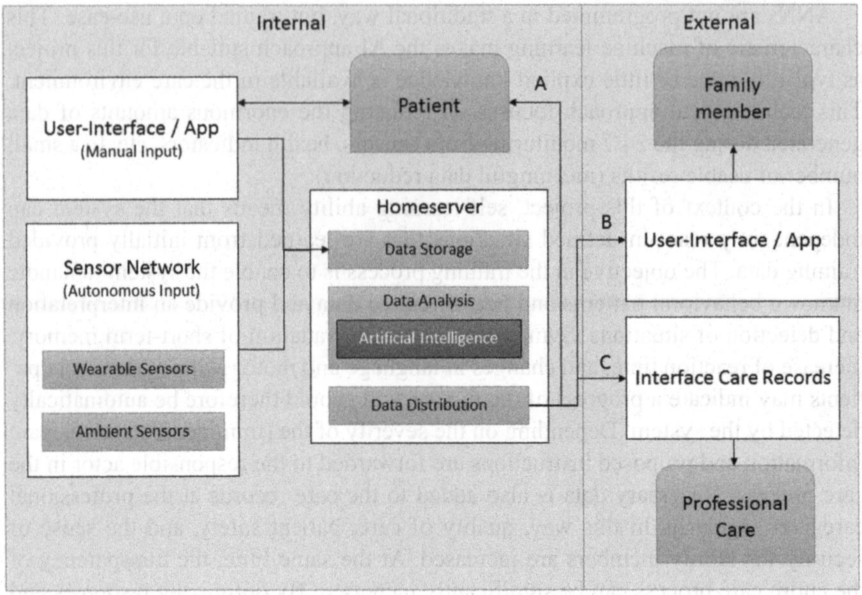

Fig. 3.4 SAKI architecture

Flex," "Withings Smart Activity Tracker" or medical solutions such as the "Vivago CARE 8000 series." This approach avoids the reinvention of existing sensors and opens the ability to include newer or improved sensors over time (Fig. 3.4).

As a result, a practical, affordable, and market-oriented hardware and software solution for outpatient care is developed. The solution is specified as follows:

- Combination of hardware and software which is able to monitor the patient's condition and to give recommendations and information according to the situation
- Sensor-based: Ambient and mobile sensors monitor parameters like blood pressure, oxygen saturation, and behavior. In order to obtain the widest possible range of input data, the development is focused on integrating existing commercial systems
- Integrated and seamless data acquisition to create an automated data collection process
- AI-based evaluation of the collected sensor data to provide situation-based recommendations and calls to action
- A database structure which includes the collected data from the stationary and wearable sensors as well as medical and nursing data
- Involve the patient in the care process and support doctors and nurses as well as family members, so they can intervene if necessary
- The system does not replace today's solutions, but rather bridges the gaps in outpatient care when multiple actors are involved in the care process.

Solutions and Impact for Consumers

The market for nursing services is one of the largest markets in the health sector. In 2013, the spending for nursing services in Germany were 58.8 billion € (Statistisches Bundesamt 2015). As part of the demographical change, the demand (and hence the market) for care services is growing.

Within the health-care domain, dementia care is one of the most widespread and most expensive diseases: According to the Robert Koch Institute, the total annual cost per patient is 43,767 € per year (Weyerer 2005). In Germany, 1.4 million people are living with dementia. By 2050, this number will increase to approximately 3 million (BMFSFJ 2013). This will raise the costs of dementia care to 45–84 billion € in the next 20 years.

A possible answer for this challenge is to reach people with mild or moderate dementia and support them to live independently while being monitored by caregivers. The German market for home emergency call systems is currently dominated by a few large welfare and care organizations such as Caritas, Social Service, or St. John of Malta Ambulance Corps. These organizations can be seen as potential buyers of the system and not as competitors as they are in need of technological support to provide their core services.

The aim of this project is to ensure the safety for patients and provide qualitative advantages over existing care solutions that are based on similar sensory approaches in the following fields:

- *Real-time disease management*: Provision of a real-time status of the patient by using mobile and stationary sensors. This means, for example, to determine whether the patient leaves the bed, is taking up food and liquid, or is in a state of confusion. In this way, the actors in the care process can intervene as needed, without being on-site permanently.
- *Long-term behavioral monitoring*: A system that applies artificial intelligence techniques has advantages by being self-learning: The system independently detects long-term behavioral changes at an early stage and recognizes deterioration before a potentially self-endangering situation arises. The long-term history of individual disease is recorded as a side product of the real-time monitoring. Long-term changes and progression of dementia are recognized by the system automatically to recommend additional measures (e.g., intensive care) in time.
- *Cooperation of caregivers*: Participants in the care process are informed about actions of all other actors and remain up-to-date on the patient's status. This enables a more transparent care process and more efficient coordination. By emphasizing usability, the software is tailored to the need of individual actors depending on the preferred device like a smartphone or tablet.
- *Connection to other health care actors*: Collected disease data can be used for following the treatment progress of the patient. For example, information about behavioral changes can be provided to the hospital or doctors to assess a progressing impairment. Data reduction is done by the AI system to ensure that the data can both be handled by the doctor as well as ensuring the patients privacy.

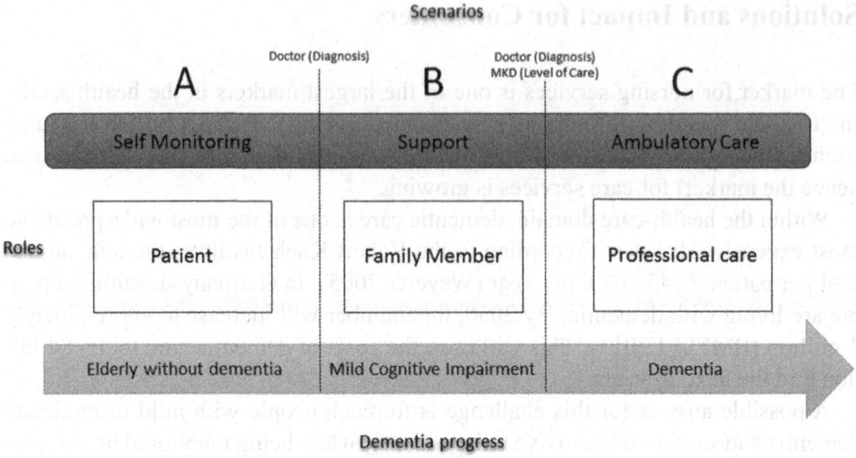

Fig. 3.5 SAKI stakeholders and scenarios

As shown below, the main user of the system might change as the dementia progresses. In early stages or even before beginning dementia, the gathered information is used for self-monitoring. In dementia stages with mild cognitive impairment, the system provides information mainly to family members. With progressing dementia, the support is extended to professional caregivers (Fig. 3.5).

By connecting all actors in the care process, the system supports the following goals:

- Prolong independent living and avoid moving to residential care facilities.
- Reduce the number of unplanned or unnecessary activities of health service providers.
- Reduce accidents by tailoring the care process to individual needs.
- Optimize resource allocation in the ambulant care sector.
- Gain additional time for personal contact through resource optimization.

This data-driven approach might leverage the impact of technology in dementia care in a changing health-care environment.

References

Aarts, E., & Wichert, R. (2009). Ambient intelligence. In H.-J. Bullinger (Ed.), *Technology guide* (pp. 244–249). Berlin: Springer.

Alert 1. (2015). Fall detection technology. https://www.alert-1.com/content/fall-detection-technology/1390.

Amoretti, M., Copelli, S., Wientapper, F., Furfari, F., Lenzi, S., & Chessa, S. (2013). Sensor data fusion for activity monitoring in the PERSONA ambient assisted living project. *Journal of Ambient Intelligence and Humanized Computing, 4*(1), 67–84. http://dx.doi.org/10.1007/s12652-011-0095-6.

Becks, T. (2007). Ambient assisted living: Neue "intelligente" Assistenzsysteme für Prävention, Homecare und Pflege.

Bick, M., & Kummer, T.-F. (2008). Ambient intelligence and ubiquitous computing. In H. Adelsberger, Kinshuk, J. Pawlowski, & D. Sampson (Eds.), *International handbooks on information systems. Handbook on information technologies for education and training* (pp. 79–100). Berlin: Springer.

Bick, M., Kummer, T.-F., & Rössig, W. (2008). *Ambient intelligence in medical environments and devices: Qualitative Studie zu Nutzenpotentialen ambienter Technologien in Krankenhäusern. ESCP-EAP working paper* (Vol. 36). Berlin: European School of Management.

Bizer, J., Spiekermann, S., & Günther, O. (2006). *Technikfolgenabschätzung: Ubiquitäres Computing und Informationelle Selbstbestimmung: TAUCIS; Studie im Auftrag des Bundesministeriums für Bildung und Forschung* (Stand: Juli 2006). Kiel.

Blasco, R., Marco, Á., Casas, R., Cirujano, D., & Picking, R. (2013). A smart kitchen for ambient assisted living. *Sensors (Basel, Switzerland), 14*(1), 1629–1653.

BMFSFJ. (2007). Möglichkeiten und Grenzen selbständiger Lebensführung in stationären Einrichtungen (MuG IV): Demenz, Angehörige und Freiwillige, Versorgungssituation sowie Beispielen für "Good Practice". http://www.bmfsfj.de/RedaktionBMFSFJ/Abteilung3/Pdf-Anlagen/abschlussbericht-mug4,property=pdf,bereich=bmfsfj,sprache=de,rwb=true.pdf.

BMFSFJ. (2013). Demenz: Lebensqualität verbessern und Pflegende unterstützen. http://www.bmfsfj.de/BMFSFJ/Aeltere-Menschen/demenz.html. Accessed 20 April 2015.

Bundesagentur für Arbeit. (2015). Der Arbeitsmarkt in Deutschland—Altenpflege. http://statistik.arbeitsagentur.de/Navigation/Statistik/Arbeitsmarktberichte/Arbeitsmarkt-Allgemein/Arbeitsmarkt-Allgemein-Nav.html. Accessed 21 April 2015.

Cardinaux, F., Bhowmik, D., Abhayaratne, C., & Hawley, M. S. (2011). Video based technology for ambient assisted living: A review of the literature. *Journal of Ambient Intelligence Smart Environment, 3*(3), 253–269. http://dl.acm.org/citation.cfm?id=2010465.2010468.

Chaaraoui, A. A., Padilla-López, J. R., Ferrández-Pastor, F. J., Nieto-Hidalgo, M., & Flórez-Revuelta, F. (2014). A vision-based system for intelligent monitoring: Human behaviour analysis and privacy by context. *Sensors, 14*(5), 8895–8925. http://www.mdpi.com/1424–8220/14/5/8895.

Chen, L., Nugent, C. D., & Hui Wang (2012). A knowledge-driven approach to activity recognition in smart homes. *IEEE Transactions on Knowledge and Data Engineering, 24*(6), 961–974.

Cucchiara, R., Prati, A., & Vezzani, R. (2007). A multi-camera vision system for fall detection and alarm generation. *Expert Systems Journal, 24*(5), 334–345.

De Silva, L. C., Morikawa, C., & Petra, I. M. (2012). State of the art of smart homes. *Engineering Applications of Artificial Intelligence, 25*(7), 1313–1321. http://www.sciencedirect.com/science/article/pii/S095219761200098X.

Dohr, A., Modre-Opsrian, R., Drobics, M., Hayn, D., & Schreier, G. (2010). The internet of things for ambient assisted living (pp. 804–809). http%3A//ieeexplore.ieee.org/lpdocs/epic03/wrapper.htm?arnumber=5501633. Accessed 20 April 2015.

Fernandez-Luque, F. J., Martínez, F. L., Domènech, G., Zapata, J., & Ruiz, R. (2014). Ambient assisted living system with capacitive occupancy sensor. *Expert Systems, 31*(4), 378–388. http://dx.doi.org/10.1111/exsy.12021.

Fleck, S., & Strasser, W. (2008). Smart camera based monitoring system and its application to assisted living. *Proceedings of the IEEE, 96*(10), 1698–1714.

Fraunhofer, A. A. L. (2009). sens@home: Notfallerkennung im häuslichen Umfeld. http://www.aal.fraunhofer.de/projects/sensathome.html.

Georgieff, P. (2008). *Ambient assisted living: Marktpotenziale IT-unterstützter Pflege für ein selbstbestimmtes Altern. FAZIT-Schriftenreihe Marktanalyse* (Vol. 17). Stuttgart: MFG-Stiftung Baden-Württemberg.

Hervás, R., Garcia-Lillo, A., & Bravo, J. (2011). Mobile augmented reality based on the semantic web applied to ambient assisted living. In J. Bravo, R. Hervás, & V. Villarreal (Eds.), *Lecture notes in computer science. Ambient assisted living* (pp. 17–24). Berlin: Springer.

Hervás, R., Bravo, J., Fontecha, J., & Villarreal, V. (2013). Achieving adaptive augmented reality through ontological context-awareness applied to AAL scenarios. *J-JUCS, 19*(9), 1334–1349.

Krähenbühl-Melcher, A., Schlienger, R., Lampert, M., Haschke, M., Drewe, J., & Krähenbühl, S. (2007). Drug-Related problems in hospitals. *Drug Safety, 30*(5), 379–407. http://dx.doi.org/10.2165/00002018-200730050-00003.

Kunze, C. (2008). Kontextsensitive Technologien und intelligente Sensorik für Ambient-Assisted-Living-Anwendungen. In *Ambient assisted living 2008: 1. Deutscher Kongress mit Ausstellung; Technologien—Anwendungen—Management; 30.1.—1.2.2008 in Berlin; Tagungsbandbeiträge*. Berlin: VDE-Verl.

Lifeline, P. (2015). AutoAlert. http://www.lifelinesys.com/content/lifeline-products/confident-home-homesafe.

Lotfi, A., Langensiepen, C., Mahmoud, S., & Akhlaghinia, M. J. (2012). Smart homes for the elderly dementia sufferers: Identification and prediction of abnormal behaviour. *Journal of Ambient Intelligence and Humanized Computing, 3*(3), 205–218. http://dx.doi.org/10.1007/s12652-010-0043-x.

Luštrek, M., Kaluža, B., Dovgan, E., Pogorelc, B., & Gams, M. (2009). Behavior analysis based on coordinates of body tags. In M. Tscheligi, B. de Ruyter, P. Markopoulus, R. Wichert, T. Mirlacher, & A. Meschterjakov, et al. (Eds.), *Lecture notes in computer science. Ambient intelligence* (pp. 14–23). Berlin: Springer.

MDS. (2008). Richtlinie zur Feststellung von Personen mit erheblich eingeschränkter Alltagskompetenz und zur Bewertung des Hilfebedarfs. http://www.mds-ev.de/media/pdf/Richtlinie_PEA-Verfahren_Endfassung.pdf.

Mulvenna, M., Carswell, W., McCullagh, P., Augusto, J. C., Huiru Zheng, Jeffers, P., et al (2011). Visualization of data for ambient assisted living services. *Communications Magazine, IEEE, 49*(1), 110–117.

Noury, N., Rumeau, P., Bourke, A., ÓLaighin, G., & Lundy, J. (2008). A proposal for the classification and evaluation of fall detectors. *5IRBM6, 29*(6), 340–349. http://www.sciencedirect.com/science/article/pii/S1959031808001243.

nox medical. (2015). Nox T3 sleep monitor. http://www.noxmedical.com/products/nox-t3-sleep-monitor.

Nugent, C., Coronato, A., & Bravo, J. (Eds.) (2013). *Lecture notes in computer science. ambient assisted living and active aging*. New York: Springer.

Patel, S., Park, H., Bonato, P., Chan, L., & Rodgers, M. (2012). A review of wearable sensors and systems with application in rehabilitation. *Journal of NeuroEngineering and Rehabilitation, 9*(1), 21. http://www.jneuroengrehab.com/content/9/1/21.

Philips. (2014). Philips medication dispensing service. http://www.managemypills.com/content/.

Planinc, R., & Kampel, M. (2011). Emergency system for elderly—A computer vision based approach. In J. Bravo, R. Hervás, & V. Villarreal (Eds.), *Lecture notes in computer science. Ambient assisted living* (pp. 79–83). Berlin: Springer.

Preventice. (2015). BodyGuardian. http://www.preventice.com/bodyguardian/howitworks/.

Radhakrishnan, S., Duvvuru, A., & Kamarthi, S. V. (2014). Investigating discrete event simulation method to assess the effectiveness of wearable health monitoring devices. *Procedia Economics and Finance, 11*(0), 838–856. http://www.sciencedirect.com/science/article/pii/S2212567114002482.

Rosas, J., Camarinha-Matos, L., Carvalho, G., Oliveira, A., & Ferrada, F. (2014). Development of an ecosystem for ambient assisted living. In Y. Rybarczyk, T. Cardoso, J. Rosas, & L. Camarinha-Matos (Eds.), *IFIP Advances in information and communication technology. innovative and creative developments in multimodal interaction systems* (pp. 200–227). Berlin: Springer.

Smartex. (2015). Wearable wellness system (WWS). http://www.smartex.it/index.php/en/products/wearable-wellness-system.

Statistisches Bundesamt. (2015). Gesundheitsausgaben nach Leistungsarten. https://www.destatis.de/DE/ZahlenFakten/GesellschaftStaat/Gesundheit/Gesundheitsausgaben/Tabellen/Leistungsarten.html. Accessed 21 April 2015.

Sütterlin, S., Hoßmann, I., & Klingholz, R. (2011). *Demenz-Report: Wie sich die Regionen in Deutschland, Österreich und der Schweiz auf die Alterung der Gesellschaft vorbereiten können.*
Tunca, C., Alemdar, H., Ertan, H., Incel, O. D., & Ersoy, C. (2014). Multimodal wireless sensor network-based ambient assisted living in real homes with multiple residents. *Sensors (Basel, Switzerland), 14*(6), 9692–9719.
Urzaiz, G., Murillo, E., Arjona, S., Hervas, R., Fontecha, J., & Bravo, J. (2013). An integral medicine taking solution for mild and moderate alzheimer patients. In C. Nugent, A. Coronato, & J. Bravo (Eds.), *Lecture notes in computer science. Ambient assisted living and active aging* (pp. 104–111). Berlin: Springer.
Valero, M., Bravo, J., García, J., López-de-Ipiña, D., & Gómez, A. (2013). A knowledge based framework to support active aging at home based environments. In C. Nugent, A. Coronato, & J. Bravo (Eds.), *Lecture notes in computer science. Ambient assisted living and active aging* (pp. 1–8). Berlin: Springer.
Vieregge, P., Stolze, H., & Deuschl, G. (2008). Stürze im Alter. *Psychoneuro, 34*(11/12), 524–527.
Vigilio. (2015). Vigi'Fall: A unique solution. http://www.vigilio.fr/solutions-4-71.html.
Weyerer, S. (2005). Gesundheitsberichterstattung des Bundes: Altersdemenz. http://edoc.rki.de/documents/rki_fv/ren4T3cctjHcA/PDF/22wKC7IPbmP4M_43.pdf.
Winkler, T., & Rinner, B. (2014). Security and privacy protection in visual sensor networks: A survey. *ACM Computing Surveys, 47*(1), 2 (1–2:42). http://doi.acm.org/10.1145/2545883.

Andreas Hamper holds a master's degree in information systems. Since 2011, he is a member of the research staff and Ph.D. student at the Institute of Information Systems at the University of Erlangen-Nuremberg. In his research, he is focusing on mobile technologies in health care.

Isabella Eigner holds a master's degree in international information systems. Since 2014, she has been a member of the research staff and a Ph.D. student at the Institute of Information Systems at the University of Erlangen-Nuremberg. In her research, she is focusing on data mining in health care.

Chapter 4
Tailored Physical Activity Promotion with Context-Based Mobile Applications

Andreas Hamper

Introduction

Preventive self-care approaches aim at involving the patient into the process of medical treatment and achieve shared responsibility with him or her (Mattila et al. 2010). While this has been used in the treatment of chronic diseases as well as preventive measures like smoking cessation and nutrition (Jepson et al. 2010), this study focused on physical activity promotion. As the user is not under permanent supervision of medical experts, the success of self-care applications depends to a large extent on the patient's compliance and long-term involvement with the preventive measures (Fogg 1999). Preventive measures work towards a behavior change on the patient's side for a healthier lifestyle (Jepson et al. 2010). Therefore, understanding the process of behavior change is vital to support patients in their self-care actions and preventive measures. If the cognitive and behavioral processes of the patient are well understood, IT systems can be designed to guide and support the user in this process (Oinas-Kukkonen 2010). To leverage the impact of such IT systems, applicable behavior change theory is needed as a foundation to guide the development process.

Traditionally, behavior change strategies have been used in human-to-human communication (Oinas-Kukkonen and Harjumaa 2009) when fitness coaches or medical advisors interacted with their customers. Today's mobile technologies enable new ways of communication which can either be computer-mediated, human-to-human communication or computer-to-human communication (Oinas-Kukkonen 2010) when the IT system itself reacts to the users behavior. Mobile technologies are personal and pervasive devices providing high penetration (Klasnja et al. 2011), high availability (Mattila et al. 2010) and high technological abilities (Holzinger et al. 2010). They close the gap between professionals in preventive care and the patient by being in arm's reach almost 24 h a day. Their potential might be leveraged

A. Hamper (✉)
University Erlangen-Nuremberg, Institute of Information Systems, 90403 Nuremberg, Germany
e-mail: andreas.hamper@fau.de

N. Wickramasinghe et al. (eds.), *Contemporary Consumer Health Informatics*,
Healthcare Delivery in the Information Age, DOI 10.1007/978-3-319-25973-4_4

when behavior theories and models "guide the development of complex interventions that adapt rapidly over time in response to various inputs" (Riley et al. 2011).

If the services provided by mobile applications are built on theoretical frameworks of behavior change, mobile services can be offered depending on the user's progress in the process of behavior change. Many users experience relapse and setbacks when trying to stick to a new fragile habit (Klasnja et al. 2011). In order to achieve long-term sustainability in adapting new habits, it is important to integrate cognitive and behavioral strategies to integrate physical activity into daily life (Bielik et al. 2012).

Related Work

Promotion of physical activity with mobile technologies, especially smartphones, was examined in many projects in the recent years (Campbell and Chau 2010; Consolvo et al. 2006a, 2008; Lin et al. 2006). While the number of fitness trackers and health accessories for smartphones are growing (Gartner 2012), the effectiveness of these solutions is in doubt. In 2014 Ledgers and McCaffrey from the strategy consulting think tank Endeavour Partners (Cambridge, MA) published a study (Ledger und McCaffrey 2014) on wearable accessories for physical activity promotion. They call it the "dirty secret of wearables" (Ledger und McCaffrey 2014) that more than 50% of customers have stopped using their fitness tracking device after 6 months after buying it. They conclude that behavioral science strategies are poorly implemented in available solutions but are needed and vital for long-term engagement (Ledger und McCaffrey 2014).

We focused on related research project which used widely available smartphone technology in their research. Borg-Roig et al. (2014) published a systematic review of the use of smartphones in physical activity promotion in 2014. In their literature review they examined papers from Web of Knowledge, Pubmed, PsycINFO, EBSCO ScienceDirect and Scopus to September 2013. Thirteen studies were selected and analyzed, how behavior change towards more physical activity is supported by the projects. While five projects were based on behavior change theories, a theoretical framework was not reported in the rest (Borg-Roig et al. 2014). The authors criticized the lack of theoretical foundation. They highlighted the importance of using smartphone features, like built-in sensors, in combination with behavior change strategies (Borg-Roig et al. 2014).

While the study of Borg-Roig et al. focused on papers from the medical and psychological area, we have found several projects published in ACM journals and conference to June 2012 (Hamper und Müller 2014). The projects were screened for their underlying theoretical framework. Two reviewers performed the evaluation of the selected projects independently. Eight projects have been identified to support physical activity with mobile applications. While one combines Goal Setting Theory with the Transtheoretical Model and three of them use the Transtheoretical Model as a background, in four projects a theoretical foundation can not be seen. It

Table 4.1 Projects on physical activity promotion

Project	Year	Underlying theory
Houston (Consolvo et al. 2006b)	2006	Transtheoretical model
Fish'nSteps (Lin et al. 2006)	2006	Transtheoretical model
UbiFit garden (Consolvo et al. 2008)	2008	Transtheoretical model
Mobile mentor (Campbell und Chau 2010)	2010	–
Fitness tour (Chuah und Sample 2011)	2011	Transtheoretical model, goal setting theory
RunWithUs (Gil-castiñeira et al. 2011)	2011	–
iDetective (Kimura 2011)	2011	–
Move2Play (Bielik et al. 2012)	2012	–

is notable that the theoretical foundation does not seem to be stronger in later projects. The identified projects are shown in the table below. (Table 4.1)

Based on these finding, we support the suggestion of Borg-Roig et al. to strengthen the theoretical foundation in persuasive technology for physical activity promotion.

Requirements Analysis

Persuasive technology, a term coined by Fogg (1999), can not be seen as a monolithic IT artifact which can be applied to anyone in order to change his or her behavior. Persuasive Technology must be tailored towards a specific user and consider medical, psychological and environmental factors that influence his or her behavior (Fogg 2003).

Persuasive Service Portfolio

This study focused on adults that are not under medical treatment for pre-existing medical conditions, but may have risk factors that can lead to chronically diseases. The goal is to increase their level of physical activity in their everyday life to meet the WHO recommendations (World Health Organization 2010). This means, based on the general WHO calculations, walking at least 10,000 steps a day, reach at least 150 min of cardiovascular exercise per week and at least 30 min of muscular exercise twice per week. Depending on the individual WHO recommendation and existing activity level, persuasive services have to guide towards the target level of physical activity in everyday life. Persuasive actions therefore have to be applied multiple times during the day, considering the users' context such as motivation, activities and habits. Two time horizons are dominant in behavior change theories.

Large timescale theories focus on cognitive and behavioral conditions, which change over a long period of time. One of the predominant theories used in behavior change support systems is the Transtheoretical Model (TTM) by Prochaska et al. (Prochaska et al. 2008). In this model, at least 6 months are needed to perform a sustainable attitude and behavior change. We use the TTM model as a basis for large time scale tailoring of persuasive measures. The TTM describes five different stages of behavior change an individual goes through: Precontemplation, contemplation, preparation, action and maintenance (Prochaska et al. 1992). In the precontemplation stage, the individual has no intention to change his or her behavior in the near future. In the contemplation and preparation stages, awareness rises and the individual takes first steps to change his or her behavior. The action and maintenance stages describe the stages in which the new behavior is performed and afterwards maintained for a long period of time. Specific strategies are suggested to support the transition from one stage to the next. Nine strategies have been identified to be important for intervention programs (Hoeger und Hoeger 2010; Prochaska et al. 2008). Strategies can be divided along the dimensions 'cognitive-affective' and 'behavioral' (Prochaska et al. 2008). Cognitive-affective strategies are aiming at a change of mind by increasing awareness for the necessity to change, point out the impact of negative behavior and the relevance of positive behavior. Therefore, cognitive-affective strategies are mainly successful in the early stages of change, namely precontemplation and contemplation. Behavioral strategies focus on supporting the actual behavior after the decision to change has been made. Therefore these strategies help the individual to perform or maintain the changed behavior. Persuasive services have to be tailored depending on the stage of change, in which the user currently is. Inactive users, or so-called couch potatoes, are starting in the first stages of behavior change (Prochaska et al. 2008). That means, that persuasive services should focus on cognitive strategies in order to raise risk awareness and change the users mind set. A well-known example of persuasive messages with cognitive strategies can be found in the field of smoking cessation. Shocking pictures of smokers' lungs are printed on the cigarette packets to create risk awareness and visualize the health consequences (Abdolahinia et al. 2010). Active users, which have progressed further in the process of behavior change, should be addressed with persuasive services that focus on behavioral strategies. A famous example is the new years' resolution problem when users are willing to change their behavior at the beginning of the New Year, but lack guidelines and tools to stick to their goal over a long period of time (Schut und Stam 1994).

Deciding When and How to Persuade

Besides the long-term behavior change, a dimension of all-day micromanagement is needed to manage the little steps of behavior change. Widely used theories, like the goal setting theory (Schut und Stam 1994) state, that target behavior and goals must be broken down into smaller, achievable goals. These goals can be tackled easier than focusing on goals that are too far away to be reached in adequate time. The goals setting theory proposes requirements ('SMART' goals) in order to be suitable for behavior change. While goals setting can be an important strategy for behavior change, this study used a broader approach to influence behavior. The Fogg Behavior Model (FBM) proposed by BJ Fogg (2003) is based on three elements that determine, whether a behavior happens or not. Fogg describes them as 'Motivation', 'Ability' and 'Trigger' while all of them have to be present at the same time. A behavior takes place when the user is motivated enough, has the ability to perform the behavior and is triggered to do it. Behavior can therefore be described as the formula:

Behavior = motivation*ability*trigger

To influence the motivation dimension, three pairs of core motivators are described: Pleasure and Pain, Hope and Fear, Social Acceptance and Rejection (Fogg 2009). While Pleasure and Pain focus on immediately perceived emotions, Hope and Fear includes expected results in the future. Social Acceptance and Rejection address the role of the individual in contact with others or in a group following inherent standards and values.

For the dimension of ability six factors are described (Fogg 2009): Time, money, brain cycles, non-routine, physical effort and social deviance.

The crucial elements whether a behavior occurs or not, are triggers. Even if the user is motivated enough and the behavior is easy to do, an additional trigger is needed as a reminder and call to action (Fogg 2009). Triggers will fail if either motivation is too low or ability is lacking.

Persuasive services can boost motivation—called sparks—or make a behavior easier—called facilitators. They can also serve as a trigger. In order to be successful in changing behavior, the services not only have to be of the right type and at the right time as proposed by Fogg (2009). We propose to also adapt the services to the current stage of change in the TTM. This means that the three types of services have to focus on cognitive strategies if the user is in the earlier stages of behavior change and should use behavioral strategies when the user has already started to change his or her behavior. The following list gives examples on how persuasive services to promote physical activity can be designed:

- Cognitive:
  - Sparks: Visualizing the health impact of increased physical activity. By showing how risk factors for cardiovascular diseases, high blood pressure and diabetes will change, the current risk level (fear) and the health benefits (hope) that can be pointed out.
  - Facilitators: Showing, opportunities for physical activity in everyday life. Building first steps guidelines can reduce the needed brain cycles and outlines, how physical activity can be integrated in the daily routine (time).
  - Triggers: Monitoring daily activity and physical parameters like weight and body fat. The daily confrontation with the existing situation brings the need for action into the users mind and helps building risk awareness.
- Behavioral:
  - Sparks: Rewarding the user, even for small steps towards a physically active lifestyle. Strategies from goal setting theory can be used here. Rewards can

be external, like monetary bonuses, or in form of virtual points and achievements. Getting rewarded for physical activity (pleasure) can also be used in social groups to make the own progress and status visible to other members of the group (social acceptance).

- Facilitators: Making physical activity easier by providing information when, where and how to do sports, and helping to prepare the right sports equipment. This reduces planning activities (brain-cycles) and avoids fallbacks like missed training days (non-routine).
- Triggers: Reminders to interrupt unhealthy behavior. They focuse on daily habits that can easily be changed, but are often too deep integrated into daily activity. While the user is mostly motivated enough and the behavior change does not require noteworthy resources, simple calls to action are needed to remind the user to change something.

Detection of Context Information

To start persuasive services in the right situation to induce a defined target behavior, a comprehensive insight into the users behavior is needed 24/7. This comprises health information as well as information about physical activity and even behavioral patterns how days are structured regularly. Human persuaders like personal fitness coaches can easily question the user or watch their behavior (Chen und Hekler 2011). To bring this to an IT based persuasive service platform, context information of the user has to be gathered in a structured way.

Context information is needed for two purposes: Information about the user's health status, like preconditions, body composition, fitness level but also performed activities like daily steps, spent calories and training routines have to be gathered for medical interpretation. Individual fitness goals are derived from WHO recommendations for different user groups (World Health Organization 2010). This defines the target behavior for each individual user. Information about the already performed activity allows a comparison of the target behavior and the actual behavior. The degree, in which users follow the medically indicated recommendations, is an indicator for compliance but also defines, if further behavior change is needed or not. Furthermore, context information is needed for psychological tailoring of persuasive services. This means, when and how persuasive services should be presented to the user. Sparks, facilitators and triggers have to react on the user's behavior in order to support the little changes in everyday life (Fogg 2009). Facilitators should react on context information such as weather information, working hours or sleeping times. Sparks can provide extra motivation when a major underperformance is predicted, based on the activity so far. Sparks can also boost motivation when a user is close to the daily goal and can reach it with just a slight increase in activity. Triggers need complex information about performed activities, like sitting, walking or sleeping, to interrupt unhealthy habits.

This leads to the need for a comprehensive detection of context information. Every persuasive service needs individual subsets of context information to be placed efficiently. Therefore, when creating new persuasive services the amount of needed context information may grow. To support this by design, the context model of Dey and Abowd (2000) is used as an underlying structure. Four categories of primary context are distinguished: Time, location, activity and identity. The so-called secondary context types provide detailed information about individual aspects of a primary context type (Dey und Abowd 2000). Examples for relevant secondary context information are shown below:

- Time: Day/Night, workday/weekend, usual training time
- Location: POIs like workplace, home or gym
- Activity: Steps, burned calories, activity types, intensity of activity
- Identity: Gender, age, body composition, heart rate, blood pressure, blood sugar, motivational state

The required types of secondary context information are defined by the persuasive services, as they need a subset of context information to be working correctly. This shows that the system work on pull mechanisms, where services demand for context information. Therefore each service has different requirements on the available information. At the current stage, the concept is restricted for the use as a virtual fitness coach. Persuasive services for treatment of chronic conditions require a lot more secondary context information, especially from the category 'identity' when monitoring blood and cardiovascular data (Bergert et al. 2014).

Concept for Context-Based Behavior Change Support Services

The concept is created on the Google Android platform ("Android KitKat | Android Developers" n.d.) and consists of three layers: Sensor framework, data analysis and service presentation. Sensor framework and data analysis are not visible to the user. All user interaction is done within the service presentation layer. The figure below shows the system architecture that is described in the following section. (Fig. 4.1)

Sensor Framework

Individual sensors have been used in many mobile IT applications since smartphones emerged. Often, the sensors are sold as fitness accessories for smartphone applications ("Nike+Fuelband SE. Aktivitätstracker & Fitnessmesser. Nike.com (DE)" n.d., "Offizielle Fitbit®-Website: Kabellose Aktivitäts- und Schlaf-Tracker Force, Flex, One und Zip" n.d.). This is suitable for e.g. step counters and corresponding smartphone applications to monitor daily steps. Thus, the approach of hardwiring sensors to applications comes to it's limits when more complex behavior has to be monitored. As shown in the previous chapter, numerous sensor information has to be gathered and combined automatically in order to give a comprehensive

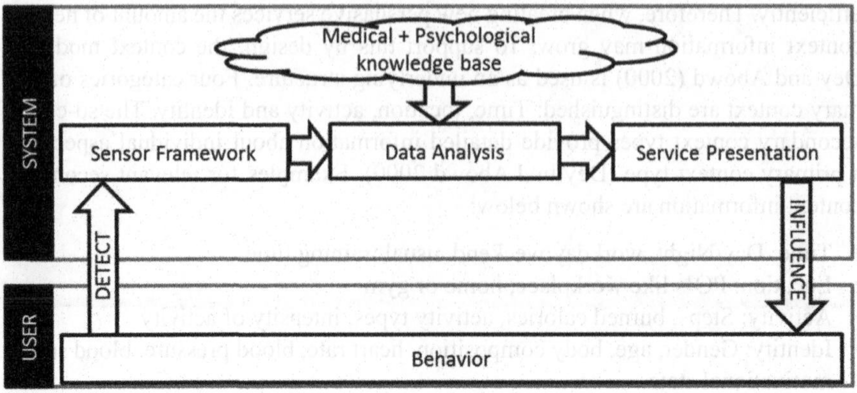

Fig. 4.1 System architecture

overview of relevant user context in all four primary context dimensions. A flexible and expandable approach is needed to collect and store sensor data from multiple devices. In addition, the quickly evolving economic environment of wearable consumer devices demands readiness for new or improved sensors in the next hardware generations. While hardware manufacturers change and precision improves, the output values of the sensors stay the same. We have seen improvements in the prevention of false positive step detection ("Android KitKat | Android Developers" n.d.) as well as heart rate monitoring which can now be done with a finger scan on the back of your smartphone ("My life powered by GalaxyS5" n.d.). However, the output data of these sensors is still the same (steps and heart rate in these examples).

To allow fixed types of context data and yet utilize improved sensor hardware, we have created a sensor framework for context information.

Two types of measurement are distinguished. Event-based measurement is used when a value does not radically change over short periods of time. This is the case for identity information like gender, date of birth, height and previous medical conditions. That information is manually entered in the user profile on the first use of the application. To evaluate the user's motivational state and his or her progress through the different stages of the TTM, the URICA-E2 (Marcus et al. 1992) standardized questionnaire for dimensional evaluation of the stages of change is used. Event-based measurement is also used for information that is collected from external sensors which are stationary installed in the household or gym. For example this is the case for a wireless body scale to measure weight, body fat and heart rate. We use the 'Withings Body Analyzer' ("Withings: Smart Body Analyzer" n.d.) which transfers measured data over inbuilt Wi-Fi to the Withings server, where the data can be accessed via a REST based API. In the next iteration of the project, we will integrate the Withings Wireless Blood Pressure Monitor ("Withings: Wireless Blood Pressure Monitor" n.d.) and blood sugar and cholesterol sensors with the same API.

In contrary to the monitoring of 'identity', which has to be event-based, information from the primary context types 'activity', 'time' and 'location' have to be recorded constantly because of their perishable nature. Interesting information does not only lie in the discrete values but also when looking at certain timespans. Therefore, information about activities and locations are recorded as time series. A recording interval of 1 min was chosen. This is an acceptable delay, before the system can react to new information but still keeps the amount of data in a manageable dimension for mobile devices. 1440 entities of continuous data measurement points are recorded per day. Each recorded entity contains information about what has happened in the minute before. Location is saved as the averaged measures from a FusedLocationProvider ("Location APIs | Android Developers" n.d.) which combines GPS, Wi-Fi triangulation with cell positioning. Activity types like walking, driving, cycling etc. are detected with an ActivityProvider ("Location APIs | Android Developers" n.d.) which uses pattern recognition algorithms to tell activities apart. Calorie expenditure, walked steps and walking distance are calculated on the basis of the user's height, weight and gender and the built-in step counter ("Android KitKat | Android Developers" n.d.) in the smartphone.

By using the concept of 'providers' to collect context information from sensors, an abstraction layer is created. This allows switching from one sensor to another (e.g. from step counter in the smartphone to a step counter wristband). Furthermore, this makes it possible to extend the sensor framework to other sensor categories by creating new providers.

The collected information is stored in a relational database. The framework and data structure is shown in the figure below. (Fig. 4.2)

Data Analysis

The set of context information, as described above, gives no direct insight into the user's behavior. Meaningful knowledge about the user has to be extracted. We use data mining techniques on the context information to gain insight in two areas: The medical interpretation of the user's health status and the psychological revealing of situations with behavior change potentials. A rule-based inference machine (Hayes-Roth 1985) is used to analyze context information.

Medical interpretation analyzes the user's health status and evaluates, if the current behavior influences the health positively or negatively. These indicators are called Health Key Performance Indicators (hKPI). While simple hKPIs like body mass index are easy to calculate (Garrouste-Orgeas et al. 2004), more complex indicators are needed to give risk assessment and recommendations. An established approach for valuating the personal cardiovascular risk for cardiac infarction and apoplectic stroke is the 'Arriba' calculator (Krones et al. 2008). General practitioners use the concept in prevention talks. 'Arriba' is based on the long term Framingham heart study. Based on gender, age, smoking habits, blood pressure and cholesterol the personal 10 year risk for suffering from cardiac infarction or apoplectic stroke is calculated. The cardiovascular risk is used as the individual health score in the system. Furthermore, when having the cardiovascular risk, the preventive

Fig. 4.2 Sensor framework

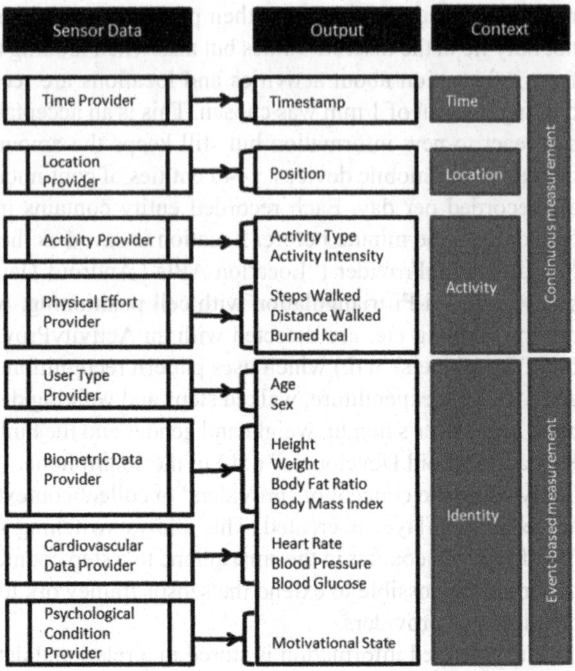

effect of physical activity can be quantified. It can be visualized as a percentage in risk reduction. To generate precise physical activity recommendation, the WHO guidelines for physical activity are used (World Health Organization 2010). Based on identity information, the appropriate WHO guidelines on cardiovascular and muscular activity for the specific user group are selected. The combination of these approaches gives an overview about the user's current health status as well as clear recommendations for behavior change.

Psychological tailoring is needed to communicate the identified need for behavior change to the user. As described in Fogg's concept, sparks, facilitators and triggers are needed at the right moment to make behavior change happen. To identify situations, in which persuasive services should be applied, expert knowledge of personal fitness coaches was collected. Personal fitness coaches guide their customers through the process of change by supporting them in their everyday life. Sometimes, 24/7 supervision is provided. Typical user stories and daily activity profiles have been evaluated with seven personal fitness coaches in expert interviews in 2013. They have identified situations, where they would influence their customers towards behavior change. This comprises methods like wake-up calls, rewards for proper training or interruptions to have active breaks during the working hours. In a second step, recorded context data was analyzed to find patterns, which are characteristic to automatically detect the situations identified by the personal fitness coach. Patterns are formalized in rule sets where the premise is derived from patterns in the context information and the conclusion is the type of intervention the

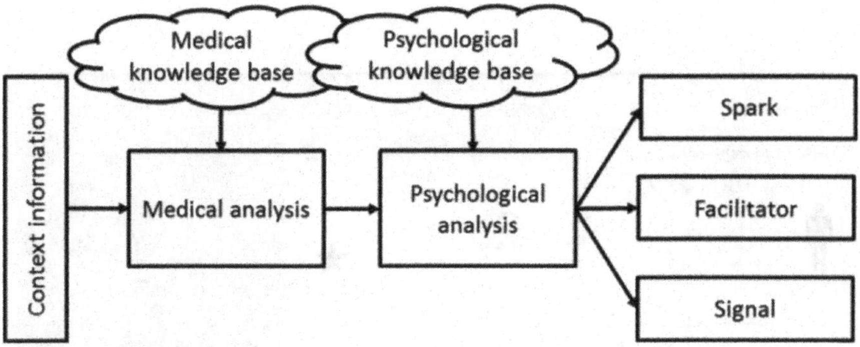

Fig. 4.3 Overview of the data analysis process

fitness coach would start. The figure below shows the two parts of the data analytics system, the medical analysis and the psychological analysis. (Fig. 4.3)

The system is monitoring new context information in real time and evaluates the rule sets for matched patterns. Triggered rules are the indicator which kind of persuasive service should be presented to the user.

So, a persuasive service can be seen like a piece of a puzzle that has one or more connectors, but fits only in certain situations.

Service Presentation

The design of persuasive services is based on the evaluation of successful services in existing mobile applications. In 2012, we conducted a market review and analyzed services in existing applications that have a high impact on the user acceptance (Hamper and Müller 2014). Services with high impact on the user acceptance and clear connection to one of the Fogg service types are used in the system. The figure below shows the user interface of the main application. (Fig. 4.4)

The application is divided into three parts. The 'performance' view on the left focuses on ex-post analysis of the user's health status, risk level and the physical activity performance in the past. Splitting the health score up into the sub scores 'cardio', 'muscular', 'balance' and 'stress' gives the user an overview, which areas of health prevention are affected by his activities. The 'goals' view on the right focuses on the target activity level that has been identified as suitable for this user by using the 'Arriba' calculation and WHO recommendations. Goals are visualized as green circles, which fill up slowly while the user performs the activity. This is used for monitoring the daily steps, calorie expenditure and gym training sessions. Besides these goals, also negative behavior can be visualized in this way. Unhealthy habits like permanent sitting are visualized as red circles which appear when the user is exceeding the acceptable time of uninterrupted sitting. Red circles can be removed by interrupting the unhealthy behavior. The graphical representation gives

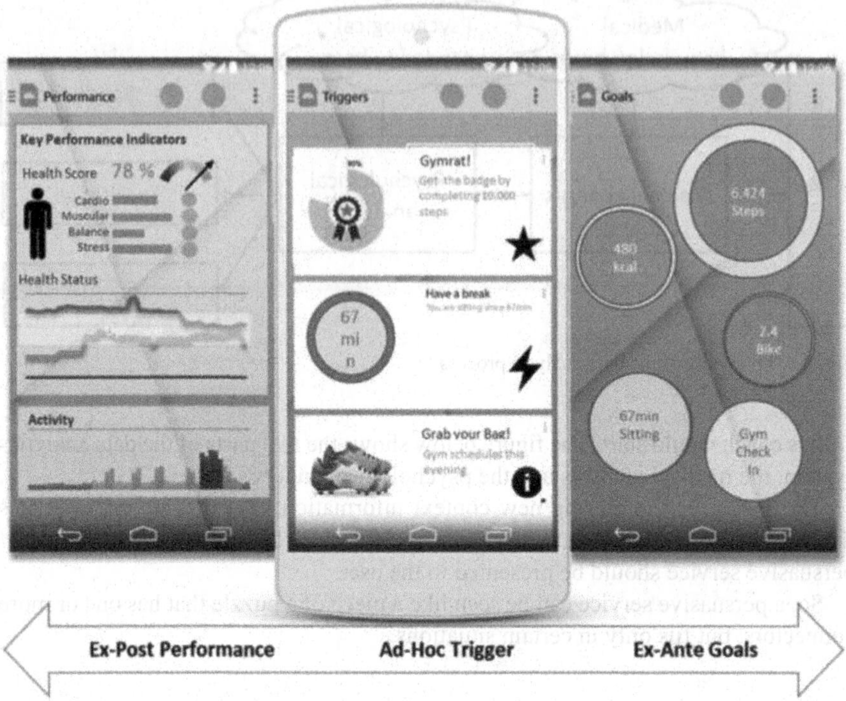

Fig. 4.4 Application overview

a quick overview about the numerous daily goals and their level of achievement without cluttering the interface.

The focus of this paper lies on the middle view, which represents the ad-hoc situation. The view is organized as a notification center where persuasive services appear, based on detected context situations. The list of services in the notification center can be seen as a to-do list for the user. Each service is triggered in certain situations and influences the user either as a facilitator, spark or trigger. By building rich notifications, we also allow interaction with the service. Feedback can be given by clicking on a persuasive service and therefore accept the challenge or swipe it away if the service is inappropriate in the current situation. This mechanism allows iterative optimization of the underlying rule base and the service design. The following list gives an excerpt of persuasive services that appear in the notification center:

- Cognitive:
  - Spark: A summary of the current health score (fear) and the achievable risk reduction (hope) is presented every morning and evening. The service is triggered by the time of the day, the first use of the smartphone and when returning to the POI 'home' in the evening.

  - Facilitators: Short-term 'driving' activities are detected. The alternatives, when using the bike or walking are calculated in terms of needed time (time) and positive health impact (non-routine, brain cycles). By showing this information, the user evaluates replacing the car with walking or cycling the next time.
  - Triggers: The user is prompted to measure his or her body weight every morning. While doing this, the step count and calorie expenditure for the previous day is shown. The connection of bodyweight and physical activity is brought to the user's mind in that moment when he or she is already thinking about the bodyweight.
- Behavioral:
  - Sparks: Rewards in form of badges can be archived by reaching the WHO recommendations for daily steps. The user is rewarded with different badges as well when achieving the daily goal for multiple days in a row (pleasure, social acceptance).
  - Facilitators: On days with scheduled gym activities, the user is reminded to pack the sports equipment in the morning. The gym reminder is triggered again as soon as the user leaves the POI 'work'. This enables the user to go directly to the gym (brain cycles, time) and avoids the situation of having to get up from the couch at home again (non-routine).
  - Triggers: During sedentary activities at the POI 'work', a persuasive message reminds the user to stand up and have an active break every 60 min. This acts as a simple, yet sufficient call to action to interrupt an unhealthy habit.

The figure below shows the ad-hoc view where persuasive services appear. (Fig. 4.5)

In further iterations, the portfolio of persuasive services will be extended. The underlying sensor framework and data analysis layer build a basis for comprehensive situational support with persuasive services.

Research Contribution and Outlook

The paper has shown a concept of a context aware system for physical activity promotion. The proposed concept for sensor frameworks provides a basis for comprehensive and automatical sensing of context information. With new mobile sensors emerging in the field of consumer centric healthcare, a structured integration of context data is possible by creating further data providers in the framework. The assessment of health data and activity with data mining methods follows the idea of learning from health and fitness practitioners with the proposed expert system. Services are proposed with strong theoretical connection and fine-grained so the persuasive impact on the user can be evaluated in detail.

We also see contribution to research in the combination of the TTM as a long-term theory with the FBM as short-term theory. As stated by Bort-Roig et al. (2014), many research projects lack a theoretical framework. Including behavior change

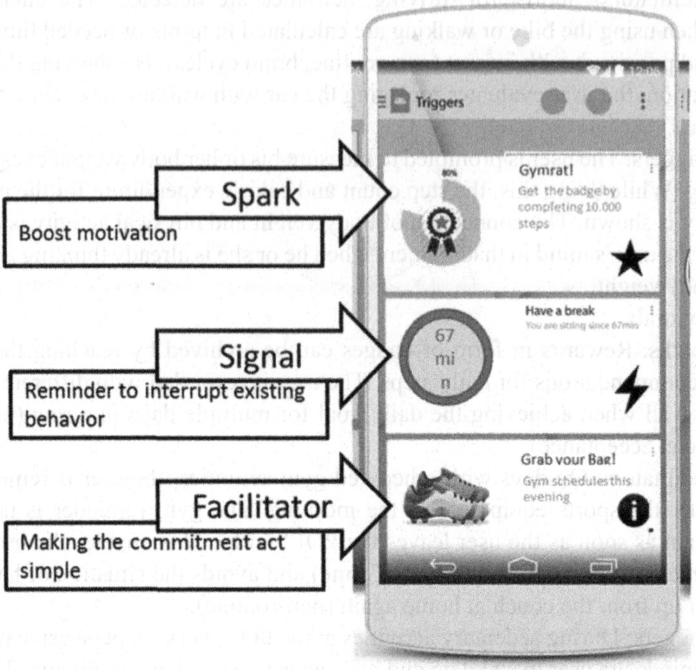

Fig. 4.5 Ad-hoc view

theory in design science projects might be easier to handle when using the combination of TTM and FBM.

In future work, evaluation of several elements is needed. The artifacts have to be evaluated, following a design science approach:

Precision and reliability: The precision and reliability of individual sensors, used in the providers, have to be evaluated. The reliability of the detected context information can then be quantified.

Rule base: The precision and quality in the detection of situations for persuasive services has to be evaluated. The intervention events from human persuader (fitness coaches) are the standard to reach.

Service-theory-fit: The individual services have to be evaluated, whether their design is following the theoretical framework. This leads to a precise characterization of each services regarding the TTM and FBM.

User acceptance: To ensure compliance, user acceptance is important. Especially the interactive nature of the system makes it necessary that the user believes in the analytical capabilities of the system.

Behavior change impact: The effect of an intervention with the proposed system on the overall behavior change process must be measured. The individual increase of physical activity and the reaching of WHO recommendation can be used as indicators. We also propose to use the time needed for the progression between the individual stages of change. Furthermore, as proposed in the TTM, the perceived self-efficacy and decisional balance should be used for measuring the behavior change process.

References

Abdolahinia, A., Maadani, M., & Radmand, G. (2010). Pictorial warning labels and quit intention in smokers presenting to a smoking cessation clinic. *Tanaffos, 9*, 48–52. http://www.sid.ir/EN/VEWSSID/J_pdf/100220100407.pdf.

Android, KitKat | Android Developers. (n.d.). https://developer.android.com/about/versions/kitkat.html. Accessed 14 June 2014.

Bergert, F., Braun, M., Clarius, H., & Ehrentahl, K. (2014). Hausärztliche Leitlinie Kardiovaskuläre Prävention Zusammenfassung. *Leitliniengruppe Hessen*. http://www.leitlinien.de/mdb/downloads/lghessen/kardiovaskulaere-praevention-lang.pdf.

Bielik, P., Tomlein, M., & Barla, M. (2012). Move2Play: An innovative approach to encouraging people to be more physically active. *Proceedings of the 2nd ACM SIGHIT International Health Informatics Symposium* (pp. 61–70). Miami, Florida, USA.

Borg-Roig, J., Gilson, N. D., Puig-Ribera, A., & Contreras, R. S. (2014). Measuring and influencing physical activity with smartphone technology: A systematic review. *Sports Medicine, 1179–2035.*

Campbell, C., & Chau, S. (2010). Mobile mentor: Weight management platform. *Proceedings of the 2010 International Conference on Intelligent User Interfaces* (pp. 409–410). Hong Kong, China.

Chen, F., & Hekler, E. (2011). Designing for context-aware health self-monitoring, feedback, and engagement. *Proceedings of the 2011 ACM Conference on Computer Supported Cooperative Work* (pp. 613–616). Hangzhou, China.

Chuah, M., & Sample, S. (2011). Fitness tour: A mobile application for combating obesity. *Proceedings of the Mobile Health 2011 Conference*. Paris, France: ACM Press.

Consolvo, S., Everitt, K., Smith, I., & Landay, J. a. (2006a). Design requirements for technologies that encourage physical activity. *Proceedings of the 24th International Conference on Human Factors in Computing Systems* (pp. 457–466). Montréal, Québec, Canada: ACM Press. doi:10.1145/1124772.1124840.

Consolvo, S., Everitt, K., Smith, I., & Landay, J. a. (2006b). Design requirements for technologies that encourage physical activity. *Proceedings of the SIGCHI conference on Human Factors in computing systems — CHI '06* (pp. 457–466). Montréal, Québec: ACM Press. doi:10.1145/1124772.1124840.

Consolvo, S., Klasnja, P., Mcdonald, D. W., Avrahami, D., Froehlich, J., Legrand, L., Libby, R., Mosher, K., & Landay, J. A. (2008). Flowers or a robot army? Encouraging awareness & activity with personal, mobile displays. *Proceedings of the 10th International Conference on Ubiquitous Computing*. Seoul, Korea.

Dey, A. K., & Abowd, G. D. (2000). Towards a better understanding of context and context-awareness. *CHI 2000 workshop on the what, who, where, when, and how of context-awareness* (Vol. 4, pp. 1–6). Citeseer. http://citeseerx.ist.psu.edu/viewdoc/download?doi=10.1.1.150.4833&rep=rep1&type=pdf.

Fogg, B. J. (1999). Persuasive technologies. *Communications of the ACM, 42*(5), 26–29.

Fogg, B. J. (2003). *Persuasive technology: Using computers to change what we think and do*. San Francisco: Morgan Kaufmann. http://books.google.com/books?hl=de&lr=&id=9nZHbxULMwgC&pgis=1.

Fogg, B. J. (2009). A behavior model for persuasive design. *Proceedings of the 4th International Conference on Persuasive Technology*. Claremont, California, USA: ACM Press. doi:10.1145/1541948.1541999.

Garrouste-Orgeas, M., Troché, G., Azoulay, E., Caubel, A., de Lassence, A., Cheval, C., Montesino, L., Thuong, M., Vincent, F., Cohen, Y., & Timsit, J.-F. (2004). Body mass index. An additional prognostic factor in ICU patients. *Intensive Care Medicine, 30*(3), 437–443. doi:10.1007/s00134-003-2095-2.

Gartner. (2012). Gartner Says Worldwide Smartphone Sales Soared in Fourth Quarter of 2011 With 47 Percent Growth. http://www.gartner.com/it/page.jsp?id=1924314. Accessed 14 March 2012.

Gil-castiñeira, F., Cid-vieytes, N., Conde-lagoa, D., & Javier, F. (2011). RunWithUs: A social sports application in the ubiquitous Oulu environment. *Proceedings of the 4th IEEE International Conference on Computer Science and Information Technology* (pp. 195–204). Beijing, China.

Hamper, A., & Müller, T. (2014). Supporting preventive healthcare with persuasive servicese. In N. Wickramasinghe, L. Al-Hakim, C. Gonzalez, & J. Tan (Eds.), *Lean thinking for healthcare*. New York: Springer.

Hayes-Roth, F. (1985). Rule-based systems. *Communications of the ACM, 28*(9), 921–932. doi:10.1145/4284.4286.

Hoeger, W. W. K., & Hoeger, S. A. (2010). *Lifetime physical fitness and wellness: A personalized program*. Cengage learning. http://books.google.com/books?id=2b5eymIvO-QC&pgis=1.

Holzinger, A., Dorner, S., & Födinger, M. (2010). Chances of Increasing youth health awareness through mobile wellness applications. *Proceedings of the 6th Symposium of the WG HCI & UE of the Austrian Computer Society* (pp. 71–81).

Jepson, R. G., Harris, F. M., Platt, S., & Tannahill, C. (2010). The effectiveness of interventions to change six health behaviours: A review of reviews. *BMC public health, 10*, 538. doi:10.1186/1471-2458-10-538.

Kimura, H. (2011). iDetective: A persuasive application to motivate healthier behavior using smart phone. *Proceedings of the 26th Symposium on Applied Computing* (pp. 399–404). TaiChung, Taiwan.

Klasnja, P., Consolvo, S., & Pratt, W. (2011). How to evaluate technologies for health behavior change in HCI research. *Proceedings of the 29th International Conference on Human Factors in Computing Systems* (pp. 3063–3072). Vancouver, BC, Canada: ACM. doi:10.1145/1978942.1979396.

Krones, T., Keller, H., Sönnichsen, A., Sadowski, E.-M., Baum, E., Wegscheider, K., Rochon, J., & Donner-Banzhoff, N. (2008). Absolute cardiovascular disease risk and shared decision making in primary care: A randomized controlled trial. *Annals of Family Medicine, 6*(3), 218–227. doi:10.1370/afm.854.

Ledger, D., & McCaffrey, D. (2014). *Inside wearables: How the science of human behavior change*. Cambridge: Endeavour Partners. http://endeavourpartners.net/assets/Wearables-and-the-Science-of-Human-Behavior-Change-EP4.pdf.

Lin, J. J., Mamykina, L., Lindtner, S., Delajoux, G., & Strub, H. B. (2006). Fish'n'Steps: Encouraging physical activity with an interactive computer game. *Proceedings of the 8th ACM international conference on Ubiquitous computing* (pp. 261–278).

Location APIs | Android Developers. (n.d.). http://developer.android.com/google/play-services/location.html. Accessed 14 June 2014.

Marcus, B. H., Selby, V. C., Niaura, R. S., & Rossi, J. S. (1992). Self-efficacy and the stages of exercise behavior change. *Research Quarterly for Exercise and Sport, 63*(1), 60–66. http://www.ncbi.nlm.nih.gov/pubmed/1574662.

Mattila, E., Korhonen, I., Salminen, J. H., Ahtinen, A., Koskinen, E., Särelä, A., Pärkkä, J., & Lappalainen, R. (2010). Empowering citizens for well-being and chronic disease management with wellness diary. *IEEE Transactions on Information Technology in Biomedicine: A Publication of the IEEE Engineering in Medicine and Biology Society, 14*(2), 456–463. doi:10.1109/TITB.2009.2037751.

Nike + Fuelband SE. Aktivitätstracker & Fitnessmesser. Nike.com (DE). (n.d.). http://www.nike.com/de/de_de/c/nikeplus-fuelband. Accessed 14 June 2014.

Offizielle Fitbit®-Website: Kabellose Aktivitäts- und Schlaf-Tracker Force, Flex, One und Zip. (n.d.). https://www.fitbit.com/de. Accessed 14 June 2014.

Oinas-Kukkonen, H. (2010). Behavior change support systems: The next frontier for web science. In *Proceedings of the Second International Web Science Conference*. Raleigh, NC, USA.

Oinas-Kukkonen, H., & Harjumaa, M. (2009). Persuasive systems design: Key issues, process model, and system features. *Communications of the Association for Information Systems, 24*(28), 485–500.

Prochaska, J. O., DiClemente, C. C., & Norcross, J. C. (1992). In search of how people change—Applications to addictive behaviors. *The American Psychologist, 47*(9), 1102–1114. http://www.ncbi.nlm.nih.gov/pubmed/1329589.

Prochaska, J. O., Redding, C. A., & Evers, K. E. (2008). The transtheoretical model and stages of change. In K. Glanz, B. K. Rimer, & K. V. Viswanath (Eds.), *Health behavior and health education: Theory, research, and practice* (Vol. 4, pp. 1–552). San Francisco: Jossey-Bass.

Riley, W. T., Rivera, D. E., Atienza, A., Nilsen, W., Allison, S. M., & Mermelstein, R. (2011). Health behavior models in the age of mobile interventions: Are our theories up to the task? *Translational Behavioral Medicine, 1*(1), 53–71. doi:10.1007/s13142-011-0021-7.

Schut, H. A., & Stam, H. J. (1994). Goals in rehabilitation teamwork. *Disability and Rehabilitation, 16*(4), 223–226. http://www.ncbi.nlm.nih.gov/pubmed/7812023.

Withings: Smart Body Analyzer. (n.d.). Retrieved June 14, 2014, from http://vitrine.withings.com/de/smart-body-analyzer.html.

Withings: Wireless Blood Pressure Monitor. (n.d.). http://vitrine.withings.com/de/blood-pressure-monitor.html. Accessed 14 June 2014.

World Health Organization. (2010). Global recommendations on physical activity for health. *Vasa*. http://medcontent.metapress.com/index/A65RM03P4874243N.pdf.

My life powered by GalaxyS5. (n.d.). http://www.samsung.com/global/microsite/galaxys5/features.html. Accessed 14 June 2014.

Andreas Hamper holds a master's degree of International Information Systems. Since 2014, he is a member of the research staff and PhD student at the Institute of Information Systems at the University of Erlangen-Nuremberg. In his research he is focusing on data mining in healthcare.

Chapter 5
A Multi-centred Empirical Study to Measure and Validate User Satisfaction with Hospital Information Services in Australia and Germany

Anke Simon, Bill Davey, Bettina Flaiz, Vass Karpathiou and Nilmini Wickramasinghe

Introduction

Australia and Germany have many similarities when we compare healthcare delivery. Both countries have two-tier health systems, that is, a mix of public and private, and are designing national e-health solutions; for Australia, it is the personally controlled electronic health record (PCEHR) and, for Germany, it is the e-health card. In addition, these countries are embracing information technology (IT) solutions to effect better healthcare delivery to try to stem escalating cost pressures. These similar health environments provide an exceptional opportunity to investigate healthcare issues, simultaneously in similar contexts to leverage the potential for shared learning and the transfer of expertise. In any application of IT, key success factor now becomes the level of user satisfaction and the rate of adoption of the various technology

N. Wickramasinghe (✉)
Deakin University and Epworth HealthCare
60 Baker Ave, Kew East 3102, Australia
e-mail: n.wickramasinghe@deakin.edu.au

A. Simon
Department of Health Sciences & Management, Faculty of Business/Economics,Cooperative State University Baden-Wuerttemberg, Tuebingerstr. 31-33, 70174 Stuttgart, Germany
e-mail: anke.simon@dhbw-stuttgart.de

B. Davey
RMIT School of Business Information Technology and Logistics,
GPO Box 2476, Melbourne, VIC 3001, Australia
e-mail: bill.davey@rmit.edu.au

B. Flaiz
Tübinger Strasse 33, 70178 Stuttgart, Germany
e-mail: Bettina.flaiz@dhbw-stuttgart.de

V. Karpathiou
School of Business IT and Logisics, Building 80 Level 7, 445 Swanston Street,
Melbourne, VIC 3000, Australia
e-mail: VASS.KARPATHIOU@rmit.edu.au

N. Wickramasinghe et al. (eds.), *Contemporary Consumer Health Informatics*,
Healthcare Delivery in the Information Age, DOI 10.1007/978-3-319-25973-4_5

solutions. In healthcare, given the multiplicity of users and their respective needs of a system, high user satisfaction is always challenging. To date, good metrics which serve to correctly capture user needs and satisfaction have yet to be developed for healthcare contexts and proxies are used from other industries which naturally at best lead to suboptimal solutions. This chapter attempts to address this important issue by designing and developing a suitable evaluation criterion for measuring user satisfaction with IT in healthcare contexts in both German and Australian hospitals and then providing a systematic framework to address the key issues identified. Given the cost to healthcare of poorly designed technology solutions and low user acceptance, this study is especially timely and its results are most beneficial and far reaching. Moreover, given the similarities between the two healthcare systems in the respective countries, such a study can leverage lessons within and between the two systems, which not only make the study truly unique but also make the findings much more robust, useful and useable in order to develop superior technology solutions that, in turn, will serve to support and enable the realisation of excellent healthcare services that address all current challenges for both countries.

Background

The healthcare sector is an information-intensive area with high information demands (Wickramasinghe and Schaffer 2010). IT provides timely and accurate information to make sure that physicians, nurses and other care professionals obtain the complete and extensive information they require to provide high-quality care (Wickramasinghe et al. 2009; Haux et al. 2003). On the other hand, hospital IT also ensures fulfilling managerial needs while improving the hospital's effectiveness and efficiency needed to support such care (Brand et al. 2012; Simon 2010). Given the rapid development of healthcare IT, many hospitals have aggressively increased their IT expenditures. Today, hundreds of information systems are used in hospitals (from widely used electronic patient records, computerised order entry systems, to modern radiology information systems, including speech recognition technology). A series of IT support, maintaining, consulting and training services usually provided by a hospital's IT department is now in high demand. Although the technology-related benefits are obvious in theory, it seems that they are not clearly associated with the operating situations in hospitals. The evidence is strong: A high number of reports are published about system flaws, poor IT usability and insufficient relation to work activities (review in Viitanen et al. 2011). Previous research indicates that a key factor affecting the successful adoption of hospital IT lies in user acceptance, perceived usability and satisfaction (Viitanen et al. 2011; Chen and Hsiao 2012; Bundschuh et al. 2011; Smelcer et al. 2009; Ash et al. 2004; Stürzlinger et al. 2009; Bleich and Slack 2009; Ludwick and Doucette 2009). Despite the increasing trend towards user satisfaction issues, relatively little systematic data have been gathered on user satisfaction with hospital information services in a comprehensive way. Usually, the successful implementation, adoption and daily use of hospital IT depends on the quality of the information systems themselves as well as on the various IT services provided by the hospital IT department (i.e. IT hotline, on-site service, on-call duty, training and advising for user, and project management, etc.). As the literature shows, previous publications focus mainly on a single project or healthcare information system (e.g. Smelcer et al. 2009; Stürzlinger et al. 2009; Bleich and Slack 2009; Ludwick and Doucette 2009; Bürkle et al. 2001; Khajouei et al. 2009; McKinlay et al. 2010), are conducted in a specified use context (e.g. Ash et al. 2004; Ludwick and Doucette 2009; Röhrig et al. 2007; Kuosmanen et al. 2010; Ammenwerth et al. 2002; Oroviogoicoechea and Watson 2009; Sánchez 2004) and involve rather a small number of participants or include only one health profession (often only physicians; e.g. Viitanen et al. 2011; Stürzlinger et al. 2009). Furthermore, whether in Germany or Australia, no national reference data exist. In addition to the data issues in current studies, there is nearly no information about the psychometric properties of the used or developed instruments and scales (i.e. validity and reliability). Hence, the quality of such study results must at least be considered as uncertain.

Aim

Physicians and nurses are key providers of healthcare services in hospitals and are main users of hospital IT. The implementation, appropriate usage and user satisfaction can improve the quality of care that health professionals provide and influence the hospital performance and outcome quality for patients. The aim of our investigation is to measure and validate user satisfaction with hospital information services in a comprehensive manner. This study will be one of the first investigations in this research area in Australia and Germany. The research outcomes will not only answer the senior hospital management's question, "How good is our hospital information service?", but will also provide hospital IT researchers and practitioners for the first time with valid and useful measurement instruments (best practice standard questionnaire).

Objective

The objective of this investigation is to measure and validate user satisfaction with hospital IT services, specifically to:

1. Understand the current state of user satisfaction with IT services in the context of clinical environments in hospitals, and provide a descriptive picture of the present situation from the subjective perspective of health professionals in Germany and Australia

2. Provide first reference values/data on user satisfaction in both countries for senior hospital management and chief information officers (CIOs), as well as a basis for benchmarking and efforts for developing quality and efficiency of IT performance in hospitals
3. Develop and implement empirical analysis and statistical validation of appropriate metrics and scales for healthcare contexts (to provide validated and appropriate standard measures)
4. Identify starting points for increasing the quality of hospital IT systems as well as IT support, and to support a more detailed evaluation processes in the future

Rationale

Healthcare costs in Australia and Germany are increasing exponentially. To address this and other healthcare challenges including the aging population and increases in chronic diseases, both countries are investing heavily in information systems (IS)/IT. Nowadays, nearly all clinical and administrative processes depend on IT systems and related services. However, without proper metrics that are designed specifically for the known challenging, multilayered dynamic environment of healthcare contexts, neither is it possible to evaluate the benefits of these technology investments nor design them to optimally meet the user needs. Thus, a key void is the existence of appropriate metrics and instruments to measure and validate user satisfaction with hospital IT services—a void that this research will address.

Achievement and Measurement of Aims

To achieve the stated aim, we have already developed a comprehensive questionnaire based on literature research and expert focus group interactions in Germany. A pretest and a preliminary study proved the validity and appropriateness of the questionnaire in Germany successfully ($n=106$, Hospital Nuernberg). Before administering the questionnaire in Australia and extending our study to the intended multicentre investigation, we will run pretests in a second pilot study (including translation/retranslation of the questionnaire). Our main purpose is to collect a sufficient national sample in Germany and Australia to analyse the current status of user satisfaction, and provide valid and useful measuring instruments and scales for hospital executives. Figure 5.1 illustrates the research design. In addition, unstructured interviews will be conducted at all data sites. Second, but equally important, aspects of this project include achieving a high level of knowledge transfer between the two countries as well as significant industry participation. The development of the comprehensive questionnaire and its subsequent administration represents a key sharing/transfer of expertise and knowledge, which will be further enhanced through the focus group discussions with key experts. Industry partners, namely the respective public and private hospitals, who have agreed to participate in this study

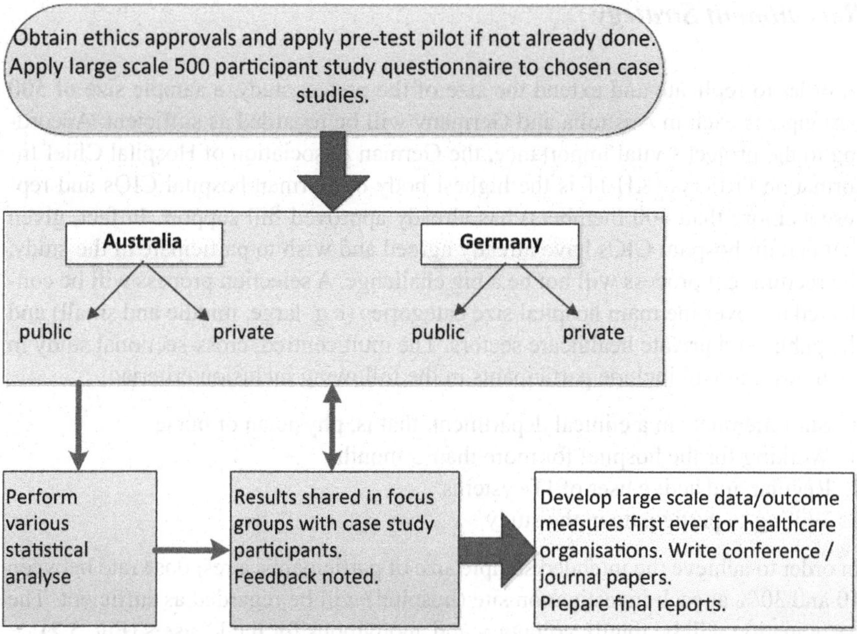

Fig. 5.1 Proposed research design highlighting key project steps

will not only benefit themselves but also represent significant industry support and participation in the study. Finally, transfer of skills and expertise especially between Early Career Researcher (ECR) and senior project team members within and across countries will occur. Given the existing track record and collaboration to date between Professors Simon and Wickramasinghe, we are confident that not only will the knowledge transfer within and between the research groups be successful but also the whole project will be completed so that all aims will be achieved and all key success factors will be met.

Data Collection

Data will be collected in multiple ways including site visits, briefing and debriefing of CIOs, senior hospital management as well as medical and nursing directors, and the administering of questionnaires completed by IT users (health professionals). The central focus of the planned investigation will be on the main occupational groups within hospitals: physicians and nurses. All data collection will be guided by healthcare and IT professionals. Visits to the respective data sites by all members of the project team (i.e. German and Australian) will ensure that replication is being conducted in a similar fashion and will also serve to facilitate learning across both data sites.

Recruitment Strategy

In order to replicate and extend the size of the pretest study, a sample size of 500 participants each in Australia and Germany will be regarded as sufficient. According to the project's vital importance, the German Association of Hospital Chief Information Officers (KH-IT is the highest body of German hospital CIOs and represents more than 400 members) has already approved full support. In fact, given that certain hospital CIOs have already agreed and wish to participate in the study, the recruitment process will not be a big challenge. A selection process will be conducted to cover the main hospital size categories (e.g. large, middle and small) and the public and private healthcare sectors. The multicentred, cross-sectional study in each hospital will include participants in the following inclusion criteria:

a. Staff members in a clinical department, that is, physician or nurse
b. Working for the hospital for more than 3 months
c. Regular and active user of IT systems
d. Willing to participate in the study

In order to achieve the intended sample size of participants, a response rate between 10 and 30% at each investigation site (hospital) will be regarded as sufficient. The participation will be totally voluntary and anonymous for the IT users (Fig. 5.2).

Study Methodology

We will apply a triangular approach to measure user satisfaction with hospital IT. Triangulation defines a research method that combines various study measurements and concepts as well as theories in one investigation. It is increasingly used to cover complex investigation objects in qualitative as well as quantitative studies (Flick 2011). Our comprehensive concept includes the measurement of four questionnaire modules (see Fig. 5.2):

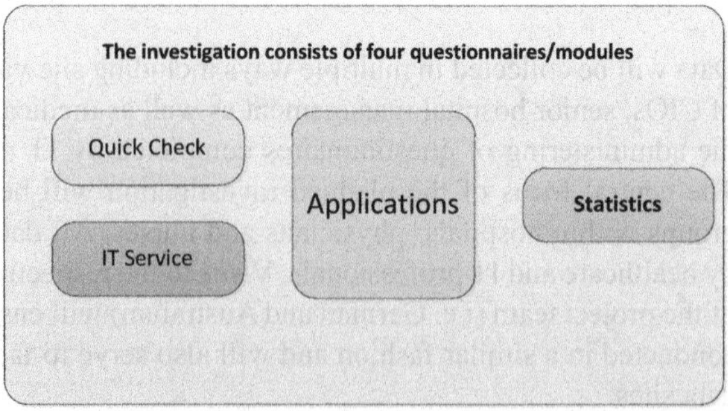

Fig. 5.2 Four-module questionnaire study

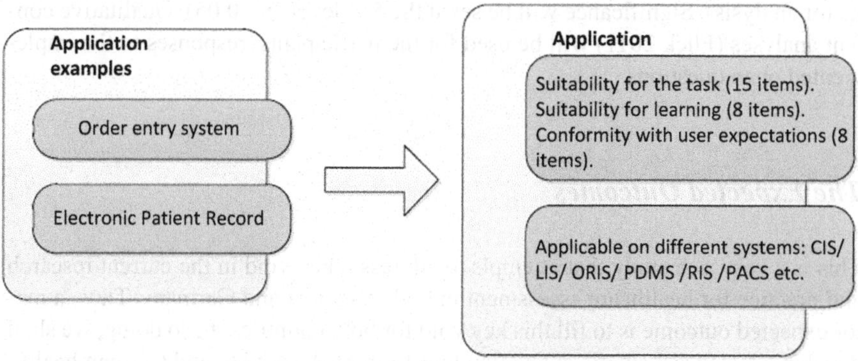

Fig. 5.3 Module IT application

1. Module Quick Check: general user satisfaction (4 items), three open questions, overall satisfaction grade
2. Module IT-Service: appropriateness of IT equipment and frequency of use, IT hotline (10 items), IT on-site service/support (7 items), IT on-call duty (at night and weekends) (7 items), IT training for users (8 items)
3. Module IT-Application: suitability for the task (15 items), suitability for learning (8 items), conformity with user expectations (8 items)[1] (see Fig. 5.3)
4. Module Statistics (socio-demographic variables)

The questionnaire will be administered as an online version (applied in Questback Unipark, EFS Survey, version 8.0). Closed and open variables will be included (e.g. user satisfaction, importance, satisfaction grade and open questions, i.e. appraisal, critical issues, statements and hints).

Data Analysis

Statistical analyses will be performed with the Statistical Package for the Social Sciences (SPSS), version 20. Descriptive statistics, including mean, standard deviation and frequency, percentage will be calculated. The differences between the subsamples from Australia and Germany will be compared using the *t*-test should the data prove to be normally distributed. Psychometric evaluation will be conducted to validate all developed instruments. The reliability of the scales (internal consistency and split-half reliability) and the validity will be reported (exploratory

[1] The IsoMetrics inventory (Bundschuh et al. 2011) will be applied based on EN ISO 9241−10. The scale is applicable to different systems: clinical information systems (CIS), laboratory information systems (LIS), radiology information systems (RIS), patient documentation and management system (PDMS), picture archiving and communication systems (PACS), nursing information systems (NIS), etc.

factor analysis). Significance will be set at the 5 % level ($p<0.05$). Qualitative content analyses (Flick 2011) will be used for the participants' responses to the implemented open questions.

The Expected Outcomes

This is a very rich study that attempts to address a key void in the current research and practice for healthcare assessment in both Australia and Germany. Thus, a major expected outcome is to fill this key void for both countries. In so doing, we shall develop a tested systematic evaluation tool for both Australian and German healthcare organisations to clearly and accurately measure the level of user satisfaction with hospital IT services and thereby enable the hospitals in the respective organisations to immediately address any/all issues with their existing IS/IT solutions, as well as be able to inform the design and development of new solutions. Thus, the value of the outcomes of this study is far reaching and potentially very large, especially in view of the millions of dollars and euros spent on developing IT solutions for healthcare delivery in the respective countries.

Innovation and Significance

According to our preliminary research and pilot project, most of the hospital CIOs in Germany and Australia do not measure user satisfaction. Among the small number of hospital CIOs with relevant data, the majority use self-developed, hands-on questionnaires with poor empirical quality. Moreover, as outlined previously, there is nearly a complete lack of national studies on user perception on hospital IT service quality in Germany, Australia or elsewhere. Hence, valid reference data covering the entire national hospital sector are not available. This research project will be one of the first, if not the first, investigations in this field. Given the huge amount of money spent on healthcare IT in both countries as well as the increasing escalating costs of healthcare expenditure for both countries, it is not possible to overstate the importance and significance of this study.

Conclusions

This chapter has served to outline a longitudinal study to investigate user satisfaction of hospital information services. Consumers of healthcare information are many and varied. In a hospital context, this includes physicians, surgeons, nurses and allied healthcare professionals, as well as various levels of healthcare managers. Clearly, all these user groups have different needs and requirements from the information they access and use. Understanding all these different user perspectives is an essential first step in the design and development of technology solutions that are, in fact, user/consumer centric. Our proposed study then serves to outline a systematic and rigorous approach to assist in gaining a better understanding of consumer needs of health information services and systems within hospital context. We conclude by calling for more research in this key area.

References

Ammenwerth, E., Ehlers, F., Kutscha, A., Kutscha, U., Eichstadter, R., & Resch, F. (2002). Supporting patient care by using innovative information technology. A case study from clinical psychiatry. *Practical Disease Management, 10,* 479–487.

Ash, J. S., Berg, M., & Coiera, E. (2004). Some unintended consequences of information technology in health care: The nature of patient care information system-related errors. *Journal of the American Medical Informatics Association, 11,* 104–112.

Bleich, H. L., & Slack, W. V. (2009). Reflections on electronic medical records: When doctors will use them and when they will not. *International Journal of Medical Informatics, 79,* 1–4.

Brand, C. A., Barker, A. L., Morello, R. T., Vitale, M. R., Evans, S. M., Scott, I. A., Stoelwinder, J. U., & Cameron, P. A. (2012). A review of hospital characteristics associated with improved performance. *International Journal for Quality in Health Care: Journal of the International Society for Quality in Health Care/ISQua, 24*(5), 483–494.

Bundschuh, B. B., Majeed, R. W., Buerkle, T., Kuhn, K., Sax, U., Seggewies, C., Vosseler, C., & Röhrig, R. (2011). Quality of human-computer interaction—results of a national usability survey of hospital-IT in Germany. *BMC Medical Informatics and Decision Making, 11,* 69.

Bürkle, T., Ammenwerth, E., Prokosch, H. U., & Dudeck, J. (2001). Evaluation of clinical information systems. What can be evaluated and what cannot? *Journal of Evaluation in Clinical Practice, 7,* 373–385.

Chen, R. F., & Hsiao, J. L. (2012). An empirical study of physicians' acceptance of hospital information systems in Taiwan. *Telemedicine and e-Health, 18*(2), 120–125.

Flick, U. (2011). *Triangulation eine Einführung*. Wiesbaden: Verlag für Sozialwissenschaften.

Haux, R., Winter, A., Ammenwerth, E., & Birgl, B. (2003). *Strategic information management in hospitals: An introduction to hospital information systems*. New York: Springer.

Khajouei, R., de Jongh D., & Jaspers, M. W. (2009). Usability evaluation of a computerized physician order entry for medication. *Studies in Health Technology and Informatics, 150,* 532–536.

Kuosmanen, L., Jakobsson, T., Hyttinen, J., Koivunen, M., & Valimaki, M. (2010). Usability evaluation of a web-based patient information system for individuals. *Journal of Advanced Nursing, 66,* 2701–2710.

Ludwick, D. A., & Doucette, J. (2009). Adopting electronic medical records in primary care: Lessons learned from health information systems implementation experience in seven countries. *International Journal of Medical Informatics, 78,* 22–31.

McKinlay, A., McVittie, C., & Reiter, E. (2010). Design issues for socially intelligent user interfaces. A discourse analysis of a data-to-text system for summarizing clinical data. *Methods of Information in Medicine, 49,* 379–387.

Röhrig, R., Beutefuhr, H., Hartmann, B., Niczko, E., Quinzio, B., Junger, A., & Hempelmann, G. (2007). Summative software evaluation of a therapeutic guideline assistance system for empiric antimicrobial therapy in ICU. *Journal of Clinical Monitoring and Computing, 21,* 203–210.

Sánchez, A. (2004). A chronic wound healing information technology system: Design, testing and evaluation in clinic. *Electronic Journal of Information Systems Evaluation, 7,* 57–66.

Simon, A. (2010). Die betriebswirtschaftliche Bewertung der IT-Performance im Krankenhaus. The economical evaluation of IT performance in hospitals. In *Steuerung der IT im Klinikmanagement. Methoden und Verfahren. IT governance in clinical management. Methods and programs* (pp. 73–88). Wiesbaden: Vieweg + Teubner Verlag.

Smelcer, J. B., Miller-Jacobs, H., & Kantrovich, L. (2009). Usability of electronic medical records. *Journal of Usability Studies, 4,* 70–84.

Stürzlinger, H., Hiebinger, C., Pertl, D., & Traurig, P. (2009). Computerized Physician Order Entry—Wirksamkeit und Effizienz elektronischer Arzneimittelverordnung mit Entscheidungsunterstützungssystemen. *GMS Health Technology Assessment, 5,* 56–63.

Viitanen, J., Hyppönen, H., Vänskä, J., Reponen, J., & Winblad, I. (2011). National Questionnaire study on clinical ICT systems proofs: Physicians suffer from poor usability. *International Journal of Medical Informatics, 6,* 708–725.

Wickramasinghe, N., & Schaffer, J. (2010). *Realizing value driven patient centric healthcare through technology*. IBM Center for The Business of Government, DC.

Wickramasinghe, N., Bali, R., Lehany, B., & Gibbons, C. (2009). *HCKM primer*. New Jersey: Routledge.

Anke Simon (Dr. rer. pol., MBA, MSc, RN) is the head of the Department of Health Sciences & Management, Baden-Württemberg Cooperative State University. She holds degrees in nursing (registered nurse), business and informatics (master of business data processing), social and healthcare management (master of business administration) and economics (PhD).

Dr. Bill Davey is a senior lecturer at RMIT University in Australia. Bill has published more than 100 papers in a range of information systems-related topics varying from design methods to applications. He is currently researching aged care with colleagues in the USA and hospital systems in Australia and Germany. Bill is particularly interested in actor–network theory and phenomenography as research methods for uncovering explanations for uptake of technology and the conceptual frameworks that are formed by people using technology.

Bettina Flaiz is a research assistant at Baden-Württemberg Cooperative State University. Bettina holds a master's degree in nursing science from the Esslingen University of Applied Sciences in Esslingen. She also holds a bachelor degree in nursing and nursing management. She is a registered nurse in Germany.

Vass Karpathiou has varied experience in academia, business, technology and engineering spanning more than 30 years. His research interests include developing business technology solutions with a social engagement outcome and value. His current research focuses on healthcare value in the interaction of business, technology and medicine.

Nilmini Wickramasinghe PhD; MBA; GradDipMgtSt; BSc. Amus.A, piano; Amus.A, violin has a well-recognised research record in the field of healthcare and IT/IS. Her expertise is in the strategic application and management of technology for effecting superior healthcare solutions. She is currently the professor director of Health Informatics Management at Epworth HealthCare and a professor at Deakin University.

Chapter 6
Social Media in Health Care

Nima Kordzadeh

Overview

People are increasingly using health-related online social networks (OSNs) and virtual communities to seek and provide social support and health information in collaboration with other users of these websites (Lau and Kwok 2009; Newman et al. 2011). A national survey conducted by the Pew Research Center revealed that one in four respondents had looked at someone else's personal health experience and medical issues posted online, and 16 % of the respondents had looked for other Internet users with similar health conditions within the past 12 months (Fox and Duggan 2013). Additionally, 40 % of the respondents indicated that they shared their health-related experiences online.

In line with this trend, health-care organizations such as hospitals, clinics, and pharmacies have also started to embark on social media strategies to directly communicate with health consumers (e.g., patients and caregivers), promote medical services and products, and enable individuals to communicate with each other and exchange social support on social media websites. Mayo Clinic, for instance, pioneered the use of social media in the USA by establishing "Mayo Clinic Center for Social Media"[1] and initiating an OSN[2] for their patients to be able to communicate with one another. They state their philosophy as:

> At Mayo, we believe individuals have the right and responsibility to advocate for their own health, and it's our responsibility to help them use social networking tools to get the best information, and connect with providers as well as one another.[3]

[1] http://socialmedia.mayoclinic.org/, retrieved November 2015.

[2] http://connect.mayoclinic.org, retrieved November 2014.

[3] http://socialmedia.mayoclinic.org/about-mccsm-smhn, retrieved November 2015.

N. Kordzadeh (✉)
Department of Informatics, College of Business, Idaho State University,
921 South 8th Avenue, Stop 8020, Pocatello, ID 83209-8020, USA
e-mail: kordnima@isu.edu

N. Wickramasinghe et al. (eds.), *Contemporary Consumer Health Informatics*,
Healthcare Delivery in the Information Age, DOI 10.1007/978-3-319-25973-4_6

Health-care providers primarily use general-purpose OSNs such as Facebook and Twitter to enhance users' awareness about health topics (Griffis et al. 2014; Rhoads 2012; Richer et al. 2014). Health-care organizations and professionals also use these OSNs to offer useful information about health-care procedures and services they provide (Lagu et al. 2008). Moreover, there are hundreds of socially integrated health-specific websites that offer collaboration platforms for health consumers (e.g., patients and caregivers). People visit these websites, exchange social support in collaboration with other individuals, and make one-to-one social ties with them (Lasker et al. 2005). Consistent with the extant literature (e.g., Demiris 2006), these social media-enabled health-care websites are referred to as virtual health communities (VHCs) in this chapter and are defined as "online environments in which users interact with one another around a set of common interests or shared purpose related to health using a variety of tools including discussion boards, chat, virtual environments, and direct messaging" (Newman et al. 2011, p. 342).

Adoption of social media technologies by health consumers will allow them to become active participants in social support and health-related information exchange activities, which are consistent with the notion of consumer health informatics (Wickramasinghe et al. 2013a). Thus, understanding various aspects of health social media will help health-care organizations, providers, and professionals utilize these systems and incorporate them into consumer health informatics practices and applications more effectively. Moreover, this understanding will allow researchers in different disciplines related to consumer health informatics direct their research efforts specifically toward health social media concepts, technologies, and applications. Therefore, in this chapter, we aim to shed light on various aspects of health social media technologies.

The remainder of the chapter is structured as follows. First, the notion of patient-centered e-health (PCEH) applications and the connection between this concept and social media in health care are discussed. Second, a distinction is made between the two major social media environments used for health-related communications. These two environments include general-purpose OSNs and VHCs. Third, a typology of social media platforms provided by VHCs and the implications of this typology are presented. Fourth, the typology is applied to analyze the types of collaboration platforms provided by a number of popular VHCs in the USA. The opportunities and future developments as well as concerns and challenges associated with the use of health social media are also discussed. The chapter is concluded with a brief recap of its contents.

Patient-Centered e-Health and Social Media

Patient-centered e-Health (PCEH) pertains to the applications that rely on the Internet technologies and revolve around patients as major actors in the health-care ecosystem (Wilson 2009). The three major characteristics of PCEH systems include patient focus, patient activity, and patient empowerment (Wilson 2009; Wilson et al.

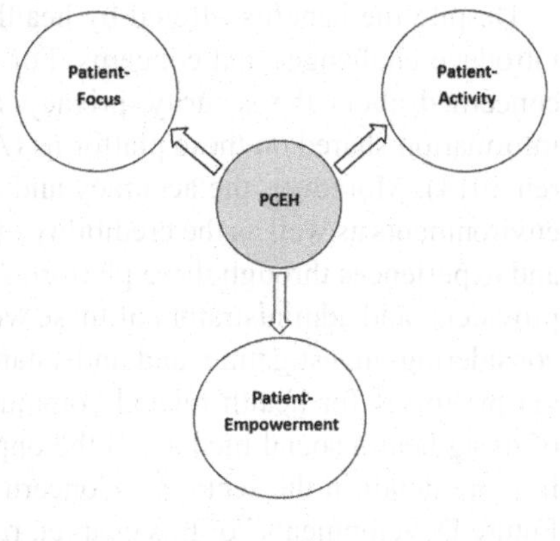

Fig. 6.1 Major characteristics of patient-centered e-health. (Adapted from Wilson **2009**)

2014). Patient focus means that PCEH applications are primarily developed to address patients' needs and perspectives. Patient activity implies that PCEH systems are designed in such a way that patients can actively participate in providing and consuming health-related information about, or of interest to, them. Patient empowerment means that PCEH systems enable patients to control some aspects of their health care via these systems. This generation of health information systems comprises various forms of technologies from personal health records (PHRs; Greenhalgh et al. 2010) and telehealth applications to Internet-based patient communication tools and platforms (Fig. 6.1; Wilson et al. 2014).

Consistent with the definition and major characteristics of PCEH systems, health-related social technologies are considered a form of, or a structural component of, these systems. The reason is that socially enabled, health-related technologies facilitate consumer-centered health care and enable health consumers (e.g., patients and caregivers) to play an active, pivotal, and meaningful role in providing and consuming health information related to them (Kordzadeh et al. 2014; Wickramasinghe et al. 2013a). These socially enabled technologies are also referred to as consumer-centered or patient-driven health-care systems by the extant literature (Lewis et al. 2005; Swan 2009).

The use of consumer-centered social technologies for health communications provides various benefits to health consumers. The benefits include empowering patients, particularly chronic disease sufferers (Merolli et al. 2013), to manage their health care through communication with their peers (Houston et al. 2002); feeling a sense of belonging and support (Kordzadeh and Warren 2014); learning from others' health-related experiences (Demiris 2006; Kordzadeh et al. 2014; Newman et al. 2011); feeling less isolated (Houston et al. 2002; Powell et al. 2003); and coping with medical conditions more effectively (Houston et al. 2002). Moreover, these technologies may help individuals manage and shape their health-related behaviors more effectively (Wickramasinghe et al. 2013). These benefits along with the relatively low costs associated with using health social media have made these platforms an appropriate tool for health communication and social support exchange activities on the Internet.

Despite the benefits offered by health social media, these virtual environments introduce challenges and concerns. For instance, users of these websites might be concerned about the security, privacy, and confidentiality of the personal health information shared on these platforms (Antheunis et al. 2013; Kordzadeh and Warren 2014). Moreover, the accuracy and quality of information shared within these environments as well as the credibility of individuals who post medical tips, advice, and experiences through these platforms may also be a source of concern for users, providers, and administrators of these websites (Hoffman-Goetz et al. 2009). Thus, considering, investigating, and understanding the negative sides of using social media platforms for health-related communications seem necessary. The drawbacks of using health social media and the opportunities provided by them are discussed in more detail in the sections “Concerns and Challenges” and “Opportunities and Future Developments” of this chapter, respectively.

Health Social Media Categories

In general, social media websites used by health consumers and professionals can be categorized into two generic types: general-purpose OSNs and VHCs.

General-Purpose OSNs

General-purpose OSNs such as Facebook, Twitter, Instagram, and YouTube provide mass collaboration platforms to Internet users to make friendships, share thoughts, videos, audios, and pictures on any subject ranging from events in daily lives to sports, music, and education. Using OSN platforms, Internet users can also provide feedback on each other’s activities on those websites. This category of social media platforms is not specifically designed for patients and health-care organizations; however, the features and functionalities provided by such websites have made them a widely used outlet for health-related communications between individuals and health-care providers.

OSNs provide an inexpensive yet effective channel through which clinics, hospitals, pharmacies, and other health-related organizations can communicate directly with their target audience that include their actual and potential patients. Health-care organizations create profile pages on general-purpose OSNs to promote their medical services and products (Bermúdez-Tamayo et al. 2013), educate health consumers, and raise public awareness on diseases, medical conditions, and treatments (Richer et al. 2014; Griffis et al. 2014). In this way, health-care organizations can manage their relationships with health consumers and also manage their brand’s image and reputation at the community and global levels.

As of November 2014, more than 1500 hospitals in the USA had a presence on general-purpose OSNs (Bennett n.d.). For instance, 93 hospitals and clinics in Texas had a social media presence, whereas this number for the state of New York was 118. Boston Children’s Hospital and Cleveland Clinic are among the prominent health-care organizations in the USA that have established a social media presence on Facebook, YouTube, or other socially enabled websites (Sharp 2012). As another example, Johns Hopkins Hospital, a world-class hospital in Baltimore, MD, has more than 225,000 users on their Facebook fan page[4]. Moreover, Johns Hopkins' YouTube channel[5] and Twitter page[6] have more than 11,000 subscribers and 260,000 followers, respectively, from all over the world. These statistics demonstrate that health-care organizations are more and more relying on social media websites for communications with individuals.

Health consumers including those who are suffering from particular medical conditions and those who have health-related questions or concerns join the OSN pages administered by health-care organizations. In this way, health consumers communicate directly with the organization's representatives on those pages, express their questions or concerns on their medical conditions, treatments, or procedures, and provide feedback on the services offered by that organization to health consumers. Individuals also read the articles and watch the videos related to health and wellness topics posted on those pages, and this may help them learn more about those topics and make better future decisions on their health and health care accordingly.

In addition to the communications between health providers and consumers on OSN websites, individuals can communicate with each other on those pages and share their opinions, experiences, and knowledge on medical topics (Greene et al. 2011). This consumer-to-consumer (C2C) form of collaboration will enable individuals to not only learn from health-care organizations but also learn from other individuals who have had similar health concerns or experiences related to themselves or their friends, families, or acquaintances (Greene et al. 2011; Newman et al. 2011). Providing and consuming health information in this way will empower health consumers and make them active participants in their health-care processes and education, and this is, in fact, the ultimate goal of PCEH applications and consumer health informatics.

Virtual Health Communities

As opposed to general-purpose OSNs, VHCs are social media websites that are specifically designed for individuals to communicate on health-related topics. These websites typically provide various functionalities and collaboration platforms to facilitate health communications and discussions. DailyStrength.org, PatientsLikeMe.com, and MedHelp.org are among the most popular VHCs in the USA. For instance, MedHelp.org states that this website "empowers more than 12 million people each month to take control of their health and find answers to their medical questions."[7] DailyStrength.org provides more than 500 support groups ranging

[4] https://www.facebook.com/Johns.Hopkins.Medicine, retrieved November 2014.

[5] https://www.youtube.com/user/JohnsHopkinsMedicine, retrieved November 2014.

[6] https://twitter.com/HopkinsMedicine, retrieved November 2014.

[7] www.Medhelp.org, retrieved October 2013.

from depression and alcoholism to pregnancy and insomnia for people to join, initiate discussions on those topics, ask related questions, and exchange informational and emotional support with other members of that website.

VHCs are different from one another in various ways. Some VHCs host users of a wide range of medical conditions. DailyStrength.org and MedHelp.org are in this group. Other VHCs host people who are somehow related to specific health-related conditions. CancerForums.net, for instance, offers collaboration platforms for individuals who are suffering from cancer or have questions or concerns related to that disease. Another difference across VHCs is the forms of collaboration platforms they provide to their users. For instance, CancerForums.net relies primarily on discussion boards and discussion threads initiated inside them, whereas MedHelp.org fosters communications between health professionals and consumers and allows individuals to ask questions and seek advice on medical issues from verified professionals on the website.

Understanding what collaboration platforms are currently provided or can potentially be offered by VHCs is important because the effectiveness, usefulness, and usability of those platforms will drive adoption and active participation of individuals on those websites, which will ultimately trigger those websites to prosper, succeed, and grow. Thus, in the next section of this chapter, a typology of collaboration platforms within VHCs will be developed, presented, and discussed. The section will start with a brief literature review on various classification schemas related to virtual communities that are proposed in the extant literature. This will be followed by explaining the method that we adapted to develop our typology. The details of the typology along with the implications of this framework will also be discussed.

A Typology of Collaboration Platforms Within VHCs[8]

Background

Researchers in different disciplines related to online communities have developed various classification frameworks and typologies of the technologies, tools, applications, and services provided by those websites. Some frameworks aimed at classifying the platforms provided by virtual communities in a general context (e.g., Porter 2004; Stanoevska-Slabeva and Schmid 2001). Porter (2004), for instance, considered two dimensions of virtual communities, establishment and relationship orientation, as well as their subdimensions to develop a general classification of online communities. He also discussed that virtual communities can be classified based on five attributes initiated with the letter "p": purpose, place, platform, population interaction structure, and profit model.

[8] This typology was originally published and discussed in the May 2013 issue of *Health and Technology:* Kordzadeh, N., and Warren, J., (2013). "Toward a Typology of Health 2.0 Collaboration Platforms and Websites," Health and Technology, 3(1), 2013, pp. 37–50.

Other researchers focused on context-specific virtual communities and provided their typology in particular for those websites. In the context of health-related online communities, researchers have made efforts to develop and present typologies and frameworks to better understand the various types of collaboration platforms as well as features and services offered by VHCs. Beijnum et al. (2009), for example, emphasized mobile virtual communities for telemedicine and discussed the different attributes and implications of this type of services. They adopted Porter's (2004) five attributes to characterize virtual communities for telemedicine. In another study, Scanfeld et al. (2010) classified and discussed various collaboration tools and platforms used for health communications through online social media. Seven types of platforms proposed in this article include blogs, microblogs, social network websites, wikis, social news and bookmarking, user reviews, and photo/video sharing. The platforms and the examples provided for each platform in this list include both health-specific websites (e.g., WebMD.com) and general-purpose OSNs (e.g., Twitter and Facebook). Scanfeld et al.'s (2010) classification, however, does not cover a set of major platforms provided by VHCs, such as physician rating, medicine rating, and ask-a-doctor. A few years later, Schein et al. (2011) added three more platforms, namely virtual worlds, news aggregators, and widgets/gadgets/badges/buttons, to the set of platforms proposed by Scanfeld et al. (2010).

Weber-Jahnke et al. (2011) adopted a three-stage typology development methodology to categorize consumer health informatics applications and services into six broad categories: (1) information aids, (2) decision aids, (3) education aids, (4) management aids, (5) health sales services, and (6) meta/rating services. They argued that various forms of health social media tools and platforms could be utilized for specific consumer health informatics applications. For example, forums, OSNs, and chat rooms can be used for management aids. A summary of the typologies discussed in this section is provided in Table 6.1.

The existing classifications in the context of health social media need an update for several reasons. First, they do not distinguish VHCs (e.g., DailyStrength.org) from general-purpose OSNs (e.g., Facebook and Twitter). Consequently, these typologies do not cover numerous state-of-the-art collaboration platforms such as physician rating and ask-a-doctor, which are provided specifically by VHCs. Second, the typologies related to health social media that are proposed by the extant literature are not built on the type of users and the forms of collaborations between them. In order to fill these gaps, we developed a specific typology of collaboration platforms within VHCs that revolves around two major types of VHC users and the interactions between them.

In order to develop the typology, a two-step method used in various typology development studies is also followed in this study. This method, known as conceptual-empirical approach (Nickerson et al. 2013), revolves around a logically supported conceptual development of a typology followed by an empirical verification. Accordingly, in the first step of the typology development process, a typology of collaboration platforms and websites within the VHC context is developed. The conceptual development is built on the prior literature on social media platforms (Scanfeld et al. 2010; Schein et al. 2011) as well as e-commerce business models

Table 6.1 Typologies of general and health-specific social media

Citation	Content	Categories/types
Porter (2004)	Virtual communities (general)	Based on the two main dimensions (establishment and relationship orientation), five major categories of virtual communities were proposed as follows:
		1) Social member-initiated communities
		2) Professional member-initiated communities
		3) Commercial organization-sponsored communities
		4) Nonprofit organization-sponsored communities
		5) Government organization-sponsored communities
		To further expand the typology, five attributes were also considered: purpose, place, platform, population interaction structure, and profit model
Beijnum et al. (2009)	Mobile virtual communities for telemedicine	Porter's 5p attributes which include purpose, place, platform, population interaction structure, and profit model were adopted to characterize different forms of mobile virtual communities for telemedicine
Scanfeld et al. (2010)	Collaboration tools and platforms used for health communications through social media, e.g., Twitter	Seven major types of collaboration platforms that can be offered by socially enabled websites were identified:
		1) Blogs
		2) Microblogs
		3) Social network websites
		4) Wikis
		5) Social news and bookmarking
		6) User reviews
		7) Photo/video sharing
Schein et al. (2011)	Social media in health care	The following three categories were added to Scanfeld et al.'s (2010) typology:
		1) Virtual worlds
		2) News aggregators
		3) Widgets/gadgets/badges/buttons
Weber-Jahnke et al. (2011)	Consumer health informatics Services and applications	Based on the purpose of using collaboration services and applications, six major types of these applications were identified:
		1) Information aids
		2) Decision aids
		3) Education aids
		4) Management aids
		5) Health sales services
		6) Meta/rating services

(Turban et al. 2010). It is followed by an empirical verification of the proposed typology. To do so, various keywords relevant to this study, such as "virtual health communities," "online patient communities," "online physician communities," "health blogs," and "health social media," are searched on Google.com to find relatively popular English language VHC websites and to make it possible to compare them with respect to the typology proposed in this study. The top-ranked VHC websites in terms of the number of users and page views are identified and included in a list. Then, that list is compared with the lists provided by ranking websites. Only those VHC websites that are consistently mentioned as top health-related social media websites used by either patients and caregivers or physicians and medical doctors are included in the final list. The final list includes 20 VHC websites. The names of those websites along with the collaboration platforms they provide are presented and discussed in the section "Typology in Action."

The Proposed Typology

Within the context of VHCs, we define collaboration platform as socially enabled computer-mediated communication environment used for contribution of health-related digital content (e.g., articles, messages, emoticons, audios, and videos). As opposed to the traditional computer-mediated communication tools and technologies such as e-mail, private messaging, and chat services, VHC collaboration platforms are more comprehensive, socially oriented systems typically built upon mass collaborations on health-related topics, making social ties among individuals and creating social support exchange relationships among them.

VHC collaboration platforms derive their structures, applications, technologies, and characteristics from a wider concept of "Web 2.0 collaboration platforms"—also known as Web 2.0 applications, functionalities, or tools—such as blogs, OSNs, and user reviews (Schein et al. 2011; Constantinides and Fountain 2008). Following this naming convention, health social media and VHC websites are sometimes referred to as Health 2.0 or Medicine 2.0 websites by researchers and practitioners (Hughes et al. 2008; Wickramasinghe et al. 2013b). Among different taxonomies proposed for Web 2.0 collaboration platforms that can be applied to the context of health care, we consider the one provided by Scanfeld et al. (2010) a starting point for our typology (Table 6.2).

In the classification proposed by Scanfeld et al. (2010), seven major collaboration platforms provided by socially enabled websites are distinguished. These platforms could be used for sharing health information among users of these websites. In our study, we revised Scanfeld et al.'s (2010) classification because they did not focus on VHCs websites, which are dedicated to health topics (e.g., DailyStrength.com). Rather, they considered general-purpose OSNs such as Facebook and Twitter. Thus, the set of social media platforms proposed by them does not cover health-specific platforms such as health forums or ask-a-doctor, which are widely provided by VHCs. Moreover, platforms such as "microblog" and "social news and

Table 6.2 A typology of Web 2.0 collaboration platforms. (Adapted from Scanfeld et al. 2010)

Collaboration platform	Definition
Blog ("Weblog")	A website that contains regularly updated entries displayed in reverse chronological order
Microblog	A form of blogging that allows users to send brief text updates or micro-media to be viewed by the public or a restricted group
Social networking website	Online communities that share interests and/or activities
Wiki	A website that enables the easy creation and editing of interlinking web pages
Social news and bookmarking	Social bookmarking enables users to save and share links to web pages organized by metadata (e.g., "tags" or keywords). Social news sites often enable users to vote on links to news, bringing the most popular stories to the top
User reviews	A website or site feature on which people can post opinions about people, businesses, products, or services
Photo/video sharing	A website that enables the publishing of a user's digital photos or video clips online, facilitating sharing with others

bookmarking," included in Scanfeld et al.'s (2010) classification, are not typically utilized by VHC websites. Therefore, we customized their classification to make it better fit in the context of health social media and VHCs. We also customized the definition of each type to make them meaningful in the context of our typology. Thus, the VHC collaboration platforms we focused on in this study along with their definitions are summarized in Table 6.3.

Table 6.3 Virtual health community (VHC) collaboration platforms

Collaboration platform	Definition
Health blog	A collaboration platform that displays postings by one or more individuals on different health-related topics such that other Internet users can post their comments on each entry (Scanfeld et al. 2010)
Physician rating	A collaboration platform through which people can post their opinions about health professionals such as doctors and dentists (Scanfeld et al. 2010)
Medicine rating	A collaboration platform through which people can share knowledge and experience about different types of medicine
Online health social network	A collaboration platform on which users can create a public or semipublic profile, share their personal information such as demographics, photos, health conditions, and feelings, and make connections with other users of the website by adding them to their friends lists (Ellison 2007)
Health discussion board/forum	A collaboration platform for the open discussion of subjects relevant to health and wellness (Wang et al. 2006)
Ask-a-doctor	A collaboration platform through which health consumers can ask their questions and receive responses from health professionals hosted on a given Health 2.0 website

The collaboration platforms listed in Table 6.3 can be incorporated into various forms of VHCs and used by different types of VHC users. In general, there are two major types of individual users/actors within the context of health social media: (1) health consumers such as patients and caregivers and (2) health professionals such as physicians, medical practitioners, and dentists. Both health consumers (C) and health professionals (P) can serve as either support provider or support recipient while interacting with other users of these websites. Accordingly, the collaborations within Health 2.0 websites can be categorized into four major types: professional-to-professional (P2P), professional-to-consumer (P2C), consumer-to-consumer (C2C), and consumer-to-professional (C2P). P2C collaborations occur when health professionals provide support for health consumers, while C2P collaborations can be realized when health consumers contribute their experience and opinions to health professionals. P2P and C2C collaborations represent interactions and support exchanges among health professionals and health consumers, respectively, on VHC websites.

This perspective toward collaborations among Health 2.0 users is very similar to the way e-commerce transactions are categorized by researchers and practitioners in different fields into C2C, consumer-to-business (C2B), business-to-business (B2B), and business-to-consumer (B2C), as well as government-to-consumer (G2C) and consumer-to-government (C2G; Turban et al. 2010). For example, in the context of e-commerce, when a product or service is provided by companies for individuals over the Internet (e.g., purchasing a laptop from Dell.com), B2C transactions occur. Similarly, when individuals sell and buy items from other individuals, (e.g., trading on ebay.com or Craigslist.com), C2C transactions are realized.

The platforms proposed in Table 6.3 can enable and support specific type(s) of collaborations within the context of health social media from P2P to C2C. For instance, OSNs can be used for both C2C and P2P communications, whereas the ask-a-doctor platform is primarily used for P2C support provisions. Thus, in the following section, the proposed typology of VHC platforms is further developed and how each type of platform supports specific types of collaborations among VHC users is discussed in detail.

Platforms Supporting P2C Collaborations

P2C collaborations occur when health professionals provide supports for health consumers through VHC channels. Two major platforms used by health professionals to provide direct support for patients are health blogs and ask-a-doctor. Health blogs have become an important source of online health information for Internet users (Hu and Shyam Sundar 2010). They are typically authored by health professionals and comprise health-related news, information, tips, and advice that can be beneficial for health consumers (Lagu et al. 2008). The Internet users who read the blogs can then post their comments and questions regarding the topics of those blogs. Other blog readers as well as the blog authors can afterward answer the questions posted on the blogs.

"Ask-a-doctor" is the second prominent P2C collaboration platform. Using this platform, any user can ask specific questions regarding medications, diseases, or any health-related topics from the health professionals approved by the website. These health professionals then provide the user with an answer that is specifically tailored based on the user's question. Unlike the P2C interactions through health blogs, the interactions based on ask-a-doctor are initiated by a health consumer. An ask-a-doctor platform can be provided as a private channel such that the answers by the health professionals cannot be viewed by any user other than the one who asks the question (e.g., DailyStrength.org). Other VHC websites (e.g., MedHelp.org) provide a more socially enabled ask-a-doctor platform such that when a user posts a question and the health professionals answer that, other users can also view the question–answer thread and engage in the discussion.

Platforms Supporting C2C Collaborations

Various collaboration platforms are provided by VHC websites to enable health consumers to interact, make social ties, and support each other on their health issues and concerns. The most widely used C2C collaboration platform is health discussion boards or forums. Health discussion boards are topic-oriented platforms used by health consumers to discuss specific diseases, treatments, or any other health-related topic (Tanis 2008). Health consumers initiate discussion threads on a topic, ask a question, and/or seek support from others on the website. In response to the thread initiator, others post comments to the thread and provide their thoughts, sympathy, information, and experience that specifically address the thread topic. Forums are typically categorized based on different criteria such as medical conditions (e.g., cancer and depression) or treatments.

OSNs of health consumers are another C2C platform widely used by VHC websites. Using this platform, users create profile pages, add profile photos, share personal information such as demographics and health status, and make connections with each other by adding individuals to their friends lists (Eysenbach 2008). This structure is very similar to the typical structure of general-purpose OSNs such as Facebook and MySpace (Ellison 2007).

Although online health social networks and health discussion boards have much in common, they have their differences. Online health social networks and the interactions based on them are basically user oriented (Ellison 2007). Consequently, social ties between users who interact based on these platforms are strong, emotional based, and long term, whereas the interactions that occur within discussion boards are inherently topic oriented (Stanoevska-Slabeva and Schmid 2001; Ellison 2007). Thus, the social ties formed between users who engage in discussion threads are more transaction based. It leads typically to short-term relationships between those who participate in discussion threads and support each other merely through these channels. The main advantage of discussion boards is that users can take advantage of others' knowledge and experience, regardless of their friendship status. This leads to an extensive knowledge base available to users, compared to situations where users seek information only from their friends within the community. Additionally, discussion boards provide a more structured platform that users can initiate, follow, or contribute to the topics that are of more interest to them.

Health blogs can also be used for C2C communications. Health consumers initiate blogs on their current health issues, concerns, or questions, and others post their supportive messages on the blog. The difference between personal health blogs and discussion threads is that health discussion threads are categorized based on specific health topics, while blogs can be on any topic of interest to the user. Thus, health blogs are usually incorporated into OSNs such that users can simply initiate their personal blogs on their profile pages (e.g., DailyStrength.org).

User reviews, which is another collaboration platform used for C2C interactions, primarily emerge in two forms: medicine rating and physician rating. Medicine-rating platforms provided by VHC websites enable health consumers to share their experience and knowledge on the effectiveness, side effects, and other characteristics of medicines. Users can also rate drugs and compare the drug ratings (e.g., AskAPatient.com). Physician-rating platforms are also among the fastest growing user reviews in the context of health social media (Lagu et al. 2010; Kadry et al. 2011). Using this form of C2C platform, health consumers post their reviews on doctors, surgeons, health practitioners, and any other health professionals. Moreover, physician-rating platforms sometimes allow the users to rate clinics and hospitals in terms of the quality of health-care services they provide for their patients. The reviews posted are useful for the patients who may potentially need to visit a specific health-care organization or health professional.

Platforms Supporting P2P Collaborations

Health professionals can also use VHC collaboration platforms to communicate with their colleagues. Discussion boards, for example, can be used by them to discuss on specific diseases, treatments, medications, surgery techniques, technologies, and other professional topics in their areas of expertise. This can enable health professionals to always be up-to-date on health-related sciences and technologies. Additionally, professional OSNs and health blogs can be utilized by health professionals for P2P interactions and peer-to-peer support provision. However, unlike C2C, P2C, and C2P collaboration platforms in which health consumers play a major role as support provider or recipient, P2P platforms and communications within them merely revolve around health professionals. Thus, consistent with the definition of consumer health informatics and PCEH applications, which emphasizes the active role of health consumers, P2P Health 2.0 platforms and websites are not considered part of consumer health informatics.

		Support Recipient	
		Health Professional	Health Consumer
Support Provider	Health Professional	**P2P (not part of consumer-centered e-health)** 1. Online Social Networks 2. Health Discussion Boards 3. Health Blogs	**P2C** 1. Health Blogs 2. Ask-A-Doctor
	Health Consumer	**C2P** 1. Physician-Rating	**C2C** 1. Online Social Networks 2. Health Discussion Boards 3. Health Blogs 4. Medicine-Ratings 5. Physician-Ratings

Fig. 6.2 The proposed typology of virtual health community (VHC) collaboration platforms. *P2P* professional-to-professional, *C2P* consumer-to-professional, *P2C* professional-to-consumer, *C2C* consumer-to-consumer

Platforms Supporting C2P Collaborations

Unlike the previous types of collaborations, C2P collaborations are not well supported by the current types of Health 2.0 collaboration platforms. However, physician-rating websites can be used by health consumers to post their reviews on health professionals for the use of these professionals and not merely for the advantage of health consumers. For example, health-care organizations can provide specific physician-rating platforms for their patients so that the organization management team can learn about the patients' opinions about the physicians who work in the organization. This can help them improve the quality of care they provide for their patients. A summary of the types of collaboration platforms that enable and support each type of collaboration within VHC websites is presented in Fig. 6.2.

Typology in Action

In order to validate the proposed typology and make it clearer, we applied our typology to a list of 20 VHC websites. Considering the different types of platforms and websites introduced in the typology, we compared these websites and the prominent platforms they provide. As mentioned earlier, to compile the list of these 20 websites, we searched various keywords relevant to health social media on Google.com to find relatively popular health-related websites that provide collaboration platforms for their users. We compared the search results with the list of the top health-related websites provided by different blogs, ranking services, and other websites. Then, we included the names of the VHC websites that appear in different rankings and that offer socially enabled services and features. The results containing the names of the websites found throughout this search process as well as the types of collaboration platforms provided by them are summarized in Table 6.4.

Table 6.4 shows that Sermo.com and Ozmosis.org are virtual communities of health professionals and, consequently, health consumers do not get involved in the communications that occur within these online communities. Thus, these two websites are not considered as a part of consumer-centered websites or consumer health inform. The other 18 websites, however, revolve around health consumers and provide platforms for their users to communicate with health professionals and/or other health consumers who are members of these websites.

Table 6.4 Virtual health communities (VHCs) websites and collaboration platforms

	Type of Health 2.0 platform					
	P2P	P2C		C2C		C2P
Website name	Professional discussion board	Blog/news group	Ask-a-doctor	Online health social network	Discussion board	Physician rating
DailyStrength.org	–	✓	✓	✓	✓	–
WebMD.com	–	✓	–	–	✓	–
Connect.MayoClinic.org	–	–	–	✓	✓	–
Drugs.com	–	–	–	✓	✓	–
AskaPatient.com	–	–	–	–	✓	–
HealthBoards.com	–	–	✓	✓	✓	–
PatientsLikeMe.com	–	–	–	✓	✓	–
MedHelp.org	–	✓	✓	✓	✓	–
Inspire.com	–	–	–	✓	✓	–
CancerForums.net	–	–	–	✓	✓	–
Breastcancer.org	–	✓	✓	✓	✓	–
KevinMD.com	–	✓	–	–	–	–
Sermo.com	✓	–	–	–	–	–
Ozmosis.org	✓	–	–	–	–	–
HealthGrades.com	–	–	–	–	–	✓
iWantGreatCare.org	–	–	–	–	–	✓

P2P professional-to-professional, *P2C* professional-to-consumer, *C2C* consumer-to-consumer, *C2P* consumer-to-professional

Opportunities and Future Developments

Despite the pervasive adoption of health social media in the health-care industry, still various opportunities exist for developers and providers of these systems as well as health-care organizations to make a better use of these technologies. Three such opportunities are synchronous collaboration platforms, social-media-enabled mobile applications, and knowledge discovery.

Synchronous Collaboration Platforms

Currently, VHC websites tend to provide asynchronous collaboration platforms, while synchronous platforms such as chat rooms, video conferencing environments, and webinars can be incorporated into those websites for the users' real-time communications. Chat rooms, for example, can be used as an alternative or as a complement to health discussion boards. If chat rooms are developed within VHCs, users can join them and discuss on specific medical topics including their current health issues, concerns, and experience in a real-time manner. VHCs can also enable the users to chat with health professionals and ask their questions through this medium. In order to enrich the interactions via chat rooms, video communication functionalities can also be added to them. Video conferencing and webinars (web-based presentations, lectures, or workshops) can also be used for educational purposes, targeting health professionals or health consumers. VHCs can offer periodic webinars each on specific health/wellness topic for their users. Webinars could be even more effective than traditional health blogs for conveying health tips and advices from health professionals to health consumers.

In future studies, the potential values that each of the aforementioned synchronous collaboration platforms can provide for VHC users can be investigated. Researchers can also study how these platforms can be combined with their asynchronous counterparts to make health consumers and professionals more inclined toward adopting and using VHC websites and participating actively within these environments.

Mobile Applications

Another type of collaboration platform that is not yet widely offered by VHC websites and, consequently, not researched adequately in the context of health social media is mobile applications. Recently, various communities such as WebMD.com have offered mobile applications for their users such that the members of those websites can communicate using their mobile devices. Other communities such as Epocrates.com have gone beyond that and based their business model solely on developing and providing mobile applications, mostly for health professionals. However, there is still a huge potential for other VHC websites to take advantage of the mobile-based emerging technologies and collaboration platforms. In future studies, researchers can investigate the attitudes and perceptions of VHC users toward using mobile devices for different types of health communications from P2C to C2C. The potential capabilities of these platforms for enriching communications within VHCs can also be researched in future.

Knowledge Discovery

Everyday millions of health-related posts are sent through various VHC websites. Each post may contain valuable information not only for the specific audience of that post but also for other health consumers and professionals. Health forums, for example, are becoming a rich repository of unstructured knowledge about health topics such as disease symptoms, medicine side effects, successful treatments, medical cases, and medications. The knowledge stored in this way can be discovered and organized to be used by future patients, caregivers, and, more importantly, by health professionals. Despite these opportunities, the application of knowledge management has still been overlooked by health-care information system researchers and practitioners. Future research can examine how knowledge management techniques and strategies can be utilized in Health 2.0 collaboration platforms and websites and how the knowledge discovered in this way can create value for health professionals and health consumers.

Concerns and Challenges

Adoption and use of social media technologies for health care have risks and drawbacks, such as possible violation of information privacy, lack of information quality and credibility, and free riding and lurking behaviors on those websites.

Information Privacy

Personal health information is sensitive information that individuals may not be willing to share and discuss through public collaboration platforms and websites (Williams 2010). Thus, adopting VHCs and active participation within them presents information privacy risks. While interacting with other Internet users, individuals may be concerned that the personal health information they reveal on a website may be misused by the website's administrator, the members of the website, or third parties such as insurance companies. Considering these privacy risks, health professionals may not be willing or allowed to discuss their patients on publicly accessible VHC websites. Nonetheless, those websites typically provide privacy policies and controls for their users.

The importance of health information privacy within the context of health social media demonstrates that researchers should focus more on this issue. Future research can assess perceived privacy risks and concerns of health consumers and professionals and provide practical guidelines for VHC providers to address user concerns more effectively. Website providers should also improve their privacy policies and utilize privacy-enhancing technologies to better protect their members' privacy, which will result in members being more willing to participate actively in the collaborative activities on the website.

Information Quality/Credibility

A major challenge which the users of health social media platforms face is the quality, reliability, and credibility of the information provided by others on the website (Antheunis et al. 2013). For example, users may share their experience of using a specific medicine on discussion boards. However, how can one trust this information that comes from a user whose real identity is probably not disclosed on the website? To what extent do people rely on this information and take advice from other users on these websites? And, if a user claims to be a medical expert, how could his/her credibility be verified? Is it the website's responsibility to approve the reliability of the health information, tips, and advice shared through collaboration platforms, or should the users be aware of the potential risks of using and relying on such information? These are all questions that can be addressed by VHC providers and by researchers in future studies.

Lurking

The success, growth, and viability of VHCs are subject to the level of user participation. The online communities within Health 2.0 websites may not survive if the vast majority of the community comprises lurkers who merely read the posts and do not actively participate in the discussions and communications (Nonnecke and Preece 2000; Panciera et al. 2010). Extant literature has addressed the reasons behind active participation and lurking within different types of online communities. However, the specific characteristics of VHC collaboration platforms and websites as well as the specific reasons for joining and participating within these websites demonstrate that researchers should particularly study the drivers and inhibitors to knowledge contribution within these environments. The results of these studies can also help online community providers to foster user participation within their websites.

Conclusion

Social media platforms and websites are becoming a major channel through which health consumers including patients and caregivers seek and provide information and emotional aid in collaboration with other users of those websites. In this way, individuals are not merely passive consumers of health information, rather they get involved in producing, sharing, seeking, and discussing health information related, or of interest, to them. This is the ultimate goal of consumer health informatics and PCEH application.

The two major health social media categories discussed in this chapter, general-purpose OSNs and VHCs, can play a crucial role in driving individuals' engagement in their health care. Accordingly, general-purpose OSNs are primarily used by health-care organizations not only to facilitate C2C communication but also as a gateway through which those organizations educate people on health and wellness-related topics and promote the services and products that they offer to health consumers. Moreover, in order to communicate with their target audience more effectively, health-care organizations need to systematically develop a social media strategy to exactly know what their intentions of using such channels are and how they want to implement those strategies. For example, some hospitals may want to use their official Facebook pages to share organizational news on achievements, awards, new facilities, and new services provided to the community. Thus, they may need to hire social media marketing experts to better communicate organizational news and promote their quality of care through those social media websites. Other hospitals may intend to use their social media pages primarily to provide tips and advice on health and wellness topics to patients and to the broader community. Therefore, this group of hospitals will need to have physicians and medical experts develop medical articles that are easy to understand for the public audience and share those articles regularly on those social pages.

The second category of health social media, which is VHCs, can also offer various collaboration platforms for health consumers that help them communicate with other users of those websites more effectively. The primary collaboration platforms offered by VHC websites include health discussion boards, online health social networks, health blogs, ask-a-doctor, physician rating, and medicine rating. Additionally, providers of VHCs can provide users with synchronous communication environments such as chat rooms and webinar sessions. Those websites can also offer social-media-enabled mobile applications.

Hospitals and clinics all over the world can develop their own social media websites and get their own patients as well as the public audience engaged in the social interactions within those websites. In this way, health-care institutions can create support groups, encourage users to post topics and respond to others' topics through discussion boards, rate physicians, services, and products through rating platforms, and seek medical consulting services through the ask-a-doctor platform. A major advantage of organization-sponsored VHCs (e.g., Mayo Clinic's social media website) against public VHCs (e.g., CancerForums.net) is that organization-sponsored VHCs are provided, administered, and controlled by a specific (or a group of specific) health-care organization(s). As a result, physicians and other medical experts sponsored by these organizations can moderate the health-related discussions and social interactions within the community to verify the quality, accuracy, credibility, and reliability of the user-generated content on the collaboration platforms such as discussion boards.

Despite the benefits of health social media for health providers and consumers, protecting the privacy of users, particularly those who intentionally or unintentionally disclose their identifiable information within VHCs, remains a major challenge for the providers of VHC websites. Providers and administrators of these websites can develop and offer comprehensive privacy policies and statements. They can also provide users with privacy setting features to enable them to adjust their identifiability and profile visibility. Training users and raising awareness on privacy topics such as why protecting health information privacy is important and how users can protect their privacy on VHCs are among other ways of mitigating privacy risks in health social media environments. Governmental agencies such as the US Department of Health and Human Services that enforce health information privacy-related acts and regulations can also address privacy risks on socially enabled environments.

Another challenge that VHC providers face is lurking, which means many users may not be willing to actively participate in online discussions. If people tend to merely read and use the information shared by others on VHCs, the overall activity level within those communities will diminish. This is not desirable and will need to be addressed through providing incentives and making policies to encourage individuals to actively provide emotional and informational support to other users of those virtual environments.

In summary, health social media including general-purpose OSNs and VHCs offer various opportunities and challenges to health-care organizations as well as health consumers. Hospitals and clinics communicate with their audience through collaboration platforms provided by health social media. Health consumers also play an active role in their health care via adopting social media to exchange medical information and knowledge in collaboration with each other and with health-care providers. Given the current trend of using social media in health care, it is expected that in the near future, social technologies will be adopted more widely, more wisely, and more effectively in that context.

References

Antheunis, M. L., Tates, K., & Nieboer, T. E. (2013). Patients' and health professionals' use of social media in health care: Motives, barriers and expectations. *Patient Education and Counseling, 92*(3), 426–431.

Beijnum, B. J. F., Pawar, P., Dulawan, C., & Hermens, H. (2009). Mobile virtual communities for telemedicine: Research challenges and opportunities. *International Journal of Computer Science & Applications, 6*(2), 19–37.

Bennett, E. (n.d.). Health care social media list. http://network.socialmedia.mayoclinic.org/hcsml-grid. Accessed 15 Nov 2014.

Bermudez-Tamayo, C., Jimenez-Pemett, J., Garcia Gutierrez, J., Yubraham-Sanchez, D., Alba Ruiz, R., & Traver-Salcedo, V. (2013). Use of social media by Spanish hospitals: Perceptions, difficulties, and success factors. *Telemedicine and e-Health, 19*(2), 137–145.

Constantinides, E., & Fountain, S. J. (2008). Web 2.0: Conceptual foundations and marketing issues. *Journal of Direct, Data and Digital Marketing Practice, 9*(3), 231–244.

Demiris, G. (2006). The diffusion of virtual communities in health care: Concepts and challenges. *Patient Education and Counseling, 62*(2), 178–188.

Ellison, N. B. (2007). Social network sites: Definition, history, and scholarship. *Journal of Computer-mediated Communication, 13*(1), 210–230.

Eysenbach, G. (2008). Medicine 2.0: social networking, collaboration, participation, apomediation, and openness. *Journal of Medical Internet Research, 10*(3), e22.

Fox, S., & Duggan, M. (2013). Health online 2013. http://www.pewinternet.org/files/old-media//Files/Reports/PIP_HealthOnline.pdf. Accessed 15 Nov 2014.

Greene, J. A., Choudhry, N. K., Kilabuk, E., & Shrank, W. H. (2011). Online social networking by patients with diabetes: A qualitative evaluation of communication with Facebook. *Journal of general internal medicine, 26*(3), 287–292.

Greenhalgh, T., Hinder, S., Stramer, K., Bratan, T., & Russell, J. (2010). Adoption, non-adoption, and abandonment of a personal electronic health record: case study of HealthSpace. *BMJ: British Medical Journal, 341,* c5814.

Griffis, H. M., et al. (2014). Use of social media across US hospitals: Descriptive analysis of adoption and utilization. *Journal of Medical Internet Research, 6*(11), e264.

Hoffman-Goetz, L., Donelle, L., & Thomson, M. D. (2009). Clinical guidelines about diabetes and the accuracy of peer information in an unmoderated online health forum for retired persons. *Informatics for Health and Social Care, 34*(2), 91–99.

Houston, T. K., Cooper, L. A., & Ford, D. E. (2002). Internet support groups for depression: A 1-year prospective cohort study. *American Journal of Psychiatry, 159*(12), 2062–2068.

Hu, Y., & Shyam Sundar, S. (2010). Effects of online health sources on credibility and behavioral intentions. *Communication Research, 37*(1), 105.

Hughes, B., Joshi, I., & Wareham, J. (2008). Health 2.0 and medicine 2.0: Tensions and controversies in the field. *Journal of Medical Internet Research, 10*(3), e23

Kadry, B., Chu, L. F., Gammas, D., & Macario, A. (2011). Analysis of 4999 online physician ratings indicates that most patients give physicians a favorable rating. *Journal of Medical Internet Research, 13*(4), e95.

Kordzadeh, N., & Warren, J. (2014). Communicating personal health information in virtual health communities: A theoretical framework. *47th Hawaii International Conference on System Sciences (HICSS)*, Waikoloa, HI.

Kordzadeh, N., Zhechao Liu, C., Au, Y. A., & Clark, J. G. (2014). A Multilevel investigation of participation within virtual health communities. *Communications of the Association for Information Systems, 34*(1), 26.

Lagu, T., Kaufman, E. J., Asch, D. A., & Armstrong, K. (2008). Content of weblogs written by health professionals. *Journal of General Internal Medicine, 23*(10), 1642–1646.

Lagu, T., Hannon, N. S., Rothberg, M. B., & Lindenauer, P. K. (2010). Patients' evaluations of health care providers in the era of social networking: An analysis of physician-rating websites. *Journal of General Internal Medicine, 25*(9), 942–946.

Lasker, J. N., Sogolow, E. D., & Sharim, R. R. (2005). The role of an online community for people with a rare disease: content analysis of messages posted on a primary biliary cirrhosis mailing list. *Journal of Medical Internet Research,* 7(1), e10.

Lau, A., & Kwok, T. (2009). *Social features in online communities for healthcare consumers—A review.* International Conference on Online Communities and Social Computing (OCSC), San Diego, CA, pp. 682–689.

Lewis, D., Chang, B. L., & Friedman, C. P. (2005). Consumer health informatics. *Health Informatics,* 1–7. http://link.springer.com/book/10.1007/0-387-27652-1#page=19

Merolli, M., Gray, K., & Martin-Sanchez, F. (2013). Health outcomes and related effects of using social media in chronic disease management: A literature review and analysis of affordances. *Journal of Biomedical Informatics, 46*(6), 957–969.
Newman, M. W., Lauterbach, D., Munson, S. A., Resnick, P., & Morris, M. E. (2011). *It's not that I don't have problems, I'm just not putting them on Facebook: Challenges and opportunities in using online social networks for health*. ACM conference on Computer supported cooperative work (CSCW), ACM.
Nickerson, R., Muntermann, J., Varshney, U., & Isaac, H. (Eds.). (2013). Taxonomy development in information systems: Developing a taxonomy of mobile applications. *European Journal of Information Systems, 22,* 336–359.
Nonnecke, B., & Preece, J. (Eds.). (2000). *Lurker demographics: Counting the silent*. ACM Conference on Human Factors in Computing Systems (CHI), ACM.
Panciera, K., Priedhorsky, R., Erickson, T., & Terveen, L. (Eds.). (2010). *Lurking? cyclopaths?: A quantitative lifecycle analysis of user behavior in a geowiki*. ACM Conference on Human Factors in Computing Systems (CHI), ACM.
Porter, C. E. (2004). A typology of virtual communities: A multi–disciplinary foundation for future research. *Journal of Computer–Mediated Communications,* 10(1), Article 3.
Powell, J., McCarthy, N., & Eysenbach, G. (2003). Cross-sectional survey of users of internet depression communities. *BMC Psychiatry, 3*(1), 19.
Preece, J., Nonnecke, B., & Andrews, D. (2004). The top five reasons for lurking: Improving community experiences for everyone. *Computers in Human Behavior, 20*(2), 201–223.
Rhoads, J. (2012) *Ready to interact: Social media use by U.S. hospitals and health systems*. CSC's Global Institute for Emerging Healthcare Practices. http://assets1.csc.com/health_services/downloads/CSC_Survey_Social_Media_Use_by_U.S._Hospitals_and_Health_Systems.pdf. Accessed 10 Nov 2014.
Richer, J. P., Muhlestain, D. B., & Wilks, C. E. A. (2014). Social media: How US hospitals use it, and opportunities for future use. *Journal of Healthcare Management, 59*(6), 447–460.
Scanfeld, D., Scanfeld, V., & Larson, E. L. (2010). Dissemination of health information through social networks: Twitter and antibiotics. *American Journal of Infection Control, 38*(3), 182–188.
Schein, R., Wilson, K., & Keelan, J. E. (2011). Literature review on effectiveness of the use of social media: A report for peel public health. Region of Peel. Peel Public Health. http://www.rop.ca/health/resources/pdf/socialmedia.pdf. Accessed 10 Sept 2014
Sharp, J. (2012). A look at social media in health care—Two years later. http://www.ihealthbeat.org/perspectives/2012/a-look-at-social-media-in-health-care-two-years-later.aspx. Accessed 15 Nov 2014
Stanoevska-Slabeva, K., & Schmid, B. F. (Eds.). (2001). *A typology of online communities and community supporting platforms*. 34th Hawaii International Conference on System Sciences (HICSS), IEEE.
Swan, M. (2009). Emerging patient-driven health care models: An examination of health social networks, consumer personalized medicine and quantified self-tracking. *International Journal of Environmental Research and Public Health, 6*(2), 492–525.
Tanis, M. (2008). Health-related on-line forums: What's the big attraction? *Journal of Health Communication, 13*(7), 698–714.
Turban, E., Lee, J. K., King, D., Liang, T. P., & Turban, D. (2010). *Electronic commerce*. Upper Saddle River: Prentice Hall Press.
Wang, J. H., Fu, T., Lin, H. M., & Chen, H. A. (2006). Framework for exploring gray web forums: Analysis of forum based communities in Taiwan (pp. 498–503). Intell Secur Inform.
Weber-Jahnke, J., Williams J. Anissa, (2011). *Consumer health informatics services—A taxonomy*. Informational Privacy Interdisciplinary Research Group (IPIRG), University of Victoria, BC, Canada.
Wickramasinghe, N., Teoh, S., Durst, C., & Viol, J. (2013a). *Insights from an investigation of the design of a consumer health 2.0 application to address the relationship between on-line social networks and health-related behaviours*. Australian Conference on Information Systems (ACIS), Melbourne, Australia.

Wickramasinghe, N., Davey, B., & Tatnall, A. (2013b). Web 2.0 Panacea or placebo for superior healthcare delivery? In R. Bali, I. Troshani, S. Goldberg, & N. Wickramasinghe (Eds.), *Pervasive health knowledge management* (pp. 317–330). Springer New York.

Williams, J. (Ed.) (2010). *Social networking applications in health care: threats to the privacy and security of health information*. ICSE Workshop on Software Engineering in Health Care, ACM.

Wilson, V. (2009). *Patient-centered E-health*. Hershey: IGI Publications.

Wilson, V., Wang, W., & Sheetz, S. D. (2014). Underpinning a guiding theory of patient-centered E-Health. *Communications of the Association for Information Systems, 34*(16), 337.

Nima Kordzadeh PhD is an assistant professor of business and health informatics at the College of Business, Idaho State University. He received his PhD in business administration from The University of Texas at San Antonio. His research areas include health informatics, data analytics, information privacy, and social media. His research has been presented at national and international conferences including Hawaii International Conference on System Sciences (HICSS), Americas Conference on Information Systems (AMCIS), and Southern Association for Information Systems (SAIS) conferences and published in such peer-reviewed journals as *Health and Technology* and *Communications of the Association for Information Systems.*

Chapter 7
Satisfaction with Health Informatics System Characteristics and Their Effect on Openness to Frequent Use

Karoly Bozan and Pratim Datta

Introduction

Health informatics systems, such as electronic health records (EHRs), offer the capacity and promise to increase the quality of patient care, to improve efficiency and effectiveness in the health-care delivery process, and to reduce care-related costs (World Health Organization 2005). EHRs are the digitized longitudinal health records of an individual that is shared across agencies and providers. The success of an EHR system implementation is often measured by the degree it is used (e.g., Devaraj and Kohli 2003) because it meets the users' expectations. Meeting expectations is an especially challenging objective to attain in a multiclient environment, such as the health-care industry. A common reason for Information Systems (IS) implementation failures is that organizations decide on a technological solution without fully understanding the underlying processes and client objectives (Sallas et al. 2007; McGowan et al. 2008).

The need for an EHR system, which delivers quality information securely and accurately across multiple health-care provider systems is urgent. Due to the nature of health-care organizations value chains, multiple clients are involved in the information flow process, whose duties and responsibilities significantly differ within the same care process (McGlynn 1997, Joss and Kogan 1995). These clients are identified as health-care providers, patients, administrators, and regulators.

The diverse client needs and use of EHR systems in a health-care organization require the system features and their characteristics to be beneficial for all users

The original version of this chapter was revised. An erratum to this chapter can be found at DOI 10.1007/978-3-319-25973-4_26

K. Bozan (✉)
Office: Room 540, 921 South 8th Avenue, Pocatello, ID 83209, USA
e-mail: bozakaro@isu.edu

P. Datta
Kent State University College of Business Administration, P.O. Box 5190, Terrace Drive, Kent, OH 44242, USA
e-mail: pdatta@kent.edu

N. Wickramasinghe et al. (eds.), *Contemporary Consumer Health Informatics*, Healthcare Delivery in the Information Age, DOI 10.1007/978-3-319-25973-4_7

by design. Clients perceive the same system characteristics differently, and what is beneficial for one group may cause workarounds for others. These varying perceptions of system characteristics by different clients result in partial use or abandonment of the system and evidence for failed EHR implementation in the literature abound (e.g., Zhang 2005; Aarts and Peel 1999; Goddard 2000). Understanding the software attributes and their effect on client system use behavior is an important tenet that needs to be understood for proper system design and selection.

Existing literature provides guidance on better understanding of user and organizational characteristics that leads to better success with acceptance and initial use of health informatics systems (e.g., Handy et al. 2001; Schectman et al. 2005; Kazley and Ozcan 2007). However, the continued usage of an information system (Bhattacherjee 2001) based on system characteristics and client groups is yet to be scrutinized and empirically tested for EHR systems.

After reviewing the relevant literature, this chapter aims to investigate and empirically test the client continued use behavior based on satisfaction with EHR system characteristics. Multiple different EHR client user groups were surveyed to answer this question, and based on the findings this study suggests a fine balance in crafting operational and regulatory policies for effective use of EHR systems across clients.

Research Design and Method

The aim of this study is to empirically validate the relationship between user satisfaction with health information system characteristics and openness to frequent use (OTU). OTU is perceived as an indicator of continued use of an EHR system and based on portability, usability, and confidentiality. The study considers the different perceptions across different client groups and the patient care processes. Ramanujam and Rousseau (2006) pointed out that this is especially challenging when often conflicting objectives and goals are involved in complex coordination of patient care.

Questionnaire Design

Following Walls et al.'s (1992) information system design theory (ISDT), 11 system features that support organizational requirements were proposed to form the base of the system-level investigation. These 11 system features are namely as follows: (1) confidentiality, (2) integrity, (3) availability, (4) efficiency, (5) effectiveness, (6) satisfaction, (7) responsibility, (8) auditability, (9) interconnectivity, (10) interconnectedness, and (11) transparency.

Health-care professionals representing four major client groups, namely (1) primary-care providers (PCPs), including nurses, (2) auditors, (3) administrators, and (4) patients, were surveyed on the perceived importance of and perceived satisfaction with the above 11 system features. The survey divided the patient-PCP encounter into four major process sequence blocks: (1) schedule and administer patient visit, (2) collect and review patient medical information, (3) diagnose and treat patient, and (4) report and follow-up.

Sample Data

A review of the literature suggests that existing studies limit their attention to conflicting client interests (Ahn and Skudlark 1997; Oz and Sosik 2000; Pan 2005), but these studies either lack empirical evidence or focus on one particular process or client group (e.g., Greenhalgh et al. 2010; Greenhalgh and Russell 2010). This study encompasses the PCP-patient encounter processes and their activities from the time of appointment scheduling until the follow-up care across all four major client groups. This approach provides a more realistic dissection of the health-care industry reflecting its multilayered and sequential processes and the levels clients are involved in each of the activities. Thus, professionals representing all four previously identified client groups across six different health-care institutions (Shi and Singh 2008) were presented an online questionnaire.

Sample Population

The sample population was from outpatient care settings and convenience sampling approach was used. Respondents comprised of health-care professionals who possessed some level of experience with some type of information system that supports the health-care organization's operations across one or multiple processes PCP–Patient encounter. The patient client group consisted of respondents, who had familiarity with patient portals and other self-managed health-care technology for online appointment booking, refilling prescriptions, accessing medical information, etc. (IRB approval #: 14–132, Kent State University).

The respondents were contacted through e-mail or asked in person to participate in the survey. While the initial contacts were all personal acquaintances of the researcher, everyone was asked to forward the questionnaire to their colleagues who represent the same client group. The personal contacts and personal references to a colleague expected the respondents to engage in the survey more than if a similar survey is requested from an unknown person. A large group of health-care administrators were contacted from a publicly available Regional Healthcare Partnership (RHP) list as well.

A relatively short deadline was given to complete the online questionnaire (2 weeks) and a reminder e-mail sent after 1 week. We did not provide random drawing for prize among those that completed the questionnaire. It reduced the possibility of unengaged responders, who complete the survey simply for the purpose of being included in the prize drawing.

The online survey software provider tracked the number of times the questionnaire was opened and the incomplete/complete questionnaires. There have been 35 incomplete questionnaires, which were eliminated due to inadequate information they included. Most abandonment happened soon after the demographics, therefore not providing valuable information about the system features; thus these incomplete responses were eliminated.

One hundred and sixty-eight completed questionnaires were received of which 43 came from the patient client group, 41 came from the PCP client group, 51 came from the health-care administrator client group, and 33 came from the health-care auditor client group. Respondents based their responses across different health-care organization and health information systems. The respondents' role and the particular care processes identified in the questionnaire ensured that responses may be generalized across the different health-care organization and health information systems that respondents represented.

Empirical Analysis

Data Reduction and Validity Check

Dependent Variables

Respondents were asked to identify their openness to more frequently using (OTU) a health-care information system because it meets their expectations of a particular system feature. All 11 system characteristics were asked separately, and factor analysis was used in Statistical Package for the Social Sciences (SPSS) version 22 for Windows to identify the "intercorrelated" observed indicators, which load under a common factor (Field 2000, p. 424). Principal component analysis (PCA) method was utilized to extract the factors and determine the interrelationships (Carr 1992; Gorsuch 1983), followed by varimax (orthogonal) rotation (Gorsuch 1983, p. 205).

Testing for multicollinearity, the Bartlett's test of sphericity was employed (χ^2 $(55)=881.13$, $p<0.001$), which indicated that PCA was adequate for the data; the correlation matrix, in fact, is not an identity matrix. The Kaiser–Myer–Olkin (KMO) measure of sampling adequacy is a high value of 0.858. This indicates that the data will factor well as the items will be able to be grouped into a smaller set of underlying factors.

Three factors were used for the dependent variables, labeled as confidentiality, usability, and portability. Their indicator variables were accountability and security, usability and portability, and portability. Table 7.1 displays the factor loadings across three indicator-dependent variables and their component loadings.

Independent Variables

Respondents were asked to identify their satisfaction with health-care system features across patient flow processes. The 44 indicators included the 11 system characteristics listed earlier across the four patient flow processes. Factor analysis and PCA were again used to determine the interrelationships.

Table 7.1 Indicator loadings of the latent dependent variables

Observed indicators		Factors			
		Confidentiality	Usability	Portability	
Accountability	OTU_Ac_Resp	0.865			
Security	OTU_S_I	0.850			
Security	OTU_S_C	0.838			
Accountability	OTU_Ac_Audit	0.831			
Usability	OTU_U_Ec		0.617		
Usability	OTU_U_Et		0.793		
Portability	OTU_P_Tr		0.670		
Usability	OTU_U_S		0.880		
Portability	OTU_P_Ic			0.784	
Portability	OTU_P_Io			0.882	
	OTU_S_A				0.876

Testing for multicollinearity, the Bartlett's test of spherity ($X2\ (351)=3021.94$, $p<0.001$) was used, which indicated that PCA was adequate for the data; the correlation matrix, in fact, is not an identity matrix. The KMO measure of sampling adequacy is a high value of 0.859. This indicates that the data will factor well as the items will be able to be grouped into a smaller set of underlying factors.

Factors with scores of >0.6 were retained in accordance with Hair et al. (2010). The reliability statistics (Cronbach's alpha) is 0.866, which indicates a high level of internal consistency for the scale and exceeds the recommended 0.7 value (DeVellis 2003; Kline 2005).

Construct validity evidence of self-reporting satisfaction with system features is supported as items loaded together measuring the same constructs, labeled as security/accountability, portability, and availability (see Table 7.2).

A scree test and eigenvalues also suggested 18 factor indicators with face validity. Seven items loaded in the first factor, labeled after the system feature, on which the conjointly loaded items suggested to measure the perceived satisfaction: *security/accountability*. The items are (1) responsibility during all four patient flow processes, (2) auditability during diagnosis/treatment and reporting processes, and (3) confidentiality during reporting. These observed variables describe the expected satisfaction with security/accountability of an existing health-care information system.

Similarly, seven items loaded on the second factor and labeled *portability* due to the communality in its factor indicators: (1) interconnectedness during all four patient flow processes and (2) interoperability during reviewing patient medical information, diagnosing and treating patients, and reporting and follow-up processes.

The third factor labeled *availability* and the following four factor indicators loaded on it: (1) data availability during reviewing patient medical history, diagnosing and treating patient, and reporting and follow-up processes and (2) efficiency during diagnosing and treating patient flow process.

Table 7.2 Indicator loadings of the latent independent variables

Observed indicators		Factors		
		Security/ accountability	Portability	Availability
Auditability	Ac_Au_S_4	0.616		
Responsibility	Ac_R_S_1	0.631		
Responsibility	Ac_R_S_4	0.653		
Auditability	Ac_Au_S_3	0.694		
Responsibility	Ac_R_S_3	0.713		
Responsibility	Ac_R_S_2	0.732		
Confidentiality	S_C_S_4	0.609		
Interconnectedness	P_Ic_S_4		0.591	
Interconnectedness	P_Ic_S_2		0.613	
Interconnectedness	P_Ic_S_3		0.617	
Interconnectedness	P_Ic_S_1		0.619	
Interoperability	P_Ic_S_3		0.624	
Interoperability	P_Ic_S_2		0.668	
Interoperability	P_Ic_S_1		0.673	
Availability	S_A_S_2			0.706
Availability	S_A_S_3			0.686
Efficiency	U_Ec_S_3			0.673
Availability	S_A_S_4			0.593

Framework

The results of the survey show that there are connections between the features and satisfaction with a system. This leads to a framework for studying what might be the relationship between satisfaction with characteristics and OTU.

The proposed framework and hypotheses with their suggested direction of effects are depicted in Fig. 7.1. The professionals to whom the survey was administered were asked to base their experiences on any existing health-care system features, not only on a particular EHR systems currently in use. EHR systems are not widely implemented, yet they are the ultimate goal of the health-care industry based on President Bush's Executive Order of 2004 (Executive Order 13335). Hence, the term "EHR system" is used to indicate any health information system.

This framework assumes that availability is positively associated with the portability system feature, and openness to use an EHR system (OTU) based on portability will increase the OTU based on usability. On the contrary, negative relationship is assumed between OTU based on portability and satisfaction with portability system feature. Similarly, negative relationship is assumed between OTU based on confidentiality and satisfaction with security/accountability. Finally, negative relationship is assumed between OTU based on usability and met expectations with confidentiality. Overall, the framework suggests that higher expectations of certain EHR characteristics will often reduce client use behavior.

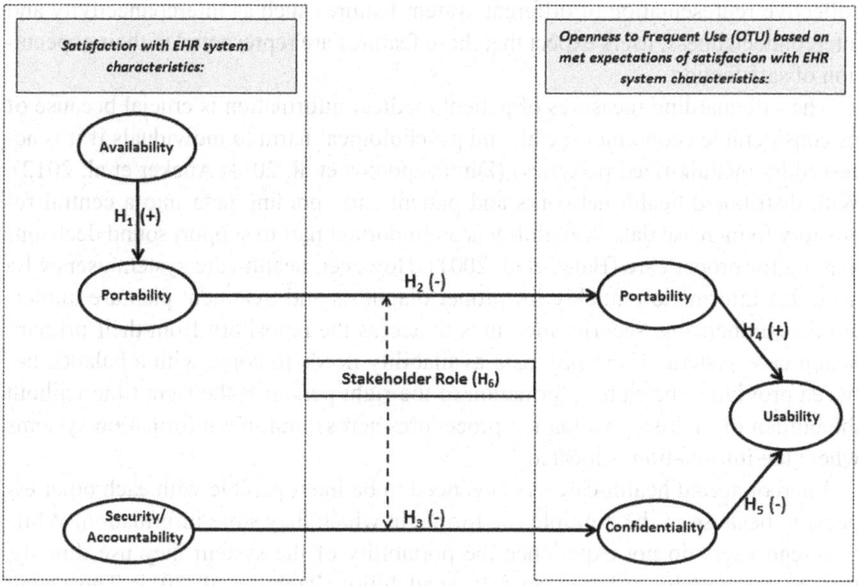

Fig. 7.1 Research framework. *EHR* electronic health record

For the independent variables, (1) availability construct is measured by data availability and efficiency, (2) portability is measured by interconnectivity and interoperability, and (3) security/accountability construct is measured by auditability, responsibility, and confidentiality system features.

For the dependent variables, (1) portability construct is measured by interconnectivity or interconnectedness; (2) usability is measured by satisfaction, effectiveness, efficiency, and transparency; and (3) confidentiality construct is measured by confidentiality, integrity, responsibility, and auditability system features.

In the next sections, the association between these constructs are investigated and their effects on client system-use behavior.

Hypotheses

The framework was tested using six hypotheses as indicated in Fig. 7.1.

Hypotheses 1 and 2 (H1 & H2)—Availability and Portability

Clients who require information shared across different systems to support their job function have expectations towards portability system characteristic. If the expectations are met, users are satisfied with data portability. Since data portability is a collective representation of different system features such as interconnectivity and interconnectedness, users expect that these features are represented to their expectation of satisfaction.

The safeguarding measures of patient medical information is crucial because of its considerable economic, social, and psychological harm to individuals if it is accessed by unauthorized party(ies) (Dimitropoulos et al. 2011; Ancker et al. 2012). With distributed health networks and patient care, pooling data into a central repository to increase data availability is an important part to support sound decision-making for proper care (Bates et al. 2001). However, health-care system users who need this information quickly for proper diagnosis and treatment plan are intolerant for cumbersome security measures to access the repository from their primary health-care system. Therefore, data availability needs to come with a balance between providing the right information to the right person at the right time without the burden of multistep validation procedures across multiple information systems where the information is located.

Interconnected health-care systems need to be interoperable with each other especially because of the multiple file format in which they store information. While front-end users do not experience the portability of the system they use directly, they assess portability based on data availability (Padhy et al. 2011; Thornewill et al. 2011).

In a health-care organization, clients need supporting information available while they may or may not be aware that the data they retrieve is pooled from internal or external repository(ies). Satisfaction with data portability is directly related to data availability since clients measure their satisfaction based on whether or not they receive the required information. Therefore, it is posited that increased satisfaction with data availability leads to increased satisfaction with data portability for clients in a health-care organization.

Hypothesis 1 Satisfaction with health records availability is positively associated with satisfaction with portability.

Dissatisfaction with a system characteristic impacts the use of the system. DeLone and McLean's widely cited work, the IS Success Model (1992), also confirms that system use is dependent on the satisfaction with the system. Therefore, if a system provides the required features to the expected satisfaction, a user group is more likely to use it. It is especially true if the user group is satisfied and the feature is important to support their job function. For example, if PCPs are concerned about not having their patient's medical records available for review, therefore dissatisfied with portability, it signals that this system characteristic is important for them, but less likely will they use a system that exhibits the portability system feature that is perceived unsatisfactory. In turn, providing a health-care system that meets the PCPs expectations of satisfaction with the portability system feature will likely result in the usage of that system. We therefore hypothesize that the decrease in satisfaction of a system feature will increase the likelihood of a system use *if that characteristic performs to the expected satisfaction* of the users, given that the feature is important to the user. Decrease in satisfaction is correlated with a level of importance, which in turn suggests openness to use if expectations of satisfaction are met (See Fig. 7.2). Therefore, we hypothesize:

				Accountability - Importance							
				Responsibility				Auditability			
				Scheduling	Reviewing	Treatment	Reporting	Scheduling	Reviewing	Treatment	Reporting
Accountability - Satisfaction	Responsibility	Scheduling	Corr.	-.321**	-.248**	-.222**	-.214**	-.263**	-.211**	-.153*	-.259**
			Sig.	.000	.001	.004	.005	.001	.006	.048	.001
		Reviewing	Corr.	-.301**	-.303**	-.201**	-.249**	-.208**	-.196*	-.182*	-.305**
			Sig.	.000	.000	.009	.001	.007	.011	.018	.000
		Treatment	Corr.	-.311**	-.217**	-.272**	-.179*	-.173*	-.147	-.179*	-.223**
			Sig.	.000	.005	.000	.020	.025	.057	.020	.004
		Reporting	Corr.	-.213**	-.122	-.186*	-0.095**	-.212**	-.201**	-.175*	-.208**
			Sig.	.006	.116	.016	.000	.006	.009	.023	.007
	Auditability	Scheduling	Corr.	-.272**	-.253**	-.232**	-.173*	-.396**	-.392**	-.224**	-.176*
			Sig.	.000	.001	.002	.025	.000	.000	.003	.022
		Reviewing	Corr.	-.200**	-.184*	-.096	-.129	-.262**	-.256**	-.261**	-.261**
			Sig.	.009	.017	.215	.095	.001	.001	.001	.001
		Treatment	Corr.	-.150	-.146	-.083	-.091	-.163*	-.159*	-.248**	-.145
			Sig.	.052	.059	.286	.242	.035	.039	.001	.061
		Reporting	Corr.	-.214**	-.140	-.110	-.116	-.211**	-.090	-.190*	-.193*
			Sig.	.005	.070	.157	.136	.006	.246	.013	.012

Fig. 7.2 Correlation sample between importance and satisfaction with a system feature

Hypothesis 2 Satisfaction with portability is negatively related to the OTU of a health record system based on met expectations of satisfaction with portability.

Hypothesis 3 (H3)—Security/Accountability and Confidentiality

Digitized patient medical records are stored and shared across departments, and patient's privacy is more prone to threats (Mercuri 2004). In this section, we establish the connection between satisfaction or dissatisfaction with security/accountability and the OTU of a health-care system if user expectations of satisfaction with confidentiality are met.

The security/accountability construct shares their indicators with OTU confidentiality; therefore, we posit that they have an effect on each other. For example, it is essential that auditors and administrators explore methods and establish policies that protect the confidentiality of patients' medical records in an accountable manner (Walker et al. 2008). In order to enforce and audit such policies, they need a support system that requires users to obey them. The importance of such features of a health-care system may be demonstrated with the lack of satisfaction, and it is shown that use of an information system is directly related to the satisfaction with it (DeLone and McLean 1992). Consecutively, to increase the OTU of a health-care information system, such as EHR, largely depends on whether or not users may expect that it will perform to their expected level of satisfaction. In regard to security and accountability, a decrease in satisfaction assumes importance, and the OTU of a health-care information system depends on whether users' expectations of satisfaction are confirmed through the confidentiality feature of the system. Hence, we hypothesize:

Hypothesis 3 Satisfaction with security/accountability is positively related to OTU of a health record system based on met expectation of satisfaction with confidentiality.

Hypothesis 4 (H4)—Portability and Usability

As we previously discussed, interconnectivity and connectedness of systems to provide the information necessary are suggested to drive the openness to use a system based on the portability system feature. The question arises: Would users consider a system usable if it meets their expectations of satisfaction with portability? While portability offers connection to other systems, a user may believe that it helps with their tasks in an efficient and effective manner. This is measured with the observed variables of portability and usability, which is tested with the hypothesis:

Hypothesis 4 OTU of a health record system based on met expectations of satisfaction with portability is positively related to OTU of a health record system based on met expectations of satisfaction with usability.

Hypothesis 5 (H5)—Confidentiality and Usability

Openness to use a system based on the expectations of satisfaction with confidentiality is measured by auditability, responsibility, confidentiality, and data integrity. These system features, however, obstruct system usability perceived by users (Yen and Bakken 2012). It might be the result that strict and compliant security measures make the system difficult to continuously use without interruption. For example, doctors criticized their health-care system's usability due to the fact that they had to swipe their security badge overly frequently or they got logged out of the system while reviewing patient information (personal interview in March 2014). This process level protection of confidentiality conforms to internal and external policies but disrupts workflow and reduces the usability of the system; therefore, we hypothesize:

Hypothesis 5 OTU of a health record system based on met expectations of satisfaction with confidentiality is negatively related to OTU of a health record system based on met expectations of satisfaction with usability.

Hypothesis 6 (H6)—Client Role as Moderator

As Dorr et al. (2007) found, EHR system designs lack multiclient support. The varying client expectations based on their work functions and objectives drive their needs differently for system features. Different processes involve clients in a different way due to their differing job functions (Ravichandran and Rai 2000; Hirschheim and Klein 1994). Therefore, we will investigate the client role as a moderator on the relationships among system characteristics and the expectations of satisfaction with system characteristics and hypothesize:

Hypothesis 6 Client role moderates the relationship between EHR system characteristics and openness to use the system.

Empirical Validation

Data from the survey were used to test each hypothesis. The constructs were measured by reflective indicators, and AMOS (Analysis of Moment Structures) software for structural equation modeling (SEM) was used to test the hypothesis. All constructs have multiple indicators as it was deduced from the survey items earlier. Layout of the model in the AMOS software is shown in Fig. 7.3.

Model Fit: We retained the unstandardized estimates as recommended for variables with unequal variance (Kline 2010) as Levene's test failed to confirm the null hypothesis that states that the groups have equal variances. Composite reliability and average variance extracted cannot be dependably computed as those values use standardized values. We take the factor loading statistical significance, chi-square values significance, and root-mean-square error of approximation (RMSEA) along with goodness-of-fit index (GFI) to ensure that the data fit our proposed model.

The RMSEA is 0.67, which is above the recommended 0.05 (Browne and Cudeck 1993) and indicates an acceptable error of approximation. The GFI is 0.853, which is above the recommended 0.8 value (Baumgartner and Hombur 1996) and also above the permissible level of 0.7 in certain model complexity and sample size combinations (Hair et al. 1998), which we agree that the sample size is not optimal ($N=168$) with the number of indicators we use in this model ($k=28$). The chi-square test yields a value of $\chi^2=686.7$ ($df=345$), $p<0.001$, which does not reject the null hypothesis of an overall good fit.

Independent Variables of the Overall Model Across All Clients

The path estimates are displayed, and the critical ratios are statistically significant ($p<0.001$) in the measurement model of the independent variables. We deduced the items to keep in the measurement model earlier in this study. Table 7.3 displays the estimate loadings of the independent variables in the measurement model.

Satisfaction with security/accountability of existing health-care systems is best indicated by responsibility during reviewing the patient medical history, and diagnosing and treating patients as their estimate loadings are 1.47 and 1.297, respectively. The highest loadings reveal that clients together expect to be satisfied with the responsibility system feature during the above processes.

Satisfaction with portability of existing health-care systems is best indicated by interoperability during the patient medical history review process and interconnect-

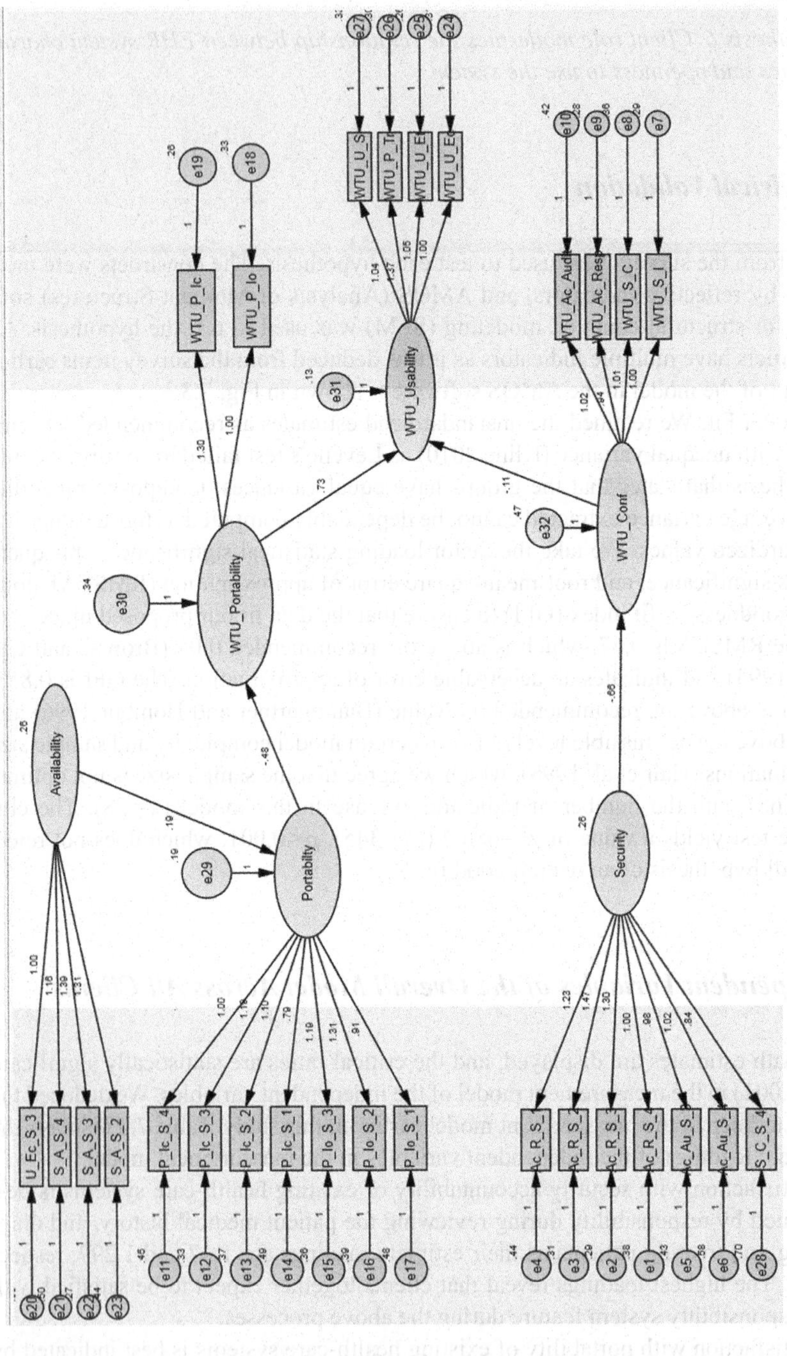

Fig. 7.3 AMOS layout for structural equation modeling (SEM) to test the hypotheses

Table 7.3 Estimate loadings of the independent variables in the measurement model

			Maximum likelihood estimates			
Constructs	Indicators	Patient flow process	Estimates	SE	CR	*p*
Security/accountability	Auditability	Diagnosing and treating patients	0.981	0.148	6.623	***
	Auditability	Reporting and follow-up	1.02	0.164	6.21	***
	Responsibility	Scheduling patient visit	1.226	0.168	7.281	***
	Responsibility	Reviewing patient medical history	1.47	0.18	8.155	***
	Responsibility	Diagnosing and treating patients	1.297	0.163	7.973	***
	Responsibility	Reporting and follow-up	1	*Fixed regression weight*		
	Confidentiality	Reporting and follow-up	0.836	0.162	5.148	***
Portability	Interconnectedness	Scheduling patient visits	0.79	0.171	4.615	***
	Interconnectedness	Reviewing patient medical history	1.102	0.189	5.846	***
	Interconnectedness	Diagnosing and treating patients	1.192	0.195	6.114	***
	Interconnectedness	Reporting and follow-up	1	*Fixed regression weight*		
	Interoperability	Scheduling patient visits	0.906	0.18	5.023	***
	Interoperability	Reviewing patient medical history	1.31	0.213	6.14	***
	Interoperability	Diagnosing and treating patients	1.195	0.198	6.022	***
Availability	Data availability	Reviewing patient medical history	1.306	0.226	5.776	***
	Data availability	Diagnosing and treating patients	1.385	0.233	5.942	***
	Data availability	Reporting and follow-up	1.162	0.211	5.514	***
	Efficiency	Diagnosing and treating patients	1	*Fixed regression weight*		

SE standard error
CR critical ratio

edness during diagnosing and treating patient. This indicates that clients find the portability system feature most important during the medical history review process and diagnosing and treating patients in regard to system portability. The dependence of data availability is clearly explained by the fact that relevant medical information during diagnosis and treatment is inevitable through interconnected systems, and clients expect more in regard to this system feature.

Satisfaction with availability of existing health-care systems is best indicated by data availability during diagnosis and treatment and reviewing patient medical history. It is in line with the expectations of "the right information at the right time for the right person," as indicated by the other two constructs' factor loadings. Clients collectively expect that a system has data available during the review of the patient medical history and diagnosis and treatment, but they are not satisfied with the current feature in existing information systems.

Measurement Model Loadings of the Dependent Variables Across All Clients

The path estimates are displayed, and the critical ratios are statistically significant ($p<0.001$) in the measurement model of the dependent variables. We deduced the items to keep in the measurement model in the first part of this study. Table 7.4 displays the estimate loadings of the dependent variables in the measurement model.

OTU based on expectation of satisfaction with usability of EHR systems is best indicated by satisfaction and transparency; their estimate loadings are 1.47 and 1.226, respectively. These indicators properly represent the clients' expectation of satisfaction with these features as they are open to frequently use a system if it is built to their satisfaction and the externally connected databases seamlessly provide

Table 7.4 Estimate loadings of the dependent variables in the measurement model

		Maximum likelihood estimates			
Constructs	Indicators	Estimates	SE	CR	*p*
OTU_Usability	Efficiency	1	*Fixed regression weight*		
	Effectiveness	1.02	0.164	6.21	***
	Transparency	1.226	0.168	7.281	***
	Satisfaction	1.47	0.18	8.155	***
OTU_Confidentiality	Confidentiality	1.005	0.092	10.945	***
	Integrity	1	*Fixed regression weight*		
	Responsibility	0.941	0.084	11.242	***
	Auditability	1.02	0.096	10.641	***
OTU_Portability	Interoperability	1	*Fixed regression weight*		
	Interconnectedness	1.304	0.153	8.532	***

SE standard error
CR critical ratio

access to data. It is aligned with the expectations of satisfaction with data availability as well.

OTU based on expectation of satisfaction with confidentiality of EHR systems is best indicated by auditability and confidentiality with estimate loadings of 1.02 and 1.005, respectively. Clients are expected to be satisfied with a system that exhibits a higher level of auditability and confidentiality.

OTU based on expectation of satisfaction with portability of EHR systems is best indicated by interconnectedness. Clients are expected to be satisfied with a system that is connected to other databases. Respondents indicated a lack of satisfaction with this system feature.

Structural Model Estimate Loadings of the Latent (Unobserved) Variables

All path estimates of the latent variables loaded statistically significantly ($p<0.001$, except $p<0.05$ for availability to portability). The associations of the latent variables are indicated through the estimates direction and magnitude. The corresponding hypotheses are reviewed whether or not the loadings support them. Table 7.5 provides a summary of the estimate loadings and the hypotheses confirmation.

Hypothesis 1 Satisfaction with availability is positively associated with satisfaction with portability.

Satisfaction with availability of existing health-care systems is an important tenet across clients. Patients want their medical records available when calling to schedule, so no delay is necessary while the provider's office collects the latest medical records from other providers. Furthermore, it can be cost saving as well, as redundant tests will not be necessary if a recent result is sufficient. Providers need data availability while reviewing the patient medical history and diagnosing. Administrators and auditors need data availability especially for reporting and auditing purposes.

Data availability itself is important, but it is expected to be portable as well, else the availability is limited. The path loading of 0.186 across all clients supports the hypothesis and can be generalized that satisfaction with availability of EHR

Table 7.5 Estimate loadings of the dependent variables in the structural model

			Maximum Likelihood Estimates			
Construct ➡	**Construct**	**Hypothesis --> supported?**	**Estimates**	**S.E.**	**C.R.**	**P**
Availability ➡	**Portability**	*H1 --> YES*	0.186	0.091	2.052	0.04
Portability ➡	**OTU_Portability**	*H2 --> YES*	-0.481	0.145	-3.32	***
Security / Accountability ➡	**OTU_Confidentia**	*H3 --> YES*	-0.662	0.144	-4.59	***
OTU_Portability ➡	**OTU_Usability**	*H4 --> YES*	0.73	0.104	7.056	***
OTU_Confidentiality ➡	**OTU_Usability**	*H5 --> YES*	-0.114	0.092	10.945	***

SE standard error

systems is positively associated with satisfaction with portability of EHR systems. Clients collectively find that satisfaction with the availability system feature leads to satisfaction with the portability system feature. It is an especially important finding in the domain of health information systems, where multiple data sources are expected to supply the information to the right person at the right time. The findings indicate that users who have access to the information when needed consider the system portable.

Hypothesis 2 Satisfaction *with portability is negatively related to the OTU of a health record system based on met expectations of satisfaction with portability.*

Portability is a construct that is measuring the satisfaction with interconnectedness and interoperability. As previously deduced, all clients have a great interest in access to information from outside of the main system, especially if patient records are needed from other providers/systems.

The importance-satisfaction correlation matrix indicated predominantly negative correlations between importance and satisfaction. Openness to use a health-care system if portability meets users' expectation is reflected by importance. Therefore, the negative correlation between satisfaction with portability and the openness to use a system if portability meets users' expectation is reflected with a negative association between the two constructs. The −0.481 factor loading confirms this negative association, and we can conclude that clients collectively find a system more appealing if a feature, with which they are currently dissatisfied, is designed to support their needs. Based on the results, it can be concluded that expectations of satisfaction with the portability system feature is negatively correlated with OTU of a system based on met expectations of satisfaction with the portability system characteristic. A less satisfied client with the portability system feature is more likely to choose to use a system if this portability meets his/her expectations of satisfaction.

Hypothesis 3 Satisfaction with security/accountability is positively related to OTU of a health record system based on met expectation of satisfaction with confidentiality.

Satisfaction with security and accountability reflects users' perceptions of existing system's capabilities in regard to auditability, responsibility, and confidentiality. These system level features represent the protection of privacy of a patient and the accountable retrieval and modification of such sensitive information. Patients are concerned that their medical information might be accessed by unauthorized parties, while doctors are held accountable for their actions with patient's information. Audit trails include detailed information about the access of patient information, and administrators ensure that proper role-based security access is in place. Auditors want to have available access logs and other audit trail information, on which they can run reports to ensure that proper security is in place in an accountable manner.

Openness to use a health-care information system based on met expectations of satisfaction with confidentiality has very similar indicators to security/accountability. Therefore, we can assume that clients, who are dissatisfied with the security/

accountability system feature, will likely be willing to use a system if it meets their expectations of confidentiality.

The negative relationship between satisfaction with security/accountability of an EHR system and the openness to use a health-care system based on met expectations of satisfaction with confidentiality, if this system characteristic meets user expectation, confirms our second hypothesis. The results indicate that confidentiality is an important system characteristic for users and more likely to use a health record system if their expectation of satisfaction with confidentiality is met. A less-satisfied client with security/accountability system feature is more likely to choose to use a system if this confidentiality meets his/her expectations of satisfaction.

Hypothesis 4 OTU of a health record system based on met expectations of satisfaction with portability is positively related to OTU of a health record system based on met expectations of satisfaction with usability.

Portability of a system also reflects its ability to retrieve information from outside systems. When information about a patient is urgently needed, quick access to such data could avoid delay in providing proper treatment and consequently save the patient's life. Therefore, it is not surprising that clients collectively deem a system usable if portability meets their expectations of satisfaction. The factor estimate of 0.73 reflects this positive association and confirms our fourth hypothesis. Increase in met expectations with portability of a health record system will drive users more likely to use a system if their expectations of satisfaction with system usability is met.

Hypothesis 5 OTU of a health record system based on met expectations of satisfaction with confidentiality is negatively related to OTU of a health record system based on met expectations of satisfaction with usability.

Protecting sensitive information requires proper security measures within an information system. Besides the back-end security, the front end or user side is also affected. When a system requires multiple log-ins and reconfirming of authority by re-swiping the access card or reentering the password every 30 s, it may increase security but reduce user positive experience with such a system.

Therefore, we hypothesized that increased expectations of satisfaction with confidentiality reduced the openness to use a health-care system based on expectations of satisfaction with usability. The negative factor loading of −0.114 lends support to this hypothesis and establishes the inverse relation between these two variables. The proper security measures will meet clients' expectations with confidentiality, but it will result in a decrease of the usability of a health record system.

Hypothesis 6 Client role moderates the relationship between EHR system characteristics and openness to use the system.

While the full model considered the clients collectively, we hypothesized that client roles moderate the relationship between satisfaction with EHR system features and openness to use the system. We argue that there is a difference between system features across processes based on the role the clients represent.

While the full model was examined for all previous hypotheses, we will break down the model into sections to test each hypothesis separately and investigate whether the client role changes the factor loadings and the direction and magnitude of loading estimates between the latent variables. Another reason for breaking down the model is the limited sample size we have for each client group.

Even though the reduced models had smaller sample size, they exhibited better GFI than the overall model; most of them had GFI>0.9 and RMSEA<0.7. All reduced models had the statistically significant chi-square test ($p<0.001$).

The hypothesis only called for client role moderation between system features and the OTU based on the expectation of satisfaction with the same feature, but we will investigate whether the client role moderates the other latent variable relationships as well.

Client Role as Moderator (H6) for Hypothesis 1

The overall model exhibited proper fit (GFI>0.9), and the estimates were statistically significant ($p<0.001$). Satisfaction with the health records availability of is positively associated with the satisfaction with the portability of existing health-care systems, which is confirmed with a factor loading of 0.22. Table 7.6 displays the highest factor loadings (highlighted) for all clients collectively and for each client separately.

The highest factor loading for satisfaction with availability of existing health-care systems has a variation across client groups. While patients and administrators exhibit interconnectedness during diagnosing and treating patient processes as the most important indicator, PCPs find interoperability during reviewing the patient medical history to be the best indicator of satisfaction with the portability of an existing health-care system. This indicator is also the best across all client groups. Auditors find interconnectedness to be the best indicator during the same process.

While there is a degree of variation in regard to highest estimates across client groups, the direction of path coefficients stayed the same, therefore, indicating positive association between satisfaction with the availability of existing health-care systems and satisfaction with the portability of existing health-care systems.

Table 7.6 Moderation effect of client role on the relationship between portability and availability

H1 - Satisfaction with availability is positively associated with satisfaction with portability.			All Client Groups	Patients	PCP's	Admins	Auditors
Constructs	**Indicators**	**Patient Flow Process**	**Estimates**				
Portability	Interconnectedness	Scheduling patient visit	0.67	0.22	0.35	0.62	0.65
	Interconnectedness	Reviewing patient medical history	0.94	0.84	0.24	0.91	1.61
	Interconnectedness	Diagnosing and treating patient	1.03	0.96	0.38	1.64	1.55
	Interconnectedness	Reporting and follow-up	0.87	0.83	0.39	0.99	0.54
	Interoperability	Scheduling patient visit	0.77	0.46	0.73	0.79	0.72
	Interoperability	Reviewing patient medical history	1.09	0.94	1.44	0.85	1.15
	Interoperability	Diagnosing and treating patient	1	1	1	1	1
Availability	Data Availability	Reviewing patient medical history	1.31	2.54	1.45	1.22	1.27
	Data Availability	Diagnosing and treating patient	1.38	2.93	1.34	1.68	0.62
	Data Availability	Reporting and follow-up	1.16	2.02	1.24	1.37	1.23
	Efficiency	Diagnosing and treating patient	1	1	1	1	1
Availability --> Portability			0.22	1.59	0.06	0.29	0.41

PCP primary-care provider

Patients exhibited the strongest path coefficient and PCPs the weakest. This signals that patients feel better cared for if all of their medical history is accessible and available at the time of their care, while PCPs seem not to associate data availability with system portability that closely. They seem to trust the internally available data and not rely on external accessibility.

It could be grounds of further investigation why PCPs do not correlate data availability with connectivity with other systems.

Client Role as Moderator (H6) for Hypothesis 2

The factor loadings of satisfaction with portability of existing health-care systems slightly vary across client groups. PCPs responses indicated that the best indicator of satisfaction with portability is interoperability during reviewing patient medical records, which is the same as the best indicator of all clients' responses collectively. PCPs need access to patient information while reviewing patient medical records. Table 7.7 displays the highest factor loadings (highlighted) for all clients collectively and for each client separately.

Patients' and administrators' responses imply interconnectedness during diagnosis and treatment the strongest indicator for satisfaction with portability. They want to ensure that the diagnosis and treatment are based on all available information to limit the possibility for improper diagnosis and treatment due to lack of information. Auditors' responses indicate that interconnectedness during reviewing a patient medical history is the best indicator for satisfaction with portability.

The negative correlation between satisfaction with availability of existing health-care systems and OTU based on expectation of satisfaction with portability is confirmed across all clients. Auditors have the strongest negative path coefficient, which may indicate that their dissatisfaction with portability of an existing health-care system has the greatest effect on their openness to use a system (such as EHR)if portability satisfies their needs. It can further be concluded that the importance of the portability system feature is rated the highest among auditor client groups. We argue that it is due to reporting reasons since auditors want to ensure that they have access to all auditable information across all systems within their practice.

Table 7.7 Moderation effect of client role on the relationship between portability and OTU_portability

H2 - Decrease in satisfaction with portability will increase the likelihood of the openness to frequent use (OTU) of an EHR system based on met expectations of satisfaction with portability.			**All Client Groups**	**Patients**	**PCP's**	**Admins**	**Auditors**
Constructs	**Indicators**	**Patient Flow Process**	**Estimates**				
Portability	Interconnectedness	Scheduling patient visit	0.68	0.29	0.32	0.6	1.07
	Interconnectedness	Reviewing patient medical history	0.92	0.78	0.2	0.94	1.95
	Interconnectedness	Diagnosing and treating patient	0.99	0.92	0.36	1.06	1.54
	Interconnectedness	Reporting and follow-up	0.84	0.82	0.35	1	0.71
	Interoperability	Scheduling patient visit	0.78	0.41	0.74	0.75	1.02
	Interoperability	Reviewing patient medical history	1.11	0.88	1.54	0.84	1.41
	Interoperability	Diagnosing and treating patient	1	1	1	1	1
OTU_Portability	Interconnectedness		1	1	1	1	1
	Interoperability		0.87	0.72	0.2	1.08	1.53
Portability --> OTU_Portability			-0.54	-0.09	-0.54	-0.58	-1.31

PCP primary-care provider, *EHR* electronic health record

The lowest loadings for patients (path coefficient of −0.09) may be due to the fact that patients did not rate portability of high importance. Therefore, their level of dissatisfaction is not significant, and they are not indicating that they are more open to use a system if their expectation of satisfaction with portability meets their expectations.

Client Role as Moderator (H6) for Hypothesis 3

Patients' and auditors' responses reveal that auditability during diagnosis and treating patients is the strongest indicator for satisfaction with security/accountability of an existing health-care system. They both want to ensure that it can be traced back who accessed or updated patient records, and auditability system feature ensures this.

PCPs and administrators share the concern that patient records are laying around and that computer screens are left open on hallways where other employees and patients walk through. Their responses indicate that the best indicator for satisfaction with security/accountability of an existing health-care system is responsibility during reviewing patient medical records and diagnosing/treating patients.

The hypothesized negative association between satisfaction with security/accountability of existing health-care systems and the OTU based on expectation of satisfaction with confidentiality of existing health-care system, if security/accountability meets users' expectations, is confirmed across all clients. The strongest negative path coefficient is represented by administrators; they indicate that they would very likely be open to use a system if it meets their need of security/accountability. It can be concluded that they are not satisfied with security/accountability in their current system and they deem this system characteristic very important. Therefore, administrators are looking for this feature in a health-care system (such as EHR) in order for them to use it.

On the other hand, the lowest level of coefficient among PCPs seems to indicate that they rated this feature as not important (importance rating $\overline{x}$ for PCPs = 2.9 vs. administrators' $\overline{x} = 4.3$); therefore, they are not likely to be open to using a health-care system that exhibits this system characteristic. Table 7.8 displays the highest factor loadings (highlighted) for all clients collectively and for each client separately.

Client Role as Moderator (H6) for Hypothesis 4

System usability has different perceptions across user groups (Jiang et al. 2002) and even within user groups, as managers seem to be less concerned about this system characteristic (Morris and Dillon 1996). In a health-care information system, openness to use based on expectations of satisfaction with usability is best indicated by transparency according to responses by all client groups but patients. It allows us to argue that while clients in the health-care organization have to access multiple in-

Table 7.8 Moderation effect of client role on the relationship between security/accountability and OTU_confidentiality

H3 - Decrease in satisfaction with security/accountability will increase the likelihood of the OTU of an EHR system based on met expectation of satisfaction with confidentiality.			All Client Groups	Patients	PCP's	Admins	Auditors
Constructs	**Indicators**	**Patient Flow Process**	**Estimates**				
Security / Accountability	Responsibility	Scheduling patient visit	1.5	1.26	1.04	5.61	1
	Responsibility	Reviewing patient medical history	1.81	1.83	2.12	6.42	0.87
	Responsibility	Diagnosing and treating patient	1.62	1.48	2.87	6.27	6.4
	Responsibility	Reporting and follow-up	1.23	1.05	2.62	3.87	4.65
	Auditability	Diagnosing and treating patient	1.23	1.91	0.91	3.74	4.95
	Auditability	Reporting and follow-up	1.25	1.23	0.55	3.79	3.41
	Confidentiality	Reporting and follow-up	1	1	1	1	1
OTU_Confidentilaity	Confidentiality		1	1	1	1	1
	Integrity		1.06	0.93	5.57	1.25	0.67
	Responsibility		1.05	1.03	2.52	0.94	0.9
	Auditability		0.26	0.97	3.92	1.26	1.2
Security / Accountability --> OTU_Confidentiality			-0.46	-0.06	-0.03	-1.58	-0.13

PCP primary-care provider, *EHR* electronic health record, *OTU* openness to frequent use

formation systems with possibly different software and log-on credentials, patients usually access their portal, and they are not facing the inconvenience of multiple log-on requests across systems. Patients' responses indicated satisfaction as the best indicator for openness to use a system based on expectations of satisfaction with usability, which probably translates to the granularity of information they are able to access and the extent to which they are able to use the system to manage their care. It is important to realize that patients use a very different depth and breadth (even though they should have access to all their medical records (Annas 2003), it remains to the discretion of a health-care provider (Reti et al. 2010))of information and the extent they can use the system is much more limited than that of users within the health-care organization. Table 7.9 displays the highest factor loadings (highlighted) for all clients collectively and for each client separately.

Administrators' path coefficient is the strongest (0.71), which suggests that if they are open to use a health-care information system based on their expectations of satisfaction with portability, they are more likely to be open to use the system based on their expectation of satisfaction with usability. In short, portability system characteristic is an indicator of usability for administrators, as they will be able to ensure that the other clients get their work done effectively and efficiently and reducing the error rate if they have access to external systems.

Conversely, PCPs openness to use a health-care information system based on satisfaction with portability is lesser of an indicator whether they are open to use a system if it meets their expectations of usability.

Client Role as Moderator (H6) for Hypothesis 5

The strongest indicator of openness to use a health-care information system based on expectations of satisfactions with confidentiality seems to be responsibility for all client groups except for auditors, whose answers suggest that the best indicator is confidentiality. It suggests that most client groups find it important that users of an information system are ensured that a dedicated process owner is in place to ensure proper policies are in place.

Table 7.9 Moderation effect of client role on the relationship between OTU_portability and OTU_usability

H4 - Increase in OTU of an EHR system based on met expectations of satisfaction with portability will increase the likelihood of OTU of an EHR system based on met expectations of satisfaction with usability.		All Client Groups	Patients	PCP's	Admins	Auditors
Constructs	**Indicators**	**Estimates**				
OTU_Portability	Interconnectedness	1	1	1	1	1
	Interoperability	0.72	4.69	0.28	0.71	0.74
OTU_Usability	Efficiency	1	1	1	1	1
	Effectiveness	1.06	0.87	1.84	1.22	0.69
	Satisfaction	1.04	2.01	0.59	0.9	0.89
	Transparency	1.37	1.43	2.63	1.22	1.2
OTU_Portability --> OTU_Usability		0.56	0.66	0.05	0.71	0.64

PCP primary-care provider, *EHR* electronic health record, *OTU* openness to frequent use

Somewhat surprising that the auditors' responses did not result in responsibility being the strongest indicator for OTU based on expectations of satisfaction with confidentiality. The strongest indicator is confidentiality, which may be because auditability's path coefficient has been fixed during model validation and it might have been the actual strongest indicator.

The strongest indicators of openness to use a system based on expectations of satisfaction with usability seems to be different for almost all client groups. Patients reveal that satisfaction is the best indicator of whether they are open to use a system. It is understandable as patients most likely will only use limited functionalities, and they want to have an easy-to-understand user interface. PCPs' answers suggest that effectiveness is the strongest indicator, which can be explained by the fact that they have limited time with the patient and they want an effective user interface that captures the relevant information properly. Administrators and auditors' answers indicate that transparency is the strongest indicator whether they are open to use a system based on expectations of satisfaction with usability. Since these two client groups are running reports, they want to have relatively simple access to information across multiple systems without constant log-ins and credibility checks.

The path coefficients reveal an interesting, yet expected, difference in the direction among client groups. While patients and PCPs indicated that they are less likely to find a system usable if it is satisfying their requirements of confidentiality, administrators and auditors expressed the contrary by indicating that they are only considering a system usable if it satisfies the expectations of confidentiality. This can be understood by knowing that while patients and PCPs understand the importance of confidentiality, they do not feel that it is positively correlated with usability as it may hinder them from achieving their goals of using the system effectively and to their satisfactions. On the other hand, administrators and auditors, who are the gatekeepers of policies and ensuring proper handling of sensitive medical information, indicate that they are only open to use a system based on usability if it is also satisfying their expectations of confidentiality. In short, it is important to have the confidentiality system characteristic in place in order to find a system usable. Table 7.10 displays the highest factor loadings (highlighted) for all clients collectively and for each client separately.

Table 7.10 Moderation effect of client role on the relationship between OTU_confidentiality and OTU_usability

H5 - Increase in OTU of an EHR system based on met expectations of satisfaction with confidentiality will decrease the likelihood of OTU of an EHR system based on met expectations of satisfaction with usability.		All Client Groups	Patients	PCP's	Admins	Auditors
Constructs	**Indicators**	**Estimates**				
OTU_Confidentilaity	Confidentiality	0.92	1.74	0.91	0.4	0.95
	Integrity	0.98	0.66	0.78	0.81	0.27
	Responsibility	1	1.8	0.93	0.93	0.28
	Auditability	1	1	1	1	1
OTU_Usability	Efficiency	1	1	1	1	1
	Effectiveness	1.06	0.86	6.81	1.25	0.67
	Satisfaction	1.06	1.08	2.36	0.94	0.9
	Transparency	1.3	0.87	3.67	1.27	1.23
OTU_Confidentiality --> OTU_Usability		-0.2	-0.04	-0.61	0.54	0.95

PCP primary-care provider, *EHR* electronic health record, *OTU* openness to frequent use

Discussion and Implications

The American health industry is lacking the technological support for information management that other industries have been utilizing and improving upon. Literature supports that EHR systems offer the capacity and promise to improved healthcare delivery across the episodes of patient care (e.g., Greenhalgh et al. 2010; Blumenthal and Tavenner 2010). However, the use of an EHR system in a multiclient environment, such as the hospitals and outpatient care providers, is often hindered by the fact that different client groups with varying client objectives use the same system. Understanding the software attributes and their effect on client system use behavior is an important tenet that needs to be understood for proper system design and selection. This will ensure that users of an EHR system will be satisfied with the characteristic that is perceived the most important for their job functions, and they will use the system. System use is the measure of EHR implementation success (e.g., Devaraj and Kohli 2003).

In this chapter, the relationships between satisfaction with system characteristics and their effect on OTU of the health record systems were investigated. EHR system users were surveyed on their satisfaction with current system characteristics and their OTU of an EHR system if their expectations were met. Respondents from outpatient care providers across the USA responded, and structural equation modeling was used to test the hypotheses. Figure 7.4 indicates the results, which is discussed below.

The empirical validation revealed several important EHR client use behaviors. First, the negative relationships between satisfaction with portability and OTU based on met expectations with portability system characteristics (H2). This confirms that clients who do not find portability system characteristics satisfactory are more likely to use an EHR system if this characteristic meets their expectations of satisfaction (H4). Client role as moderator was used to understand which client group has the strongest need for a particular system characteristic. The findings revealed that auditors are the least satisfied with system portability, while administrators are more likely to use an EHR system if portability meets their expectations of satisfaction.

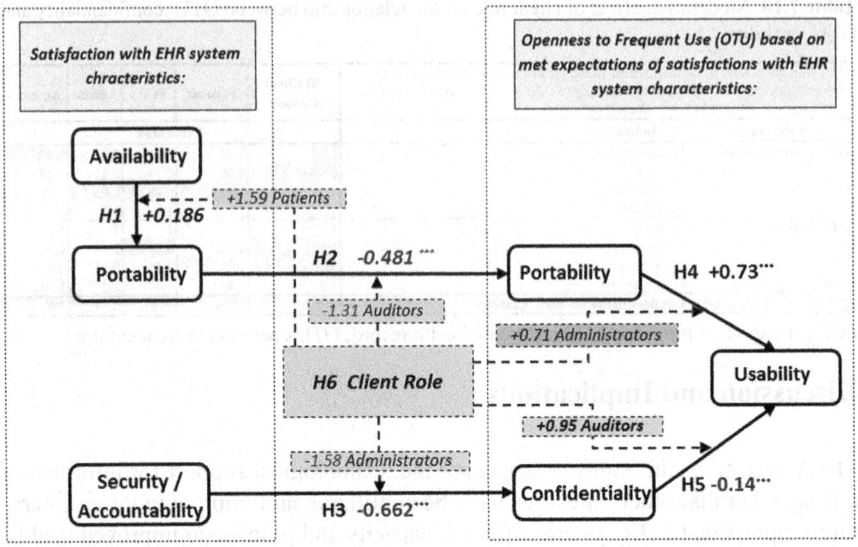

Fig. 7.4 Research framework with estimate loadings and client role moderating effect on the relationships. *EHR* electronic health record

Similarly, another interesting client use behavior was exposed through testing H3. Users that are unsatisfied with security/accountability of and EHR system are more likely open to frequent use of the system if the confidentiality EHR system characteristic meets their expectations of satisfaction. This negative relationship is present in all client groups but is the strongest in the administrators client group, which confirms their EHR system characteristic preference for their job function.

The surprising negative relationship between confidentiality and usability (H5) shows that an EHR with more confidentiality is perceived as less usable by all clients collectively. However, if client role is considered as a moderator, auditors and administrators perceive the system more usable if confidentiality meets their expectations. On the other hand, PCPs and patients find an EHR system less usable, the more confidentially meets their expectations of satisfaction. The findings suggest that higher expectations of EHR characteristics can often reduce client use behavior. Furthermore, our discoveries highlight that aspects of portability, security/accountability, and confidentiality serve as a double-edged sword and suggest a fine balance in crafting operational and regulatory policies for effective use of EHR systems across clients.

These findings support the fact that clients of an EHR system understand the importance and demand the regulatory drives of the safeguarding measures of patient health information (Wiljer et al. 2008). However, certain client groups find an EHR system less usable, and they would less likely continue to use an EHR system when these regulatory policies are implemented in a way that hinders clients to perform their job duties. Customizable user interface and client group specific training and manuals would likely lessen the perceived usability issues, which may negatively impact client intention of continued use of an EHR system.

The framework presented in this chapter provides a very clear understanding of the importance of an EHR system feature and its effect on the OTU based on the expectations of satisfaction of this system feature. Understanding the implication of dissatisfaction with an EHR system feature may prevent failed implementations and increase the plummeting EHR use.

Providing EHR system features to the users in a form that they will find that they meet their expectations of satisfactions will reduce the numerous workarounds they may maintain. It not only increases efficiency and effectiveness but also will reduce the risk of privacy and compliance breaches for capturing patient information outside of the secure EHR system.

Limitations and Future Directions

This study is limited in scope and not free of shortcomings. These limitations may provide directions for future research within and beyond the domain of this research.

We have collected information through a questionnaire from a decent sample population representing each client group. However, due to the large number of variables we observed, exploratory factor analysis may have experienced "underfactoring," where large enough discrepancies between the model and data may not be significant (Humphreys and Montanelli 1975). Consequently, the model fit in confirmatory factor analysis (CFA) had to follow a more relaxed cut-off value than the literature-suggested limit. Future studies may want to consider smaller number of variables or increase the sample population.

Similarly, we ran the CFA on a simplified model to test the hypotheses on the client level due to decreased sample size once we used client role as a grouping variable. It would be preferable to run the model in its entirety while observing estimates on the region level. We were, however, able to observe the expectations across client groups within a hypothesis in regard to what indicator variable turned out to be the strongest and also the variation on path coefficient intensities.

We were unable to utilize the collected information on regions, which might have provided further direction on expectations from clients based on what region they operate. It is an interesting objective to test whether regional regulations influence clients' expectations from an EHR system characteristic. It can be the focus of a future research itself. Additionally, due to the same reason, we were unable to capitalize on the health-care institution type that we also collected.

As we investigated the moderating effect of client role, some path coefficients revealed surprising magnitude. It would be worthwhile to investigate the underlying reason behind it, whether it is correlated to regions of the institute type from where data were collected.

References

Aarts, J., & Peel, V. (1999). Using a descriptive model of change when implementing large scale clinical information systems to identify priorities for further research. *International Journal of Medical Informatics, 56*(1–3), 43–50.

Ahn, J., & Skudlark, A. (1997). Resolving conflict of interests in the process of an information system implementation for advanced telecommunication services. *Journal of Information Technology 12,* 3–13.

Annas, G. J. (2003). HIPAA regulations – a new era of medical-record privacy? *New England Journal of Medicine, 348*(15), 1486–90.

Ancker, J. S., Edwards, A. M., & Miller, M. C. (2012). Consumer perceptions of electronic health information exchange. *American Journal of Preventive Medicine, 43*, 76–80.

Bates, D. W., Cohen, M., Leape, L. L., Overhage, J. M., Shabot, M. S., & Sheridan, T. (2001). Reducing the frequency of errors in medicine using information technology. *Journal of the American Medical Informatics Association, 8*(4), 299–308.

Baumgartner, H., & Hombur, C. (1996). Applications of structural equation modeling in marketing and consumer research: A review. *International Journal of Research in Marketing, 13*, 139–161.

Bhattacherjee, A. (2001). Understanding information systems continuance: An expectation-confirmation model. *MIS Quarterly, 25*(3), 351–370.

Blumenthal, D., & Tavenner, M. (2010). "The Meaningful Use" regulation for electronic health records. *New England Journal of Medicine, 363*(6), 501–504.

Browne, M. W., & Cudeck, R. (1993). Alternative ways of assessing model fit. In K. A. Bollen & J. S. Long. (Eds.), *Testing structural equation models* (pp. 136–162). Beverly Hills: Sage.

Carr, S. C. (1992). A primer on the use of Q sort technique factor analysis. *Measurement and Evaluation in Counseling and Development, 25*, 133–138.

DeLone, W. H., & McLean, E. R. (1992). Information systems success: The quest for the dependent variable. *Information Systems Research, 3*(1), 60–95.

Devaraj, S., & Kohli, R. (2003). Performance impacts of information technology: Is actual usage the missing Link? *Management Science, 49*, 273–289.

DeVellis, R. F. (2003). *Scale development: Theory and applications* (2nd ed). Thousand Oaks: Sage.

Dimitropoulos, L., Patel, V., & Scheffler, S. A. (2011). Public attitudes toward health information exchange: Perceived benefits and concerns. *The American Journal of Managed Care, 17*, 111–116.

Dorr, D., Bonner, L. M., Cohen, A. N., Shoai, R. S., Perrin, R., Chaney, E., & Young, A. S. (2007). Informatics systems to promote improved care for chronic illness: A literature review. *Journal of the American Medical Informatics Association: JAMIA, 14*(2), 156–163.

Field, A. (2000). *Discovering statistics using SPSS for Windows*. London: Thousand Oaks. (New Delhi: Sage publications).

Goddard, B. L. (2000). Termination of a contract to implement an enterprise electronic medical record system. *Journal of the American Medical Informatics Association, 7*, 564–568.

Gorsuch, R. L. (1983). *Factor analysis* (2nd ed). Hillsdale: Lawrence Earlbaum Associates.

Greenhalgh, T., & Russell, J. (2010). Why do evaluations of eHealth programs fail? An alternative set of guiding principles. *PLoS Medicine, 7*(11), e1000360. doi:10.1371/journal.pmed.1000360.

Greenhalgh, T., Hinder, S., Stramer, K. et al. (2010). Adoption, non-adoption, and abandonment of a personal electronic health record: Case study of Health Space. *British Medical Journal, 341,* 10.1136/bmj.c5814

Hair, J. F. Jr., Anderson, R. E., Tatham, R. L., & Black, W. C. (1998). *Multivariate data analysis* (5th ed). Upper Saddle River: Prentice Hall.

Hair, J., Black, W. C., Babin, B. J., & Anderson, R. E. (2010). *Multivariate data analysis* (7th ed). Upper saddle River: Pearson Education International.

Handy, J., Hunter, I., & Whiddett, R. (2001). User acceptance of inter-organizational electronic medical records. *Health Informatics Journal, 7*(2), 103–107.

Hirschheim, R., & Klein, H. (1994). Realizing emancipatory principles in information systems development: The case for ETHICS. *MIS Quarterly, 18*(1), 83–109.

Humphreys, L. G., & Montanelli, R. G. Jr. (1975). An investigation of the parallel analysis criterion for determining the number of common factors. *Multivariate Behavioral Research, 10*(2), 193–205.

Jiang, J., Klein, G., & Carr, C. (2002). Measuring information systems service quality: SERVQUAL from the other side. *MIS Quarterly, 26*(2), 145–166.

Joss, R., & Kogan, M. (1995). *Advancing quality: Total quality management in the National Health Service*. Buckingham: Open University Press.

Kazley, A., & Ozcan, Y. (2007). Organizational and environmental determinants of hospital EMR adoption: A national study. *Journal of Medical Systems, 31*(5), 375–384.

Kline, R. B. (2005). *Principles and practice of structural equation modeling* (2nd ed). New York: Guilford.

Kline, R. B. (2010). *Principles and practice of structural equation modeling* (3rd ed). New York: Guilford.

Mercuri, R. T. (2004). The HIPAA-potamus in health care data security. *Communications of the ACM, 47*(7), 25–28.

McGlynn, E. A. (1997). Six challenges in measuring the quality of health care. *Health Affairs, 16*, 7–21.

McGowan, J. J., Cusack, C. M., & Poon, E. G. (2008). Formative evaluation: A critical component in EHR implementation. *Journal of American Medical Association, 15*(3), 297–301.

Morris, M. & Dillon, A. (1996). The role of usability in the organizational standards setting process. *International Journal of Human-Computer Studies, 45*(2), 243–258.

Oz, E., & Sosik, J. J. (2000). Why information systems are abandoned: A leadership and communication theory and exploratory study. *Journal of Computer Information Systems, 41*(1), 66–78.

Padhy, R. P., Patry, M. R., & Satapathy, S. C. (2011). Cloud computing: Security issues and research challenges IRACST. *International Journal of Computer Science and Information Technology & Security (IJCSITS), 1*(2), 136–146.

Pan, G. S. C. (2005). Information system project abandonment: A stakeholder analysis. *International Journal of Information Management, 25,* 174.

Ramanujam, R., & Rousseau, D. M. (2006). The challenges are organizational not just clinical. *Journal of Organizational Behavior, 27*(7), 811–827.

Ravichandran, T., & Rai, A. (2000). Quality management in systems development: An organizational system perspective. *MIS Quarterly, 24*(3), 381–415.

Reti, S., Feldman, H., Ross, S., & Safran, C. (2010). Improving personal health records for patient-centered care. *Journal of the American Medical Informatics Association, 17*(2), 192–195.

Sallas, B., Lane, S., Mathews, R., Watkins, T., & Wiley-Patton, S. (2007). An iterative assessment approach to improve technology adoption and implementation decisions by healthcare managers. *Information Systems Management, 24*, 43–57.

Schectman, J. M., Schorling, J. B., Nadkarni, M. M., & Voss, J. D. (2005). Determinants of physician use of an ambulatory prescription expert system. *International Journal of Medical Informatics, 74*(9), 711–717.

Shi, L., & Singh, D. A. (2008). *Delivering health care in America: A systems approach* (4th Ed). Sudbury: Jones & Bartlet Publishers.

Thornewill, J., Dwling, A. F., Cox, B. A., & Esterhazy, R. J. (2011). Information infrastructure for consumer health: A health information exchange client study. *American Journal of Preventative Medicine, 40*(5), 123–133.

Walker, J. M., Carayon, P., Leveson, N., Paulus, R. A., Tooker, J. et al. (2008). EHR safety: The way forward to safe and effective systems. *Journal of the American Medical Informatics Association, 15*, 272–327.

Walls, J., Widmeyer, G., & El Sawy, O. (1992). Building an information system design theory for vigilant EIS. *Information Systems Research, 3*(1), 36–59.

Wiljer, D., Urowitz, S., Apatu, E., DeLenardo, C., Eysenbach, G., Harth, T., & Leonard, K. J. (2008). Patient accessible electronic health records: Exploring recommendations for successful implementation strategies. *Journal Of Medical Internet Research, 10*(4), 6. doi:10.2196/jmir.1061.

World Health Organization. (2005). eHealth: Report by the Secretariat. http://www.who.int/gb/ebwha/pdf_files/WHA58/A58_21-en.pdf. Accessed 12 Jan 2015.

Yen, P. Y., & Bakken, S. (2012). Review of health information technology usability study methodologies. *Journal of the American Medical Informatics Association, 19*(3), 413–422.

Zhang, J., Dawes, S. S., & Sarkis, J. (2005). Exploring clients' expectations of the benefits and barriers of e-Government knowledge sharing. *The Journal of Enterprise Information Management, 18*(5), 548–567.

Dr. Karoly Bozan is an associate professor of informatics and computer science at Idaho State University. Dr. Bozan's research interest encompasses system design in the health domain in the multistakeholder context. Prior to joining academia, Dr. Bozan held numerous technical and management consulting positions in a variety of industries.

Pratim Datta (Ph.D.) is a two-time Farris Family Research Innovation Fellow and an Associate Professor of IS and Supply Chains at Kent State University. Ranked among the top 40 researchers internationally, Datta has over 55 journal articles and conference proceedings with multiple best paper awards. Datta focuses on IS and supply chain use, performance and security as well as cross-functional corporate decision-making. He has won the Paul Pfeiffer Professional and Teaching Award. He has also received the Outstanding MBA Professor Award and he is the showcased professor for the Executive MBA Program.

Chapter 8
A Context-Aware Remote Health Monitoring Service for Improved Patient Care

Christopher Doss, Mohd Anwar and Nadine Manjaro

Introduction

We have been observing a paradigm shift in terms of the delivery of health care. Health status monitoring is at the center of this new paradigm that has the following characteristics:

1. *Wellness promotion:* The health-care industry has increased its focus on wellness. A health-care system that only focuses on treating illness is costly and ineffective. Mobile technologies are leading the way to support wellness (Daniel et al. 2011; Na and Choi 2013; Tollmar et al. 2012). Many mobile applications have been developed to motivate people to exercise (Stevens and Bryan 2012; Ho et al. 2012),eat healthy (Anwar et al. 2013; Andrew et al. 2013; Lopes et al. 2011), and relax (Ahtinen et al. 2010). However, we are still a long way from building a comprehensive wellness support system. Tethered to a health monitoring system, a wellness support system can timely inform users about their wellness status and recommend wellness-promoting activities.
2. *Patient-centered care:* Patient-centered care involves patients and their families in the care (Bloom 2002). Patient-centered care requires partnership with the caregivers, and, as a result, an improved communication channel needs to be established. A remote health monitoring system should facilitate the participation of patients and their communication channel.

M. Anwar (✉)
Department of Computer Science, North Carolina A&T State University, Greensboro, NC, USA
e-mail: tanjosep@mcmaster.ca

C. Doss
Department of Electrical and Computer Engineering, North Carolina A&T State University, Greensboro, NC, USA
e-mail: tanjosep@mcmaster.ca

N. Manjaro
Tech Mahindra, New York, NY, USA
e-mail: tanjosep@mcmaster.ca

N. Wickramasinghe et al. (eds.), *Contemporary Consumer Health Informatics*, Healthcare Delivery in the Information Age, DOI 10.1007/978-3-319-25973-4_8

3. *Anytime and anyplace care:* Patient mobility across providers and across regions is a very common thing (Brekke et al. 2014). A monitoring system needs to support monitoring anytime and at any place. The monitoring system also needs to be respectful to individual choices and preferences.

Today's health-care market is full of personal health devices (PHDs) that measure vital signs, blood pressure, blood glucose, respiratory activity, and other physiological information. Besides, personal mobile devices such as smartphones come with many embedded sensors that can be used to capture an individual's health status. The novel concept of Internet of Things (IoT) shows the potential in taking health status monitoring to a different level that is more context aware, ubiquitous, patient centered, and can assist in clinical decision support. The IoT (Gubbi et al. 2013; Coetzee and Eksteen 2011; Hu et al. 2013) is a global concept that underpins machine-to-machine (M2M) technologies (Wu et al. 2011; Kim et al. 2014). The M2M technologies enable wired, cellular, wireless, or hybrid communication modalities between machines.

Our contributions in this chapter are as follows:

1. We propose a set of requirements for an improved remote health monitoring system.
2. We develop a functional prototype of a remote monitoring system.

In the section "Proposed Remote Health Monitoring System," we elicit the requirements of a remote health monitoring system. The section "Architecture" presents the architecture of a functional prototype followed by the implementation details in the section "Implementation." The section "Results" describes how we validate the functionalities of the system. Our concluding remarks are in the section "Discussion."

Materials and Methods

Proposed Remote Health Monitoring System

Tele-health is primarily concerned with the remote delivery of health care. Traditional health-care systems, tele-health or otherwise, are reactive that respond to ailments of patients. However, proactive health care responds to any health status anomalies (vital signs or other measurements), implicit or explicit, that may lead to an ailment. Therefore, it is important to watch for health status irregularities in individuals. Remote health monitoring is an essential component of a proactive tele-health system that transmits vital signs and other physiological measurements to health-care providers. To ensure proactive care, a remote health monitoring system needs to offer the following capabilities:

- *Context awareness:* Contexts refer to conditions in which something occurs. A context-aware system takes advantage of contextual information. Any information to characterize the situation of an entity is contextual information (Dey 2000). This may include user context (such as knowledge about the user profile, social situation, and location) or time context (such as time of the day and season). The system should anticipate what the user wants and needs and act on it. A user may not want monitoring in a certain situation due to privacy reasons, or certain monitoring may not be needed due to other conditions. Context information may be inextricably linked to physiological measurements and, therefore, necessary to understand physiological measurements. For example, contextual information of how long ago an individual had his meal helps interpret the blood glucose level of that individual. A user needs to have control over their monitoring system based on the contextual information and over who may gain access.
- *Ubiquitousness:* Anytime, anyplace health monitoring is a prerequisite for proactive healthcare. Monitoring services need to be accessible at any time and from any place. This is especially critical for people with chronic health conditions. Networks, mobile devices and embedded sensors, M2M communication protocols, and geo-location and positioning technologies form the underlying technologies to support ubiquitous health monitoring services. Although limited, ubiquitous monitoring is already in use for home-bound elderly care. However, the IoT paradigm, where small, inexpensive, networked devices are distributed throughout the everyday life, can be leveraged to making health monitoring more pervasive. Using Web services, physiological measurements can easily be transmitted directly to the Web, and Web portals can show that information to caregivers and patients. Mobile devices and wireless standards (Wi-Fi, Bluetooth, Zigbee, etc.) can make that information accessible from any place.
- *Clinical decision support:* A working definition of clinical decision support has been proposed by Robert Hayward of the Centre for Health Evidence: "Clinical Decision Support systems link health observations with health knowledge to influence health choices by clinicians for improved health care" (Hayward 2014). Rich, relevant, and easy-to-understand data are expected to translate into better diagnosis and patient care. Therefore, a health monitoring system should be able to fuse data from disparate sources (multiple medical devices) and customize the monitoring activities according to clinical decision support needs. Furthermore, the system needs to convert raw sensor information into application-understandable/human-consumable health status information.
- *Just-in-time patient care:* Patient care, when rendered right on time, is more effective. The near-real-time delivery of vital signs or monitored data is essential for just-in-time care. The health monitoring system requires efficient data transfer with minimal or no human interventions. Therefore, choices of appropriate network technology and data capturing algorithms need to consider near-real-time transfer of data to caregivers.

Architecture

A remote health monitoring service needs an architecture that can support the following tasks:

1. *User authentication:* Clinicians and patients need to be properly authenticated. Each user will have a different role and, consequently, access to different types of information. The patient has access right to their own information. The clinician will need to be able to see a list of their patients as well as the history of monitored data for each of their patients. Therefore, user authentication is required to allow different permissions for each user type.
2. *Data capture:* Patients will need to be able to seamlessly allow or deny their health data to be captured. This data capture must support a variety of medical devices.
3. *Electronic health record (EHR) integration:* Data captured from the medical devices must be stored in EHRs at the hospital or clinic. Therefore, the data must be transformed into a format that can be consumed by the EHR.
4. *Data analysis:* There should be automated data analysis to alleviate data overload on the clinicians.
5. *Anomaly detection:* The system should automatically detect if a patient's vital signs are above or below acceptable ranges.
6. *User notification:* If a measurement is outside of the acceptable range, the clinician should be notified.

Figure 8.1 shows the architecture of the remote health monitoring system, which allows capturing data from a variety of Bluetooth-enabled medical devices. The medical devices (weight, glucose, and blood pressure sensors) communicate

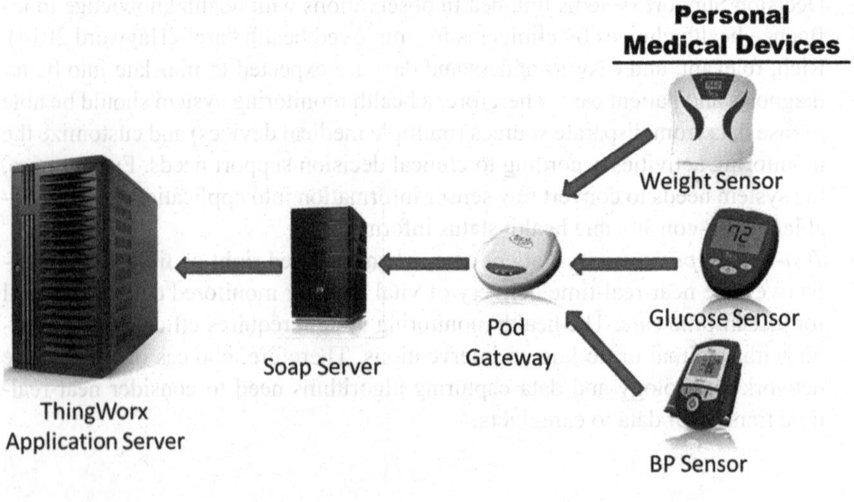

Fig. 8.1 Architecture of remote health monitoring service

measurement information to the Pod Gateway. The Pod, connected to the Internet via Ethernet, is capable of transmitting this information to a simple object access protocol (SOAP) server. The SOAP server then transmits information to the ThingWorx application server, which is responsible for running the health monitoring service. The application also contains a graphical user interface, which allows interaction with the service. The following subsections provide details of the architecture.

Medical Devices

In our implementation, the medical device elements include an IDEAL Life weight scale, a blood pressure device, and a glucose meter. The weight scale is capable of measuring weight in pounds or kilograms. The blood pressure device is capable of measuring systolic and diastolic pressure and pulse. The glucose meter is capable of assessing blood sugar levels. Each device transmits measurement information to the Pod Gateway via Bluetooth.

ThingWorx Platform

ThingWorx[19] is a platform for developing M2M communications and IoT applications. The platform includes a run-time environment that allows for mashups that can be deployed over the Internet. ThingWorx supports an object-oriented or "Thing-oriented" paradigm. A ThingWorx implementation consists of Things, ThingTemplates, and ThingShapes (ThingWorx 2014; Miller and Chung 2013). Things are the equivalent of objects in object-oriented languages. Each Thing contains properties and business logic, and can be used to model a physical asset such as a vending machine, a truck, or a medical device.

ThingShapes are used to define Things. ThingShapes specify the properties, services, events, and subscriptions for the Things. ThingShapes can be viewed as an abstract class. ThingTemplates provide the basis for Things by implementing one or more ThingShapes. Thus, a ThingTemplate can be viewed as a class or an interface.

The properties within a ThingWorx ThingShape, ThingTemplate, or Thing describe the current state of Things, similar to fields in some object-oriented languages. An example would be the *current temperature of a vending machine* or the *current Global Positioning System (GPS) position of a truck*. Services, similar to methods or functions, provide functionality to Things. An example would be *log the current temperature*, or *update the driver of the current address*. Events provide similar functionality to that of object-oriented events. An example of an event would be a *change in temperature* or a *change in position*. Each event contains associated information in the form of a DataShape. Subscriptions, which are similar to event-listeners, allow Things to be notified when an event is dispatched. An example of a subscription would be *listen for all changes in temperature* or *listen for all changes in GPS position*.

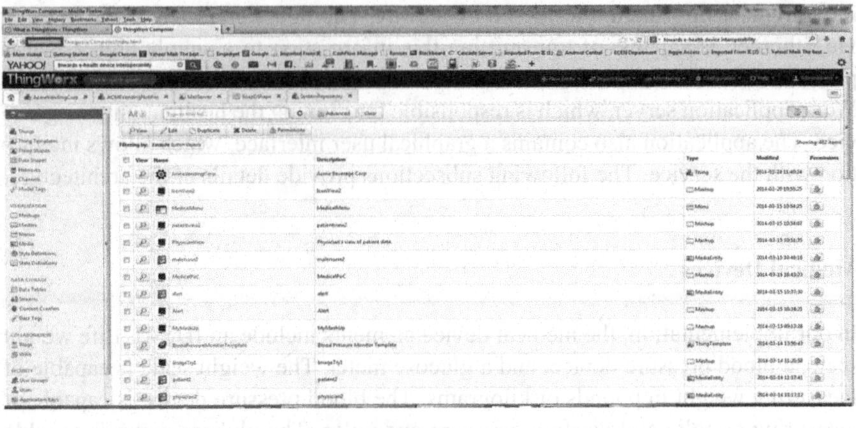

Fig. 8.2 ThingWorx development environment

The ThingWorx integrated design environment (IDE) is deployed on a Tomcat server as a Web archive (WAR file). Figure 8.2 shows the home screen of the IDE for ThingWorx. The left-hand part of the home screen provides links to view all items within the IDE. For instance, clicking on the Things link will bring up all Things that have been implemented. The creation and/or editing of an element within ThingWorx occur in a separate dedicated tab within the IDE. The successful implementation requires modeling the hardware, implementing the underlying services, and connecting these together within the graphical user interface, known as a Mashup. The section "Implementation" discusses these steps in detail.

Communication Middleware

The communication middleware consists of a Pod Gateway and a SOAP server. The Pod Gateway captures data from the corresponding medical devices. It connects to the medical devices via Bluetooth. It then transmits the data to a remote server via Ethernet connection.

The remote server in this implementation is a SOAP server. It captures the data from the Pod Gateway and translates the data into SOAP format. The parameters of a server request are customerID, accountNo, and memberID. The customerID is based on the serial number of the Pod Gateway. The accountNo is the account of the current user. The memberID specifies the type of the M2M device.

Graphical User Interface

The graphical user interface has separate views for clinicians and patients. The clinician is able to see their list of patients, as shown in Fig. 8.3. This list contains the

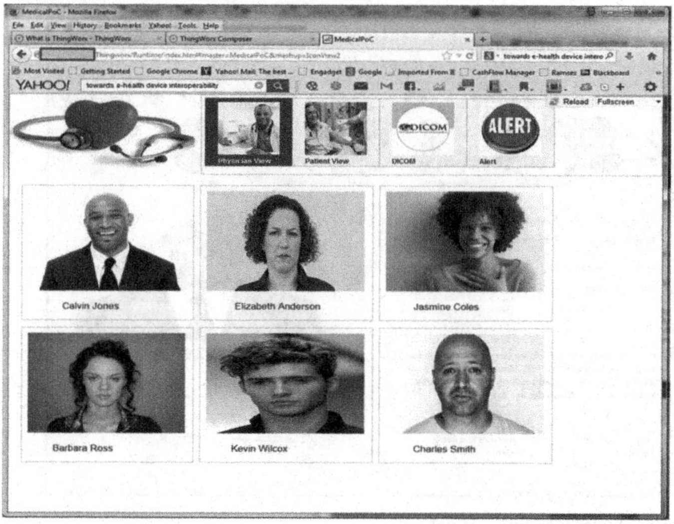

Fig. 8.3 Graphical user interface for clinicians

patient's picture along with their name. Each item in the list can be clicked to access details of the patient, as shown in Fig. 8.4.

The patient details screen contains four sections. The top-left section contains general information about the patient, including patient name, number, age, and height. The top-right section contains a picture of the patient. The lower-left section contains recent summaries of the patient's status. The lower-right section contains

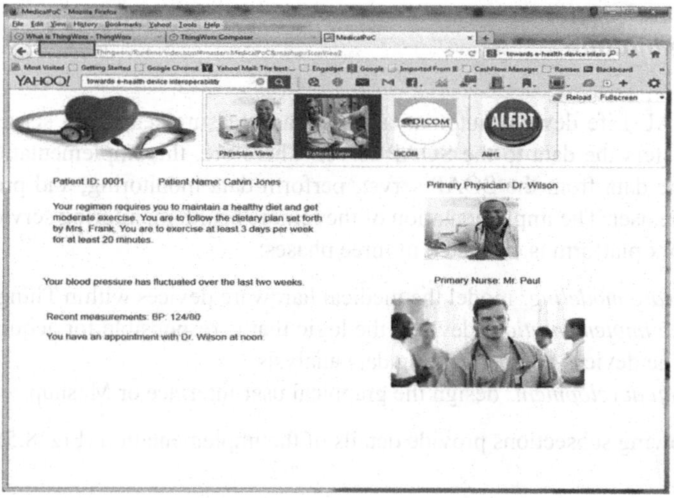

Fig. 8.4 Graphical user interface for patient details

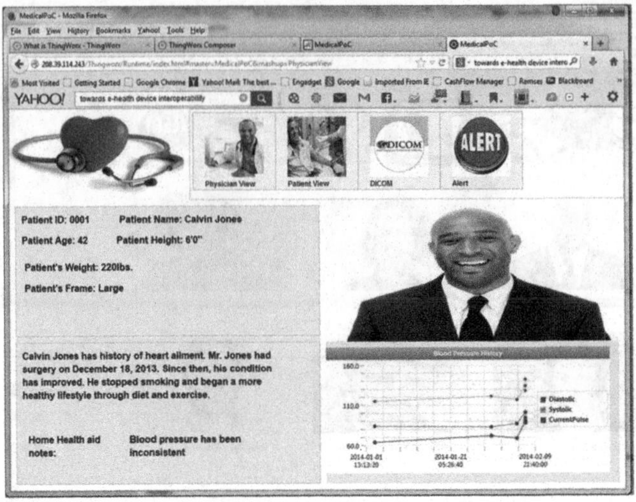

Fig. 8.5 Graphical user interface for patients

graphs of the patient's vital signs. This information is captured as discussed in the section "Mashup Development."

The patient view screen contains four sections. The top-right and bottom-right sections contain information about the patient's primary physician and primary nurse, respectively. These sections include the clinicians' names and pictures. The top-left section contains instructions from the clinician, such as the regimen or diet the patient should follow. The lower-right section contains summaries of the patient's recent measurements.

Implementation

The IDEAL Life devices automatically upload measurements to a server, which then transfers the data to the SOAP server. Therefore, this implementation needs to pull the data from the SOAP server, perform data monitoring, and present the data to the user. The implementation of the remote health monitoring service on the ThingWorx platform is consisted of three phases:

1. *Hardware modeling:* model the medical hardware devices within ThingWorx
2. *Service implementation:* develop the logic that is responsible for acquiring data from the devices and performing data analysis
3. *Mashup development:* design the graphical user interface or Mashup

The following subsections provide details of the implementation (Fig. 8.5).

Hardware Modeling

The hardware modeling phase of the ThingWorx implementation creates a representation of the hardware elements. The first step of modeling the hardware was to create the ThingShapes for the medical devices within ThingWorx. This required creating a BloodPressureMonitorShape, a WeightScaleShape, and a GlucoseMeterShape. The BloodPressureMonitorShape models the blood pressure sensor and consists of the following properties:

- *DiastolicPressure:* a number that represents the diastolic blood pressure of the patient
- *SystolicPressure:* a number that represents the systolic blood pressure of the patient
- *Pulse:* a number that represents the pulse of the patient
- *MeasurementTime:* a DateTime that represents when the measurement was taken

The WeightScaleShape models the weight scale and consists of the following properties:

- *Weight:* a number that represents the weight of the patient in pounds
- *MeasurementTime:* a DateTime that represents when the measurement was taken

The GlucoseMeterShape models the glucose meter shape and consists of the following properties:

- *BloodGlucoseLevel:* a number that represents the measured glucose level of the patient
- *MeasurementTime:* a DateTime that represents when the measurement was taken

The next step was to create the ThingTemplates. This required creating a BloodPressureMonitorTemplate, a WeightScaleTemplate, and a GlucoseMeterTemplate. Several additional properties were added to each ThingTemplate to allow for the triggering of alert conditions. The BloodPressureMonitorTemplate contains the following additional properties:

BPSystolicSomewhatHigh, BPSystolicSomewhatLow, BPSystolicVeryHigh, BPSystolicVeryLow: Boolean values that indicate corresponding alert condition for the systolic pressure.

- *BPSystolicSomewhatHighLimit, BPSystolicSomewhatLowLimit, BPSystolicVeryHighLimit, BPSystolicVeryLowLimit:* Numbers that indicate the value at which the corresponding alert condition is triggered. (For example, if BPSystolicVeryHighLimit is 140, BPSystolicVeryHigh is set to true if SystolicPressure is above 140).
- *BPDiastolicSomewhatHigh, BPDiastolicSomewhatLow, BPDiastolicVeryHigh, BPDiastolicVeryLow:* Boolean values that indicate corresponding alert condition for the diastolic pressure.

- *BPDiastolicSomewhatHighLimit, BPDiastolicSomewhatLowLimit, BPDiastolicVeryHighLimit, BPDiastolicVeryLowLimit:* Numbers that indicate the value at which the corresponding alert condition is triggered.
- *BPPulseHigh, BPPulseLow:* Boolean values that indicate corresponding alert condition for the pulse.
- *BPPulseHighLimit, BPPulseLowLimit:* Numbers that indicate the value at which the corresponding alert condition is triggered.

The GlucoseMeterTemplate and WeightScaleTemplate have similar properties.

The last step was to create the Things. Each thing represents a medical device. Therefore, to represent three physical blood pressure monitors, three Things must be created within ThingWorx. Although there was only one physical blood pressure monitor, weight scale, and glucose meter, three of each were created within ThingWorx. The three blood pressure Things were named BPM-001, BPM-002, and BPM-003. The three weight scales were named WS-001, WS-002, and WS-003. The three glucose meters were named GM-001, GM-002, and GM-003.

Service Implementation

The service implementation phase adds business logic to each of the elements (Things, ThingTemplates, and ThingShapes). These can be written in JavaScript inside the ThingWorx IDE. This required implementing a service to access the SOAP server, a service for sending alerts, and a timer service. There is a separate SOAP access service for each medical device type.

The *SOAPAccess* service is responsible for implementing a SOAP client for capturing data from the SOAP server. This service initiates a SOAP request to the SOAP server, which contains all the readings from the devices. The SOAPAccess service filters the data to retrieve the elements associated with the corresponding device. For example, the *SOAPAccess* service for the blood pressure monitor filters the data to retrieve the blood pressure data.

Once the data have been retrieved, they are placed into a DataTable for storage. This allows the data to be shown in a Mashup. The *SOAPAccess* service also identifies if any of the measurements are outside of acceptable ranges. If they are, an alert is sent using the *SendAlert* service.

The *SendAlert* service is responsible for sending a text message to the clinician if the user's information should be noted. The parameters for this service are the phone number and the message body. This service uses e-mail to send a corresponding text message.

The *Timer* service is a service that identifies whether a predetermined amount of time has elapsed. ThingWorx provides a Timer ThingTemplate for building a customized timer. The *Timer* service indicates when 60 s have elapsed and is used to start the *SOAPAccess* service.

Mashup Development

The Mashup development phase ties the Things, including services and events, to the graphical user interface. Each Mashup is a self-contained window, capable of having sub-elements, known as widgets. Each Mashup has its own URL, meaning a user can navigate directly to each using a standard browser. The graphical user interface requires three screens. This requires creating four components: the *Mashup Master*, the *Physician View Mashup*, the *Patient Detail View Mashups,* and the *Patient View Mashup.*

The *Mashup Master* is a base Mashup that can contain other Mashups. The top of the Master contains a logo and a menu that allows the user to select the Mashup they would like to navigate to. The menu contains four buttons for navigating to the Physician View Mashup, the Patient View Mashup, the DICOM Viewer Mashup, and an Alert View Mashup.[1]

The *Physician View Mashup* contains a list of panels, each containing an image widget and a label widget. Each panel is overlaid with a navigation widget. The navigation widgets are links to the corresponding *Patient Detail View Mashup*. The *Physician View Mashup* is also linked to the *Mashup Master*. Therefore, users navigating to the *Physician View Mashup* will also see the menu, allowing navigation to the other Mashups.

The *Patient Detail View Mashup* allows the clinician to view the details of the patient. This Mashup contains a layout with two columns, each with two rows to create four sections. The upper-left section contains label widgets that indicate general information about the patient. The upper-right section contains an image widget that is linked to a picture of the patient. The lower-left section contains label widgets that indicate summaries of the patient's status. The lower-right section contains a time series chart widget that is linked to the *SOAPAccess* service. The *SOAPAccess* service is triggered once the *Patient Detail View Mashup* is loaded. This populates a DataTable linked to the Time Series Chart. As with the *Physician View Mashup,* the *Patient Detail View Mashup* is linked to the Mashup Master.

The *Patient View Mashup* allows the patient to view information about their clinicians as well as recent information on their medical status. This Mashup contains four sections in a 2×2 grid. The upper-left section contains label widgets that provide patient status information. The lower-left section contains label widgets that provide information on their recent results. The upper-right section contains an image widget and a label widget that indicate the primary physician. The lower-right section contains an image widget and a label widget that indicate the primary nurse. The *Patient View Mashup* is linked to the *Mashup Master*.

[1] The DICOM View and Alert View were created for testing and for identifying future functionality. Therefore, their details are not presented in this chapter.

Results

As a proof of concept, we implemented the following essential scenarios of a health monitoring system. A doctor needs to monitor three patients with chronic conditions. The doctor desires to improve the wellness of these patients and to be able to quickly respond when the patient's condition changes. In order to facilitate this, the doctor needs to be able to remotely monitor the patients' conditions.

These patients have been asked to take regular blood pressure measurements and weight measurements. The doctor would like to be notified when the patients perform measurements, and whether any of these measurements are outside of acceptable ranges. Each patient has been given a measurement device and instructions on how often to take measurements.

Validation The remote monitoring service was validated with an IDEAL Life blood pressure sensor and a weight scale. There were two types of alert conditions for blood pressure: low priority and high priority. Low-priority alerts were sent if the user's blood pressure was 120–139 systolic or 80–90 diastolic. High-priority alerts were sent if the user's blood pressure was 140–159 systolic or 90–99 diastolic.

Several blood pressure measurements were taken over the course of several days. Weight scale measurements were also taken over the course of several days. The SOAP server received the information and stored the measurement time of each recording. The ThingWorx application retrieved the information and successfully isolated the measurements based on measurement time and measurement type. Figure 8.6 shows the data stream from the blood pressure monitor. As can be seen, there were several measurements that triggered alerts. It was then able to display this information in the corresponding Mashup (Fig. 8.5). The ThingWorx server was

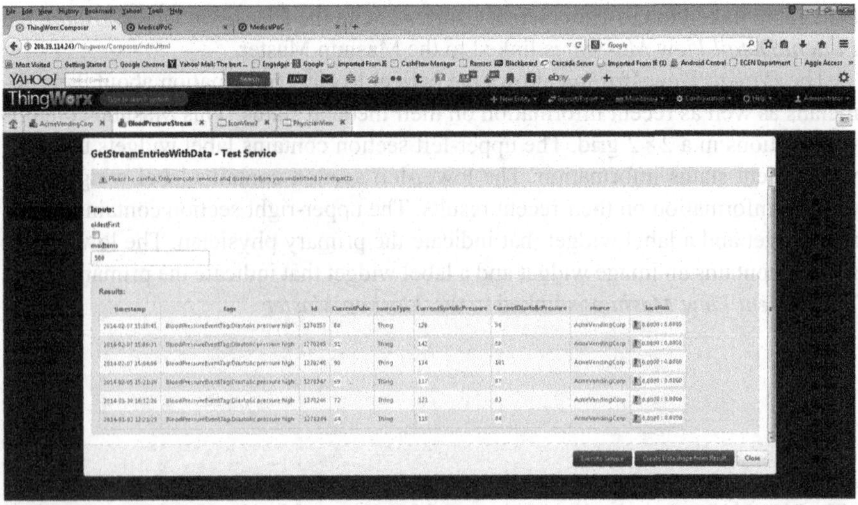

Fig. 8.6 Data stream of blood pressure measurements

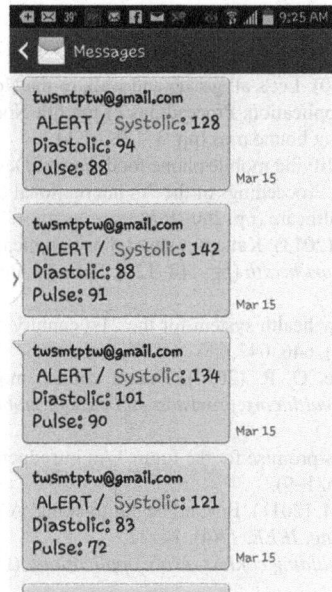

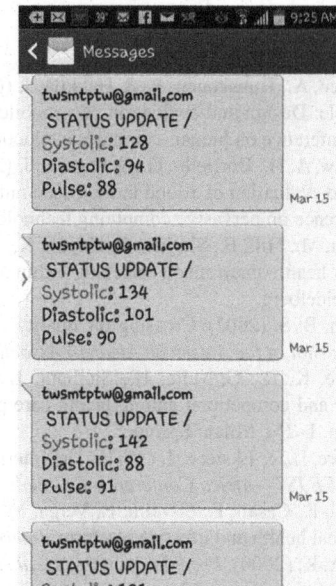

Fig. 8.7 Text alerts sent to caregiver

also able to identify measurements that were in a range that could cause concern. Alerts were sent to the sample cell phones indicating these conditions. Figure 8.7 shows the text message alerts, as well as status updates, that were sent to the sample cell phone.

Discussion

This chapter presented a context-aware, remote health monitoring service that is capable of capturing measurements from Bluetooth-enabled medical devices. The data are transferred from the device to a central server and are made available for external consumption via SOAP. A ThingWorx application service captures the information from the SOAP server and presents information to patients and clinicians via a graphical user interface Mashup. The application monitors patient measurements and sends alerts if the conditions are outside of acceptable ranges. The application was tested and verified over the course of several days using a blood pressure sensor and a weight scale.

The system currently supports user authentication, data capture, data analysis, anomaly detection, and user notification. The data analysis is currently limited to identifying if a measurement is within or outside of a given range. Future work will allow integration into EHR systems as well as additional capabilities for data analysis. Also, support for additional medical devices, including pulse oximeters, will be included.

References

Ahtinen, A., Huuskonen, P., & Häkkilä, J. (October 2010). Let's all get up and walk to the North Pole: Design and evaluation of a mobile wellness application. Proceedings of the 6th Nordic conference on human-computer interaction: Extending boundaries (pp. 3–12). ACM.

Andrew, A. H., Borriello, G., & Fogarty, J. (2013). Simplifying mobile phone food diaries: Design and evaluation of a food index-based nutrition diary. Proceedings of the 7th international conference on pervasive computing technologies for healthcare (pp. 260–263).

Anwar, M., Hill, E., Skujins, J., Huynh, K., & Doss, C. (2013). Kalico: A smartphone application for health-smart menu selection within a budget. *Smart health* (pp. 113–121). Springer Berlin Heidelberg.

Bloom, B. S. (2002). Crossing the quality chasm: A new health system for the 21st century. *The Journal of the American Medical Association, 287*(5), 646–647.

Brekke, K. R., Gravelle, H., Siciliani, L., & Straume, O. R. (2014). Patient choice, mobility and competition among health care providers. *Health care provision and patient mobility* (pp. 1–26). Milan: Springer.

Coetzee, L., & Eksteen, J. (2011). The Internet of Things-promise for the future? An introduction. *IEEE IST—Africa Conference Proceedings, 2011* (pp. 1–9).

Daniel, F., Casati, F., Silveira, P., Verga, M., & Nalin, M. (2011). Beyond health tracking: A personal health and lifestyle platform. *Internet Computing, IEEE, 15*(4), 14–22.

Dey, A. K. (2000). *Providing architectural support for building context-aware applications*. (Doctoral dissertation, Georgia Institute of Technology).

Gubbi, J., Buyya, R., Marusic, S., & Palaniswami, M. (2013). Internet of Things (IoT): A vision, architectural elements, and future directions. *Future Generation Computer Systems, 29*(7), 1645–1660.

Hayward, R. (2014). Clinical decision support system. http://en.wikipedia.org/wiki/Clinical_decision_support_system. Accessed 1 Nov 2014.

Ho, Y., Tanaka, K., Ishiguro, S., Sato-Shimokawara, E., & Yamaguchi, T. (2012). Applying user model as the basis for daily exercise support application. IEEE conference on technologies and applications of artificial intelligence (TAAI), (pp. 250–255).

Hu, F., Xie, D., & Shen, S. (August 2013). On the application of the Internet of Things in the field of medical and health care. IEEE international conference on and IEEE cyber, physical and social computing (pp. 2053–2058).

Kim, J., Lee, J., Kim, J., & Yun, J. (2014). M2M service platforms: Survey, issues, and enabling technologies. *Communications Surveys & Tutorials, IEEE, 16*(1), 61–76.

Lopes, I. M., Silva, B. M., Rodrigues, J. J., Lloret, J., & Proenca, M. L. (2011). A mobile health monitoring solution for weight control. IEEE conference on wireless communications and signal processing (WCSP) (pp. 1–5).

Miller, R., & Chung, P. (2013). ThingWorx fundamentals. ThingWorx, 2013.

Na, H., & Choi, Y. (2013). Conceptual design of personal wellness record for mobile health monitoring. IEEE 2nd global conference on consumer electronics (GCCE) (pp. 410–411).

Stevens, C. J., & Bryan, A. D. (2012). Rebranding exercise: There's an app for that. *American Journal of Health Promotion, 27*(2), 69–70.

ThingWorx. (2014). What is thingworx @ONLINE. http://www.thingworx.com/platform/key-features. Accessed 1 April 2014.

Tollmar, K., Bentley, F., & Viedma, C. (2012). Mobile health mashups: Making sense of multiple streams of wellbeing and contextual data for presentation on a mobile device. IEEE international conference on pervasive computing technologies for healthcare (PervasiveHealth) (pp. 65–72).

Wu, G., Talwar, S., Johnsson, K., Himayat, N., & Johnson, K. D. (2011). M2M: From mobile to embedded internet. *Communications Magazine, IEEE, 49*(4), 36–43.

Dr. Christopher Doss received his B.S. degree from the University of South Florida in spring 1994 and M.S. and Ph.D. degrees from North Carolina State University in spring 1997 and 2001, respectively—all in computer engineering. While working on his Ph.D., Dr. Doss served as an instructor at Wake Technical Community College, where he worked until summer 2001. Dr. Doss currently holds an associate professor position at North Carolina A&T State University. His current research interests focus on the design and implementation of applications on reconfigurable and embedded computing systems for bioinformatics, assistive domotics, mobile health, and telemedicine. His work also focuses on utilizing mobile technology for science, technology, engineering, and mathematics (STEM) education, centering on developing interactive systems that provide educational tools on several platforms, including smartphones, tablets, and desktops. His research also includes the development of new tools.

Dr. Mohd Anwar is an assistant professor of computer science at North Carolina A&T State University (NCAT). At NCAT, he directs the Secure and Usable Social Media & Networks (SUSMaN) Lab. Prior to joining NCAT, he was a research assistant professor at the University of Pittsburgh. Dr. Anwar has experience and interest in designing usable secure, privacy-preserving, and trusted infrastructures, systems, and applications in different online contexts, especially in online social networks (OSNs) and mHealth domains. His research applies methods from software engineering, human–computer interaction, and artificial intelligence, as well as theories from social sciences to understand and solve problems in cybersecurity and health-care domains.

Nadine Manjaro is currently working as a director of the Internet of Things (IoT) Program with Tech Mahindra. In this role, she is responsible for machine-to-machine (M2M) presales, solutions, and North America ecosystem partner development. Nadine Manjaro has more than 18 years of experience in wireline and wireless networking. She has worked for tier 1 operators including Sprint for more than 7 years and Verizon for more than 3 years. Nadine also worked as an industry analyst for ABI Research for 3 years providing global coverage of the wireless infrastructure market. She has written extensive research on long-term evolution (LTE), WiMAX, IMS, global spectrum, managed services, cell site infrastructure, and mobile backhaul. She has been quoted as an industry expert in the Wall Street Journal, Barrons, International Data Group (IDG), RCR Wireless, Fierce Wireless, and several other publications. Ms. Manjaro holds a bachelor of science degree in industrial engineering and a bachelor of arts degree in economics and statistics, both from Rutgers University. She completed the 2-year AJI Network Business Leaders Program and holds a master of science degree in engineering management from the University of Kansas.

Chapter 9
Evaluating NDF-RT's Comprehensiveness as a Drugs Classification Standard: Drug Interaction Checker

Awatif Alotaibi and Mona Alkhattabi

Introduction

Drug–drug interactions (DDIs) happen when the effect of a specific drug changes due to another drug taken with it. DDI is a serious problem and happens to a patient when he/she has two conflicting drugs. A substance of one drug can affect the activity of another when both are taken together. Over-the-counter (OTC) drug labels contain information about ingredients, uses, warnings, and directions; in addition, this label has important information about drug interactions. In the warning section, there is information about drugs or ingredients that cause interactions with their current drug. When the physician prescribes a new drug, he/she should explain about OTC and prescription drugs and discuss other drugs to prevent any DDIs. Also, the patient should ask the pharmacist about the issue and declare any other medications being taken. As can be noticed, this responsibility lies with physicians and pharmacists. However, it is better for the patient to manage his/her medications because no one can take better care than himself/herself. So, the patient has to have a good knowledge and be aware of his/her medication to preserve his/her life (The New Over-the-Counter Medicine Label: Take a Look 2014).

The project intends to serve patients who receive more than one prescribed medication and who have a little knowledge about the names of drugs. The necessity to implement a solution comes from a need to increase and improve patients' knowledge of drug interactions and the possibility of human mistakes by physicians and pharmacists, and also from the shortage of electronic solutions in health organizations.

A. Alotaibi (✉)
King Fahad Medical City (KFMC), Riyadh, Saudi Arabia
e-mail: kmalotaibi@gmail.com

M. Alkhattabi
College of Computer Sciences and Information, Al-Imam Mohammad Ibn Saud University, Riyadh, Saudi Arabia
e-mail: monaalkhattabi@ccis.imamu.edu.sa

N. Wickramasinghe et al. (eds.), *Contemporary Consumer Health Informatics*, Healthcare Delivery in the Information Age, DOI 10.1007/978-3-319-25973-4_9

The research asks a simple question, which is based on a discussion of the efficiency and the benefits of the proposed solution (Drug Interaction Checker) on the population (30 patients from KFMC) based on the comprehensiveness of the source data (National Drug File-Reference Terminology application program interface, NDF-RT API). The question is: Does the Drug Interaction Checker increase and improve the patients' awareness and knowledge, if an NDF-RT API is comprehensive?

Unified Medical Language System

The Unified Medical Language System (UMLS) is a set of files and software that assembles and uses health, biomedical vocabularies and standards to enable interoperability between different electronic systems. The purpose of the UMLS is to connect medical information, medical terminologies, drug names, and diagnosis codes across diverse electronic systems. The UMLS tools are (1) Metathesaurus: terms and codes from several vocabularies, including RxNorm, International Classification of Diseases, 10th Revision, Clinical Modification (ICD-10-CM), Logical Observation Identifiers Names and Codes (LOINC), Medical Subject Headings (MeSH), Current Procedural Terminology (CPT), and Systematized Nomenclature of Medicine (SNOMED); (2) Semantic Network: comprehensive categories (semantic types) and their relationships (semantic relations); and (3) Specialist Lexicon and Lexical Tools: natural language processing tools (Unified Medical Language System 2014).

RxNorm

RxNorm is "a normalized naming system for generic and branded drugs, and a tool for supporting semantic interoperation between drug terminologies and pharmacy knowledge base systems." RxNorm is produced by the National Library of Medicine (NLM). Hospitals, pharmacies, and other organizations use electronic systems to record and process drug information; however, drug names are diverse, so the systems cannot communicate with each other. Therefore, RxNorm provides normalized names and unique identifiers for medicines and drugs. NLM gets drug names from numerous data foundations, evaluates and routes the data, and produces the data, which RxNorm stores in a standard format. There are various steps involved in RxNorm production. However, these five elementary steps explain one way in which an RxNorm is produced:

> Group source data into collections of synonyms (called concepts). Create an RxNorm normalized name for each concept (if the concept is in scope and unambiguous). Assign an RxNorm concept unique identifier (RXCUI) to each concept and an RxNorm atom unique identifier (RXAUI) to each atom. Include relationships and attributes from the source data. Create related RxNorm names and relationships.

RxNorm receives drug names from 12 source terminologies, for example Veterans Health Administration National Drug File—Reference Terminology, US Edition of SNOMED CT (drug information) and Veterans Health Administration. (Unified Medical Language System, RxNorm 2014)

National Drug File-Reference Terminology

National Drug File-Reference Terminology (NDF-RT) is an enhancement of NDF built on a core of RxNorm. RxNorm is a more formal representation that lists every drug in a hierarchical classification and can support many applications and systems to retrieve drug information. NDF-RT was created by the NLM and Veterans Affairs (VA). Each NDF-RT entry for a drug or a drug component is joined to its exact copy in RxNorm. RxNorm and NDF-RT are built together. NDF-RT has expanded the RxNorm entries. NDF-RT was developed using description logics (DL) and can be downloaded in different formats, including Extensible Markup Language (XML) and Ontology Web Language (OWL) formats (Unified Medical Language System—2012AB National Drug File—Reference Terminology Source Information 2014).

National Drug File-Reference Terminology Application Program Interfaces (NDF-RT APIs)

The NDF-RT API is a Web service for retrieving the NDF-RT data set. The license does not state that it is mandatory to use the NDF-RT API. There are two different approaches to retrieving data from the NDF-RT data set. The first approach is through representational state transfer (RESTful) Web services. The NDF-RT RESTful Web API is a Web service that is executed using hypertext transfer protocol (HTTP) and an assembly of *resources*, stated as uniform resource identifiers (URIs) to the base URI for the Web service, which is http://rxnav.nlm.nih.gov/REST/Ndfrt. REST-style architectures involve clients and servers and support a multipurpose Internet mail extension (MIME) type of XML, so drug data are returned in XML format. The second approach is the Simple Object Access Protocol (SOAP)-based NDF-RT API Web service, which is a Web service that can access and retrieve NDF-RT data sets from customized implemented solutions via SOAP/Web Services Description Language (WSDL). This approach needs an initial setup to set the appropriate environment and develop the code. The steps include obtaining a (SOAP) 1.2 compatible engine for Web service message routing, downloading the WSDL for the NDF-RT API Web service, and generating the client side ends for WSDL to start writing the code. Instead of using URI resources, as with RESTful Web services, SOAP uses *functions* to retrieve NDF-RT data sets. Resources and functions have the same purpose, as can be seen below (NDF-RT API 2014).

NDF-RT API's Resources and Functions

NDF-RT API has many resources or functions; although they have different retrieving approaches, they have the same inputs and outputs. Resources can supply the end users with many meaningful data if calling by appropriate uniform resource locators (URLs) and inputs. Each resource has its own extension included in the basic NDF-RT URL. In addition, functions can supply the appropriate outputs when an accurate setting has been put in place and the appropriate inputs are entered. Each resource and function has specific inputs and outputs, and every function and resource has the same purpose, as seen below (NDF-RT API 2014; Table 9.1).

XML Parser

XML parser is a software library that provides methods or resources via an interface for client applications to retrieve data from XML files. This software checks the format of the files by using appropriate methods. It is a great way to shelter the end user from the complexities. There are two types of XML parser: Document Object Model (DOM) and Simple API for XML (SAX) parsers. A DOM is an object that has all the information of an XML file and is composed of a tree of nodes; these nodes are connected with other nodes, even if they are not included on the same DOM tree. The most important types of nodes are elements and text. The DOM parser is tree based and creates its own file structure in memory once the customized applications have got the information from the original XML file by appealing methods on this file object. This approach is more efficient when random access to commonly disconnected parts of a file is necessary. Also, because it has the ability to create its own structure, it supports both read and write operations. A SAX parser

Table 9.1 Resources with corresponding functions in National Drug File-Reference Terminology

SOAP function	REST resource	Description
findConceptsByID	/idType=*{idType}*&idString=*{idString}*	Get the NDF-RT concept for a specified identifier
findConceptsBy-Name	/search?conceptName=*{conceptName}* &kindName=*{kindName}*	Get the concepts for a specified name and kind
findDrugInteractions	/interaction/nui=*{nui}*&scope=*{scope}*	Get the drug concepts that interact with a given drug
getAllInfo	/allInfo/*{nui}*	Get concept information
getAllConcepts-ByKind	/allconcepts?kind=*kindNames*	Get concept information for specified kinds
getAllInfo	/allInfo/*{nui}*	Get concept information for specified kinds

NDF-RT National Drug File-Reference Terminology, *SOAP* Simple Object Access Protocol

is event based, where the parser reads the elements from the start-tag, end-tag as an event. When an end user enters inputs then calls, the methods or resources of the API place it in the source code. Therefore, when the events happen, the handler automatically appeals particular methods built by the developer. Then, the methods are returned to the appropriate output. A SAX parser is simple and it is memory efficient because it does not create its own structure (SAX and DOM Parser 2014).

NXML Parser

NXML parser is one of the SAX parsers. NXML parser exists in iOS software development kit (SDK), which is provided by Apple. It is used as an Objective-C for development. It is event based and informs the delegate about the element in the document. It is created as an object with methods to parse the element (iOS Developer Library 2013).

Lexicomp Inc.

Lexicomp is a provider of clinical information and technical solutions for the health-care industry. It provides new medical technology to improve patient safety and to share knowledge about medical and drug information; this includes reference handbooks, mobile applications, and online Lexicomp.

Lexicomp Online is an Internet-based technical solution that gives end users the authority (via a subscribing method) to access clinical and drug information. The users are divided into community groups: hospital community, academic community, pharmacy community, group practice multiuser community, and dentistry community. Each community has its own portal, which is customized according to its type of subscription (Lexi comp 2013).

From previous studies (which will be discussed in more detail in another publication), it is obvious that there are capabilities which could enable the construction of a technical solution for end users (patients) in order to gain benefits from drug data resources. This will be possible through utilizing source information, such as NDF-RT API, which comprises finding drug interactions and concepts by name resources, represented by URLs, to explore information about drug interactions, in order to guarantee safety and awareness. In addition, this solution enables the evaluation of NDF-RT to use it as a drug classification standard based on appropriate utilized resources (Asuncion et al. 2013; Barrière and Gagnon 2011; Bodenreider et al. 2010; Boyce et al. 2013; Fry 2005; Karaiskos 2013; Mortensen 2010; Mortensen and Bodenreider 2010; Mougin et al. 2012; Nelson et al. 2011; Pathak and Chute 2011; Pathak et al. 2011a, b; Petersa et al. 2013; Zhu et al. 2012, 2013).

The Proposed Solution

The objective of the proposed solution is to deliver a search tool that enables the end user to quickly search for drug interaction information using appropriate Web services. In addition, based on this prototype, we would like to evaluate the chosen drug data sources.

The basic requirements that should be considered important to the implementation of the Drug Interaction Checker and used to test and evaluate the drug data source are:

1. *SR 1*: The prototype should rely on international classification standards to avoid any shortages or missing values to build the local drug database—*System Requirement*.
2. *SR 2*: The prototype should be portable to enable the end user to use it anytime and anywhere—*System Requirement*.
3. *FR 1*: The prototype should enable the end users to enter two drugs—*Functional Requirement (Process Oriented)*.
4. *FR 2*: The prototype should provide drug interaction information to the end user—*Functional Requirement (Information Oriented)*.
5. *NFR 1*: The prototype should provide the output within 2 s—*Nonfunctional Requirement (Performance)*.

The proposed application needs to retrieve and present Web services information, but retaining any processed information is not part of the requirements. Therefore, the project does not have to build a database for storage. The first important issue involves gaining access to specific classification standards and retrieving the necessary information. The second issue covers interface design and data presentation.

Access to Classification Standard APIs

The classification standards are different from each other with regard to their structure, fees, and techniques used to access them. The greatest difficulties faced in searching are the following:

- Most of the classification standards APIs are not free.
- The classification standards are represented in different formats: XML format, WSDL format, and plain format.
- Searches for appropriate resources or functions in order to retrieve necessary drugs information is a challenge.

Fortunately, NDF-RT has a Web service that contains the necessary resources for drugs and corresponding interaction information; it is a free Web service and their data are stored in XML format.

Table 9.2 Utilized resources from National Drug File-Reference Terminology application program interfaces (NDF-RT APIs) representational state transfer (RESTful)

	REST resource	Description
	/	Resource base
R1	/search?conceptName= *{conceptName}*&kindName=*{kindName}*	Get the concepts for a specified name and kind
R2	/interaction/nui=*{nui}*&scope=*{scope}*	Get the drug concepts that interact with a given drug

Retrieving Drug Data and Interaction Information

These services allow the retrieval of drug information from NDF-RT servers to end-user applications through HTTP. The response is presented in XML format, while access to the NDF-RT RESTful services is executed through URIs. NDF-RT RESTful APIs provide many resources—the base URI for the Web service is http://rxnav.nlm.nih.gov/REST/Ndfrt.

Two resources are chosen and added to the base URI for retrieval of the appropriate information upon which the proposed solution depends; these are R1 and R2 and can be seen in Table 9.2.

The NDF-RT returned the drug data in XML format. The schema files for R1 look as illustrated in Fig. 9.1.

In schema file for R2, it can be noticed that the drug has six drug interactions, but only one is shown below (Fig. 9.2).


```
http://rxnav.nlm.nih.gov/REST/Ndfrt/search?conceptName=morphine&kindName=DRUG_KIND

(returns)

<ndfrtdata>
  <responseType>
    <inputConceptName>morphine</inputConceptName>
    <inputKindName>DRUG_KIND</inputKindName>
  </responseType>
  <groupConcepts>
    <concept>
      <conceptName>MORPHINE</conceptName>
      <conceptNui>N0000145914</conceptNui>
      <conceptKind>DRUG_KIND</conceptKind>
    </concept>
  </groupConcepts>
</ndfrtdata>
```


Fig. 9.1 An Extensible Markup Language (XML) format for R1

```
http://rxnav.nlm.nih.gov/REST/Ndfrt/interaction/nui=N0000145914&scope=2

(returns)

<ndfrtdata>
  <responseType>
    <inputNui1>N0000145914</inputNui1>
  </responseType>
  <groupInteractions>
    <interactions>
      <comment>MORPHINE is resolved to MORPHINE and MORPHINE has 6 interaction(s)</comment>
      <concept>
        <conceptName>MORPHINE</conceptName>
        <conceptNui>N0000145914</conceptNui>
        <conceptKind>DRUG_KIND</conceptKind>
      </concept>
      <groupInteractingDrugs>
        <interactingDrug>
```

Fig. 9.2 An Extensible Markup Language (XML) format for R2

Interface Design Data Presentation

NDF-RT was chosen as the international classification standard to meet SR1 with respect to the difficulties faced when searching for the best one. NDF-RT was the chosen APIs Web service to meet NFR 1. NDF-RT RESTful was chosen because it returns data in XML format. XML format is the appropriate format for XML parser, which is the simplest and most elegant technique used to retrieve data. Parser techniques have two approaches: SAX parsers and DOM parsers. To parse drug information, a SAX parser was chosen because it is the appropriate choice for iPhone applications. NSXML parser is the most popular type of SAX parser, which is fortunately, by default, included in iPhone SDK tools; all these factors meet the mobility requirements of SR 2, as explained in Tables 9.3and 9.4.

Table 9.3 The platform for the Drug Interaction Checker

iPhone environment	
Programming language	Objective C
Software tool	Xcode
Operating system	iOS
Tools	SDKs including SAX parser

SDK software development kit, *SAX* Simple Application Program Interface for Extensible Markup Language

Table 9.4 The requirements with corresponding meeting design choices

Requirements	Specifications met
SR 1	NDF-RT
SR 2	NDF-RT APIs web services
FR 1	Objective C/Xcode/iOS/SDKs
FR 2	NDF-RT API/RESTful/XML parser/SAX parser ⇔SDKs/Objective C/Xcode/iOS
NFR 1	NDF-RT APIs Web services

NDF-RT National Drug File-Reference Terminology, *API* application program interface, *RESTful* representation state transfer, *XML* Extensible Markup Language, *SAX* Simple API for XML, *SDK* software development kit

Design Architecture Framework

Drug Interaction Checker is a mobile application that uses the NDF-RT API Web service via HTTP program elements, using URLs. The Drug Interaction Checker uses a SAX parser (NSXML parser for mobile environment) to request information about drugs from the RESTful Web service to call methods and get responses. Figure 9.3 shows the framework of the proposed solution:

Web Service Resources Composition

Drug Interaction Checker utilizes two resources from NDF-RT API. It is built using a workflow composition of the resources. When the end user enters the name of

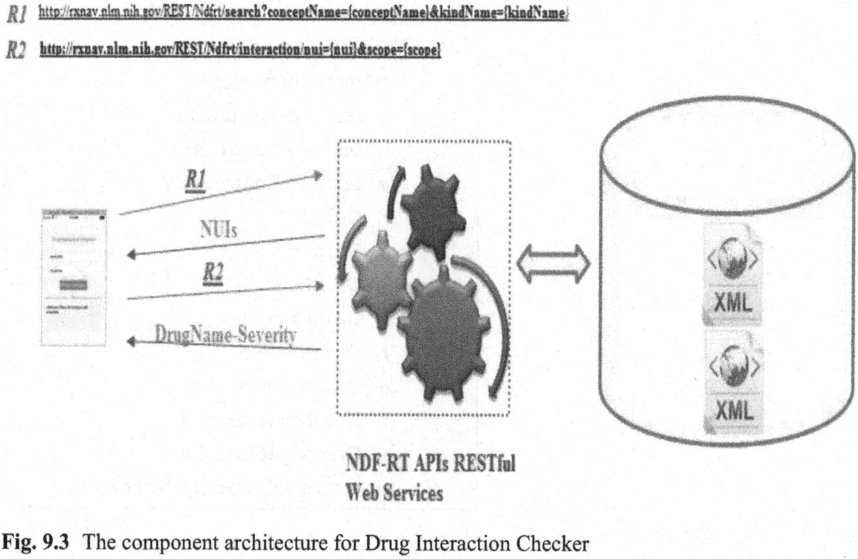

Fig. 9.3 The component architecture for Drug Interaction Checker

Table 9.5 Illustration of the request and responses for utilized resources

Request (input)	Response (output)
R1 (Name1)	R1 (NUI 1)
R1 (Name2)	R1 (NUI 2)
R2 (NUI 1, NUI2)	F (does interact with/does not interact with) + R2 (Name1, F, Name2, severity)

NUI natural user interface

the drug, it is considered as the input for the first resource. To retrieve the output, which is a natural user interface (NUI), the same resource is used for the second drug. Then, these two outputs are used as inputs for the second resource to give the output through a customized function that searches for the intersection between the two drugs in specific drug names to provide interaction information ("does" or "does not") in addition to the output of R2 (name and severity). The composition of resources and their inputs and outputs are illustrated in Table 9.5.

The application (Drug Interaction Checker) was built to enable interaction with the end users in that they could enter their drugs and obtain interaction information. Furthermore, the application constructs the functions mentioned in the requirements section, develops the software, and codes the program. The organization of the files used for implementing the mobile application is listed in Fig. 9.4.The functionality of each file is explained in Appendix 1.

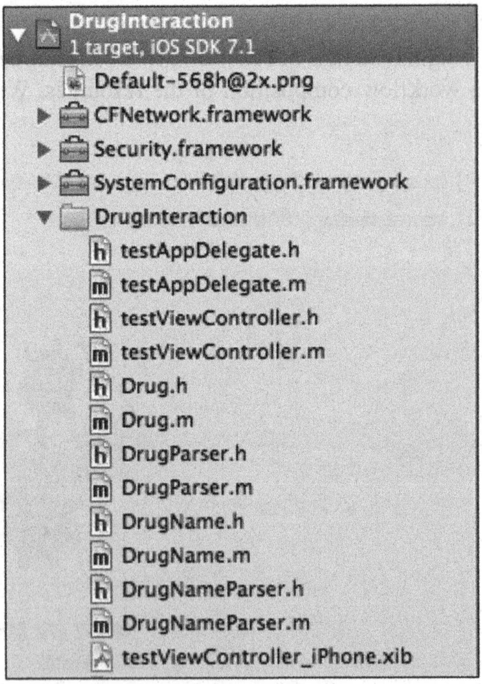

Fig. 9.4 The structure for the files used to implement the Drug Interaction Checker

```
#import <Foundation/Foundation.h>

@interface DrugName : NSObject {

  NSString *Name;
    NSString *Nui;
    NSString *Kind;

}
@property (nonatomic, retain) NSString *Nui;
@property (nonatomic, retain) NSString *Kind;
@property (nonatomic, retain) NSString *Name;

@end
```

Fig. 9.5 DrugName.h creates the objects for drug 1 and drug 2 for R1

```
#import "Drug.h"
@implementation Drug

@synthesize Name;
@synthesize Nui;
@synthesize Kind;
@synthesize Severity;

- (void)dealloc {
    [Name release],Name=nil;
    [Nui release],Nui=nil;
    [Kind release],Kind=nil;
    [Severity release],Severity=nil;
    [super dealloc];
}
@end
```

Fig. 9.6 DrugName.m allocates and deallocates the objects for drug 1 and drug 2 for R1

The application creates objects for R1, R2, and their NXML parsers. First, the object of R1 is created by the DrugName.h and DrugName.m. Actually, it creates two objects: one for drug 1 and the other for drug 2, as shown in Figs. 9.5 and 9.6.

These attributes, Name, NUI, Kind, and Severity, are the outputs retrieved from R1. Every attribute is parsed during the creation of the NXML parser object. This object has been created by DrugNameParser.h and DrugNameParser.m. The NXML parser parses each attribute using parser methods (streams), as can be seen in Fig. 9.7.

```
#import <Foundation/Foundation.h>
#import "DrugName.h"

@interface DrugNameParser : NSObject <NSXMLParserDelegate> {
    NSString *currentElementName;
    NSString *currentElementValue;
    NSMutableArray *DrugArray;
    BOOL beginNewObj;
}

@property (nonatomic, retain) NSMutableArray *DrugArray;
@property BOOL beginNewObj;

- (void)parserDidStartDocument:(NSXMLParser *)parser;
- (void)parserDidEndDocument:(NSXMLParser *)parser;
- (void)parser:(NSXMLParser *)parser didStartElement:(NSString *)elementName
    ;
- (void)parser:(NSXMLParser *)parser didEndElement:(NSString *)elementName n
- (void)parser:(NSXMLParser *)parser foundCharacters:(NSString *)string;

@end
```

Fig. 9.7 DrugNameParser.h creates the objects for the NXML parser

The parsed data are held in NSMutableDrugArray and take into account that the only output needed to be retrieved is NUI. In addition, by following the same processes, two objects are initiated: one for the output for R2 and the other for the NXML parser. The object for R2 defines the attributes Name, NUI, Kind, and Severity in Drug.h, while Drug.m is defined to allocate and deallocate the object (Figs. 9.8 and 9.9).

```
#import <Foundation/Foundation.h>

@interface Drug : NSObject {

    NSString *Name;
    NSString *Nui;
    NSString *Kind;
    NSString *Severity;
}
@property (nonatomic, retain) NSString *Nui;
@property (nonatomic, retain) NSString *Kind;
@property (nonatomic, retain) NSString *Name;
@property (nonatomic, retain) NSString *Severity;

@end
```

Fig. 9.8 Drug.h creates the objects for R2

Fig. 9.9 DrugName.m to allocate and deallocate the objects for R2

```
#import "Drug.h"
@implementation Drug

@synthesize Name;
@synthesize Nui;
@synthesize Kind;
@synthesize Severity;

- (void)dealloc {
    [Name release],Name=nil;
    [Nui release],Nui=nil;
    [Kind release],Kind=nil;
    [Severity release],Severity=nil;
    [super dealloc];
}
@end
```

All attributes are parsed with their own NXML parser object, as defined in DrugParser.h and DrugParser.m (Fig. 9.10).

After defining the objects for each of the outputs of R1 and R2 and defining an NXML parser for each them, two necessary functions are defined, F1 and F2. F1 is FindConceptByName, while F2 is GetDrugInteraction (Fig. 9.11).

Each function calls its URL to parse their attributes (drug data). F1: FindConceptByName calls its R1, which is represented by the URL, as shown in Fig. 9.12. This technique is used to retrieve appropriate outputs or attributes by entering the name of the drug as an input. These attributes come through the parsing processes.

```
#import <Foundation/Foundation.h>

#import "Drug.h"

@interface DrugParser : NSObject <NSXMLParserDelegate> {
    NSString *currentElementName;
    NSString *currentElementValue;
    NSMutableArray *DrugArray;
    BOOL beginNewObj;
}
@property (nonatomic, retain) NSString *currentElementName;
@property (nonatomic, retain) NSString *currentElementValue;
@property (nonatomic, retain) NSMutableArray *DrugArray;
@property BOOL beginNewObj;


- (void)parserDidStartDocument:(NSXMLParser *)parser;
- (void)parserDidEndDocument:(NSXMLParser *)parser;
- (void)parser:(NSXMLParser *)parser didStartElement:(NSString *)elementName
  ;
- (void)parser:(NSXMLParser *)parser didEndElement:(NSString *)elementName na
- (void)parser:(NSXMLParser *)parser foundCharacters:(NSString *)string;

@end
```

Fig. 9.10 DrugParser.h creates the objects for the NXML parser

```
@interface testViewController : UIViewController  <UITextFieldDelegate>
{
    IBOutlet UITextView *output;
    NSString *drug1;
    NSString *drug2;

    IBOutlet UITextField *tefield1;
    IBOutlet UITextField *tefield2;

    NSMutableArray *myArray;
}
@property(assign,nonatomic) NSMutableArray *myArray;
-(IBAction)Checkname;
-(BOOL)isInternetAvailable;
-(NSString*) FindConceptByName: (NSString*) dNui;
-(NSString*) getDrugInteraction: (NSString*) d1 With:(NSString*) d2;

@end
```

Fig. 9.11 Defining F1 and F2 to implement R1 and R2

```
-(NSString*) FindConceptByName: (NSString*) dNui{
  NSString *outputString1=@"";
  if ([self isInternetAvailable]) { // Check If Internet is available
    NSString *urlString1=[NSString stringWithFormat:@"http://rxnav.nlm.nih.gov/REST/Ndfrt/search?conceptName=%@&kindName=DRUG_KIND",dNui];
    NSMutableURLRequest *request1 = [[NSMutableURLRequest alloc] initWithURL: [NSURL URLWithString: urlString1]];
    NSData *returnData1 = [NSURLConnection sendSynchronousRequest: request1 returningResponse: nil error: nil];
    DrugNameParser *xmlParser = [[DrugNameParser alloc] init];
    NSXMLParser *parser = [[NSXMLParser alloc] initWithData:returnData1];
    [parser setDelegate:xmlParser];
    [parser setShouldProcessNamespaces:NO];
    [parser setShouldReportNamespacePrefixes:NO];
    [parser setShouldResolveExternalEntities:NO];
    [parser parse];
    [parser release];
    [request1 release];
    NSMutableArray *tmp= [[NSMutableArray alloc]initWithArray:[xmlParser DrugArray]];
    self.myArray=tmp;
    if (self.myArray.count>0) {
      Drug *entry = nil;
      int i=0;
      for (entry in self.myArray) {
        i++;
          outputString1=entry.Nui;
      }
    }
    [tmp release];
    [xmlParser release];
  }
```

Fig. 9.12 F1-retrieved drug name using R1

When the parsing processes are completed and successful, the application obtains the necessary outputs, which are Name, NUI, and Kind. In this situation, NUI is the only one used as input for R2.

```
-(IBAction)Checkname{
[self.view endEditing:TRUE];
drug1=tefield1.text;
drug2=tefield2.text;
NSString *drug1Nui=[self FindConceptByName:drug1];
NSString *drug2Nui=[self FindConceptByName:drug2];
output.text=[self getDrugInteraction:drug1Nui With:drug2Nui];
}
```

Fig. 9.13 F2 calls F1 for drug 1 and drug 2

```
-(NSString*) getDrugInteraction: (NSString*) d1 With:(NSString*) d2{
    NSString *outputString=[NSString stringWithFormat:@"%@ Does Not Interact with %@",drug1,drug2];
    [UIApplication sharedApplication].networkActivityIndicatorVisible = YES;
    if ([self isInternetAvailable]) { // Check If Internet is available                 (1)

        NSString *urlString=[NSString stringWithFormat:@"http://rxnav.nlm.nih.gov/REST/Ndfrt/interaction/nui=%@&scope=2",d1];
        NSMutableURLRequest *request = [[NSMutableURLRequest alloc] initWithURL: [NSURL URLWithString: urlString]];
        NSData *returnData = [NSURLConnection sendSynchronousRequest: request returningResponse: nil error: nil];
        DrugParser *xmlParser = [[DrugParser alloc] init];
        NSXMLParser *parser = [[NSXMLParser alloc] initWithData:returnData];
        [parser setDelegate:xmlParser];
        [parser setShouldProcessNamespaces:NO];
        [parser setShouldReportNamespacePrefixes:NO];
        [parser setShouldResolveExternalEntities:NO];
        [parser parse];
        [parser release];
        [request release];
        NSMutableArray *tmp= [[NSMutableArray alloc]initWithArray:[xmlParser DrugArray]];
        self.myArray=tmp;                                                                (3)
        if (self.myArray.count>0) {

            Drug *ddmm;
            int i=0;
            for (ddmm in self.myArray) {
                i++;
                if([ddmm.Nui isEqualToString:d2]){
(2)                 outputString= [NSString stringWithFormat:@"%@ Interact with %@ and the Severity is %@",drug1,drug2,ddmm.Severity];
                }}
        [tmp release];
        [xmlParser release];
    }
```

Fig. 9.14 F1-retrieved drug name using R1

Then, F2 calls the parsed output NUIs from F1 for each drug name as shown in Fig. 9.13.

When F2 calls the second URL (1), NUIs come through the R2 parsing processes to derive a result of the drug name and the severity (2). In addition, to find out the drug interaction information, F2 searches for the drug interactions for the first drug, and then compares it with the drug information for the second drug (3) to discover the certain interactions of drugs, as shown in Fig. 9.14).

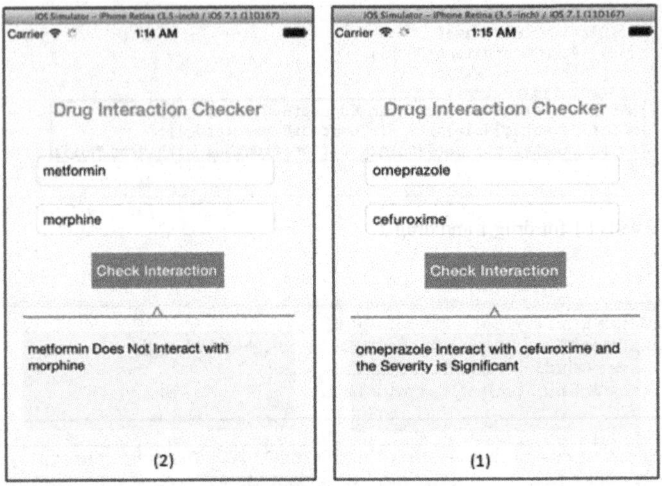

Fig. 9.15 Drug Interaction Checker interface with two possible outputs

Demonstrate the Prototype in the Final Interface

As shown in Fig. 9.15, the project presents two possible outputs for the Drug Interaction Checker: Does Not Interact and Does Interact. Two entered drug names are defined in F1 to convert DrugName to the corresponding NUI. F2 calls F1 for each entered drug name (e.g., metformin and morphine), then uses the outputs of F1 as an input for F2 (only uses NUIs), which are N0000145914 and N000002198, respectively, to retrieve the second drug data, which is defined as the object drug for F2. So, the outputs will be as shown in Fig. 9.15: (1) when entering (metformin) and (morphine) with interaction. The output will be as (2) when entering (omeprazole) and (cefuroxime) with no interaction.

Theoretical Framework

There are three main variables. The independent variable (IV) is the main purpose of the study (Drug Interaction Checker), while the dependent variable (DV; improves patient's awareness) influences the IV positively or negatively. In addition, a moderate variable (MV) affects the relationship between the IV and the DV. The MV is "the comprehensiveness of NDF-RT as a classification standard" because the comprehensiveness of this standard increases the success of the Drug Interaction Checker. The theoretical framework is illustrated in Fig. 9.16.

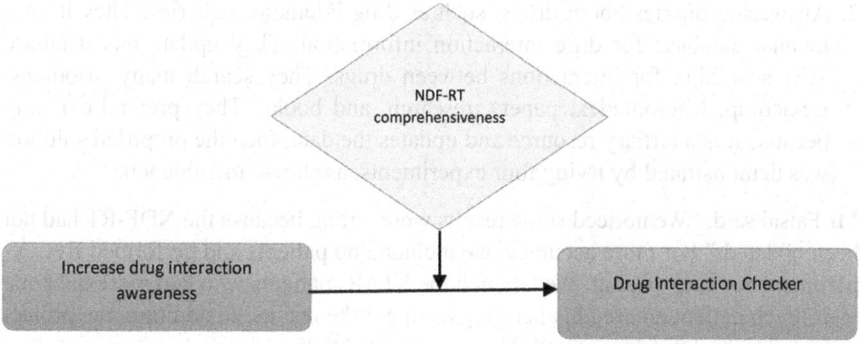

Fig. 9.16 Theoretical framework

Hypothesis

The project has one simple hypothesis, which is H1: The Drug Interaction Checker will improve awareness if the NDF-RT is comprehensive (data are complete and up to date).

Hypothesis Testing

The project intends to outline the benefits of establishing a Drug Interaction Checker to complement biomedical health services by evaluating NDF-RT as a comprehensive database. The project intends to focus on the moderate variable, comprehensiveness of NDF-RT, because it affects the relationship between the awareness of patients with regard to their drug interaction information and Drug Interaction Checker implementation based on two pillars: the NDF-RT classification standard can cover most drugs (completeness) and the NDF-RT classification standard updates their drug interaction information (modernization).

Pilot Study

The Drug Interaction Checker was presented to the Drug Information Services Department. Faisal Aledi, Drugs Informatics Specialist, evaluated the proposed solution. In addition, the current situation for a drug database for King Fahd Medical City (KFMC) and the Drug Information Services Department, which has many roles, was discussed. The most important roles are:

1. Drug database owner: They feed the drug database by adding or updating drug information. KFMC does not use any international classification standards.

2. Answering queries about drugs, such as drug interaction queries: They have a manual database for drug interaction information. They update this database after searching for interactions between drugs. They search many resources: Lexicomp, Micromedex, papers, research, and books. They prefer Lexicomp because it is a tertiary resource and updates the data; then the proposed solution was demonstrated by trying four experiments, as shown in Table 9.6.

Mr Faisal said, “We noticed some results were wrong because the NDF-RT had not been updated.” For more accuracy, we included 60 patients and performed five experiments for each patient. We targeted the KFMC patients who had more than one visit. Each patient entered his/her drugs and got the results. In addition, the project expected to find the drugs that have two or more NUIs.

Initial Work

Data were prepared and studied on two levels. The first level involved checking the availability of drugs on the NDF-RT to evaluate R1, while the second level involved checking drug interaction information to evaluate R2 and see whether the NDF-RT is up to date.

For the first level, drugs in the experiment were filtered to become 116 distinct drugs entered by the patients, as can be seen in Appendix 2. Seven distinct drugs were not found by NDF-RT. When compared to the Lexicomp used by KFMC, 16 distinct drugs were not found by Lexicomp.

To evaluate the completeness of NDF-RT, the precision, recall, and accuracy were calculated. NDF-RT drug data are represented by oval (A), while Lexicomp drug data are represented by oval (B), and the total data set is represented by rectangle (Z), as shown in Fig. 9.17.

Table 9.6 Primitive experiments demonstrated for first testing

Drug 1	Drug 2	Result	Evaluation
Warfarin	Bactrim	No	Incorrect
Acyclovir	Rifampin	Yes	Correct
Sildenafil	Warfarin	No	Correct
Sildenafil	Cimetidine	No	Incorrect

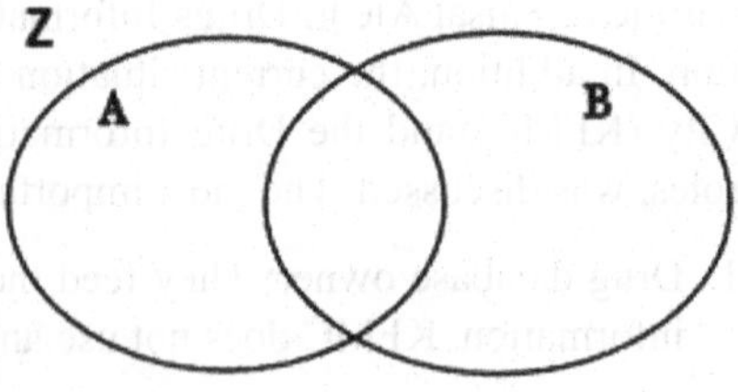

Fig. 9.17 Diagram to represent precision, recall, and accuracy for Drug Interaction Checker

Table 9.7 True positive, true negative, false positive, and false negative defined variables for the first level

	Retrieved by NDF-RT (relevant)	Retrieved by Lexicomp (irrelevant)
Retrieved	109 drugs (TP)	100 drugs (FP)
Not retrieved	7 drugs (TN)	16 drugs (FN)

NDF-RT National Drug File-Reference Terminology, *TP* true positive, *TN* true negative, *FP* false positive, *FN* false negative

Are precision, recall, and accuracy good measures for assessing the retrieved data from NDF-RT? These measures are considered appropriate for analyzing the results for retrieved data. Precision is the retrieved data from NDF-RT divided by the retrieved data from NDF-RT and the retrieved data by Lexicomp, to establish how much of the relevant data was retrieved. Recall is the retrieved data by NDF-RT divided by the retrieved data by NDF-RT and the not retrieved data by Lexicomp, to establish how much of the whole data was retrieved. The accuracy is calculated by the retrieved data from NDF-RT divided by the retrieved data from NDF-RT and Lexicomp, added to the not retrieved data from NDF-RT and Lexicomp. Table 9.7 reviews the discovered drugs and non-discovered drugs from NDF-RT and Lexicomp.

In addition, true positive (TP), true negative (TN), false positive (FP), and false negative (FN) were calculated for the previous measures. A total of 116 distinct drugs were tested, and of those, 109 drugs were true relevant positive and 7 drugs were relevant negative by NDF-RT. Then, 100 drugs were irrelevant positive and 16 were irrelevant negative by Lexicomp.

All variables were obtained for the precision, recall, and accuracy calculations. They were calculated based on these formulas:

$$Recall = \mathrm{TP} / (\mathrm{TP} + \mathrm{FN}) = 109 / (109 + 16) = 0.87 => 87\%.$$

$$Precision = \mathrm{TP} / (\mathrm{TP} + \mathrm{FP}) = 109 / (109 + 100) = 0.52 => 52\%.$$

$$\begin{aligned} Accuracy &= (\mathrm{TP} + \mathrm{TN}) / (\mathrm{TP} + \mathrm{TN} + \mathrm{FP} + \mathrm{FN}) \\ &= (109 + 7) / (109 + 7 + 100 + 16) = 0.50 => 50\%. \end{aligned}$$

At the second level, the data were classified into compatible and different results categories between NDF-RT and Lexicomp. The "different category" data were studied to evaluate the modernization of NDF-RT (i.e., how up to date it is). Also, if the result was "yes" for one resource, but corresponded with a "no" answer with the other resource, the one with the "yes" answer is the most updated one. Again, the precision, recall, and accuracy were calculated. After 300 experiments, the results were analyzed, as can be seen in Appendix 3.

Table 9.8 True positive, true negative, false positive, and false negative defined variables for the second level

	Retrieved by NDF-RT (relevant)	Retrieved by Lexicomp (irrelevant)
Retrieved	1 experiment (TP)	63 experiments (FP)
Not retrieved	61 experiments (TN)	3 experiments (FN)

NDF-RT National Drug File-Reference Terminology, *TP* true positive, *TN* true negative, *FP* false positive, *FN* false negative

The result showed that there was 1 true relevant positive and 63 relevant negatives (2 were "unfound" and 61 were "no" answers) by NDF-RT. Then, 61 were irrelevant positive and 3 were irrelevant negative (with "no" answers) by Lexicomp, as can be seen in Table 9.8.

By substituting the variables to calculate:

$$\begin{aligned} Accuracy &= (\mathrm{TP}+\mathrm{TN})/(\mathrm{TP}+\mathrm{TN}+\mathrm{FP}+\mathrm{FN}) \\ &= (1+61)/(1+61+63+3) = 0.48 \Rightarrow 48\% \end{aligned}$$

$$Recall = \mathrm{TP}/(\mathrm{TP}+\mathrm{FN}) = 1/(1+3) = 0.25 \Rightarrow 25\%$$

$$Precision = \mathrm{TP}/(\mathrm{TP}+\mathrm{FP}) = 1/(1+63) = 0.015 \Rightarrow 1.5\%$$

Results and Discussion

The optimal result for any retrieved data is high precision, high recall, and high accuracy. Actually, this result will rarely happen; therefore, it is acceptable to achieve high precision or high recall. The research was concerned with achieving high precision to avoid the risk of not retrieving data (low recall; Table 9.9).

Precision and *recall* are the two measures upon which the system accuracy metrics are based. They are illustrated together to represent the overall effectiveness, or accuracy, of retrieved data based on their value. The matrix has four regions to explain the situation for any given result. The research provided the following results, as shown in Fig. 9.18.

1. R1 has high recall and moderate precision: This result is fair to prove that NDF-RT-R1 is near the optimal result. So, this means that NDF-RT retrieved the most relevant drug data.
2. Unfortunately, R2 has very low recall and very low precision. This result suggests that NDF-RT-R2 is far from the optimal solution because even though the NDF-RT retrieved relevant drug data, the drug interaction information for these data was not updated continuously. This is considered the greatest defect for the NDF-RT database.

Table 9.9 Results conclusion of the measure for R1 and R2

	R1	R2
Precision	52 %	1.5 %
Recall	87 %	25 %
Accuracy	50 %	48 %

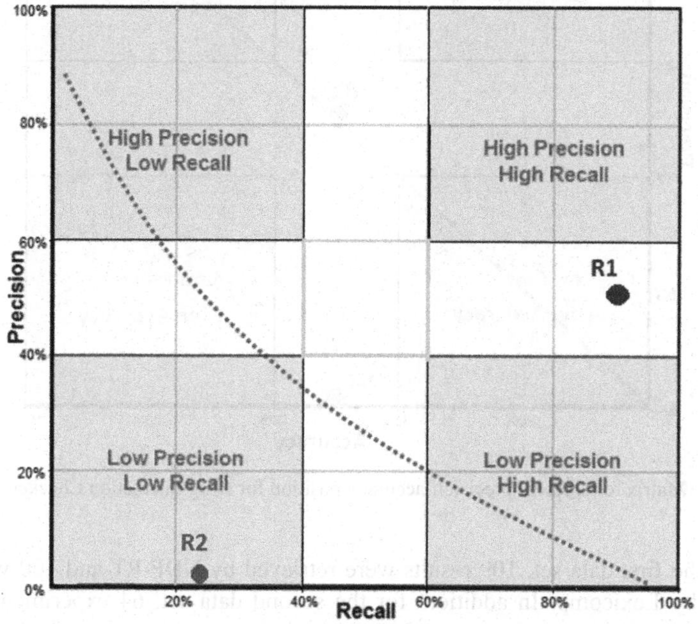

Fig. 9.18 Matrix to represent precision–recall position for Drug Interaction Checker

To guarantee the validity of the result, the optimal result is high precision and high accuracy, as can be noticed in Fig. 9.19, where:

1. R1 had moderate accuracy and moderate precision. So, this result is sufficient to prove that NDF-RT-R1 is near the optimal result. So, NDF-RT retrieved the most relevant drug data.
2. R2 has very low accuracy and very low precision. This result is sufficient to show that NDF-RT-R2 is far from the optimal solution for the same reasons shown above.

Summary

After collecting 300 experiments from end users, they became 116 filtered drugs as a data set used to evaluate R1. The results from NDF-RT and Lexicomp were compared and then were classified into "compatible" and "different" categories; then the "different" category was chosen as the data set for R2.

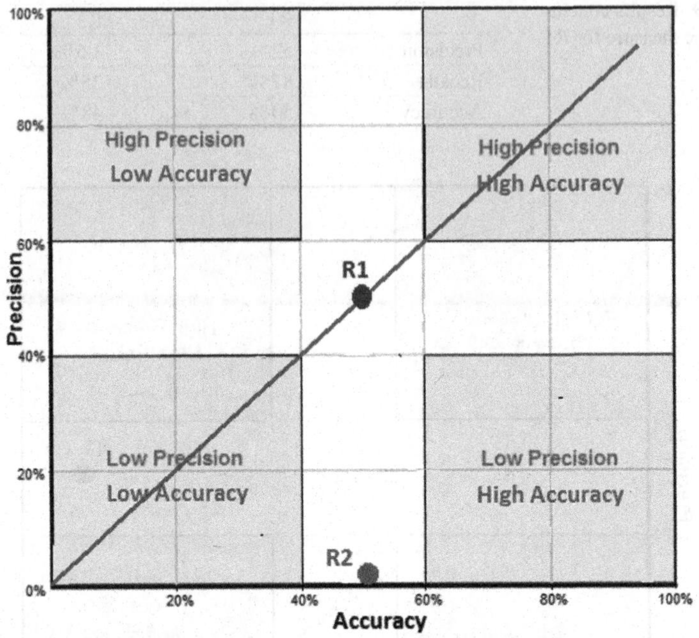

Fig. 9.19 Matrix to represent precision-accuracy position for Drug Interaction Checker

For the first data set, 109 results were retrieved by NDF-RT and 100 were retrieved by Lexicomp. In addition, for the second data set, 64 experiments from the "different" category were tested. One retuned a "yes" answer and 63 returned "unfound drug" (2) or "no" answers (61) by NDF-RT, while Lexicomp returned 61 "yes" answers and 3 "no" answers to evaluate R2.

Precision, recall, and accuracy were calculated to evaluate R1 and R2. To get the best results, all of these measures need to be high. The results for R1 showed high recall, moderate precision, and moderate accuracy; therefore, R1 was near to the optimal result. However, the result for R2 was low recall, low precision, and low accuracy; therefore, R2 was far from the optimal result.

Limitations of NDF-RT

1. This study was a pilot work and was on a limited scale; therefore, the generalizability of this study is unreliable, but at least, it presents the basic trends for NDF-RT.
2. Drugs that had more than one NUI were excluded due to the limitations of time and the fact that the concept that some drugs had more than one NUI was not discovered until evaluation time, which forced the project to exclude them.

3. The information for drugs interaction was not updated. This could lead to serious problems if the end users relied on the information.
4. NDF-RT API Web services do not provide functions to retrieve the brand name of drugs because it is the common language for all end users.
5. Saudi Arabia has different drug databases (Food and Drug Association, Ministry of Health, and Medical Cities) leading to different drug names for specific drugs; this leads to difficulty in connecting to NDF-RT APIs Web services.

Recommendations

1. NLM and VA must update R2 and keep up to modernization of these resources.
2. Try connecting a barcode reader to the Drug Interaction Checker to read drugs instead of entering manually.
3. Include all drugs that have more than one NUI.
4. Check interaction information for more than two drugs.

Conclusion

The project aimed to trial a technical solution to utilize international databases and enable end users to gain benefits from them. NDF-RT API Web services provide different functions by creating workflows to provide the necessary output using two or more functions. The output of the first resource is used as an input for the second resource. In addition, the study evaluated the comprehensiveness (the completeness for R1 and the modernization for R2) of NDF-RT. The project collected 300 experiments and utilized 116 distinct drugs in the trial. The results demonstrated that NDF-RT returned the greatest number of drug names, but the interaction information was not updated regularly enough.

Appendix 1

The description for the .h/.m/.Xib files used to implement Drug Interaction Checker.

File	Description
Drug.h	A file for a header class defines the object of the output for R2
Drug.m	A file for implement class to allocate and deallocate the object of the output for R2
DrugParser.h	A file for a header class defines the object of NXML Parser with their stream methods for the output of R2

File	Description
DrugParser.m	A file for implement class to allocate and deallocate the object of NXML Parser of the output for R2
DrugName.h	A file for a header class defines the object of the output for R1
DrugName.m	A file for implement class to allocate and deallocate the object of the output for R1
DrugNameParser.h	A file for a header class defines the object of NXML Parser with their stream methods for the output of R1
DrugNameParser.m	A file for implement class to allocate and deallocate the object of NXML Parser of the output for R1
testAppDelegate.h	A file defines the view as an object
testAppDelegate.m	A file used to add the view to window. Also to allocate and deallocate the object
testViewController.h	A file defines class to manage the views. Contains all of the IBOutlets and IBAction methods for the view
testViewController.m	A file for implement class defines IBOutlets and IBAction methods with several methods created automatically customized based on the needs
testViewController-iPhone.xib	Graphic file for the mobile application interface

Appendix 2

A data set for first level R1.

Distinct drugs data set		
Acarbose	Enoxaparin	Memantine
Alfacalcidol	Escitalopram	Metformin
Amitriptyline	Esomeprazole	Metoclopramide
Amlodipine	Etoposide	Miconazole
Amoxicillin	Fentanyl	Mirtazapine
Aprepitant	Filgrastim	Morphine
Aspirin	Fluticasone	Moxifloxacin
Atenolol	Folic acid	Naproxen
Atomoxetine	Furosemide	Nifedipine
Atorvastatin	Fusidate sodium	Nitrofurantoin
Azithromycin	Gabapentin	Nystatin
Benzaclin	Glibenclamide	Octreotide
Bisacodyl	Glimepiride	Ofloxacin
Bisoprolol	Glipizide	Omeprazole
Brimonidine	Haloperido	Ondansetron
Budesonide	Hydralazine	Pegfilgrastim
Calcium	Hydrocortisone	Perindopril
Candesartan	Ibuprofen	Phosphate
Capecitabine	Ipratropium	Potassium
Captopril	Irbesartan	Potassium chloride
Carboxymethylcellulose	Isoniazid	Prednisolone

Distinct drugs data set		
Carvedilol	Isosorbide	Pregabalin
Cefuroxime	Isosorbide dinitrate	Pyridoxine
Cholecalciferol	Lactulose	Rabeprazole
Ciprofloxacin	Lamotrigine	Ranitidine
Clopidogrel	Lapatinib	Rivaroxaban
Dabigatran	Levetiracetam	Rosuvastatin
Dasatinib	Levocabastine	Salbutamol
Dexamethasone	Levothyroxine	Senna
Diclofenac	Lidocaine	Sevelamer
Digoxin	Linezolid	Simethicone
Diltiazem	Lisinopril	Sodium bicarbonate
Diphenhydramine	Loperamide	Sodium chloride
Docusate	Loratadine	Spironolactone
Domperidone	Magnesium	Timolol
Dorzolamide	Meclizine	Trimethoprim
Doxycycline	Megestrol	Ursodeoxycholic
Enalapril	Meloxicam	Vitamin B
		Warfarin

Appendix 3

The drugs found by Drug Interaction Checker (retrieved—relevant).

Experiment no.	Experiment no./user	User no.	Drug 1	Drug 2	Answer
81	1	17	Fluticasone	Warfarin	Yes

The drugs not found by Drug Interaction Checker (not retrieved—relevant).

Experiment no.	Experiment no./user	User no.	Drug 1	Drug 2	Answer
3	3	1	Clopidogrel	Atorvastatin	No
6	1	2	Amitriptyline	Hydralazine	No
7	2	2	Aspirin	Hydralazine	No
18	3	4	Glimepiride	Perindopril	No
22	2	5	Levothyroxine	Metformin	No
25	5	5	Rabeprazole	Aspirin	No
26	1	6	Furosemide	Hydralazine	No
28	3	6	Amlodipine	Aspirin	No
31	1	7	Furosemide	Hydralazine	No
33	3	7	Aspirin	Bisoprolol	No
41	1	9	Ciprofloxacin	Ibuprofen	No
47	2	10	Digoxin	Spirnoolactnoe	No

Experiment no.	Experiment no./ user	User no.	Drug 1	Drug 2	Answer
48	3	10	Digoxin	Bisoprolol	No
52	2	11	Bisoprolol	Diclofenac	No
53	3	11	Rabeprazole	Clopidogrel	No
55	5	11	Aspirin	Lisinopril	No
59	4	12	Clopidogrel	Dabigatran	No
62	2	13	Bisoprolol	Aspirin	No
63	3	13	Diclofenac	Irbesartan	No
64	4	13	Moxifloxacin	Diclofenac	No
69	4	14	Warfarin	Rabeprazole	No
71	1	15	Aspirin	Digoxin	No
77	2	16	Lisinopril	Aspirin	No
86	1	18	Bisoprolol	Aspirin	No
89	4	18	Meloxicam	Bisoprolol	No
97	2	20	Bisoprolol	Levothyroxine	No
104	4	21	Aspirin	Rabeprazole	No
105	5	21	Nifedipine	Lisinopril	No
111	1	23	Atenolol	Furosemide	No
112	2	23	Digoxin	Captopril	No
120	5	24	Aspirin	Spirnoolactnoe	No
122	2	25	Lisinopril	Aspirin	No
123	3	25	Furosemide	Bisoprolol	No
125	5	25	Linezolid	Bisoprolol	No
126	1	26	Warfarin	Escitalopram	No
128	3	26	Candesartan	Aspirin	No
131	1	27	Metolaznoe	Bisoprolol	No
132	2	27	Aspirin	Amlodipine	No
135	5	27	Metolaznoe	Rabeprazole	No
139	4	28	Ciprofloxacin	Levothyroxine	No
147	2	30	Bisoprolol	Furosemide	No
150	5	30	Spirnoolactnoe	Aspirin	No
151	1	31	Aspirin	Atomoxetine	Drug 2 not found
158	3	32	Metformin	Carvedilol	No
162	2	33	Irbesartan	Nifedipine	No
164	4	33	Meloxicam	Furosemide	No
167	2	34	Diclofenac	Furosemide	No
169	4	34	Clopidogrel	Aspirin	No
171	1	35	Aspirin	Bisoprolol	No
173	3	35	Enalapril	Nifedipine	No
176	1	36	Amlodipine	Aspirin	No
185	5	37	Metformin	Ranitidine	No
186	1	38	Amlodipine	Carvedilol	No
194	4	39	Haloperido	Levetiracetam	No

Experiment no.	Experiment no./user	User no.	Drug 1	Drug 2	Answer
195	5	39	Levetiracetam	Haloperido	No
200	5	40	Diclofenac	Moxifloxacin	No
213	3	43	Metformin	Morphine	No
250	5	50	Timolol	Ibuprofen	No
261	1	53	Dexamethasnoe	Diclofenac	No
282	2	57	Aprepitant	Metoclopramide	Drug 1 not found
286	1	58	Escitalopram	Micnoazole	No
287	2	58	Mirtazapine	Fentanyl	No
296	1	60	Dexamethasnoe	Lactulose	No

The drugs found by Lexicomp (retrieved—irrelevant).

Experiment no.	Experiment no./user	User no.	Drug 1	Drug 2	Lexicomp
3	3	1	Clopidogrel	Atorvastatin	Yes
6	1	2	Amitriptyline	Hydralazine	Yes
7	2	2	Aspirin	Hydralazine	Yes
18	3	4	Glimepiride	Perindopril	Yes
22	2	5	Levothyroxine	Metformin	Yes
25	5	5	Rabeprazole	Aspirin	Yes
26	1	6	Furosemide	Hydralazine	Yes
28	3	6	Amlodipine	Aspirin	Yes
31	1	7	Furosemide	Hydralazine	Yes
33	3	7	Aspirin	Bisoprolol	Yes
41	1	9	Ciprofloxacin	Ibuprofen	Yes
47	2	10	Digoxin	Spirnoolactnoe	Yes
48	3	10	Digoxin	Bisoprolol	Yes
52	2	11	Bisoprolol	Diclofenac	Yes
53	3	11	Rabeprazole	Clopidogrel	Yes
55	5	11	Aspirin	Lisinopril	Yes
59	4	12	Clopidogrel	Dabigatran	Yes
62	2	13	Bisoprolol	Aspirin	Yes
63	3	13	Diclofenac	Irbesartan	Yes
64	4	13	Moxifloxacin	Diclofenac	Yes
69	4	14	Warfarin	Rabeprazole	Yes
71	1	15	Aspirin	Digoxin	Yes
77	2	16	Lisinopril	Aspirin	Yes
86	1	18	Bisoprolol	Aspirin	Yes
89	4	18	Meloxicam	Bisoprolol	Yes
97	2	20	Bisoprolol	Levothyroxine	Yes
104	4	21	Aspirin	Rabeprazole	Yes

Experiment no.	Experiment no./user	User no.	Drug 1	Drug 2	Lexicomp
105	5	21	Nifedipine	Lisinopril	Yes
111	1	23	Atenolol	Furosemide	Yes
112	2	23	Digoxin	Captopril	Yes
120	5	24	Aspirin	Spirnoolactnoe	Yes
122	2	25	Lisinopril	Aspirin	Yes
123	3	25	Furosemide	Bisoprolol	Yes
125	5	25	Linezolid	Bisoprolol	Yes
126	1	26	Warfarin	Escitalopram	Yes
128	3	26	Candesartan	Aspirin	Yes
131	1	27	Metolaznoe	Bisoprolol	Yes
132	2	27	Aspirin	Amlodipine	Yes
135	5	27	Metolaznoe	Rabeprazole	Yes
139	4	28	Ciprofloxacin	Levothyroxine	Yes
147	2	30	Bisoprolol	Furosemide	Yes
150	5	30	Spirnoolactnoe	Aspirin	Yes
158	3	32	Metformin	Carvedilol	Yes
162	2	33	Irbesartan	Nifedipine	Yes
164	4	33	Meloxicam	Furosemide	Yes
167	2	34	Diclofenac	Furosemide	Yes
169	4	34	Clopidogrel	Aspirin	Yes
171	1	35	Aspirin	Bisoprolol	Yes
173	3	35	Enalapril	Nifedipine	Yes
176	1	36	Amlodipine	Aspirin	Yes
185	5	37	Metformin	Ranitidine	Yes
186	1	38	Amlodipine	Carvedilol	Yes
194	4	39	Haloperido	Levetiracetam	Yes
195	5	39	Levetiracetam	Haloperido	Yes
200	5	40	Diclofenac	Moxifloxacin	Yes
213	3	43	Metformin	Morphine	Yes
250	5	50	Timolol	Ibuprofen	Yes
261	1	53	Dexamethasnoe	Diclofenac	Yes
286	1	58	Escitalopram	Micnoazole	Yes
287	2	58	Mirtazapine	Fentanyl	Yes
296	1	60	Dexamethasnoe	Lactulose	Yes

The drugs not found by Lexicomp (not retrieved—irrelevant).

Experiment no.	Experiment no./user	User no.	Drug 1	Drug 2	Lexicomp
81	1	17	Fluticasone	Warfarin	No
151	1	31	Aspirin	Atomoxetine	No
282	2	57	Aprepitant	Metoclopramide	No

References

Asuncion, G.-P., Marcos, M.-R., Alejandro, R.-G., Guillermo, V., & Jose, M. V.-N. (2013). Ontologies in medicinal chemistry: Current status and future challenges. *Current Topics in Medicinal Chemistry, 31*(5), 576–590.

Barrière, C., & Gagnon, M. (2011). *Drugs and disorders: From specialized resources to Web data.* Paper presented at the Workshop on Web Scale Knowledge Extraction at the 10th International Semantic Web Conference.

Bodenreider, O., Mougin, F., & Burgun, A. (2010). *Automatic determination of anticoagulation status with NDF-RT.* Paper presented at the 13th ISMB Special Interest Group Meeting on Bio-Ontologies.

Boyce, R., Horn, J., Hassanzadeh, O., de Waard, A., Schneider, J., Luciano, J., et al. (2013). Dynamic enhancement of drug product labels to support drug safety, efficacy, and effectiveness. *Journal of Biomedical Semantics, 4*(1), 5.

Fry, C. (2005). U.S. Patent Patent No.: B. CA.

iOS Developer Library. (2013). https://developer.apple.com/library/ios/documentation/Cocoa/Reference/Foundation/Classes/NSXMLParser_Class/Reference/Reference.html. Accessed 29 April 2014.

Karaiskos, C. (2013). Enhanced ontological searching of medical scientific information. University of Manchester.

Lexi comp. (2014). http://www.lexi.com. Accessed 29 April 2014.

Mortensen, J. (2010). *Evaluating NDF-RT.* Paper presented at the Fourth International Symposium on Semantic Mining in Biomedicine (SMBM).

Mortensen, J., & Bodenreider, O. (2010). *Comparing pharmacologic classes in NDF-RT and SNOMED CT.* Paper presented at the Fourth International Symposium for Semantic Mining in Biomedicine.

Mougin, F., Burgun, A., & Bodenreider, O. (2012). *Comparing drug-class membership in ATC and NDF-RT.* Paper presented at the the 2nd ACM SIGHIT International Health Informatics Symposium, Miami, Florida.

NDF-RT API. (2014). http://rxnav.nlm.nih.gov/NdfrtAPIs.html. Accessed 22 March 2014.

Nelson, S., Zeng, K., Kilbourne, J., Powell, T., & Moore, R. (2011). Normalized names for clinical drugs RxNorm at 6 years. *Journal of American Medical Informatics Association, 18*(4), 441–448.

Pathak, J., & Chute, C. (2011). Analyzing categorical information in two publicly available drug terminologies: RxNorm and NDF-RT. *Journal of American Medical Informatics Association, 17*(4), 432–439.

Pathak, J., Murphy, S., Willaert, B., Kremers, H., Yawn, B., Rocca, W., et al. (2011a). *Using RxNorm to extract medication data from electronic health records in the Rochester Epidemiology Project.* Paper presented at the International Conference in Biomedical Ontology, Buffalo, NY, USA.

Pathak, J., Weiss, L., Durski, M., Zhu, Q., Freimuth, R., & Chute, C. (2011b). Integrating VA's NDF-RT drug terminology with PharmGKB: Preliminary results. *Pacific Symposium on Biocomputing* (PubMed.), *200*(4), 400–409.

Petersa, L., Mortensen, J., Nguyena, T., & Bodenreidera, O. (2013). Enabling complex queries to drug information sources through functional composition. *Lister Hill National Center for Biomedical Communications, 192*(6), 692–696.

SAX and DOM Parser. (2014). http://www.cs.nmsu.edu/~epontell/courses/XML/material/xml-parsers.html. Accessed 22 March 2014.

The New Over-the-Counter Medicine Label: Take a Look. (2014). http://www.fda.gov/drugs/emergencypreparedness/bioterrorismanddrugpreparees/ucm133411.htm. Accessed 22 March 2014.

Unified Medical Language System. (2014). http://www.nlm.nih.gov/research/umls/quickstart.html. Accessed 22 March 2014.

Unified Medical Language System, RxNorm. (2014). https://www.nlm.nih.gov/research/umls/rxnorm. Accessed 22 March 2014.

Unified Medical Language System—2012AB National Drug File—Reference Terminology Source Information. (2014). http://www.nlm.nih.gov/research/umls/sourcereleasedocs/current/NDFRT/. Accessed 1 April 2014.

Zhu, Q., Jiang, G., & Chute, C. (2012). Profiling structured product labeling with NDF-RT and RxNorm. *Journal of Biomedical Semantics, 3*(1), 16.

Zhu, Q., Jiang, G., Wang, L., & Chute, C. (2013). Standardized drug and pharmacological class network construction. *Studies in Health Technology and Informatics* (PubMed.), *192*(1125), 9626–9630.

Awatif Alotaibi is a health informatics specialist at King Fahad Medical City since 5 years. His full name is Awatif Khalid Alotaibi. Under the umbrella of Health Informatics and Information Technology Management in the E_Health department, he had the responsibility to automate the health services for the patients (e.g., eDrugs and iEHR for the patients and EMR for the physicians) besides automating education and continuing training services for external and internal students of the Medical City. He has a Master's certificate in Computer Science from Al-Imam Muhammad Ibn Saud Islamic University, College of Computer and Information Sciences, Information Systems Department. Based on his education and experience, he came up with his work to find a solution that can serve the patients and enhance the technical quality services by utilizing existing drug data source. It is placed at the intersection of the bioinformatics, RESTful Web services, mobile application, and XML parser technique to retrieve drug information. He lives in Riyadh City, Saudi Arabia.

Dr. Mona Alkhattabi completed her PhD from the School of Computing, Informatics and Media, University of Bradford, in 2010. In the same year, she joined as an assistant professor in the Department of Information System, College of Computer and Information Sciences, Al-Imam Muhammad Ibn Saud Islamic University. Dr. Mona is currently the Vice-Dean of E-learning and Distance Education Deanship at Al-Imam Muhammad Ibn Saud Islamic University, Saudi Arabia. She has more than 5 years of educational experience in the field of mathematics, with a bachelor degree from Education College in Riyadh, Saudi Arabia. After she was awarded an M.Sc. in computing with distinction from the University of Bradford in 2006, she started her research in the quality of e-learning content. She has a number of published research papers in her field of specialization. Also, she works as a reviewer for a number of scientific publishing houses.

Chapter 10
Accessibility Issues in Interoperable Sharing of Electronic Health Records: Physician's Perspective

Shalini Bhartiya and Deepti Mehrotra

Introduction

An Electronic Health Record (EHR) is defined as an archive of patient's clinical data processed by a computer. With many hospitals implementing EHRs and other IT systems, the amount of patient data stored in electronic formats continues to grow quickly. This opens an easy and quick channel of communication between two or more independent hospitals and clinics for sharing and accessing patients' records through a common medium.

The users of healthcare domain communicate with the healthcare application in various ways, as described in Fig. 10.1. The channels of the communication (Filipa et al. 2009) are divided into three levels. Level 1 is a stand-alone single-user communication with the healthcare application or hospital information system (HIS). Level 2 is sharing of the patient's EHR between different applications, that is, two independent healthcare entities are referring to the same EHR simultaneously. Level 3 is a more advanced and complex communication that is dynamic in nature. Today, open-source EHR systems (Webster 2011) are proliferating throughout the world, and the nations are developing collaborative programs to promote global and open EHRs for the betterment of healthcare services. EHRs link consumers and providers across the continuum of care and provide relevant information to these groups. Patient privacy becomes a major concern in such environments.

Security is not really about technology, it is about people. Safeguarding the confidentiality, integrity and availability of patient data is no longer a goal, it is a legal requirement (Wyne and Haider 2007). Complying with the meaningful use rules,

S. Bhartiya (✉)
ED-94, Tagore Garden, New Delhi 110027, India
e-mail: shalinibhartiya69@gmail.com

D. Mehrotra
Amity School of Engineering and Technology, Amity University Uttar Pradesh, Sector-125, Noida, Uttar Pradesh, India
e-mail: mehdeepti@gmail.com

N. Wickramasinghe et al. (eds.), *Contemporary Consumer Health Informatics*, Healthcare Delivery in the Information Age, DOI 10.1007/978-3-319-25973-4_10

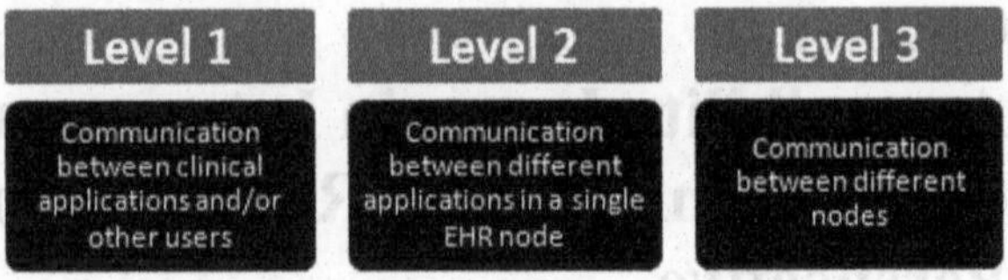

Fig. 10.1 The different levels of communication of an electronic health record *(EHR)*. (Source: Filipa et al. 2009)

which are typically a project for IT departments, hospital administrators are required to take stringent steps to protect electronic information while communicating and sharing it with independent agencies. The degree of need for access, an express statutory mandate, articulated public policy or other recognizable public interest militating towards access is sought. The way users, in this case physicians, interact with available IT resources will determine how successful privacy and security initiatives are.

This study presents the viewpoints of the physicians on certain critical issues that prevail while sharing data with their counterparts. The content of this chapter majorly revolves around accessibility of the EHR in interoperable sharing between hospitals and independent clinics. This analysis would broaden the vision and give better understanding of the relevant checkpoints before accessing confidential health information by any legitimate user. Access to patient information is a key for the most effective and efficient care. It would facilitate the researchers in designing the secured framework for sharing of EHRs in an interoperable healthcare domain.

HIS has many synonyms mentioned throughout the chapter—healthcare management system, hospital management system, clinical management system and electronic healthcare management systems, all contributing to a similar interpretation.

Major Security Aspects to Electronic Health Record Sharing

Interoperability

Interoperability allows information and resource exchange between defined subsystems. Information sharing involves various issues when exchanged in distributed environment. An analysis of various dimensions (Carmagnola et al. 2012), such as languages, protocols, approaches and standards, identifies the challenges pertaining to data exchange. Healthcare interoperability is the sharing of information between medical devices and information systems electronically. Interoperability and deployment of standards for data exchange are technological challenges for which increasingly demanding expectations are being set within the healthcare industry. EHRs formats need to be compatible among all providers to maximize the benefits of the technology. Apart from disparate systems, applications, formats, interfaces and vocabularies, many crucial and relevant clauses affect the establishment of interoperable systems in the healthcare environment.

Confidentiality

Confidentiality refers to the disclosure of EHR between hospitals or other organizations, only to intended and authorized users. The number of issues (Bhartiya and Mehrotra 2013)affects the confidentiality of data during storage and transmission over the network, namely frequent sharing of health records using various media such as compact discs (CDs), web portals, e-mails and physical copies carried by the patient. It exposes the data to various risks and threats. The CD can be lost, copied or damaged; portals can be hacked; e-mail spoofing is common and data can be stolen. Complete access or physical transfer of records might result in full access of health details to the doctor which is highly vulnerable to confidentiality.

Integrity

Integrity assures that the data are accurate all the time. Many factors affect the integrity of health records during their use. Poor documentation or typographical errors (Bhartiya and Mehrotra 2013), use of shortcut keys and drop-down menus, are a few of them. The contributing factors to integrity loss can be direct or indirect. To understand the direct loss to integrity of an EHR, let us take two scenarios as example.

Scenario 1 The patient is discharged from the hospital. The administrative technician generates his discharge report and carries it to the concerned doctor for signature. The doctor makes some changes to the report. The technician applies the said changes and gets the approval of the doctor. Once okayed by the doctor, the technician takes the final print but forgets to save the changes.

Scenario 2 The patient visits the outpatient department (OPD). The doctor treats the patient but could not record the observation due to power failure, delayed response from the system, heavy rush of patients outside or record not available. This study reveals various factors that indirectly affect the integrity of EHRs.

Availability

Doctors visit various hospitals or clinics requiring health records of their patients at varied locations. Moreover, there are referral cases where patient's records are transferred from one hospital to the other. The care providers need to access these records accordingly. The issue of discussion is: *How should data be made accessible to the doctors?* Should data be accessed directly from the data store, be available in read-only format or some other robust method needs to be discovered for secured transit of data over the network? Many factors (Bhartiya and Mehrotra 2013), as stated below, significantly correlate with this issue resulting in poor decision-making:

Multiplicative extension of access right overtime, access to complete data of the patient, different identification methods for the patients (resulting in inconsistent or duplicate records), disparate access methods, lack of decision-making policies on the amount of data to be transferred, need for monitoring and controlling of the data by IT and hospital staff jointly, effects of stringent security policies, frequency of unavailability of data and augmented chances to data breach due to interoperable sharing of EHRs over the network.

Literature Study

It is essential that information can be accessed from anywhere in the health system, even in remote locations, to facilitate seamless communication between care providers. Health Insurance Portability and Accountability Act (HIPAA) Privacy and Security Rules (ONCHIT 2012) clearly emphasize the need of privacy of health information of the patient while sharing among different agencies. It is mandatory for the system to identify any security gaps while accessing EHRs and fulfil its responsibilities for both the HIPAA Privacy Rule (Cheng and Hung 2006) and other applicable laws.

This chapter takes past surveys as the basis for further research on this topic. The surveys considered are those conducted by various national and international bodies, thus giving an authenticated platform for appropriately and correctly analysing the environment under study. The literature surfed broadly encircles the usability, adoptability, security and uniformity of EHRs during exchange.

The growth of data exchange (HIMSS and GETF 2010) clearly indicates an upward trend. It is higher in smaller organizations with number of employees less than 10. Many issues (HIMSS and GETF 2010) such as cost, EHR controlling authority, organization's size and percentage of transactions contribute to the management of well-defined, secured and organized data exchange. Survey (Davis 2009) provides an understanding of the current adoption rates of key electronic medical record (EMR) applications in US hospitals and how effectively the American Recovery and Reinvestment Act (ARRA) funding requirements are met. It provides a review of market relative to 2011, 2013 and 2015 measurements. Electronic Medical Record adoption model (EMRAM) has been divided into eight stages, with stage 0 having nothing installed and stage 7 having a fully EMR system. Privacy and security relative to the HIPAA is required for all stages of the EMRAM model. According to this survey, 2013 measurements need a clinical data warehouse that could store the data for de-identification and aggregation as per specific security requirements.

Furthermore, 2015 measures concentrate on providing patients, on request, with a timely accounting of disclosures for treatment, payment and healthcare operations in compliance with applicable law(s), and incorporate and utilize technology to segment sensitive data.

Requiring a means to transport data among different clinical information systems makes sense only after EHRs can generate standard elements to share and process. The Certification Commission for Healthcare Information Technology (CCHIT 2009) has established a minimum set of criteria for certification, emphasizing a uniform and secure method of transporting EHR from one place to another. The current focus of the commission's interoperability blueprint is on preparing EHRs to use recently identified national standards such as Continuity of Care Document (CCD) and Cross Enterprise Document Sharing (XDS) for representing a patient summary, comprising the types of information that physicians typically ask of others when assuming responsibility for the care of an individual.

The Planning Commission of India (HLEG 2011) recommends a system of universal health coverage (UHC) in India that would ensure the protection of patient's rights and choice of portability and continuity of care. British Standard and European Standard (ISO/IEC 27002 2008) state clear and concrete definitions of various security terminologies. It brings out the security measures required for health information and identifies the significance of risk assessment that can properly determine the level of effort needed to protect confidentiality, integrity and availability.

A watermark encoding and decoding scheme (Kamran and Farooq 2011) on EHR ensures information privacy preserving from malicious attacks, but the health data are heterogeneous in nature. More dynamic and customized techniques need to be developed to ensure patient safety and care, increase efficiencies and improve exchange of information. Moreover, the data are also vulnerable to internal threats. There is a need (Wainer et al. 2008) of designing a robust data-sharing model that would enable smooth and secured sharing between independent but interrelated organizations. New systems and practices are needed to protect the privacy and security of EHRs and ensure compliance with various international compliance regulations.

Researchers and observers around the world have identified the need of standardized healthcare applications that would easily enable the movement of data from one platform to another. A lot has been searched and identified on security issues in such movement of EHRs. Nations are continuously engaged in designing national frameworks to be adopted by all the healthcare agencies for uninterrupted and undisputed health data exchange. Organizations such as the International Organization for Standardization (ISO)/International Electrotechnical Commission (IEC), European Committee for Standardization (CEN) and Certification Commission for Health Information Technology (CCHIT) responsible for designing and developing standards for different domains have given various guidelines such as HIPAA, Health Information Technology for Economic and Clinical Health (HITECH) and Health Level-7 (HL7), catering to the security issues in accessing EHR by the healthcare providers. With all the standards, principles and guidelines at hand, there still arises a need of in-depth understanding of the issues and difficulties faced by the prime stakeholders of EHRs. This encouraged us to conduct a survey on the physicians to capture and analyse their opinions on the security aspects of EHR access in interoperable health data exchange.

Methodology

This is a questionnaire-based system study with an objective of identifying security issues in sharing EHRs in an interoperable environment. This is in continuity with another survey (Bhartiya and Mehrotra 2013) conducted on security issues in sharing of EHRs in stand-alone hospitals or clinics. This survey gave us a basic knowledge about the threats and challenges to secure sharing of health data in an inter-department of a hospital. It also highlights many realistic scenarios that are specific constraints in achieving best-possible security mechanisms in this domain.

The questionnaire produced is fine-grained on the basis of the previous questionnaire. An initial survey, a pilot study, was conducted on ten respondents from various departments. The objective was to further refine the questionnaire in terms of contents, language and sequence. A stratified random sampling was used to identify the sample population. The respondents, that is, physicians ($n=70$), were grouped in a manner to involve each stratum of healthcare departments, namely, general medicine, cardiology, gynaecology, oncology, pathology, orthopaedic, ear, nose and throat (ENT) and dental. The survey includes the observations from private and government hospitals, nursing homes and independent clinics. Only those hospitals that have one or the other HIS installed and where at least some part of the EHR is managed through these systems are selected. The data collected are analysed using statistical techniques applied through an automated statistical tool, Statistical Package for the Social Sciences (SPSS). The result generated is based on the varied usage of the automated system by the doctors.

The questionnaire was distributed and collected personally from the hospitals and clinics. It was also loaded on Google Docs whose link was mailed to more than 100 physicians. The response received online was 25 %.

The basis of analysis is identification of security flaws mainly during accessing of the data from multiple locations. We are interested in observing the relationship of each security control, that is, confidentiality, integrity and availability. The observations show that if we increase one of them, it adversely affects the others, thus making room for security gaps to emerge.

It has been observed that the privacy and confidentiality of patient's data are perceived differently by each doctor. Keeping this in mind, the questionnaire was distributed to 12 different specializations with an objective of recording opinions and mindsets of the physicians from each branch. Table 10.1 shows the count of physicians selected from hospitals and clinics using the convenience random sampling technique for the purpose.

The questionnaire is categorized on four parameters, namely, availability, integrity, confidentiality, and security policies and awareness. In total, there were 30 questions, subdivided into each category. Table 10.2 identifies the number of questions asked under each category.

Table 10.1 Categorization and contribution of each respondent to the survey

Physicians	Government hospitals	Government–public partnership hospitals	Corporate hospitals	Nursing homes	Independent clinics
Cardiologists	2	2	1	2	–
ENT specialists	1	1		2	3
Surgeons	–	2	2	2	–
General physicians	2	2	2	2	3
Oncologists	1	2	1	–	1
Psychologists	1	1	–	–	2
Pathologists	2	1	2	–	–
Radiologists	–	1	-	–	–
Gynaecologists	2	2	2	3	3
Orthopaedic surgeon	–	2	1	2	–
Dentist	1	–	–	2	2
Paediatricians	–	–	–	2	1
Total (n=70)	12 (17 %)	16 (23 %)	11 (16 %)	17 (24 %)	15 (21 %)

ENT ear, nose and throat

Table 10.2 Weightage of each security parameter in the questionnaire

Security parameter	Number of questions
Confidentiality	7 (23 %)
Integrity	8 (27 %)
Availability	9 (30 %)
Security policies and awareness	6 (20 %)

Each security parameter consists of subtopics to extract relevant information from the respondents and to further strengthen the analysis and confidence of research. Table 10.3 lists these topics along with the question number as marked in the questionnaire. Each stated question is based on a previous survey (Bhartiya and Mehrotra 2013) conducted on an independent set of hospitals with an objective of identifying the present working scenarios and issues due to automated healthcare systems. We have picked only few subtopics out of each category for the sake of enabling a unique and clear understanding of each issue and also for limiting the length of the chapter (Table 10.3).

Table 10.3 Questionnaire detailing of each security parameter

Security parameter	Related subtopic
Availability	Sharing of passwords
	Access during transition of the doctor from one hospital to another
	Data unavailability percentage
	Rating the satisfaction level of using HIS
Integrity	Gaining of additional access over time
	Patient's control over his EHR
	Access controls
	Authorization
	Monitoring of data access
Confidentiality	Access to specialists and others
	Inconsistency in storage of EHRs from different locations
	Security breaches experienced
	Patient's awareness
Security policies and awareness	Policies for monitoring the flow of data
	Usage of international security standards
	Security policies and rules
	Satisfaction level

HIS hospital information system, *EHR* electronic health record

Physician's Perspective

Patient records may contain more than just text. Combined with other healthcare applications, they can cause critical slowdowns, impacting patient care and staff efficiency. As more and more critical patient information migrates to the network, it must provide adequate security and data availability to ensure timely delivery of patient information to medical staff and doctors. HIPAA, for example, mandates the confidentiality of patient information, and this in turn impacts a wide range of network services that must be tailored to the secure transport and storage of patient electronic records.

Availability Versus Confidentiality and Integrity

In addition to the importance of privacy, confidentiality and security, the EHR system must address the integrity and availability of information. We concentrate on the need of making EHR timely available to the doctor. On the contrary, we assume that if the data are frequently shared, it would eventually give full access rights to the doctors. The assumption is based on the observation of various hospitals where the role-based access controls (RBACs) are frequently modified to perform assigned duties. Doctors' opinions were gathered on this assumption and the following hypothesis was generated.

H_0 *with high frequency of sharing of EHR between hospitals, the doctors will not gain full access to the patient's records*

H_1 *with high frequency of sharing of EHR between hospitals, the doctors will gain full access to the patient's records*

Cardiologist	ENT	Surgeon	General physician	Oncologist	Psychologist	Pathologist	Gynaecologist	Orthopaedic surgeon
47	14	17	15	40	50	20	17	20

ENT ear, nose and throat

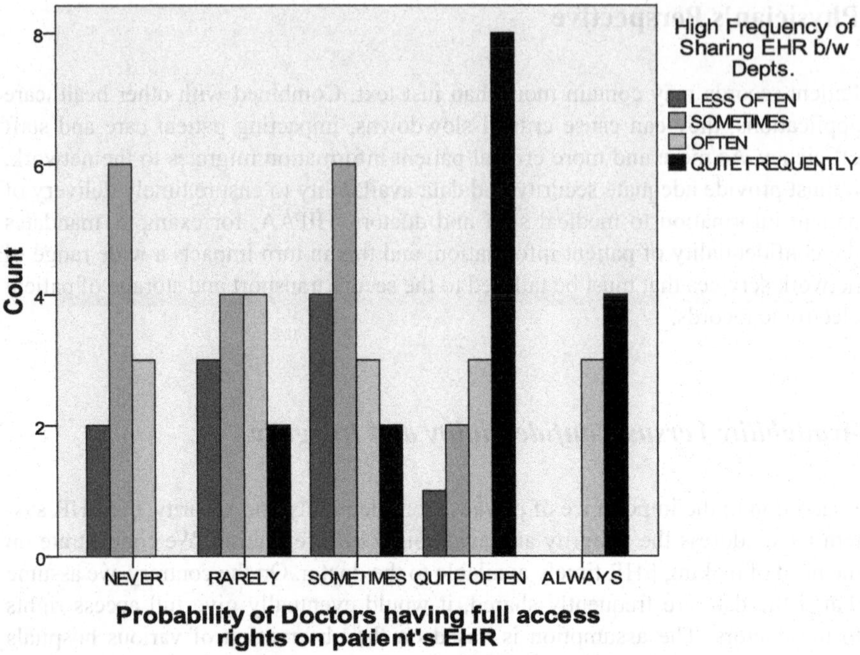

The doctors' opinion collected on this issue identifies a positive correlation between these factors, that is, the higher the frequency of sharing is, the greater are the chances of doctors acquiring full access rights on the patient's records. The table above lists the percentage of physicians of each specialization agreeing to the stated fact.

The Pearson's R is 0.52, significantly correlated at 0.01 level with $P<0.001$, hence rejecting the null hypothesis.

There is no unanimous opinion of doctors on this issue. While cardiologists, oncologists and psychologists strongly agreed about the probability of the data exposed to undue access rights, dentists, ENT specialists and general physicians gave an average nod to this reason.

Inference

The analysis reveals that though it adversely affects the confidentiality of the patient's information, but availability of both personal and diagnostic data enhance the efficiency of care providers. The threat to confidentiality of health information is the highest in psychological cases (50 %), where the patient discusses much personal information with the doctor, usually required for the treatment. Not every treatment that a patient undergoes requires identical level of security. This is reflected in our respondents' answers as well. Doctors such as dentists and ENT specialists do not find additional access to health records due to the frequent sharing between different hospitals, whereas psychologists and oncologists find the same posing confidentiality and privacy threat to the data. The results also vary between different categories of hospitals, namely, public, government-aided, corporate and private hospitals. The sharing is usually high between governments and corporate hospitals, with the latter mostly receiving the referral cases. Doctors at the government hospitals recognize a greater rate of risk of exposure of EHR as compared to responses received from the corporate hospitals.

Availability and Integrity Loss

Time is a critical factor in healthcare services. The study of real-time hospital environment shows a huge rush of patients during OPDs and especially in public-sector hospitals. The doctors have to deal with 50–100 patients in just 3 h. The EHR system must respond to the doctor's query in a timely manner. Hence, the doctors were asked to give their satisfaction level of using the HIS and whether it does somewhere affect the efficiency of their services. The following hypothesis was framed keeping this issue in mind.

H_0 *The response time of the system does not cause dissatisfaction among doctors and depletes their efficiency and interest*

H_1 *The response time of the system causes dissatisfaction among doctors and depletes their efficiency and interest*

The question was framed to identify if doctors are reluctant to use the automated system over the paper-based system because of slow response and non-timely availability of data. The table below lists the number of respondents who are either a few or not satisfied with the response time of the application.

Cardiologists	ENT specialists	Surgeons	General physicians	Oncologists	Psychologists	Pathologists	Radiologists	Gynaecologists	Orthopaedic surgeon	Dentist
5/7	5/7	3/6	7/13	2/5	3/4	3/5	1/1	7/12	3/5	3/5

ENT ear, nose and throat

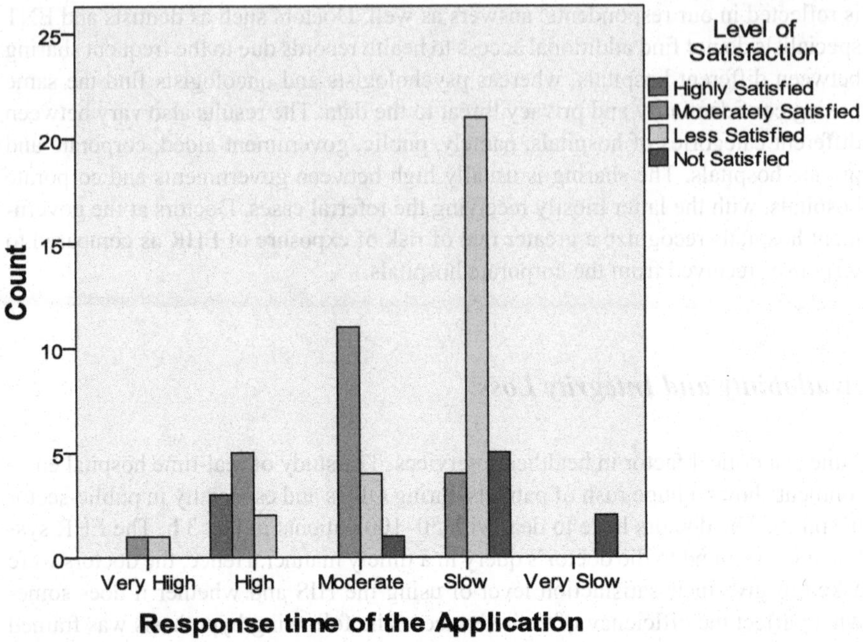

The response shows the Pearson's R as 0.61 with $P<0.001$ at 0.01 significance level. Not all the doctors are equally dissatisfied using an automated system for treating the patient. The average response from all the specializations is about 60 %, which is worth noting especially in healthcare environment.

The above figure shows that due to the slow response time of the application doctors do not want to use the automated systems and hence stick to traditional paper-based methods for recording patient's health details.

Inference

Slow response time of the application obstructs and delays doctors' work. This forces a doctor to rely on paper-based records due to their handy access. Untimely availability of data thus results in loss of integrity and consistency of EHR. It has the least impact on confidentiality as either the system is not at all used by the care providers or they usually view incomplete records. Another factor that affects the integrity of EHR is 'high number' of patients in OPD, especially in government and charitable hospitals. The doctors have to toggle between interfaces each holding some information required for further diagnosis. This takes more time to come to a conclusion as compared with the paper-based records. Scrolling papers is much easier than scrolling web pages.

Confidentiality Versus Availability

As stated, confidentiality means data should be accessed to legitimate and authorized users only. The IT team is always in a continuous process of designing and developing robust security rules and algorithms. This generated the need to identify the relationship between robust but complex security and the timely availability of records during patient visits, that is, whether complex and multilayered security adversely affects the performance of the system in terms of speed and time.

H_0 *Stringent security policies do not result in degradation of performance in terms of speed and time*

H_1 *Stringent security policies result in degradation of performance in terms of speed and time*

Vendors such as the Centre for Development of Advanced Computing (C-DAC) and Western India Products Limited (WIPRO) are the initial designers and developers of HIS. Risk analysis and monitoring are the prime concern while designing such applications. HIS incorporated with stringent security policies, namely, single sign-on, encrypted data in storage as well as in transit, encrypted mail service and firewalling, has some side effects. It deploys multiple and complex layers of authentication and access controls causing an overhead over time and speed of the system. The performance and efficiency decrease if the data are not timely available.

The question as to *how many times do they experience unavailability of data and do stringent security policies affect the availability of health records* was asked from the physicians. As the question is of no direct concern to the physicians, the majority had no opinion and very few ($n=26$) responses were received. The responses received were from those physicians who have been acting as connecting nodes between the IT team and the hospital administration. The table below distributes the responses in four categories: strongly agree, agree, somewhat agree and disagree.

	Experience	Cardiologists	ENT specialists	Surgeons	General physicians	Oncologists	Psychologists	Pathologists	Radiologists	Gynaecologists	Orthopaedic surgeons	Dentists
Unavailability of data security policies												
Strongly agree		2	0	0	7	1	1	0	0	1	0	1
Agree		2	0	0	1	0	1	2	1	1	1	0
Somewhat agree		0	0	1	0	1	0	0	0	1	0	0
Disagree		0	0	0	0	0	0	0	0	0	1	0

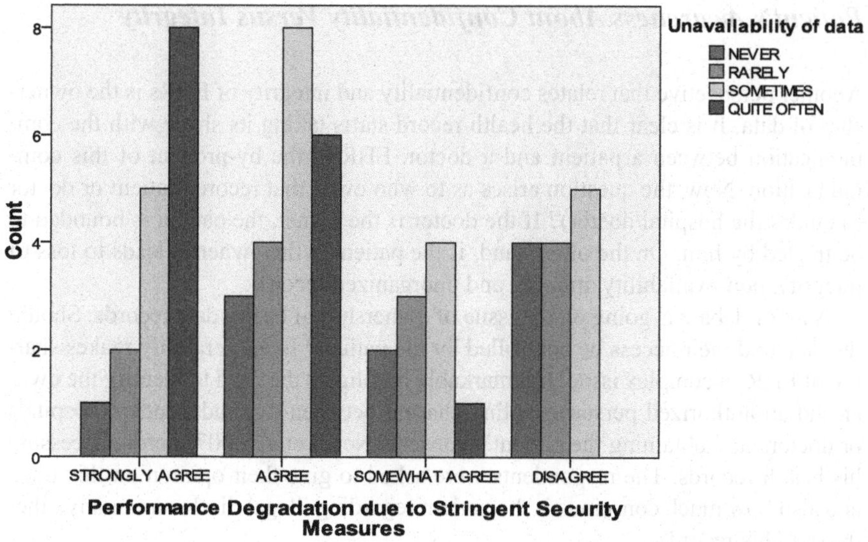

General physicians (attending maximum number of patients) have many times experienced delay in non-availability of records. The security controls include multilayer authentication, biometric, session-based data availability, patient-dependent data access, etc.

The Pearson's R of -0.54 with $P<0.001$ at 0.01 significance level signifies that with the refinement of security policies the non-availability would reduce. The result obtained is opposite to what doctors have experienced where they believe strict security would disallow timely access to EHRs. The hypothesis that stringent security policies result in degradation of performance in terms of speed and time is rejected.

Inference

Increasing complexities and layers of security do not adversely affect the accessibility of data. Thus, with confidentiality measures in place, availability is enhanced.

Security rules and policies ensure confidentiality and privacy of EHRs but can cause distress and discomfort in interoperable environment. The security policies and rules sometimes conflict with each other, disabling the access of EHRs even to authorized users. Doctors are reluctant to use the system and demand more customization and standardization in designing such systems for better and timely availability of records.

Patient's Awareness About Confidentiality Versus Integrity

Another perspective that relates confidentiality and integrity of EHRs is the ownership of data. It is clear that the health record starts taking its shape with the communication between a patient and a doctor. EHR is the by-product of this communication. Now, the question arises as to who owns that record: patient or doctor (includes the hospital/doctor)? If the doctor is the owner, the patient is bounded to be treated by him. On the other hand, if the patient is the owner, it leads to loss of integrity, non-availability, missing and unorganized records.

A lot of debate is going on the issue of ownership of health data records. Should the data and their access be controlled by the patient? Interoperability makes sharing of EHRs a complex issue. It remarkably highlights the need to identify the owner and an authorized person enabling sharing between two independent hospitals or doctors and obtaining the patient's consent (Nepal et al. 2007) before accessing his health records. The respondents were asked to give their opinion on this issue and also how much conscious is the patient regarding illegal disclosure or any other threat to his records.

H_0 *Complete control with the patient does not affect his awareness on confidentiality and integrity of data*

H_1 *Complete control with the patient increases his awareness on confidentiality and integrity of data*

Physician's Opinion on Should patient own his EHR?		Patient's Awareness					Total
		NEVER	*RARELY*	*SOMETIMES*	*QUITE OFTEN*	*ABSOLUTELY*	
Patient's Control	*DISAGREE*	2	6	10	1	0	19
	SOMEWHAT AGREE	3	2	7	2	3	17
	AGREE	4	0	7	2	5	18
	STRONGLY AGREE	2	3	6	4	1	16
Total		11	11	30	9	9	70

HIPAA makes it mandatory for a hospital to take the patient's consent before accessing his records. The null hypothesis states that the patient given the ownership and control of his record would not increase his awareness for maintaining its confidentiality and integrity. Furthermore, awareness is dependent on various factors, such as literacy, attitude, social status and disease. The table above lists the outlook of the physicians on the patient's holding the control of his health records and his concern for ensuring confidentiality and privacy of the records. The physicians predict that with more and more control lying with the patient, his responsibility and awareness of organizing and monitoring his records would increase.

The results illuminate that there is a significant relationship between patient's awareness and acquiring complete rights on the data. An increase in one definitely increases the probability of the other. The physicians view that with the patient made responsible for providing access of his health data to anyone, the current scenario where a very low percentage of patients bother about the circulation of their health records would change. The Pearson's R is 0.51 with $P<0.001$, thereby rejecting the null hypothesis. The trend in this analysis also shows the patient's awareness moving from 'never' to 'sometimes' irrespective of who is controlling the data.

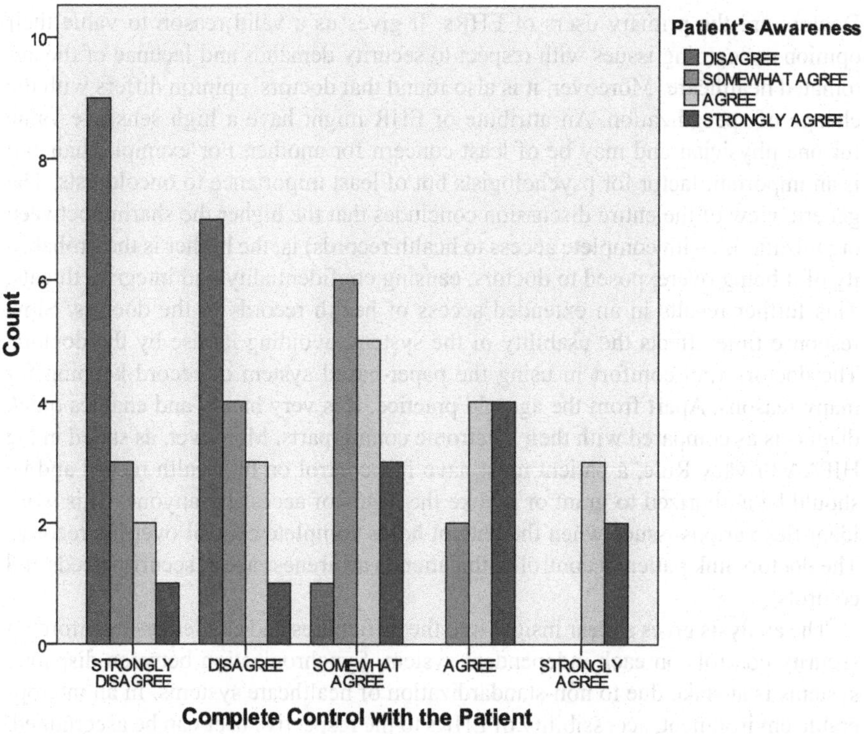

Inference

These results are contradictory. The analysis strengthens the belief that the patient should be the owner of his medical records and should be the authority of providing access rights to anyone he/she wants the records to share with. In reality, doctors (>60 %) disagree on enabling complete authority of EHRs to the patient.

Full control of data lying in the hands of the patient authorizing sharing of the same ensures robust confidentiality and privacy; however, achieving integrity and availability is not ascertained. The patient needs to be present in such a scenario, which is not always possible due to varied reasons of illness. Doctors handling emergencies and accidental cases have no medium of accessing records, and thus the treatment provided remains unrecorded, leading to incomplete documentation of EHRs.

Conclusion

Doctors are the primary users of EHRs. It gives us a valid reason to value their opinion concerning issues with respect to security demands and lacunae of the automated healthcare. Moreover, it is also found that doctors' opinion differs with the change of specialization. An attribute of EHR might have a high sensitive value for one physician and may be of least concern for another. For example, hair fall is an important factor for psychologists but of least importance to oncologists. The generic view of the entire discussion concludes that the higher the sharing between organizations (with complete access to health records) is, the higher is the probability of it being overexposed to doctors, causing confidentiality and integrity threats. This further results in an extended access of health records to the doctors. Slow response time affects the usability of the system, avoiding its use by the doctors. The doctors find comfort in using the paper-based system of record-keeping for many reasons. Apart from the age-old practice, it is very handy and enables quick diagnosis as compared with their electronic counterparts. Moreover, as stated in the HIPAA Privacy Rule, a patient must have full control on his health record and he should be authorized to grant or revoke the rights of access by anyone. This work identifies various issues when the patient holds complete control over his records. The doctors link patient's control with patient's awareness about security needs and controls.

The analysis gives a clear insight into the difficulties and challenges in enforcing security controls on each independent system. Synchronization between disparate systems is at stake due to non-standardization of healthcare systems. In an interoperable environment, accessibility of EHRs to the respective user can be ascertained, but ensuring its safety in terms of maintaining confidentiality and privacy of information and identity is beyond control.

Future Scope

This chapter draws the analysis only from the doctors' perspective. Patients' opinions are equally important. This work can be extended to gather patient's opinions on similar issues. It would generate an equilibrium of thoughts from both perspectives and enable the developers and administrators to design and implement useful and successful security controls, maybe more dynamic, for seamless but secured sharing of EHRs in between independent healthcare organizations. It would further form as a basis in designing a security framework for sharing the EHRs in an interoperable healthcare environment.

Acknowledgments For this work, we are extremely grateful to various hospitals located in Delhi National Capital Region (NCR), India-Rockland, St. Stephen, Max and Employees' State Insurance Corporation (ESIC), and many independent clinics and nursing homes for giving their consent to approach the physicians for their valuable opinions. We are highly thankful to all the doctors who spared their valuable time for filling up the questionnaire.

References

Bhartiya, S., & Mehrotra, D. (2013). Threats and challenges to security of electronic health records. *Social Informatics and Telecommunications Engineering, LNICS, 0115*, pp 543–559. ISBN: 978-3-642-37948-2.

Carmagnola, F., Cena, F., & Gena, C. (2012). User model interoperability, trends in health information exchange organizational staffing. AHIMA/HIMSS.

Certification Commission for Health Information Technology (CCHIT). (2009). Interoperability: Supplying the building blocks for a patient-centered EHR.

Cheng, V. S., & Hung, P. C. (2006). Health Insurance Portability and Accountability Act (HIPPA) Compliant access control model for web services. *International Journal of Healthcare Information Systems and Informatics, 1*(1), 22–39. doi:10.4018/jhisi.2006010102.

Davis, M. W. (2009). *The State of U.S. Hospitals relative to achieving meaningful use measurements*. Chicago: HIMSS Analytics.

Filipa, A., et al. (2009). OpenEHR in Healthcare—A review. http://www.medicina.med.up.pt/im/trabalhos08_09/.../INTROMEDII_Artigo_t14.doc.

Health informatics—Information Security Management in Health using ISO/IEC 27002. (2008). (ISO 27799:2008), BS EN ISO 27799:2008, ISO 27799:2008(E).

High Level Expert Group (HLEG) Report on Universal Health Coverage for India. (2011). Instituted by Planning Commission of India.

HIMSS Enterprise Systems Steering Committee and Global Enterprise Task Force (GETF). (2010). Electronic health records: A global perspective. http://www.himss.org/files/HIMSSorg/content/files/Globalpt1-edited%20final.pdf.

Kamran, M., & Farooq, M. (2011). An Information-Preserving Watermarking Scheme for Right Protection of EMR Systems. *IEEE Transactions on Knowledge and Data Engineering, 24*, 1950–1962.

Nepal, S., Zic, J., Jaccard, F., & Kraehenbuehl, G. (2007). A trusted system for sharing patient electronic medical records in autonomous distributed health care systems. *International Journal of Healthcare Information Systems and Informatics, 2*(1), 14–35. doi:10.4018/jhisi.2007010102.

The Office of the National Coordinator for Health Information Technology (ONCHIT). (2012). Guide to privacy and security of health information. Version 1.2.

Wainer, J., Campos, J. R., Salinas, M. D. U., & Sigulem, D. (2008). Security requirements for a lifelong electronic health record system: An opinion. *The Open Medical Informatics Journal, 2*, 160–165.

Webster, P. C.(2011), The rise of open-source electronic health records. Vol 377. http://www.thelancet.com.

Wyne, M. F., & Haider, S. N. (2007). HIPAA compliant HIS in J2EE environment. *International Journal of Healthcare Information Systems and Informatics, 2*(4), 73–89. doi:10.4018/jhisi.2007100105.

Shalini Bhartiya is a research scholar at Amity University, Noida, India. She has more than 10 years of teaching experience and has published more than 10 papers in national and international conference proceedings and refereed journals. Her areas of research are information security, software engineering and data mining.

Dr. Deepti Mehrotra is a gold medallist and has a Ph.D. from Lucknow University, India. Currently, she is working as a professor in Amity School of Engineering and Technology (ASET), Amity University Uttar Pradesh. She has more than 19 years of experience in teaching, research and content writing. She has published more than 50 papers in international refereed journals and conference proceedings. Her areas of research are information security, data mining and knowledge management.

Chapter 11
Health Information Technology to Support the Delivery of Chinese Medicine: The Design of a Chinese Medicine Clinic System

Catherine Han Lin, Angela Wei Hong Yang, Siddhi Pittayachawan and Nilmini Wickramasinghe

Introduction

Given today's healthcare challenges, most, if not all, Organization of Economic Co-operation and Development (OECD) countries are focusing on ways to incorporate information systems/information technology (IS/IT) to facilitate superior healthcare delivery. In particular, they are looking to design and develop suitable e-health solutions (Wickramasinghe and Schaffer 2010). However, to date, these solutions have solely focused on supporting the delivery of Western medicine.

Healthcare, though, is not only restricted to Western medicine practice. In the twenty-first century, we are witnessing an increased global trend of treatments in complementary and alternative medicine (Lu et al. 2004). One such development is in the area of Chinese medicine (CM) which now is considered to be a scientifically and clinically approved form of medicine that has considerably less side effects and complications as compared to Western medicine (Shi and Lu 2006). Moreover, Chinese herbs such as ginseng (or RenShen) are widely sold and used by many Western physicians and many Western medical practitioners have taken courses in Chinese acupuncture (Kaptchuk 2000). Despite the rapid growth in the embracement of CM, research and study into the role for IS/IT implementations to support and enable

C. Han Lin (✉)
185-187 Hoddle Street, Richmond, VIC 3121, Australia
e-mail: catherinehan76405.lin@gmail.com

A. Wei Hong Yang
60 Baker Ave, 3102 Kew East, Australia
e-mail: angela.yang@rmit.edu.au

N. Wickramasinghe
Deakin University and Epworth HealthCare, 60 Baker Ave, Kew East 3102, Australia
e-mail: n.wickramasinghe@deakin.edu.au

S. Pittayachawan
Building 80, Level 7, 445 Swanston Street, 3000 Melbourne, Australia
e-mail: siddhi.pittayachawan@rmit.edu.au

N. Wickramasinghe et al. (eds.), *Contemporary Consumer Health Informatics*, Healthcare Delivery in the Information Age, DOI 10.1007/978-3-319-25973-4_11

CM practices is at best very limited. To address this void, this chapter reports on a research in progress that serves to focus on examining the potential for using IS/IT tools and techniques to assist CM clinics and thereby support enhancing the delivery of CM practices. As healthcare processes heavily depend on both information and knowledge (Lenz and Reichert 2007), we will look into the field of knowledge management (KM) to identify IS/IT involvements in healthcare processes.

Why IS/IT Can Support Superior Healthcare Delivery

Voluminous data and information permeate a physician's clinic or a hospital and processing these data manually has and continues to negatively impact healthcare costs as well as make the healthcare system inefficient and ineffective (Wickramasinghe and Schaffer 2010). Hence, IS/IT systems that coordinate organizational tasks, provide information at the point of care, reduce clinical and/or hospital cost, and support quality healthcare delivery are being embraced (Lenz and Reichert 2007). Such IS/IT solutions are now playing a critical role in healthcare delivery because they offer several advantages over manual approaches as follows: (1) *Facilitate delivery of care*: IT can help deliver care to people who are located in remote areas, and who do not have access to hospitals or clinics. For example, doctors may use telemedicine equipment such as Tele-stethoscope, Tele-biologic diagnosis equipment, Tele-radiology, and Tele-surgery to diagnose and treat patients because they provide greater accessibility and availability to healthcare solutions (Hojabri and Manafi 2012). (2) *Improve quality of care*: IT can help to provide easier, safer, and faster access to patient data including laboratory results, therapeutic procedures, medication administration, clinic notes, and billing. This allows the healthcare professionals to access the right data and information at the right time (Austin and Boxerman 2003). This results in information-based diagnosis, acceleration of communication, and reduction in medical errors (COCIR 2012). Furthermore, computerized physician order entry (CPOE) systems, for example, allow bar code reading to match patients to their prescribed medications (Bernstein 2007), which in turn can serve to reduce medical errors (Ball and Lillis 2001; Bates 2000). (3) *Reduce cost and save time*: IT can help healthcare professionals to access health information in a timely manner. This reduces the issue of staff shortage as well as increases efficiency. Clinical and administrative costs can be reduced by avoiding the duplication of medical examinations and unnecessary visits. For example, by embracing cloud technology, the Swedish Red Cross was able to save 20 % on their IT operating costs. This action led to freeing 25 % of people's time to focus on more strategic tasks, better supporting the core missions of the organization (Microsoft 2011). (4) *Support better management and monitoring*: Patients learn how to control and manage their diseases correctly with the help of online disease management systems. This is particularly important in the context of chronic diseases. Features like "Ask a physician", web-based nurse line, or call centre assist patients to take control of their disease rather than solely relying on a doctor (Ball and Lillis 2001).

(5) *Provide decision support*: Web-based clinical decision support (CDS) systems can give automatic alerts and warnings to physicians. For example, a community hospital in USA used a computerized alert system to target 37 drug-specific adverse reactions. They detected opportunities to prevent injury at a rate of 64 per 1000 admissions; 44 % of the true positive alerts had not been recognized by the physician (Bates 2000). Thus, there is strong evidence in the literature to show that IS/IT can provide and enable superior healthcare delivery. Hence, we contend that IS/IT can also support the delivery of CM. To demonstrate this, it is first important to identify key aspects of CM.

Chinese Medicine

CM began in China thousands of years ago at the time when Chinese philosophy, astronomy, and literature were developed to maturity (Liao 2011). At that time, key individuals gained experiences in how to deal with human diseases by natural methods, such as acupuncture, Qigong (mind controlling), and herbs (Wang et al. 1999). Furthermore, many of these individuals began to summarize these practices and thereby developed a theory based on their philosophical and social knowledge, which in turn formed the origins of CM (Wang et al. 1999). Succinctly, CM follows two philosophies: (1) A homeostasis perspective that focuses on the integrity of human body, and emphasizes the close relationship between human body and its social and natural environment; and (2) A dynamic balance perspective with an emphasis on the movement in the integrity (Lu et al. 2004). Table 11.1 summarizes the key aspects of CM. As can be observed from this table, CM is different and distinct from Western medical practice but also heavily, perhaps even more, reliant on tacit knowledge and expertise of the practitioner—a point that is made more apparent when we look at the processes involved with CM diagnosis.

Table 11.1 Five elements of CM. (adapted from Liu and Liu 2009, p. 23)

Five elements	Five Zang (principal) organs	Five Fu organs	Five sense organs	Five body tissues	Five passions	Five fluids	Five pulses
Wood	Liver	Gallbladder	Eyes	Tendons	Anger	Tears	Taut
Fire	Heart	Small intestine	Tongue	Vessels	Joy	Sweat	Surging
Earth	Spleen	Stomach	Lips	Muscles	Thought/Anxiety	Saliva	Moderate
Metal	Lung	Large intestine	Nose	Skin and hair	Sorrow	Nasal discharge	Deep and thin
Water	Kidney	Urinary bladder	Ears	Bones	Fear/Fright	Spittle	Deep

CM Diagnosis

CM practitioners use four basic methods for diagnosis: inspection, auscultation and olfaction, inquiring, and palpation (Huang and Chen 2007; Zhao et al. 1994). Diagnosis and treatments are based on an overall analysis of the patient's symptoms and signs. This process is called "bian zheng" (differentiation of syndrome). "bian" means discrimination or classification, whereas "zheng" means syndrome (Zhao et al. 1994). Inspection begins with the physician understanding and predicting the pathological changes of internal organs by observing abnormal changes in the patient's vitality, colour, appearance, secretions, and excretions (Huang and Chen 2007). The second method, auscultation and olfaction, includes listening and smelling. The physician listens to the patient's voice, breathing, coughing, and sounds emanating from the internal organs. Ear and stethoscope may also be used in this process (Huang and Chen 2007). A patient's "stinky" smell, for example, usually indicates heat syndromes while foul and sour smell implies retention of food (Huang and Chen 2007). Inquiring is about getting information from a patient about his or her disease condition. Examples of common inquiries are chills and fever, perspiration, appetite and thirst, and pain (Huang and Chen 2007). Regarding palpation, the physician would put his or her first three fingers on the radial artery of a patient's wrist. A trained and skilled physician can detect over 30 different pulse qualities (e.g. floating, sunken, weak, and bounding) on each of the 12 pulses (Zhu and Wang 2011). The pulse qualities help the physician to identify the condition of the related organs. These four approaches are used in combination in every diagnosis and cannot be separated or omitted (Zhu and Wang 2011). A correct diagnosis can only be made based on a comprehensive and systematic analysis of a patient's condition.

CM treatments can include any of the following: Chinese herbs (i.e. leaves, seeds, roots, flowers, fruits, minerals, and animal products), acupuncture and moxibustion, tuina (Chinese remedial massage), cupping, qigong and taichi, and diet therapy (Xue and O'Brien 2003). All treatments aim to increase human body's resistance to diseases and prevention by improving the inter-connections among self-controlled systems (Lu et al. 2004).

Problems and Challenges of CM

Today, CM clinics still follow the manual administration method in recording and managing its clinical information. Although these CM practitioners are experts in their skills, some of them are not good at English. So it is often that patients' records and treatments are written on paper and in the practitioners' first language. This creates language difficulties for others. It is also hard to implement standards, and to encourage an internationally recognized and registered practice. A patient with some medical history record can come in many forms including films, images, telegraphs, and electronic medical record (EMR). CM doctors found it difficult to store these crucial evidences in assisting, analyzing, and diagnosing the patient without the proper and adequate technology and equipment.

Capturing and transforming the voluminous information and knowledge in Chinese herbs, acupuncture, syndromes, and treatments to an IS/IT system is challenging. Some research has attempted to build and transfer these tremendous information and knowledge to an information knowledge-based system that can be retrieved online or through Intranet. Dasherb, a joint Sino-German venture since 2002 (Dasherb 2013), has a herb database that contains lists of common Chinese herbal medicines that can be searched by Latin name, English name, and Pinyin Name (a pronunciation of Chinese characters). Complementary and Alternative Healing University (CAHU), California, USA has developed a comprehensive online Dictionary of Chinese Herbs. Each herb is explained in detail including pharmaceutical name; botanical name; Japanese, Korean, and Cantonese pronunciations; distribution of the herb; properties (characteristics); channels (meridians) entered; medical functions; actions and indications; chemical ingredients; recommended dosage; samples of formulae, toxicity, and cautions (CAHU 2013). A similar development has been done in Australia by the CM team at the Royal Melbourne Institute of Technology (RMIT) University. The RMIT Chinese Medicine Portal (CMP) is an online CM knowledge pool where information and clinical data can be retrieved and accessed (Yang et al. 2009). Some CM expert systems and applications are developed for certain diseases or particular treatment. For example, a Chinese acupuncture expert system can assist physicians on acupuncture prescription, needle insertion position, and usage of acupuncture points (Lam et al. 2012). These developments have few limitations: (1) Incomprehensive: Most development and resources only include limited or small amount of Chinese herbs with no or limited resources in Chinese acupuncture or vice versa (Yang et al. 2009). (2) Lack of evidence support on information production and synthesis (Yang et al. 2009). (3) Not an IS/IT system solution for CM clinics and practitioners to handle their daily key processes. (4) No standards and compliances to government regulations and assessments. (5) No system functions and features on clinical stock control and management. (6) Lack of system integration. Most expert systems and applications are designed as a stand-alone with limited integration with others.

In Australia, the Chinese Medicine Board of Australia (CMBA) was established in 2011 (CMBA 2013). CMBA provides guidelines, standards, registrations, and assessments to the CM practitioners in Australia. It is important to CMBA that an IS/IT solution is available and used by CM patients and practitioners. For many CM clinics and doctors, an IS/IT solution is essential for the following reasons: (1) To be registered and practice CM in Australia following CMBA regulations, assessments, and standards. (2) Transfer the paper process of managing clinic information to an electronic system. (3) Facilitate access to healthcare, share health information, especially patient information.

In this chapter, we propose that the solution lies in the design and development of a Chinese medicine clinic system (CMCS). The idea of such a system is to help CM clinics and practitioners with their daily key processes and activities. The system will have functions and features such as create and store patients' records; generate reports and forms with built-in templates to meet governments' regulations and guidelines. It is anticipated that such system should have multi-lingual capabilities and would require a unique sub-system to facilitate better management of the vast CM stocks.

What Areas Can IS/IT Help in CM

To develop the proposed CMCS, it is first necessary to map the processes that take place in CM clinics. This is done in Fig. 11.1.

In these processes, after consultation and diagnosis, a CM doctor may give the patient a treatment plan: the patient is given Chinese herbal medicine and/or other kinds of treatments; the patient may be referred to a specialist for more specialized treatments or be transferred to the hospital for an emergent care. It is very common that the doctor asks the patient to come back for a subsequent treatment.

The CM processes in Fig. 11.1 are a close match to the western medicine clinics. A typical Western physician clinic patient process is analyzed and modelled by Swisher et al. (2001) and include: (1) Registration, (2) Check-in, (3) Examination (including pre-examination and post-examination), (4) Exit interview, and (5) Check-out (Swisher et al. 2001). In the registration process, a patient interacts with a clinical staff prior to treatment. In Check-in, clinical staff spends time with the patient collecting initial medical information prior to examination. In the examination process, the physician collects more extensive medical information from the patient (pre-examination) if necessary; diagnoses the patient and prescribes treatments (examination); and collects any additional medical information (post-examination). The exit interview is a process where a physician performs the final consultation and diagnosis. A patient may interact with the clinical staff before exiting the clinic in the final check-out process (Swisher et al. 2001). Compared with the above-mentioned processes, Swisher's registration process matches the 1.0 process in Fig. 11.1. The check-in and examination processes match Fig. 11.1 process 2.0. Swisher's post-examination is really the 3.1, 3.3, 3.4, 3.5 processes in Fig. 11.1. Instead of having exit interview and check-out, we realize that the processes can flow back and be repeated for some patients. This may suggest that we can expect as much benefit from the proposed IS/IT solution in the context of CM scenarios as we are now witnessing when IS/IT solutions are applied to Western medical clinics.

The differences between CM and Western medicine clinic processes are, however, in the methods of diagnosis, ingredients in the medicine, the treatment

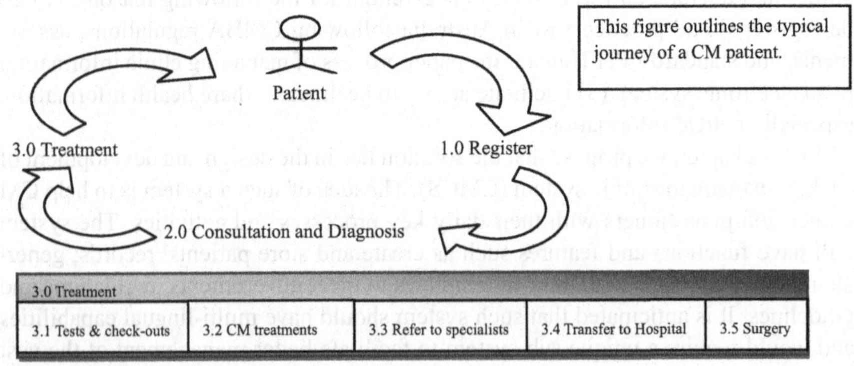

Fig. 11.1 CM patient diagnosis and treatment processes

approaches, and the philosophies of human disease. Furthermore, CM doctors and clinics do not perform surgeries, lab tests, and check-outs. Therefore, IS/IT involvements and implementations in these processes between CM and Western medicine practice are similar.

Based on the CM clinic processes shown in Fig. 11.1, we can identify the following IS/IT involvements:

- When a patient makes a scheduled visit or walks in a CM clinic for a treatment, the patient triggers the registration process. A scheduling resources or facilities system manages registration, which includes booking and scheduling. This system coordinates scheduling of resources to all care providers, identifies conflicts with other appointments for patients or provider resources that include clinical staff, materials like diagnostic equipment, and preparation requirements such as anaesthesia consultation (COCIR 2012). This system is usually a part of a Patient Administration System (PAS) that administers patient personal information, admission, discharge, and transfer (COCIR 2012).
- EMR information systems. The purpose of this system is to record and host information of patients' electronic files. EMR is a patient medical record in digital format generated and maintained in a healthcare institute such as a hospital or a clinic (Hannan 1996). EMR includes data and information such as demographics, medical history, medication and allergies, immunization status, lab test results, and radiology images (Hannan 1996).
- Medical Document Management (MDM) information system. MDM manages and supports different electronic and digital patient medical documents and files (Mitamura 2010). These files contain data and information such as scanned pdf files, care episodes, test results, diagnosis, and referrals. Functions of MDM include computer-assisted document/file entry, indexing, administration, file/document storage, access/retrieval, and archive (Mitamura 2010).
- Clinical Knowledge Management (CKM) and Clinical Decision Support (CDS) system. CKM is a repository that contains codified knowledge such as a practical set of rules and guidelines derived from experts (Wyatt 2001). CKM often comes together with CDS, as it is the back-end database where CDS depends on or gets reference from. CDS is a program assisting healthcare professionals and physicians with decision-making tasks by linking dynamic individual patient health observations (Wyatt 2001). For example, a drug–drug interaction checker requires a database of drug names and their interactions (Sittig et al. 2010). In CM, when a CKM such as the CMP is available, it can assist CM practitioners in checking/confirming a Chinese herb's toxicity and cautions, and hence better decisions can be made on the amount of usage of such a herb.
- Finance and Accounting Systems (FAS). This refers to patient billing, insurance claims, activity analysis, and cost accounting (COCIR 2012). This system is usually a built-in of PAS either directly or through EMR. The system can assist clinical staff to find a medical procedure, diagnosis, treatment and their prices with codes to optimize billing and reimbursement.
- Logistic and Resource systems. This includes Human Resources Management System (HRM), Facility and Equipment Management System (FEMS), and Supply Chain Management (SCM) or Materials Management System (MMS).

HRM manages clinic personnel. This includes: clinic staff planning, staff details and scheduling; employee time and attendance; payroll and controlling (COCIR 2012). FEMS controls and monitors clinic facility and equipment; describes and tracks their deployment, inspects and maintains the clinical equipment by clinic policies and procedures (COCIR 2012). MMS or SCM assists in planning, implementing, and controlling all movement and storage of materials and inventory from point-of-origin to point-of-consumption. Functions of MMS are: ordering purchase, stock management, warehouse/materials management, and supplier management/sourcing (COCIR 2012).

- Integrated healthcare network/system and security systems. Although some of the systems mentioned above can be stand-alone, most of the above sub-systems are built-in or connected with others. An integrated network or system to support the exchange, processing, and storage of information and knowledge in between these systems is essential.
- Security is another essential area in the design of a suitable CMCS. Key areas to consider should include protecting patient and health information through access control and passwords, encryption, and firewalls; system backup, archive, and recovery; secure database with implementation of authorization.

Another final difference between CM clinics and practices compared to Western medicine is the amount and reliance on expert tacit knowledge. A study on a group of six people with stomach pain who were diagnosed by a western medicine doctor and then by a CM physician has shown a significant difference. Based on the knowledge and theory of Western medicine practice of analyzing tendency to narrow diagnosis of an underlying entity, the Western medicine doctor used upper gastrointestinal x-rays or endoscopy by means of a fiberscope, and diagnosed all six patients as having peptic ulcer disease. According to the Western medicine doctor, all six patients suffered from the same disorder and were given the same prescription. However, the CM physician found the differences in each patient, diagnosed six different syndromes and prescribed six different herbal formulas (Kaptchuk 2000). The CM physician's expert knowledge and comprehensive analysis of each patient's unique health condition set the differences of the diagnosis and treatments. Therefore, we consider that the proposed CMCS should also incorporate the techniques and strategies of KM, and in particular evoke key knowledge transformations.

Knowledge Management

KM is a process of continually managing knowledge of all kinds to meet existing and emerging needs, to identify and exploit acquired knowledge assets and to develop new opportunities (Quintas et al. 1997). KM is about designing and implementing processes, tools, structures, systems, and culture to facilitate knowledge capture, sharing and re-use to enhance organizational performance (Gottschalk 2005).

Long and Lai (2005) summarized KM as a set of systematic actions that include establishing strategies and procedures with proper utilization of technologies. This ensures that the acquisition, storage, conversion, sharing, application, and generation of knowledge can be effectively performed.

Integral to KM is of course the knowledge construct. Nonaka (1994, p. 14) notes that "knowledge is created and organized by a flow of information, anchored on the commitment and belief of its holder". Goodson (2005, p. 148) refers to knowledge as an "insight, experience, and creativity that exist within people expressed through explicit and tacit communication events". Polanyi (1966) further categorized knowledge into two types: tacit and explicit. Tacit knowledge is gained from experiences and "by doing". It is accumulated through individual's experiences, actions, ideas, or values he or she embraces (Polanyi 1968). This type of knowledge is very hard to express and formalize; hence, it is also difficult to share with others. Explicit knowledge, in contrast, can be expressed in words, numbers, and diagrams; hence, it is easier to be captured, used, and shared. Organizations must be aware that these two types of knowledge are equally important.

The form of the knowledge can be changed in several ways. In particular, Nonaka et al. (1998) defined key transformations as: tacit to tacit through socialization; tacit to explicit through externalization; explicit to tacit through internalization; and explicit to explicit through combination. This process is known as the knowledge spiral. When people share experiences, like a master passes his or her knowledge to the apprentice through an apprenticeship, tacit knowledge can be transferred to tacit. Through a combination or conversion, explicit knowledge can be edited and systemized into more complex sets of explicit knowledge. This usually happens in a formal learning of facts (Nonaka et al. 1998). Tacit knowledge is transferred to explicit knowledge that can be understood by the others through the use of metaphors and analogies (Nonaka et al. 1998). Wickramasinghe et al. (2006) use this in a healthcare context and explain, for example, that a surgeon answers the questions of why he does a particular procedure in a certain way. The tacit knowledge of the surgeon is captured and can be used and made available for the others. Explicit to tacit occurs as conversion of new explicit to tacit knowledge of individuals. Examples of this are on-the-job-training, simulations, and experiments (Nonaka et al. 1998).

It is important to note that knowledge do not get transferred automatically by itself. Socialization, Externalization, Internalization, and Combination (Nonaka et al. 1998) involve participants' interaction, cooperation, collaboration, reflection, and management. It is equally important to note that knowledge transformation is not a one-way street. Tacit knowledge can be transferred to explicit, and the newly formed explicit knowledge can be transferred to either tacit or explicit knowledge. Hence, managing knowledge and knowledge transfer is important. Wickramasinghe et al. (2006) illustrated the generation of these two types of knowledge during the healthcare process. We would like to take a step further here to show the knowledge transfer through some examples. Moreover, we identify the IS/IT involvements in these processes in Table 11.2 below.

Table 11.2 Healthcare knowledge transfer

Healthcare process	Knowledge transfer	Example	IS/IT involvement
Symptoms	Explicit to tacit	A well, medical, self-educated patient may claim that he or she is suffering from diabetes (explicit), as some of the symptoms he or she has experienced closely match to the disease (tacit)	A patient is well medically educated by browsing medical information on the Internet. These medical information were prepared and made available for the public with the use of IT
Primary diagnosis	Explicit to explicit	A doctor listens and records the patient's symptoms (explicit) and diagnoses the patient's illness is diabetes (explicit)	A doctor records the patient's symptoms through an electronic device. Patient's records are stored at the clinic level or as an EMR that can be accessed nationally
Referral	Tacit to tacit	A doctor will refer (tacit) the patient to do a set of tests, or seeing a specialist (tacit)	An electronic referral letter can be generated and sent to a specialist or laboratory for testing with details of testing items
Second opinion	Explicit to explicit/tacit to explicit	The test results will show some data and/or information (explicit) to confirm if the patient is diabetic (explicit). A specialist may find that the patient has additional illness (tacit) and further tests may be required (explicit)	Test results are updated automatically through electric medical equipment. These results are transferred to the doctor or specialist electronically
Confirmation	Explicit to tacit/tacit to tacit	All test results (explicit) confirm the patient's illnesses (explicit). A specialist confirms the original diagnosis from the doctor (tacit to tacit)	Confirmation of a patient's illness is recorded in patient's file or EMR

Why KM Is Important?

Healthcare is one of the most complicated systems in our society today. It has many dimensions and involves many parties to collaborate to deliver a quality care to a patient, such as clinical/hospital administrations, physicians, specialists, nurses, radiologic technology technicians, psychologists, lab technicians, financial clerks, insurance companies, and department of health of the country. It is unarguably important that knowledge is captured and created from all parties and participants. It is equally important that all these knowledge are made available to all others to deliver quality healthcare to a patient at the point of need. Research has shown that KM can increase performance, develop partnership, evaluate risks, organize management, and enhance economic value (Morr and Subercaze 2010). Through the use of proper KM tools and techniques, knowledge can be formalized, shared, structured, and organized so that organization knowledge assets will not be lost. A human mind can only obtain limited information and knowledge. A Western medicine physician must be aware of hundreds of medical references, biological tests, thousands of imagery tests, and surgical interventions (Wickramasinghe et al. 2006). Additionally, they must know the potential effects and prices of medicines. KM helps healthcare professionals to focus on acquisition, knowledge storage, and retrieval, as well as other activities such as learning, strategic planning, and decision making. Thus, we will incorporate a KM focus on the design and development of the CMCS.

Chinese Medicine Clinic System

The proposed structure for the CMCS is anticipated to be a system structure that contains multiple sub-systems. Furthermore, the CMCS should be an integrated system where information and knowledge can be stored, shared, retrieved, managed, and processed. In addition, the CMCS should contain functions as detailed in Table 11.3.

Based on the proposed CMCS system structure and functions, a system prototype will be built, tested, and validated. CM clinics and practitioners will participate

Table 11.3 CM system functions

Functions	Systems
Clinic staff personal information, available working time & date, provider number	HRM
Clinic bookings, scheduling, cancellation	PAS, HRM, FEMS
Patient personal information (must follow CMBA's guidelines), including: Patient agreement (scan and upload signed clinical statements) patient medical history, insurance details, etc.	EMR
Consultation	EMR, MDM, CKM, CDS
Syndromes CM syndromes (pre-diagnosed with suggested treatments)—link with its symptoms and signs	EMR, MDM, CKM, CDS
Diagnosis Clinical conditions (pre-diagnosed with suggested treatments)—link with its commonly seen syndromes Medicinal formulae—link with its analysis and modern research	EMR, MDM, CKM, CDS
Treatment—Chinese herbal medicine Link and search with herbal monograph database Link and search with stock control and price Link and search with patient accounts (for calculation and invoice) Alert practitioners restricted herbs before prescription Herbal prescription of each diagnosis and treatment—must be written in multi-lingual (PinYin, Chinese characters, English, Latin)	EMR, MDM, CKM, CDS, SCM, FAS
Treatment—Acupuncture Assistance in acupuncture methods, points, acupuncture needles and time Link and search with acupoint monograph database Link and search with stock control and price Link and search with patient accounts (for calculation and invoice) Acupuncture prescription of each diagnosis and treatment—must be written in multi-lingual (PinYin, Chinese characters, English, Latin)	EMR, MDM, CKM, CDS, SCM, FAS

Table 11.3 (continued)

Functions	Systems
Massage (TuiNa) Assistance in massage methods, points/area, time Link and search with patient accounts (for calculation and invoice)	EMR, MDM, CKM, CDS, FAS
Reports & forms with templates Tax invoice includes specials, discounts and GST Sick leave, referral letter, herbal preparation instructions for patients Reports for government and authorities Case report—must be written in multi-lingual (English and Chinese)	EMR, MDM, FAS
Upload & scan external files (pdf, image, X-ray films, medical reports etc.)	EMR, MDM
Stock (medicine) management Herbs (including dry raw herbs, pills, tablets, powder, etc.) Acupuncture needles, points—link to monograph database Other stocks: treatment equipment, moxa, devices Stock tracking—reorder alert, reorder list/report Add/subtract stock and export to MS Excel	SCM
System network LAN access—multi location, multi user System security—access control, virus management, information security Mobile access to the system Back-up with reminder function (hard disc, USB, etc)	Integrated healthcare system, security system

in the testing and evaluation, and their feedback will be taken to further refine and enhance the system. For the CMCS to be implemented in CM clinics not only must it have user support but it is also very important that it is modified and governed by international policies and standards. For example, CMCS must follow CMBA patient records guidelines and principles when recording patients file using EMR. Fig. 11.2 depicts the proposed design and key elements.

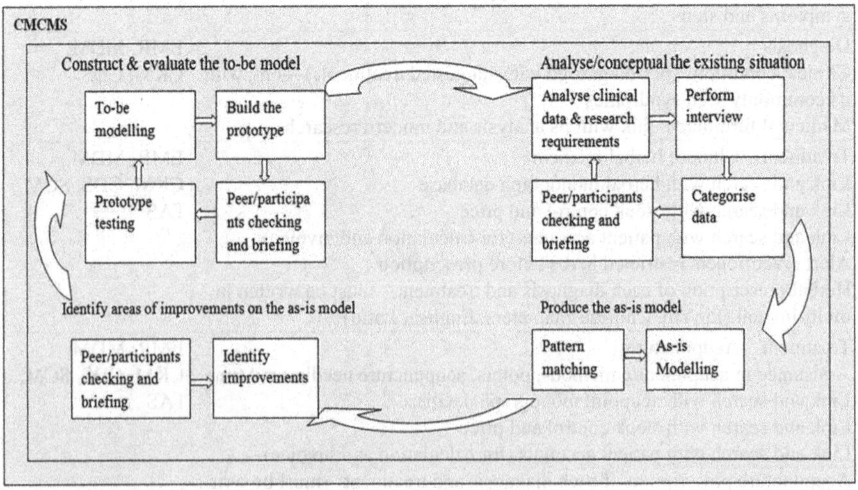

Fig. 11.2 Proposed design (adapted from Han-Lin et al. 2015)

Conclusion

Today, consumers in healthcare are also looking to alternate therapies such as CM to assist them in their care and wellness management. While the fundamental aspects of CM have not changed, we proffer that there is scope to incorporate IS/IT to facilitate its delivery. This chapter reports on a research in progress study to design and develop an appreciate CMCS. Specifically, it has served to identify the importance and advantages of using IS/IT CM healthcare contexts. Furthermore, we have identified the key activities in the processes of CM clinical practice that can benefit from IS/IT. The chapter also draws attention to the need to map key KM concepts in transferring CM knowledge and practice for clinical usage. This study is the first step in developing the CMCS. Next steps will include creating the CMCS and its sub-systems, using mobile and/or cloud technology in CM practice, and IS/IT in CM education.

References

Austin, C. J., & Boxerman, S. B. (2003). *Information systems for healthcare management*. Chicago: Health Administration Press.

Ball, M. J., & Lillis, J. (2001). E-health: Transforming the physician/patient relationship. *International Journal of Medical Informatics, 61*(1), 1–10.

Bates, D. W. (2000). Using information technology to reduce rates of medication errors in hospitals. *BMJ: British Medical Journal, 320*(7237), 788–791.

Bernstein, M. L., McCreless, T., & Cote, M. J. (2007). Five constants of information technology adoption in healthcare. *Hospital Topics, 85*(1), 17–25.

CAHU, Complementary and Alternative Healing University. (2013). Dictionary of Chinese herbs. http://alternativehealing.org/chinese_herbs_dictionary.htm. Accessed 27 Nov 2015.

CMBA, Chinese Medicine Board of Australia. (2013). Chinese medicine board of Australia, about us. http://www.chinesemedicineboard.gov.au. Accessed 27 Nov 2015.

COCIR European Coordination Committee of the Radiological, Electromedical and Healthcare IT Industry. (2012). COCIR eHealth toolkit contributing to the European digital agenda second edition May 2012. http://www.cocir.org/site/fileadmin/Publications_2011/ehealth_toolkit_link2.pdf. Accessed 27 Nov 2015.

Dasherb Corp. (2013). Dasherb herb database. http://www.dasherb.com/database/index.html. Accessed 27 Nov 2015.

Goodson, B. (2005). *Ready for take-off: Knowledge management infrastructure at easyjet. Knowledge management tools and techniques practitioners and experts evaluate KM solutions* (pp. 147–154). Amsterdam: Elsevier.

Gottschalk, P. (2005). *Strategic knowledge management technology*. Hershey: Idea Group Publishing.

Han-Lin, C., Yang, A. W. H., Pittayachawan, S., & Wickramasinghe, N. (2015). An analysis on the utilisation of health information technology to support clinical operation of Chinese medicine.

Hannan, T. J. (1996). Electronic medical records. Health informatics: An overview, pp 133–148. http://www.achi.org.au/docs/HNI_Book/Chapter_12.pdf. Accessed July 2015.

Hojabri, R., & Manafi, M. (2012). Impact of using telemedicine on knowledge management in healthcare organizations: A case study. *African Journal of Business Management, 6*(4), 1604–1613.

Huang, M. J., & Chen, M. Y. (2007). Integrated design of the intelligent web-based Chinese medical diagnostic system (CMDS)—systematic development for digestive health. *Expert Systems with Applications, 32*(2), 658–673.
Kaptchuk, T. J. (2000). Chinese medicine—the web that has no weaver. An Imprint of Elbury Press, Random House, Rider.
Lam, C. F. D., Leung, K. S., Heng, P. A., Lim, C. E. D., & Wong, F. W. S. (2012). Chinese acupuncture expert system (CAES)—a useful tool to practice and learn medical acupuncture. *Journal of Medical Systems, 36*(3), 1883–1890.
Lenz, R., & Reichert, M. (2007). IT support for healthcare processes—premises, challenges, perspectives. *Data & Knowledge Engineering, 61*(1), 39–58.
Liao, Y. Q. (2011). *Traditional Chinese medicine*. Cambridge: Cambridge University Press.
Liu, Z. W., & Liu, L. (2009). *Essentials of Chinese Medicine*. New York: Springer.
Long, I., & Lai, A. (2005). Knowledge management for Chinese medicines: A conceptual model. *Information Management & Computer Security, 13*(3), 244–255.
Lu, A. P., Jia, H. W., Xiao, C., & Lu, Q. P. (2004). Theory of traditional Chinese medicine and therapeutic method of diseases. *World Journal of Gastroenterology, 10*(13), 1854–1856.
Microsoft. (2011). Manifesto for a Ehealthier Europe. http://www.microsoft.com/nl-be/healthcare/knowledge-centre/microsoft-manifesto-for-a-e-healthier-europe.aspx. Accessed 27 Nov 2015
Mitamura, Y. (2010). Electronic document management system, medical information system, method for printing sheet of chart paper, and sheet of chart paper. U.S. Patent, February.
Morr, C. E., & Subercaze, J. (2010). *Handbook of research on developments in e-health and telemedicine: Technological and social perspectives*. Hershey: IGI Global.
Nonaka, I. (1994). A dynamic theory of organizational knowledge creation. *Organization Science, 5*(1), 14–37.
Nonaka, I., Reinmoeller, P., & Senoo, D. (1998). Management focus the 'art' of knowledge: Systems to capitalize on market knowledge. *European Management Journal, 16*(6), 673–684.
Polanyi, M. (1966). The logic of tacit inference. *Philosophy, 41*(155), 1–18.
Polanyi, M. (1968). Life's irreducible structure. *Science, 160*(3834), 1308–1312. doi:10.1126/science.160.3834.1308. PMID 5651890.
Quintas, P., Lefrere, P., & Jones, G. (1997). Knowledge management: A strategic agenda. *Long Range Planning, 30*(3), 385–391.
Shi, J., & Lu, L. (2006). Traditional Chinese medicine in treatment of opiate addiction. *Acta Pharmacologica Sinica, 27*(10), 1303–1308.
Sittig, D. F., Wrightb, A., Simonaitisc, L., Carpenterd, J. D., Allene, G. O., Doebbelingc, B. N., Sirajuddinf, A. M., Ashg, J. S., & Middletonb, B. (2010). The state of the art in clinical knowledge management: an inventory of tools and techniques. *International Journal of Medical Informatics, 79*(1), 44–57.
Swisher, J. R., Jacobson, S. H., Jun, J. B., & Balci, O. (2001). Modeling and analyzing a physician clinic environment using discrete-event (visual) simulation. *Computers & Operations Research, 28*(2), 105–125.
Wang, Z. G., Chen, P., & Xie, P. P. (1999). *History and development of traditional Chinese medicine*. Beijing: Science Press.
Wickramasinghe, N., & Schaffer, J. L. (2010). Realizing value driven patient centric healthcare through technology. IBM Center for The Business of Government, DC.
Wickramasinghe, N., Geisler, E., & Schaffer, J. L. (2006). Realising the value proposition for healthcare by incorporating KM strategies and data mining techniques with the use of information and communication technologies. *International Journal of Healthcare Technology and Management, 7*(3), 303–318.
Wyatt, J. C. (2001). Management of explicit and tacit knowledge. *Journal of the Royal Society of Medicine, 94*(1), 6–9.
Xue, C. C., & O'Brien, K. A. (2003). *A comprehensive guide to Chinese medicine chapter 2: Modalities of Chinese medicine*. River Edge: World Scientific Publishing.
Yang, A. W., Allan, G., Li, C. G., & Xue, C. C. (2009). Effective application of knowledge management in evidence-based Chinese medicine: A case study. *eCam, 6*(3), 393–398.

Zhao, Y. K., Tsursui, T., Endo, A., Minato, K., & Takahashi, T. (1994). Design and development of an expert system to assist diagnosis and treatment of chronic hepatitis using traditional Chinese medicine. *Informatics for Health and Social Care, 19*(1) 37–45.
Zhu, B., & Wang, H. C. (2011). *Basic theories of traditional Chinese medicine.* London: Jessica Kingsley Publishers.

Catherine Han Lin has worked in the information systems/information technology (IS/IT) profession for more than 20 years with many well-known international companies at various positions including: System Analyst, BI/BA, ICT Manager, Research Assistant, and IS/IT Lecturer. Her research interests include: Information Systems, Information Management, Health Informatics, and IS/IT in Complementary and Alternative Medicine.

Dr. Angela Wei Hong Yang has been teaching, researching, and practicing Chinese medicine for 20 years. Her research specialty is to investigate the quality, safety, and effectiveness of Chinese medicine for chronic diseases and apply the interdisciplinary approach (e.g. information systems) to promote, manage, and analyze Chinese medicine knowledge.

Dr. Siddhi Pittayachawan is a senior lecturer of Information Systems and Supply Chain Management, School of Business IT and Logistics, RMIT University. His primary research interests focus on trust, information system adoption, information security behaviour, sustainable business, supply chain management, and business education.

Prof. Nilmini Wickramasinghe (PhD; MBA; GradDipMgtSt; BSc. Amus.A, piano; Amus.A, violin) has a well-recognized research record in the field of healthcare and IT/IS. Her expertise is in the strategic application and management of technology for effecting superior healthcare solutions. She is currently the Professor Director of Health Informatics Management at Epworth HealthCare and a professor at Deakin University.

Chapter 12
The Prevalence of Social Question Answering in Health-Care Social Media

Blooma John, Raj Gururajan and Nilmini Wickramasinghe

Introduction

Health-care social media blends technology and social interaction to engage people in health-care activities (Denecke and Stewart 2011). Health professionals, patients, pharmacists, and insurance agents are embracing health-care social media to share facts, experiences, and opinions. Health-care social media applications such as wiki (AskDrWiki), social networks (PatientsLikeMe), and social question answering (SQA) portals (Netdoctor) are revolutionizing the way people seek and exchange health-related information. Furthermore, they augment various aspects of traditional health-care delivery (Wickramasinghe et al. 2012).

We focus on SQA services in health-care social media. SQA services are dedicated platforms for users to respond to, rate other users' questions, and build a community (Blooma et al. 2013). People use SQA services in health-care social media to seek health-related information (BabyHub), share remedy (MedHelp), discuss medical issues (JustAnswers), and offer emotional support (SmartPatients).

On a review of past studies in health-care SQA services, Denecke and Nejdl (2009) performed content analysis on health-related information in medical SQA services, medical Weblogs, medical reviews, and wikis to gain an overview on the content. The results evidenced substantial differences in the content of various health-related Web resources and users. For example, blogs and SQA services main-

B. John (✉)
Business Information Technology and Logistics, RMIT International University Vietnam, 702 Nguyen Van Linh Blvd., District 7, HCMC, Vietnam
e-mail: Blooma.john@rmit.edu.vn

R. Gururajan
University of Southern Queensland, 60 Baker Ave, Kew East 3102, Australia
e-mail: gururaja@usq.edu.au

N. Wickramasinghe
Deakin University and Epworth HealthCare, 60 Baker Ave, Kew East 3102, Australia
e-mail: n.wickramasinghe@deakin.edu.au

N. Wickramasinghe et al. (eds.), *Contemporary Consumer Health Informatics,* Healthcare Delivery in the Information Age, DOI 10.1007/978-3-319-25973-4_12

ly dealt with diseases and medications, while wiki and the encyclopedia dealt with anatomy and procedures. Moreover, patients and nurses described personal aspects of their life, while doctors aimed at present health-related information. However, the information type classification was restricted to Weblogs. Rozenkranz et al. (2013) provided a literature review of health-care social media. The study classified stakeholder groups of health-care system based on their interconnections as individuals and organizations. Although the study highlighted the patient centeredness as well as the dissemination of different types of health information, one of the limitations of the study was that literature review was restricted in terms of its selection of sources, and no databases from the medical context were used. Other studies related to health-care social media focused on data mining (Goeuriot et al. 2012; Tang and Yang 2012; Yang et al. 2012). However, there is no study yet that focused on prevalence of SQA services in health-care social media.

Therefore, we aim to develop a deeper insight into the prevalence of SQA services in health-care social media. The main contribution of this study is to inform the business of health care and provide an understanding of the critical aspects pertaining to SQA services. This is significant because users and their media content have a vital impact on other users and the overall health outcome in a society (Durst et al. 2013). To achieve the stated objective, our research question is: *To what extent is SQA service prevalent in health-care social media?*

The following section presents the framework used to evaluate prevalence of SQA in health-care social media. The next section details the methodology used to analyze SQA services. The results section discusses our findings and recommendations. We conclude with implications and future work.

Literature Review

Consumer health informatics is becoming the key differentiator for health-care delivery in the twenty-first century (Fig. 12.1; Eysenbach 2000) and Medicine 2.0 embodies this approach (Eysenbach 2008). Health-care social media facilitates the creation and exchange of user-generated content which stands for information age health care as shown in Fig. 12.1. Health-care SQA service is a type of social media widely used (Tang and Yang 2012) and offers prevention and self-help or self-care in cyber medicine (Fig. 12.1). On SQA services, consumers and professionals in health-care communities generate content particularly in the form of questions, answers, comments, and ratings. Hence, to address the research question, we review and present theories related to characteristics of social media (Kaplan and Haenlein 2010) and Medicine 2.0 themes (Eysenbach 2008) in the following sections. Based on the review, we developed a framework to evaluate the prevalence of SQA in health-care social media.

Kaplan and Haenlein (2010) classified social media based on media research and social process. Media research dimension included social presence (Short et al. 1976) and media richness theory (Daft and Lengel 1986). Following media research dimension, we use attributes of medium (Daft and Lengel 1986) to evaluate the

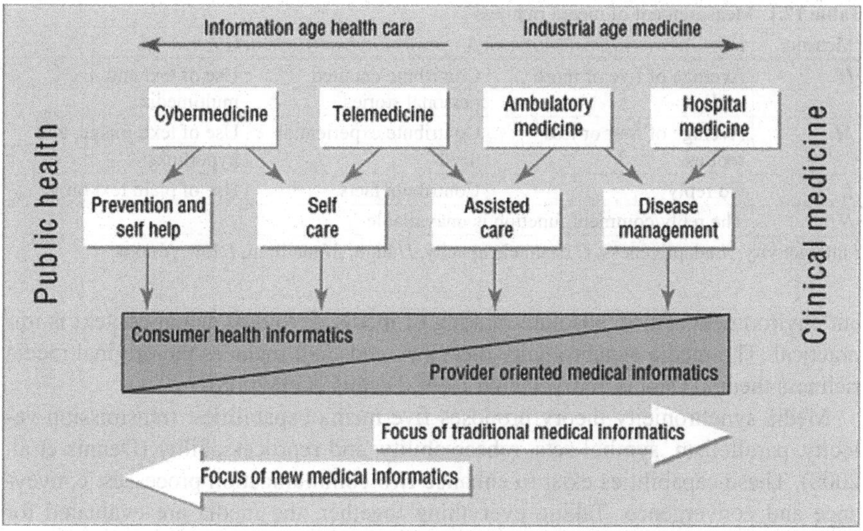

Fig. 12.1 The changing face of health-care delivery. (Source: Eysenbach 2000)

prevalence of SQA services in the angle of communication effectiveness (Dennis and Valacich 1999). Social processes dimension includes self-presentation and self-disclosure. Anchoring on the social process dimension, we use Medicine 2.0 themes (Eysenbach 2008) to understand the reasons for the prevalence of SQA services in the angle of consumer empowerment (Wickramasinghe et al. 2012).

Attributes of Medium

The concept of media richness was first introduced by Daft and Lengel (1986) to improve problem-solving in an organization. They argue that uncertainty and equivocality influence information processing in an organization. High uncertainty is the shortage of data to make informed decisions. On the other hand, equivocality, or ambiguity, arises from different interpretations and understanding of the same problem. Reduction in uncertainty involves increase in the quantity and reduction in equivocality requires rich information. Richness correlates with learning capacity of communication channels. The follow-up study provides four features relevant to the richness of medium: immediacy of feedback, multiple cues, language variety, and personal focus (Daft et al. 1987). They rank the richness of various media in a descending order: face-to-face, telephone, personal documents, impersonal written documents, and numeric documents.

Three major limitations stand against the traditional use of media richness theory (Dennis et al. 1998). First, no medium is the richest across all dimensions. Second, the same medium can take different values depending on its configuration in differ-

Table 12.1 Measurement of media richness

Measure	I	A	C
H	Average of five or more replies	Contribute detailed personal stories	Use of text and multimedia
M	Average of four or less replies	Contribute experiential need	Use of text, image, and hyperlinks
L	No reply	Contribute facts	Use of plain text only
N	The reply/comment function is unavailable		

I interactivity, *A* adaptiveness, *C* channel capacity, *H* high, *M* medium, *L* low, *N* none

ent environment. Third, absolute ranking of media devoid of actual context is impractical. The media synchronicity theory extends and replaces the original media richness theory (Dennis and Valacich 1999; Dennis et al. 2008).

Media synchronicity theory proposes five media capabilities: transmission velocity, parallelism, symbol sets, rehearsability, and reprocessability (Dennis et al. 2008). These capabilities exist to enhance two communication processes: conveyance and convergence. Taking everything together, the media are evaluated for communication and task performance. Although the theory provides a comprehensive framework, it is complex for the scope of this research and might overfit observations from limited samples. Instead, we use the media richness theory (Daft et al. 1987) adapted for new electronic media, which include health-care social media (Te'eni 2001; Zack 1993). To avoid the three major limitations above, we compare social media types based on individual characteristic and interpret the result in the context of health-care consumers. The three media characteristics are interactivity, adaptiveness, and channel capacity (Table 12.1; Te'eni 2001). Interactivity is the potential for immediate feedback from the receiver in the form of continuous exchange of information. Therefore, interactivity requires bidirectional communication where two or more people actively respond to each other. Adaptiveness is the potential to adapt (personalize) a message to a particular receiver. In specific, how one person tailors her message to the contextual experience of another person. Channel capacity is the potential to transmit a high variety of cues and languages. It is proportional to the amount of tools and service features available at the disposal of users.

Medicine 2.0 Themes

Medicine 2.0 is redefining health-care delivery and supporting patient empowerment. Medicine 2.0 evolves from traditional hospital-based medicine towards the future where consumers take responsibility of their own health by providing personalized health care at their fingertips (Wickramasinghe et al. 2012). In Medicine 2.0 applications, users connect with patients and professionals without time and space boundary to seek and share health-care-related information using applications and technologies that facilitate *social networking, participation, apomediation, collaboration, and openness* (Eysenbach 2008).

Social Networking

Social networking evokes a practice of actively seeking connections between users (Ellison and Boyd 2013). Social networking results in complex network of relationships that enable users to see, collaborate, share, and shape the opinions and information of their social peers (Eysenbach 2008; Kaplan and Haenlein 2010). A recent study on social networking states that social media networks possess four features: digital profile, search and privacy, relational ties, and network transparency (Kane et al. 2014). Among the four features, digital profile and relational ties are the features that represent social process dimension.

Digital profile ensures that the platform provides the tools for users to construct their unique profile. Digital profile has three attributes listed as content, trace, and third-party contributions. Existence of digital profile is important with respect to SQA services in health-care social media because it represents social presence. Relational ties provides insight into the intensity of social networking in SQA services as it highlights the mechanisms for users to articulate a list of other users with whom they share a connection. Four relational tie types proposed by Borgatti et al. (2009) are proximity, social relations, interactions, and flows. With respect to SQA services in health-care social media, relational ties is how users publicly articulate connections and how users interact with streams of user-generated content provided by their connections on the site.

Participation and Collaboration

Participation is the multifaceted interactions and negotiations of users in various levels. Users and their network play a vital role in the quality and quantity of participation. A deeper insight into the participation and their motivation will result in better user empowerment and involvement (Gimpel et al. 2013). Moreover, participation result in collaboration that connects groups of people with each other who before would have not been able to (Bacigalupe 2010).

Among various Information System theories, Actor Network Theory (ANT) focuses on users and their attempts to adopt and negotiate in actor network, which in turn improves participation and collaboration (Latour 1999). Applying ANT to analyze the underlying complex user interactions as they participate in health-care SQA services is important for two reasons (Troshani and Wickramasinghe 2014). First, to understand the action-oriented roles taken by consumers in health-care SQA services. Second, to recognize the multiple networks formed by actors at multiple time points, which eventually results in participation and collaboration.

ANT is a research method that analyzes the relationship between human and nonhuman objects termed as actants. The actants and their interactions form a network (Latour 2005). ANT emphasizes the symmetrical influence and power of both types of actants. Researchers in health-care technology have successfully applied ANT to investigate impact of technical solutions (Cresswell 2010; Troshani and Wickramasinghe 2014).

ANT has two fundamental concepts: inscription and translation (Troshani and Wickramasinghe 2014). Inscription states that actants continually imprint their ideas and interests onto each other. Translation consists of four sequential processes to achieve inscription: problematization, interessement, enrollment, and mobilization. During problematization, the initiating actants define the problem and articulate their interest in a solution. In interessement, the actants invite other actants by aligning their interest. Actants take up roles in the network during enrollment and finally maintain their roles in mobilization.

Health-care consumers participate and collaborate to create and consume questions and answers in SQA services. These digital artifacts serve as proxies of participants, and they too play a role in the SQA services. Each question models an emerging network where posts interact and participants influence each other. ANT is specifically suitable to analyze such dynamic interplay between human and digital artifacts.

Apomediation and Openness

Apomediation introduced by Eysenbach (2007) is an information-seeking strategy for users to identify trustworthy and credible information and services. It is social mediation of information where apomediaries (people, tools) standby to provide and guide a consumer towards relevant and high-quality information in an altruistic notion with limited power to alter the information. On the contrary, traditional approach to identify relevant information is to use intermediaries such as health-care professionals who advice a patient online or offline. Alternatively, disintermediation is a process by which the consumers bypass intermediaries to seek relevant information directly from personal health information or general health information available. While disintermediation might result in getting lost or ending up in wrong information, apomediation is a type of disintermediation where apomediaries take the role of intermediaries and guide consumers to accurate information. Apomediation support the users to navigate through the plethora of information (Boncella et al. 2013).

Apomediation dimensions, stated by Eysenbach (2008), are environment, power, dependence, nature of information consumption, nature of interaction, information filtering, learning, cognitive elaboration, and user as detailed in Fig. 12.2. We use apomediation dimensions to further understand how health-care SQA service fits in the apomediation model.

Finally, openness implies that health-care transactions and treatments should be visible and transparent. While open interface, transparency, and interoperability weigh on one side of the scale (Wickramasinghe et al. 2012), trust, ownership and privacy issues in health-care data weigh on the other side (Moumtzoglou 2011). The full treatment of these topics is beyond the scope of this study. Thus, we limit the evaluation of openness to the type and accessibility of data (Eysenbach 2008).

Analysis

For analysis, we selected popular health-care social media sites to understand the prevalence of SQA services in health-care social media. The popularity reflects the contemporary development trend of social media sites from both perspectives of

Fig. 12.2 Dimensions of apomediation environment. (Source: Eysenbach 2008)

Dimension	Apomediation Environment
Environment	Autonomous
Power	Decentralized; empowerment of information seekers
Dependence	Information seekers are emancipated from intermediaries as apomediaries (peers, technology) provide *guidance;* apomediaries are *optional*
Nature of Information Consumption	Consumers are "prosumers" (i.e., co-producers of information)
Nature of Interaction	Complex individual- and group-based interactions in a networked environment
Information Filtering	"Downstream filtering" with bottom-up quality assurance mechanisms
Learning	More informal; learning through participation, application, and information production
Cognitive Elaboration	Higher elaboration required by information seekers; higher cognitive load unless assistance through intelligent tools

health-care consumers and Web developers (Shirkley 2006). The Web usage and design in these sites represent major global trends. The two measures for popularity are Web award nomination for developer trend (webbyawards.com) and Web traffic for user trend (alexa.com). From the 15 Web sites listed by each of the above sources, we selected 5 health-care social media sites for further analysis based on three criteria.

The first criterion is the presence of user profile. To engage in meaningful long-term interaction, users need to establish and maintain their social presence through digital profile. Second, presence of SQA services, blogs and videos are mandatory according to the scope of this study. Third, the site is popular for both developer trend and user trend. The five popular health-care social media sites selected for this study are BHF.org.uk, MayoClinic.org, Drugs.com, WebMD.com, and LiveStrong.com. A sample data collected from MyoClinic.org is given in Fig. 12.3.

We adopted mixed method approach in two phases (Venkatesh et al. 2013). In the first phase, we employed qualitative content analysis to compare different social media types in the selected sites based on media richness (White and Marsh 2006). To maintain consistency, analysis of Web sites starts at the homepage (Damman

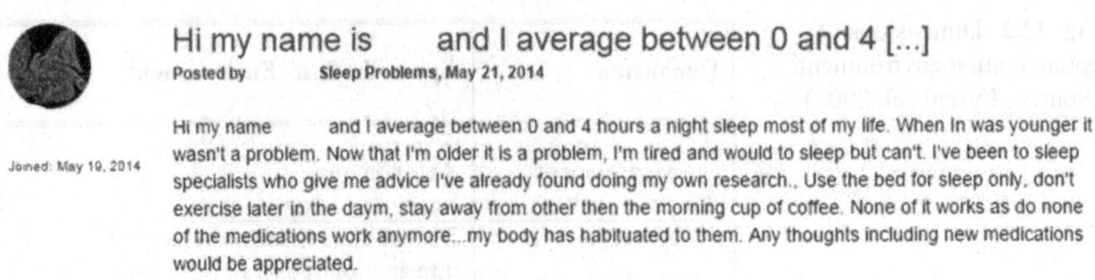
Hi my name is and I average between 0 and 4 [...]
Posted by Sleep Problems, May 21, 2014
Joined: May 19, 2014
Hi my name and I average between 0 and 4 hours a night sleep most of my life. When In was younger it wasn't a problem. Now that I'm older it is a problem, I'm tired and would to sleep but can't. I've been to sleep specialists who give me advice I've already found doing my own research., Use the bed for sleep only, don't exercise later in the daym, stay away from other then the morning cup of coffee. None of it works as do none of the medications work anymore...my body has habituated to them. Any thoughts including new medications would be appreciated.

Fig. 12.3 A sample collected from MayoClinic.org

et al. 2010; Petch 2004). However, the homepage in a large Web site fails to reflect the depth and breadth of the whole Web site. It provides Web site summary and links to other specific Web pages on the same site that contain the rich content relevant to research (Petch 2004). We used drill-down approach to expand systematically from the homepage to locate target content on the sites evaluated (Damman et al. 2010; Petch 2004). One drill-down includes all distinct and relevant Web pages within one hyperlink from the starting point, while two drill-downs reach Web pages within two hyperlinks.

To compare different social media types based on media richness, we scoped our study to blogs, videos, and SQA services. To locate the display list of blogs, videos, and SQA services, we used two drill-downs from home page or search results. Different entry points for drill-down provide better coverage of entire Web site. We select the drill-down path based on two criteria: popularity and visibility. First, the selected path leads to the most popular video, blog, or SQA service. Second, the selected path is the first on the display list. Health-care social media sites support different health conditions, and they structure the display list around these conditions. Search result pages are different for each Web site. If a popular list is absent, this criterion reduces selection bias of a particular health condition.

We performed the analysis in May 2014. For each media type, we analyzed two units based on three media richness criteria: *interactivity, adaptiveness, and channel capacity*. Each criterion has four levels of rating: High (H), Medium (M), Low (L), and None (N). Table 12.1 describes each level and its three different measures. An important distinction is that the rating of Interactivity measures the average number of bidirectional replies where people interact back and forth to exchange information; it does not measure the total number of replies. Section "Comparison of Media Richness" discusses the findings of first phase.

In the second phase, we conducted an interpretive analysis to evaluate SQA services based on the five themes of Medicine 2.0 as detailed in Table 12.2 based on literature review. We evaluated three discussions from each SQA services. The inclusion criteria are the same as in previous phase: popularity and visibility. The evaluation of the first SQA services returns baseline result. We recorded and interpreted the similarities and differences between SQA services. Section "Evaluation of SQA Services" discusses the findings of second phase.

Table 12.2 Framework for Medicine 2.0 themes

Medicine 2.0 themes	Features	References
Social networking	Digital profiles	Ellison and Boyd 2013; Kane et al. 2014
	Relational ties	
Participation	Actant	Latour 1999; Troshani and Wickramasinghe 2014
	Inscription	
Collaboration	Problematization	
	Interessement	
	Enrolment	
	Mobilization	
Apomediation	Environment	Eysenbach 2008
	Power	
	Dependence	
	Nature of information consumption	
	Nature of interaction	
	Information filtering	
	Learning	
	Cognitive elaboration	
	User	
Openness	Data and information access	

Result

Comparison of Media Richness

This section details the analysis of all five health-care social media sites and explains the rating for each medium (Table 12.3). To summarize the findings, Drugs.com, MayoClinic, and WebMD use videos to supplement the news articles and lack comment area whereas BHF and LiveStrong provide self-contained videos. BHF host all videos on Youtube but embed a few onsite as supplemental material. LiveStrong provides videos about fitness exercises with a Facebook comment section. Videos of BHF and LiveStrong generate many comments, and users engage

Table 12.3 Media richness in health-care social media

<table>
<tr><th rowspan="2">Site</th><th colspan="3">SQA</th><th colspan="3">Blog</th><th colspan="3">Video</th></tr>
<tr><th>I</th><th>A</th><th>C</th><th>I</th><th>A</th><th>C</th><th>I</th><th>A</th><th>C</th></tr>
<tr><td>Drugs.com</td><td rowspan="5">H</td><td rowspan="5">H</td><td rowspan="2">L</td><td rowspan="5">L</td><td rowspan="5">M</td><td rowspan="5">M</td><td rowspan="3">N</td><td rowspan="3">N</td><td rowspan="5">H</td></tr>
<tr><td>MayoClinic.org</td></tr>
<tr><td>WebMD.com</td><td rowspan="3">M</td></tr>
<tr><td>BHF.org.uk</td><td rowspan="2">M</td><td rowspan="2">M</td></tr>
<tr><td>LiveStrong.com</td></tr>
</table>

SQA social question answering, *I* interactivity, *A* adaptiveness, *C* channel capacity, *H* high, *M* medium, *L* low, *N* none

in light conversations but are not as engaged as in SQA services. Videos are more suitable for information where visual cues are necessary such as life-saving cardiopulmonary resuscitation (CPR) in BHF. Compared to blogs or other media types, videos aim to present information in a more dynamic way especially with animation. Users respond to videos as they would to blogs. Blogs are more suitable for regular news update and consumption such as healthy living tips in LiveStrong.

SQA services are found to be more interactive than videos and blogs. In SQA services, users create content for each other. Users respond to each other and in more diverse ways than in videos or blogs. SQA services have conversations and discussions where subsequent participants build upon the previous content (Blooma et al. 2013). The direction is many to many between all participants. On the other hand, for videos and blogs, the direction is many replies to one video or blog. Content creators of blogs and videos do not respond to users' comments. Thus, SQA services have highest interactivity, and posts are longer and more detailed.

SQA services are found to be more adaptive than videos and blogs. In videos and blogs, the content creators are experts or Web site staff, and users only comment on the content. In fact, three Web sites lack the comment function for their videos and consequently prevent user interaction. Based on users' participation, both content creators and users prefer plain text communication. If comment function is available in blogs and videos, the communication mode is strictly plain text. Among three social media types, blogs receive fewest comments. This is probably because most blogs take the role of news articles or opinions. Experts write to present new information, guide to good practice, anecdotal evidence, or motivational stories of other users. They do not focus on sharing their personal life stories as in traditional blogs. There are no user blogs. In all cases, users go beyond basic recitation of facts and information in their response and attempt to adapt to others at an emotional level by showing care and concern. In SQA services and blogs, they also detail their own personal stories (Bacigalupe 2010). Both videos and blogs contextualize their content to address common emotional concerns of users regarding health conditions. They reassure and encourage users and provide advice on how to deal emotionally with the health conditions. Users respond to show their support, agreement, or gratitude to the content (Short et al. 1976). As blogs are only for experts, users start to discuss and share their own stories in SQA services as they would in normal blogs (Gazan 2010). They even update their stories in the same discussion if there are other interested participants. Across five Web sites, SQA services are the most consistent, and blog is the least consistent in terms of interactivity and adaptiveness rating. Furthermore, SQA services have potentially the highest impact to users due to high interactivity and adaptiveness.

With respect to channel capacity, if blogs and SQA services provide medium channel capacity, content creators and users fail to use the extra tools. They dominantly favor plain text even though they can embed images or use formatting functions (bold, underline, colors, etc.) to deliver their messages more effectively. In the rare case that users applies the extra tools in their first post, they apply the tools again on subsequent posts in the same discussion (Weiss and Campion 2007). Moreover, due to the asymmetrical roles in videos and blogs, users have fewer tools to interact. This design lowers the channel capacity on user side. Channel capacity currently favors content creators over users. Content creators have more tools such as the ability to embed image in blogs and produce videos. Both blogs and videos focus on presenting and delivering information to the public. With the same content, video production and editing process generally require more time and resources than the process of writing short blogs. As users neglect the extra tools, the impact of asymmetry in channel capacity to users is insignificant. In this regard, videos, blogs, and SQA services operate at relatively equal capacity for users.

Evaluation of SQA Services

The characteristics of social networking, participation, collaboration, apomediation and openness are relatively homogeneous across SQA services. The main difference between SQA services lies in social networking characteristics. This section describes evaluation result.

Social Networking

We evaluated social networking by looking at digital profile and relational ties as given in Table 12.2. All five SQA services evaluated have basic information in digital profile. They also track user activities. WebMD and British Heart Foundation (BHF) stay at this basic level. MayoClinic records users' interests to optimize news feed content. LiveStrong and Drugs.com have the most comprehensive tracking. LiveStrong stores user-provided data related to fitness, weight loss, and food. Drugs.com automatically gathers data about users' participation. Table 12.4 gives shared results of digital profile and relational ties for all five SQA services.

Participation

We measured participation by identifying possible actants in SQA services and evaluated possible inscriptions that the actants create in SQA services. Four main actants identified in SQA are questioner, answerer, question, and answer (Latour 1999). The emerging network is the discussion eventuating from asking and answering question. Figure 12.4 illustrates the network built by the four actants in SQA service.

The questioner is the topic creator in SQA service. In WebMD, MayoClinic, LiveStrong, and BHF, the question is the first post in the discussion. The first post does not necessarily contain a question; however, it explicitly expresses the interest of the creator and types of discussion the creator desires. In Drugs.com, the

Table 12.4 Evaluation of social networking in social question answering (SQA) services

Features	Shared result
Digital profile	Basic information includes avatar, user name, and brief self-description
Relational ties	Users interact with others by joining the same community. Friend list similar to the ones in social networking sites such as Facebook is uncommon. Users can interact with stream of user-generated content provided by their connections

Fig. 12.4 Actants in social question answering (SQA) service

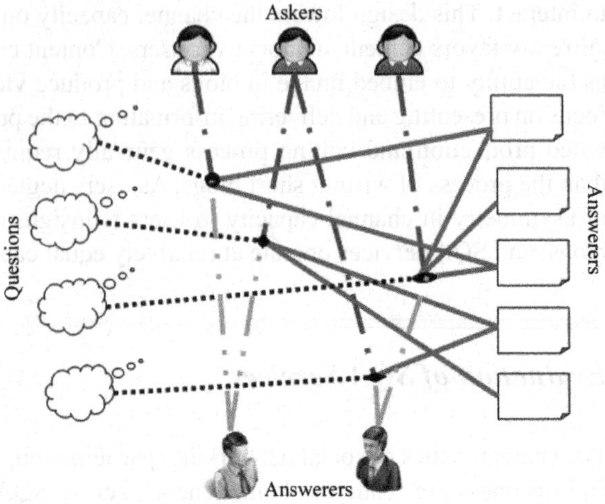

questioner has to ask an explicit question and optionally expresses interest as in other four health-care SQA services. The answerers are participants who reply to the questioner, and the answers are the participants' replies to the original question or to others' answers. Therefore, the questioner and the question are the focal actants, and the network emerges from replies of participants to each other (Gazan 2010). On analysis, actants have four symmetric general inscriptions: seek new information, support opinion and affirmation, share hints and tips, and finally receive answers to their information need. Participation results in collaboration which is discussed in the following section.

Collaboration

We evaluated collaboration through the lens of problematization, interessement, enrolment, and mobilization. In problematization, the questioner defines the problem through personal experience and history, and answerers critically expand the problem through alternative perspective. The popular discussion samples contain personal introduction and motivation of the questioners (Short et al. 1976). As answerers join and contribute their experience, the collective story of the discussion grows and branches. For example, a mother in WebMD seeks advice on applying Ritalin to treat attention deficit hyperactivity disorder (ADHD) of her son, and soon other participants join the discussion with stories of their own children. The original question about a son of a mother grows into the question about children with ADHD. Participants continually refine and develop the original question.

Interessement is highly evident in SQA collaboration. The four actants attempt to build dynamic relationships by influencing the interest of each other and outside observers. Questions invoke empathy, sense of duty to help, or curiosity. Answers invite new perspectives. In an advice against a veterinary product in Drugs.com, the questioner appeals to empathy for animals of other participants. As subsequent answers agree with this sentiment, outside observers with matching concern might become interested. There might be a small snowball effect through empathetic answers. In the

WebMD example, the new answer challenging the original question might expand the scope enough that outside observers with alternative perspective might join.

In enrolment, actants take on different roles to maintain the discussion. They initiate, support, argue, and manage the sessions in SQA services. Supporting is the most common role across the five SQA services. Participants build upon the story and experience of each other. Although arguing is the least common role, participants who object other answers also try to contribute their alternative view in a helpful manner. LiveStrong has a question doubting the merit of cardio exercises, and the very first answer argues against the negative notion in the question by providing benefits of the exercises. By default, the questioners take the managing role; however, other enthusiastic human actants also take this role such as initiating more follow-up discussions (bump the topic).

In mobilization, although human actants can change their roles in new answers, they tend to keep their initial roles. Over the course of the SQA services, a participant can interact with many answers. However, an answer has exactly one role when it replies to the original question or another answer. This allows the discussion to exist independently of human actants once there are enough answers. In WebMD, new users participate in discussions that have been inactive for months or years. Thus, some discussions span years with dozens of posts clustered around different points of time.

Apomediation

Members have full autonomy over the course of their interaction in SQA services. They decide for themselves which discussion to participate, whom to reply, and which answers meet their need. All SQA services provide a public list of available discussions often grouped by a common theme such as introduction of new members in (BHF), quit smoking in LiveStrong, or various health conditions in WebMD, MayoClinic, and Drugs.com. In each discussion, members can reply directly to an answer that branches off into a sub-conversation, as in MayoClinic, or addresses the recipient member with the notation "@username" at the beginning of their reply. Once the questioner feels satisfied, he either explicitly announces his gratitude through "thank you" replies or silently leaves the discussion to current participants.

The full autonomy empowers members (Connor 2010). There are community guidelines, moderators and experts in SQA services, but they play the support role to ensure a pleasant experience for members such as initiating the first answer in a discussion in MayoClinic or providing feedback on accuracy of other answers in WebMD. Members are free from adhering to a central dogma or authority figures (Durst et al. 2013).

Throughout a discussion, members coproduce information through group interaction. As more members participate, the number of different information sources increase, which ultimately lowers reliance on a single central information source. The ADHD example in WebMD from previous section illustrates these features. Members from that discussion coproduce a collective story of applying medication to ADHD children. Thus, if an outside observer shares the same concern, she now has real case studies to cross check with her personal information sources such as family members or doctor of her children.

The accumulative knowledge allows members to learn from each other. However, since there is no central authority, members have to judge credibility and quality of the answers based on personal heuristics. Such inference and validation lead to higher cognitive load than traditional interaction with doctors. In a question about the classification of Tramadol in Drugs.com, a member cites fact from the USA Food and Drug Administration to support her answers. The same member takes a step further to interpret and explain the fact in details. As the quality of the answer evidently rises, the credibility of the answerer becomes more important.

Across all five SQA services, members are information literate. They can articulate their problem with correct terminology such as drug name, health condition and symptom, or typical experience associated with a heart attack.

Openness

All textual data in discussion forums are open to the public. Experienced practitioners can dig and structure the data to provide meaningful insights to users (Denecke and Nejdl 2009). All SQA services track and present an activity list updating new posts of members. The level of tracking details varies between SQA services. Drugs.com presents details of each question and answer and their extra statistics. LiveStrong tracks discussions and replies separately but does not provide the statistics. WebMD, BHF, and MayoClinic only have the basic activity list.

To summarize, phase one of this study recommends to theory and practice that SQA services are rich in medium with respect to interactivity and adaptiveness. SQA services were found to be a medium where users go beyond basic recitation of facts and information in their response. Users attempt to adapt to others at an emotional level by showing care and concern. On an in-depth analysis of SQA services based on the social networking, participation, collaboration, apomediation, and openness, we conclude on three important findings for theory and practice. First, all five health-care SQA services evaluated are rich in social networking by creating digital profiles and relational ties that eventually build a community. Second, the four main actants identified in SQA services are questioner, answerer, question, and answer. The four actants participate and collaborate in SQA services. The initial findings on problematization, interessement, enrolment, and mobilization of actants in SQA services are promising. In future work, there is a need to analyze the implications of participation and collaboration in SQA services and how it affects the health-related behaviors of the society. Apomediation and openness of SQA services are evidenced in this study that sheds light to the designers of health-care Web sites on the role played by SQA services.

Conclusion

Health-care delivery in today's twenty-first century must change due to external pressures faced by all Organisation for Economic Cooperation and Development (OECD) countries including escalating costs, higher expectations from patients, and changing patient demographics including age and chronic diseases. Medicine 2.0 is enabling patient empowerment and the better transfer of pertinent information and germane knowledge with the potential result being superior health-care delivery. Further, regarding the nature of chronic disease where prevention is a key factor, Medicine 2.0 has a major role to play in supporting healthier lifestyle practices. The pervasive nature of Medicine 2.0 technologies means that this is a benefit that most if not all people can enjoy. In many ways, Web 2.0 has the potential to revolutionize current health-care delivery practices and/or roles. In addition, it has a key role to play regarding public health and enabling education and change of lifestyle for all.

In this chapter we have highlighted some of the key aspects regarding health-care SQA Services. We analyzed health-care SQA services to understand the extent to which they are prevalent in health-care social media. First, we compare blogs, videos, and SQA services in five popular health-care social media sites using media richness features. Second, we interpretively analyze SQA services using Medicine 2.0 themes. We propose an integrated framework to evaluate Medicine 2.0 themes.

With respect to media richness, SQA services are overall more interactive and adaptive than blogs and videos in health-care social media. This factor contributes to the success of SQA services with respect to health-care community. Interactivity and adaptiveness empower consumers and professionals to share personal aspects and reach relevant health-related information. However, channel capacity was low in SQA services when compared to videos and that is evident.

SQA services were rich in social process. The consumers maintained digital profile for social presence. Participation and collaboration resulted in building up the community network and sharing knowledge. SQA services apomediate consumers to the information they need and empower them to make their own decisions.

We present our findings for consumers and professionals to understand the role of SQA services for improving user-centered services and directing users to appropriate knowledge sources. Decision-makers and health-care Web developers may benchmark their own efforts in deploying SQA services by understanding its prevalence in health-care social media.

References

Bacigalupe, G. (2010). Is there a role for social technologies in collaborative healthcare? *Families, Systems, and Health, 29*(1), 1–14.

Blooma, M. J., Kurian, J. C., Chua, A. Y. K., Goh, D. H. L., & Lien, N. H. (2013). Social question answering: Analyzing knowledge, cognitive processes and social dimensions of micro-collaborations. *Computers and Education, 69*, 109–120.

Boncella, R., Sun, W., & Boncella, C. (2013). *Research model to identify the characteristics of an Effective Medicine 2.0 Application*. Proceedings of SAIS 2013.

Borgatti, S. P., Mehra, A., Brass, D. J., & Labiance, G. (2009). Network analysis in the social sciences. *Science, 323*(5916), 892–895.

Connor, D. O. (2010). Apomediation and ancillary care: Researchers' responsibilities in health related online communities. *International Journal of Research Ethics*, 3(12), 87–103.

Cresswell, K. M. (2010). Actor-network theory and its role in understanding the implementation of information technology developments in healthcare. *BMC Medical Informatics and Decision Making, 10*(67), 1–11.

Daft, R. L., & Lengel, R. H. (1986). Organizational information requirements, media richness, and structural design. *Management Science, 32*(5), 554–571.

Daft, R. L., Lengel, R. H., & Trevino, L. K. (1987). Message equivocality, media selection, and manger performance: Implications for information systems. *MIS Quarterly, 11*(3), 355–366.

Damman, O. C., van den Hengel, Y. K. A., van Loon, A. J. M., & Rademakers, J. (2010). An international comparison of web-based reporting about health care quality: Content analysis. *Journal of Medical Internet Research, 12*(2), e8.

Denecke, K., & Nejdl, W. (2009). How valuable is medical social media data? Content analysis of the medical web. *Information Science, 179*(12), 1870–1880.

Denecke, K., & Stewart, A. (2011). Learning from medical social media data: Current state and future challenges. In B. White, I. King, & P. Tsang (Eds.), *Social computing in higher learning environments: How media, tools, and platforms change learner's behaviour*. Heidelberg: Springer.

Dennis, A. R., & Valacich, J. S. (1999). *Rethinking media richness: Towards a theory of media synchronicity*. Proceedings of the 32nd Hawaii Conference on System Sciences, IEEE.

Dennis, A. R., Valacich, J. S., Speier, C., & Morris, M. G. (1998). *Beyond media richness: An empirical test of media synchronicity theory*. Proceedings of the 31st Hawaii Conference on System Sciences, IEEE.

Dennis, A. R., Fuller, R. M., & Valacich, J. S. (2008). Media, tasks, and communication processes: A theory of media synchronicity. *MIS Quarterly, 32*(3), 575–600.

Durst, C., Viol, J., & Wickramasinghe, N. (2013). Online social networks, social capital and health related behaviors: A state-of-the-art analysis. *Communications of the Association for Information Systems, 32*(5), 134–158.

Ellison, N. B., & Boyd, D. (2013). Sociality through social network sites. In W. H. Dutton (Ed.), *The Oxford handbook of internet studies* (pp. 151–172). Oxford: Oxford University Press.

Eysenbach, G. (2000). Consumer health informatics. *British Medical Journal, 320*(7251), 1713–1716.

Eysenbach, G. (2007). From intermediation to disintermediation and apomediation: New models for consumers to access and assess the credibility of health information in the age of Web2.0. *Studies in Health Technology and Informatics, 129*, 162–166.

Eysenbach, G. (2008). Medicine 2.0: social networking, collaboration, participation, apomediation, and openness. *Journal of Medical Internet Research, 10*(3), e22.

Gazan, R. (2010). Microcollaborations in a social Q&A community. *Information Processing and Managament, 46*(6), 693–702.

Gimpel, H., Niben, M., & Gorlitz, R. A. (2013). *Quantifying the quantified self: A study on the motivation of patients to track their own health*. Proceedings of the 34th International Conference on Information Systems.

Goeuriot, L., Na, J. C., Kyaing, W. Y. M., & Khoo, C. (2012). *Sentiment lexicons for health-related opinion mining*. Proceedings of ACM SIGHIT International Health Informatics Symposium.

Kane, G. C., Alavi, M., Labianca, G. J., & Borgatti, S. P. (2014). What's different about social media networks? A framework and research agenda. *MIS Quarterly, 38*(1), 275–304.

Kaplan, A. M., & Haenlein, M. (2010). Users of the world, unite! The challenges and opportunities of social media. *Business Horizons, 53*(1), 59–68.

Latour, B. (1999). *Pandora's hope: Essays on the reality of science studies*. Cambridge: Harvard University Press.

Latour, B. (2005). *Reassembling the social: An introduction to actor-network theory*. Oxford: Oxford University Press.

Moumtzoglou, A. (2011). Health 2.0 and Medicine 2.0: Safety, ownership and privacy issues. In A. Chryssanthou, A. Ioannis, & I. Varlamis (Eds.), *Certification and security in health-related web applications: Concepts and solutions*. Hershey: IGI Global.

Petch, T. (2004). *Content analysis of selected health information websites: Final report*. Vancouver: Simon Fraser University.

Rozenkranz, N., Eckhardt, A., Kuhne, M., & Rozenkranz, C. (2013). Health information on the internet: State of the art and analysis. *Business and Information Systems Engineering, 4*, 259–274.

Shirkley, C. (2006). Power laws, weblogs, and inequality. In J. Dean, J. W. Anderson, & G. Lovink (Eds.), *Reformatting politics: Information technology and global civil society* (pp. 35–42). London: Routledge.

Short, J., Williams, E., & Christie, B. (1976). *The social psychology of telecommunications*. Hoboken: Wiley.

Tang, X., & Yang, C. C. (2012). Ranking user influence in healthcare social media. *ACM Transactions on Intelligent Systems and Technology, 3*(4), 73.

Te'eni, D. (2001). Review: A cognitive-affective model of organizational communication for designing IT. *MIS Quarterly, 25*(2), 251–312.

Troshani, I., & Wickramasinghe, N. (2014). *Tackling complexity in e-health with actor-network theory*. Proceedings of the 47th Annual Hawaii International Conference on System Sciences. IEEE, 2994–3003.

Venkatesh, V., Brown, S. A., & Bala, H. (2013). Bridging the qualitative-quantitative divide: Guidelines for conducting mixed methods research in information systems. *MIS Quarterly, 37*(1), 21–54.

Weiss, J. B., & Campion, T. R. (2007). Blogs, wikis, and discussion forums: Attributes and implications for clinical information systems. *Studies in Health Technology and Informatics, 129*, 157–161.

White, M. D., & Marsh, E. E. (2006). Content analysis: A flexible methodology. *Library Trends, 55*(1), 22–45.

Wickramasinghe, N., Davey, B., & Tatnall, A. (2012). Web 2.0 Panacea or Placebo for Superior Healthcare Delivery? *Pervasive health knowledge management* (pp. 317–330). New York: Springer.

Yang, C. C., Yang, H., Jiang, L., & Zhang, M. (2012). *Social media mining for drug safety signal detection*. Proceedings of ACM CIKM International Workshop on Smart Health and Wellbeing.

Zack, M. H. (1993). Interactivity and communication mode choice in ongoing management groups. *Information Systems Research, 4*(3), 207–239.

Dr. Blooma John is a lecturer at RMIT International University, Vietnam. She completed her Ph.D. from Nanyang Technological University (NTU), Singapore. Her research interest is in the area of text mining, question answering services, and health-care social media. Her research has been published in journals such as the *Online Information Review, IEEE Internet Computing*, and *Computers and Education*. Blooma has published in various international conferences. Blooma has international experience in teaching leading information systems and business analytics courses in Middle East, Singapore, India, and Vietnam at both undergraduate and postgraduate level.

Prof. Raj Gururajan has been researching and teaching in the information systems domain for 25 years. He focuses much of his research in the area of health informatics and has over 200 publications. Currently Raj is a professor at University of Southern Queensland (USQ).

Prof. Nilmini Wickramasinghe Ph.D., M.B.A., GradDipMgtSt, B.Sc., Amus.A, piano, Amus.A, violin has a well-recognized research record in the field of health care and IT/IS. Her expertise is in the strategic application and management of technology for effecting superior health-care solutions. She currently is the professor director of Health Informatics Management at Epworth HealthCare and a professor at Deakin University.

Chapter 13
Translating Social Comparison Elements into a Mobile Solution to Support Weight Loss

Farruch Kouliev, Carolin Durst and Nilmini Wickramasinghe

Introduction

Today, overweight and obesity are considered to be a chronic disease that is widespread and has evolved into a serious public health problem for modern society. Since 1980, obesity has nearly doubled worldwide (WHO 2013). The World Health Organization (WHO) defines people with a body mass index (BMI) greater than or equal to 25 as overweight, while those with a BMI of 30 or greater are obese. According to WHO, in 2008, 1.4 billion adults (>20 years) were overweight (WHO 2013). Globally, this makes 35 %. However, in the same year: (1) 11 % of adults were obese (WHO 2013). (2) Forty-two million children under the age of 5 were counted to be overweight in 2010 (WHO 2014). And (3) nearly 83 % of them live in developing countries. In the same year, the United Nations Population Division estimated that around 642 million children under the age of 5 existed worldwide (UN 2013). This means that more than 6 % of human beings who generally do not decide what food is served were overweight. In 2011, the number decreased minimally to more than 40 million, with more than 30 million living in developing countries (WHO 2013). Since overweight and obese children are very likely to become overweight or obese adults (WHO 2014), the high ratio of overweight and obese children will become a serious issue for public health in the near future. Therefore, this study focuses on children and adolescents, also known as Generation Z (Looper 2014). The WHO names a greater caloric intake than calories expended as the main

F. Kouliev (✉)
12, Speyerer Street, 90443 Nuremberg, Germany
e-mail: farruchk@yahoo.de

C. Durst
Institute for Information Systems, Friedrich-Alexander University of Erlangen-Nuremberg, Lange Gasse 20, 90403 Nuremberg, Germany
e-mail: carolin.durst@fau.de

N. Wickramasinghe
Deakin University and Epworth HealthCare, 60 Baker Ave, Kew East 3102, Australia
e-mail: n.wickramasinghe@deakin.edu.au

N. Wickramasinghe et al. (eds.), *Contemporary Consumer Health Informatics*, Healthcare Delivery in the Information Age, DOI 10.1007/978-3-319-25973-4_13

cause for overweight and obesity (WHO 2013). There are several other organizations which support this theory (AIHW 2014; NHLBI 2012), but there are also critics who say that the human body is a complex ecosystem and weight gain or loss cannot be simplified in the just mentioned way (De Vany 2012a, b). Thus, it appears that individual behaviors and lifestyle choices shaped by the social environment drive and significantly impact the global obesity epidemic (Huffman 2011). Nevertheless, there is a wide agreement on the consequences of overweight and obesity, including sleep apnea, stroke, coronary heart disease, respiratory problems, type 2 diabetes, liver and gallbladder disease, hypertension, and osteoarthritis (NHLBI 1998). The American Institute for Cancer Research (AICR) has published an infographic, which displays that overweight and obesity increase the risk for the following types of cancer: esophageal, postmenopausal, gallbladder, pancreatic, kidney, ovarian, colorectal, and endometrial (AICR 2014). Taking a closer look at the target group of this study, the GLOBALHealthPR has found that in 2012, one in ten children were obese worldwide (GLOBALHealthPR 2012). Members of Generation Z were born and raised in a world with instant access to a huge amount of data and can be seen as digital natives (Looper 2014). In contrast to the previous generations, Generation Z accesses the Internet predominantly with smartphones, which allow them to communicate anywhere, at anyplace, and anytime (Boulos 2011; Park and Chen 2007; Capita 2013). VISA Australia found that members of Generation Z show a greater use of social media than previous generations (Kalra 2012). Interestingly, globally there were only 15,189 online conversations on the topic "obesity" in 1 month, which makes 1 per 23,400 obese children. Comparing to that, "Justin Bieber" was mentioned 6,653,854 times in 1 month (GLOBALHealthPR 2012). According to Arnaboldi et al. (2011), online social networks have a high similarity to offline social networks, since they provide similar functionalities and it can be assumed that social mechanisms, like social comparison, work in a similar way online. The beneficial impact of online social networks on health was already investigated in previous research (Wickramasinghe 2013). In this research in progress paper, we develop the mobile application CarepariZn that translates social comparison elements into different application functionalities to support weight loss.

Social Comparison Theory

The roots of the social comparison theory lie in Leon Festinger's article "A Theory of Social Comparison Processes" (Festinger 1954). The main idea is the natural behavior of humans to evaluate themselves (Festinger 1954). Generally, there are four motives for social comparison (Sedikides and Strube 1997). They are self-enhancement, self-assessment, self-verification, and self-improvement (Sedikides and Strube 1997). Self-enhancement implies the criticism of others to improve well-being (Sedikides and Strube 1997). If a person aims at getting an accurate and objective evaluation of the self, it is called self-assessment (Sedikides and Strube 1997). People who compare themselves to verify preexisting self-concepts have self-verification as a motive (Sedikides and Strube 1997). Self-improvement as a motive includes the improvement of "traits, abilities, skills, health status, or well-being" (Sedikides and Strube 1997). Festinger (1954) provides nine hypotheses and explains how and with whom people evaluate their opinions and abilities, as well as the restrictions of opinions and abilities (Festinger 1954). The key findings can be summarized in the following statements (Festinger 1954):

- Self-evaluation is done by comparison with others with similar opinions and abilities.
- Discrepancies in a group with respect to opinions or abilities will result in action on the part of members to reduce/resolve these.
- The importance of an opinion or ability has an impact on the drive for evaluation.
- Unidirectional drive upward exists mostly in the case of abilities.
- Nonsocial restraints make it very hard or even impossible to change one's ability.

In the past years, Festinger's theory has undergone several revisions and extensions. However, while Festinger assumed that people drive to compare with others who are superior (Festinger 1954), Brickman and Bulman (1977) introduced the downward comparison, where individuals compare themselves with individuals whom they consider to be worse than them in order to feel better about their self or personal situation. Brickman and Bulman (1977) argued that an upward comparison, as described by Festinger, can be threatening. Thus, comparisons like these are often avoided, especially by individuals with a fragile character (Brickman and Bulman 1977). Based on this, Wills (1981) expanded the concept of downward comparison in the context of health care. He argues that people will make use of the downward comparison in order to improve well-being (Wills 1981). McFarland et al.'s research on downward comparison shows that the effect can boost as well as lower self-esteem (McFarland et al. 2001). They refer to Tesser's self-evaluation maintenance (SEM) model (Tesser 1988) where they describe the former's impact on self-esteem. If a person sees another person who is similarly struggling, this could also lower his or her self-esteem because the person assumes to have difficulties too, since they are similar to each other (McFarland et al. 2001). Apart from self-esteem, upward and downward comparison can have an impact on the motivation of a person (Boyd 2014). Boyd (2014) says that a downward comparison reduces the motivation of a person to become better, whereas an upward comparison inspires to do better. According to Tesser's SEM, an upward comparison will only inspire individuals to do better or increase competitive behavior if the comparison dimension is relevant to the individual (Tesser 1988). For example, an amateur basketball player will feel more competitive toward other amateurs than toward professional basketball players. Goethals and Darley (1977) have a different view on Festinger's theory regarding similarity. They argue that being similar to another person means having a high similarity in the attributes related to the performance that should be compared. Olson et al. (1986) refer to this theory and suggest age, sex, and experience as related attributes. They provide an example of a tennis player who wants to compare himself with others based on attributes like physical condition and general athletic ability (Olson et al. 1986). Moreover, Mueller et al. (2010) in their experiment with overweight girls assumed weight to be a related attribute for comparisons. Nevertheless, in some situations, people tend to compare themselves with dissimilar rather than similar others (Wills 1981; Goethals and Nelson 1973; Mettee and Smith 1977; Kruglanski and Mayseless 1987). So far, social comparison theory research is mainly used to explain behaviors with regard to income and unemployment (Carrieri 2012). However, Carrieri (2012) has done a study on the relation between social comparison and well-being, which he operationalized as happiness and subjective health. For his study, he used data from the Italian Health Condition survey, and showed that well-being is negatively affected by reference groups with "high incidence of chronic conditions and disability" (Carrieri 2012). Furthermore, it is mentioned that among people in the same condition these effects are stronger (Carrieri 2012). While Carrieri focused his study on effects on health in general, Halbesleben and Buckley (2006) conducted a study on social comparison and burnout. In their study, they found that upward comparison led to increased and downward comparison to decreased levels of burnout. Mueller et al. (2010) have done a research on social comparison and weight control of adolescent girls in a school context. In their study, they aimed at finding out how girls' own weight control is affected by weight control and body sizes of their classmates. They stated that their most important finding was that similar peers are the most influential group "within the school context for girls because both their physical BMI status and their behaviors matter to individual girls of a similar weight status" (Mueller et al. 2010). Jones (2002) investigated relations between body image satisfaction and social comparisons to either same-sex peers or media models. In two studies of teenaged boys and girls, she found that social comparisons on personal and social attributes were done more likely with same-sex peers, while comparisons on physical attributes were done with same-sex peers as well as media models. Interestingly, weight comparisons were primary correlates of body dissatisfaction for both genders (Jones 2002). In this context, Smeesters et al. (2010) examined how advertisements of thin and heavy models affect the self-esteem of human beings with different BMIs. They found that the social comparison processes as well as the self-evaluative and behavioral results differentiate between people with different BMIs. Social media applications offer individuals new means of social comparison. Facebook, for instance, provides the possibility to share the latest achievements such as a new high-paid job, high graduation, expensive vacations, or exotic food instantly through a text message or a photo. In contrast to offline social networks, members of online social networks have the possibility to share a good performance with their whole friends list without extra effort. This leads to the phenomenon that "the Facebook Newsfeed turns into a parade of good news about other people's life" (Pappas 2012). However, having a large number of friends also increases the risk of getting depressed by others showing off in Facebook (Pappas 2012). Jay (2012), "a therapist who works primarily with people in their 20s and 30s", reports of a high number of clients who are unsatisfied because of upward comparison with their Facebook friends. Furthermore, a study has found that Facebook provides a new medium for men to compare themselves with others and compete with them (Pappas 2012). Consolvo et al. (2006) presented a prototype application for a Nokia 6600 that counted users' total amount of steps per day. This app aimed to increase the activity level of users in order to improve their health. However, the app named *Houston* "provided a daily goal, progress toward and recognition for meeting the goal" (Consolvo et al. 2006). Furthermore, it included social features such as (1) sending and requesting step counts to/from fitness friends, (2) seeing their friends' progress according to goals, (3) seeing the comments and goals and averages of all fitness buddies in the past 7 days, and (4) sending messages. They reported overall positive results and increased physical activity of several users (Consolvo et al. 2006). Oliveira and Oliver (2008) introduced a mobile-phone-based application called *TripleBeat* that could assist runners to achieve preset goals. One of its main features was the social competition. Users could choose their competitor manually or automatically by the system. Since the application's goal was to support users with achieving their goals, the winner of the competition was not the fastest runner or the one who crunched the most calories, but the one who achieved the predefined goal best. Eight men and two women participated in the study and tested the application. A statistical analysis showed that *TripleBeat* could effectively help runners to achieve their goals, and the social feature had a significant positive impact on the enjoyment (Oliveira and Oliver 2008). The social features of the apps described above are related to social comparison theory and can be used for one or more self-evaluation motives. The results of these studies indicate that the combination of social comparison theory and technology has the potential to influence the individual health status—which supports the assumption of our research. We assume that—similar to offline social networks—elements of social comparison can support overweight and obese people in losing weight. Our target group is the Generation Z, which communicates via social media using smartphones. Therefore, our goal is to develop an application that offers different features for social comparison. To enable social comparison, individuals have to be grouped with regard to certain attributes. As already mentioned, Goethals and Darley found that people want to compare themselves with others who have high similarity in the related attributes to a performance (Goethals and Darley 1977). Therefore, the following attributes have been identified to be relevant for establishing similarity among individuals in groups: gender, experience, and BMI. Since exercising is a key construct in our study, we also want to include motives for exercising in our grouping algorithm. According to Deforche et al. (2006), motives such as improve health and physical condition, lose weight, and feel or look better are most important to obese adolescents. Previous research has shown that losing weight is a main reason for women for exercising, while men are more concerned about their physical fitness/muscle-related issues (Fisher et al. 2002; Furnham et al. 2002; McDonald and Thompson 1992; Silberstein et al. 1988). These motives will be included in our grouping algorithm if the number of individuals will be greater than 2000. Having divided users into groups with similar others, we will provide features which offer users the possibility (1) to monitor their progress, (2) to be grouped with similar others, (3) for self-evaluation regarding all the four social comparison motives (self-assessment, self-enhancement, self-improvement, and self-verification), (4) for down- and upward comparison, (5) to compare oneself with similar and dissimilar others, and (6) to use social media features, such as share functionality, to get motivated by friends and relatives.

The CarepariZn App

This study focuses on the design and development of a mobile app, which facilitates weight loss, while implementing social comparison elements. Therefore, the main research question is: how can we translate social comparison elements into technical features of a mobile app to support weight loss online?

Basic Implementation Issues

Having the main goal in mind, the following questions have to be answered: (1) Which type of application is most suitable for the study: native, web, or hybrid? (2) Which social media platform should we use to address our target group? There are several articles that pit development technologies against each other (e.g., Budiu 2013; Kiran 2013). There are also different infographics available, with different focus, such as on the average usage of several technologies in different continents (Zakkas 2013) or on functionalities and budget (O'Dell 2013). The amount of different sites underlines the importance of the topic for every developing project. In fact, the way how the app should be implemented is a long-term decision. Therefore, decision-makers should take enough time to evaluate the benefits and disadvantages of the three possible solutions. However, the main questions that have to be asked are the following:

- Which platform(s) are we going to serve?
- How much money are we willing to spend?
- What level of interaction will be implemented?
- Which technologies are compulsory?

In our project, we will implement a web app mainly for two reasons. First, we want to guarantee platform independence and, second, we will not use any special device features. Thus, a web app is the best option for our study. The most frequently used social media application of the Generation Z is Facebook (Palley 2012). Therefore, the CarepariZn app will include a Facebook login as a basic social feature. Furthermore, we will implement additional Facebook features, such as the "invite friend" and "share" functionality. The former feature assures that users will be able to share our app and encourage their friends in order to try it out and start living a healthier life. The latter feature is an important mechanism to share individual achievements on their walls and receive likes from their friends to stay motivated.

Social Comparison Features Development

Peffers et al. (2007) developed and introduced the design science research methodology process model, which is one of the most influential design science research methodologies for information systems research. This model is also consistent with the principles and guidelines of design science research established in previous research studies such as Hevner et al. (2004). For the design and development of the CarepariZn app, we followed Peffers et al.'s design science research methodology process. The steps demonstration and evaluation has been processed in February 2015. The design and development requirements of the mobile application are determined through our literature review on social comparison theory.

Creating User Profiles

Before using the CarepariZn app for the first time, users have to create a profile. To make things easier and to enable a Facebook connection, the app provides a Facebook login to get personal information such as name, age, gender, e-mail, and profile picture. The data are verified before being saved in the database. Furthermore, we save the user's friends list. In the next step, the user is asked to give information on his weight and height and to evaluate his/her level of experience in sports and nutrition. In our application, we describe experience as a level of knowledge and practice. However, the user can choose between beginner and advanced in each category. There will be a logical AND connection between those two attributes which will result in his or her individual level of experience (see Fig. 13.1). Then, the user will prioritize the following sport motives: improve health condition, improve physical condition, weight loss, strength, and appearance (see Fig. 13.1). In the final registration step, the user has to choose what type of sports he or she is doing.

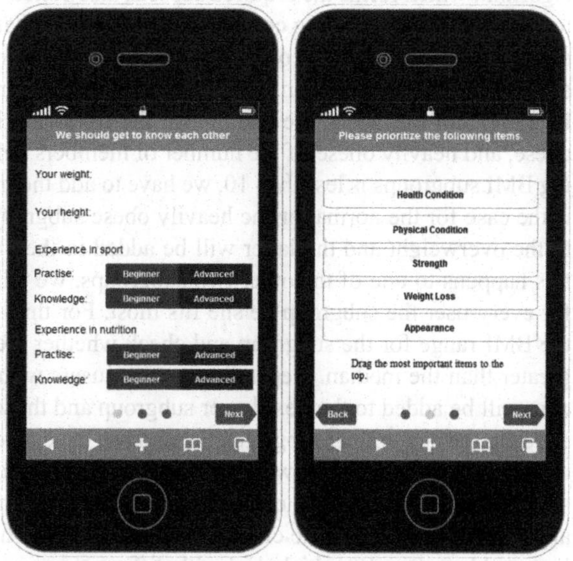

Fig. 13.1 User details and sport motives

Progress Monitoring

For a successful tracking of the users' fitness and health-related behavior, they have to regularly update their caloric intake, whether they exercise or not, the duration of exercising, and their weight. However, it makes sense to update the first three points daily whereas the last point, weight, could be updated at least once a week (VanWormer et al. 2009). For a better user experience, we implemented a connection to the existing app "myfitnesspal," which provides a huge database on products' nutritional value, so users can easily calculate their caloric intake. Furthermore, we will use the metabolic equivalent (MET), which represents the energy cost of an activity, to calculate the caloric consumption based on the activity and its duration (Jetté et al. 1990). With these updates, we will be able to derive variables such as weight change, actual BMI, regularity, and caloric expenditure in order to display users' progress.

Grouping

Having the information which was mentioned in the previous chapter, we provide a ranking system which actually implements the social comparison elements. First, users have to be grouped and divided into subgroups in order to guarantee a comparison with similar others. For this, we relate to the arguments of Darling and Goethals (Goethals and Darley 1977) and will use their BMI, experience, and their sport motives prioritization as related attributes. As mentioned before, in some situations people tend to compare themselves with dissimilar rather than similar others. To include this functionality, we offer the possibility to switch between groups with the same gender and mixed groups. In order to group users, we have developed an algorithm which forms the required subsets, also called buckets, efficiently. In order to allow a well-functioning comparison, we assume that the smallest bucket should not contain less than 10 people, while we strive to form bucket of 25 members to allow for social comparison. First, we differentiate our users by their BMI levels. However, for our study, we distinguish the following levels: normal, overweight, obese, and heavily obese. If the number of members belonging to one of the resulting BMI subgroups is less than 10, we have to add them to another subgroup. If this is the case for the normal or the heavily obese subgroup, the former will be added to the overweight and the latter will be added to the obese subgroup. However, if this happens to one of the other two subgroups, we will have to decide iteratively for every user the subgroup he/she fits most. For this, we calculate the median of the BMI range for the subgroup and check whether the user's BMI is less than or greater than the median. Depending on that, users with a BMI lower than the median will be added to the next lower subgroup and those with a higher BMI will be added to the next higher subgroup. Second, we have to look at the experience matrix of the users. Table 13.1 shows the experience matrix and the possible combinations.

At this point, we have to count: how many users of the different experience types are members of each of the created BMI subgroups. The following steps will be illustrated by examples which deal with different cases.

In the first example, the experience matrix for overweight might look similar to the data presented in Table 13.2. There are 25 BEGBEG users, 9 BEGADV users, 8 ADVBEG users, and 25 ADVADV users. In this case, it does not make sense to us to differentiate between BEGADV and ADVBEG. We would join these two sets together and form three buckets in total.

In the second example, the overweight subgroup might contain 78 BEGBEG users, 25 BEGADV users, 25 ADVBEG users, and 25 ADVADV users (see Table 13.3). As mentioned before, we strive to get buckets of 25 people. Thus, the BEGADV, ADVBEG, and ADVADV buckets are perfectly formed. So, there will be one bucket with the size of 25 for BEGADV, ADVBEG, and ADVADV of the overweight subgroup. The BEGBEG set will need more than 3 buckets of 25 users. In this case, to form equally big buckets, we will use the modulo operator (78 mod 25 = 3). Since the remainder is less than 10, we will not form a new bucket but enlarge the 3 BEGBEG buckets evenly by 1. Thus, in the worst case, a bucket can enlarge to a set of 34 users.

In the third example, the overweight subgroup might contain 25 BEGBEG users, 25 BEGADV users, 18 ADVBEG users, and 7 ADVADV users (see Table 13.4). Here, we have less than 10 members in the ADVADV sub-subgroup. In a case like that, we are going to add the members to the BEGADV or ADVBEG sets, depend-

Table 13.1 Experience matrix

	Sport		
Nutrition		*Beginner*	*Advanced*
	Beginner	BEGBEG	BEGADV
	Advanced	ADVBEG	ADVADV

Table 13.2 Case 1

	Sport		
Nutrition		*Beginner*	*Advanced*
	Beginner	25	9
	Advanced	8	25

Table 13.3 Case 2

	Sport		
Nutrition		*Beginner*	*Advanced*
	Beginner	78	25
	Advanced	25	25

Table 13.4 Case 3

	Sport		
Nutrition		*Beginner*	*Advanced*
	Beginner	25	25
	Advanced	18	7

ing on their bucket sizes. In this particular case, we would add it to the ADVBEG group to form a bucket with a size of 25 in the ADVBEG sub-subgroup. Finally, having calculated the sizes of every bucket every BMI subgroup, users will be assigned iteratively to the buckets. This algorithm has been tested on a data set of a previous study with 1000 participants and resulted in satisfying outcomes. However, if the number of participants is greater than 1000, we extend our grouping algorithm, and match our users also by the sports motives attribute.

Self-Evaluation Motives and Down- and Upward Comparison

The ranking feature consists of several items which represent different social comparison elements (see Fig. 13.2). First, users can see their statistics, including weight loss, BMI, regularity, and kilocalories burned. It makes sense to represent weight loss in percentage to compare users, since heavier people used to drop more weight (Donner 2013). However, the BMI will be derived from the updated weight attribute. Regularity shows how often users worked out in the last calendar week and the burned calories represent the difference between the caloric intake and expenditure. Since these statistics give an objective overview of users' progress, they can be used for self-assessment reasons. Second, a smiley is used to show users how good or bad they are doing. We implemented five different smileys which display the following progress levels: very good, good, not sure, bad, and very bad.

The type of smiley is derived from the stats of the user. We use an algorithm to map stats on a single index and define a range for every type of the possible smileys.

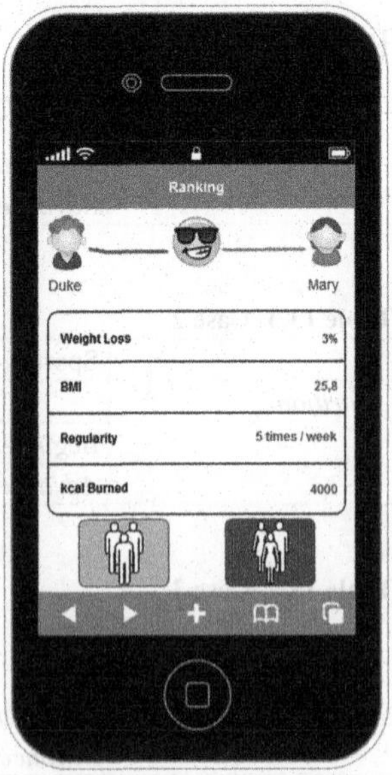

Fig. 13.2 Ranking feature

This functionality serves as self-verification possibility. Third, we show users only one user directly above and under them on the rank list. We show only one user because experiments have shown that users want to compare themselves with others who are slightly better or worse (Wheeler 1966). This functionality provides the possibility of upward comparison and self-improvement or downward comparison and self-enhancement. If a user clicks on the picture of the other user, the app shows the stats of both users next to each other. This feature supports a direct individual comparison. In addition, motivational quotes will be displayed for the downward comparisons to prevent low self-esteem and the possibility to become demotivated (see Fig. 13.3).

Finally, the user is linked via a dynamic line to his or her above- and under-ranked user. The line visualizes the distance to the other person who is better or worse than oneself. However, the distance depends on the difference between the users' stats.

Comparison with Similar/Dissimilar Others

As already mentioned earlier, we give users the possibility to compare themselves with similar and dissimilar others. Therefore, the app provides a button to switch between the same and mixed gender comparisons (see Fig. 13.3).

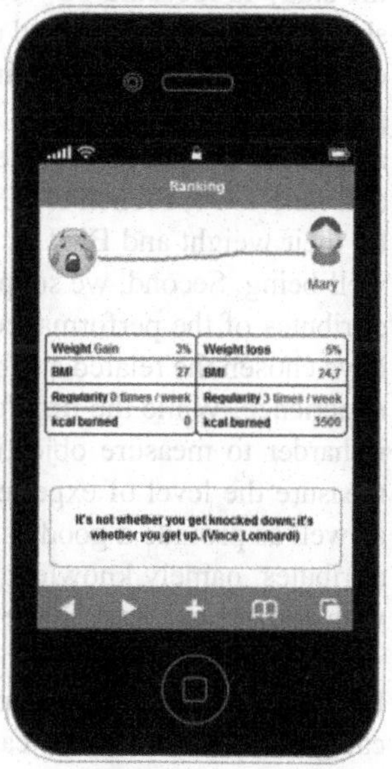

Fig. 13.3 Direct comparison between users

Social Media Features

Mainly to enlarge our community, we provide the possibility to every user to invite his or her friends. Furthermore, we give users the possibility to share their achievements with their Facebook friends via wall postings. Whenever a user types in his or her new weight, he or she becomes able to share the new weight with his or her friends. Also, when a user switches to a better BMI subgroup, a pop-up comes up, which asks whether to share the new success or not. Users can share their calories consumption and the duration of the last training. Additionally, the information of an achieved higher rank within a group can be shared as well. Social media features are provided, so users can get motivation by their own online social network, for example, via likes.

Discussion

During the development of the app design, we have faced several challenges. First, there are no best practices for social comparison studies. Furthermore, contradictions exist about the similarity or dissimilarity of the comparison partner. However, we focused on the theory (Festinger 1954) that people want to compare themselves with similar others for several reasons: (1) To evaluate one's progress, it does not make sense to compare oneself with someone who is very different. However, since the study is focusing on weight loss, and not the improvement in performance or skills of the sport, it seemed unnecessary to distinguish between types of sports and use it as an additional grouping attribute. (2) More studies exist, where people compared themselves with similar others than with dissimilar others. (3) Overweight and obese people have generally lower self-esteem (Franklin et al. 2006; Pierce and Jane 1997; French et al. 1995); therefore, it seemed reasonable to group users by their weight and BMI to guarantee a similar environment and establish a good well-being. Second, we support the theory (Goethals and Darley 1977) that related attributes of the performance are relevant for similarity. As mentioned before, we have chosen the related attributes gender, weight, BMI, motives for exercising, and experience. While the first four attributes can be measured easily, the last attribute is harder to measure objectively. However, we wanted to avoid long surveys to measure the level of experience of the user and thus guard against survey fatigue as well as provide a good usability. Hence, we divided experience into two further attributes, namely knowledge and practice, and offer users to evaluate themselves with respect to these. Since our participants will be mostly overweight or obese, we decided to have only two categories for every attribute: beginner and advanced. However, we decided to implement the Boolean AND operator between these two categories since someone can only be seen as advanced if he or she has advanced knowledge and experience. There was also the thought of adding the attribute waist size to the stats and monitor it. In the end, we decided not to add it because the measurement is time-consuming and would harm the usability of the app. Third, we had to make an early decision whether we will implement a native, web, or hybrid app. We decided to implement a web app for its major benefit: platform independence. Furthermore, we do not need any special device feature in our application. Fourth, we decided to choose Visual Studio to implement a web app for three reasons: (1) It provides a comfortable development environment. (2) We already had experience in working with it. (3) Libraries such as jQuery and bootstrap are available and can be used to implement a responsive user interface (UI). In this context, we decided to use Model-View-Controller (MVC) pattern to implement the application in order to guarantee separation of concerns. Finally, we had to decide whether we will implement the grouping and ranking features as web services. We will not implement web services, since these features do not have general public interest. Key next steps include the following: First, we have to do research on how the range for our smileys should look like and what is an appropriate technique. Second, we will further research on possibilities to map a number of variables on one index to implement the ranking feature. However, if there are different algorithms, we will have to evaluate them and pick the most suitable for our purpose. Third, we will have to implement the ranking feature and run functional tests as well as test it with some users. Fourth, we will have to find trial subjects for our field experiment to collect the needed data. Fifth, the collected data will have to be analyzed and the results will be used to (1) improve the web application and (2) see if social comparison affects health-related behavior and, if so, in what way(s). While this study has clearly showed the great potential of a positive impact of social comparison combined with technology on health, there are several limitations inherent in this study. As mentioned in the beginning of this chapter, we had to make decisions and assumptions in controversial areas in order to create an appropriate grouping algorithm and design the ranking feature. Based on this, the results of the field experiment cannot be generalized and are highly related to our understanding of social comparison. Furthermore, we see our target group as users who are IT natives. Even though we aim at providing an application with high usability, some of the participants could see the mobile dependency as a problem. In this context, as mentioned before, we want to make use of MET to calculate the caloric expenditure in order to improve the user experience. The calculated value seems to be adequate for our purpose, but we still have to mention and understand that it is not an exact value. Finally, we are not going to implement any compliance features. Thus, there is a risk that people try to cheat to get a higher rank position. Since it is a research in progress paper, we cannot rate any of our decisions so far. In addition, we have to be aware of several issues that might occur during or after our experiment. First, there is a risk that users can go from one extreme to another. In our case, this would mean that they may become anorexic. One driver could be social pressure, which forces one to become better than others, and thus people could choose an unhealthy way of dieting instead of a healthy way, just to achieve their goal faster. However, as we choose obese individuals and monitor the progress frequently, we believe that this is unlikely to occur; and if we do see such a change, we can initiate countermeasures at an early stage. Second, there is a chance that users can fall into depression if they see that others do better than them. We try to prevent this case by providing a motivational quote for upward comparisons. Still, we need to identify further actions that can be taken to minimize this risk.

Conclusion

Overall, we believe the risks are negligible, especially given the choice of individuals and the close and continued monitoring of changes. In contrast, we see the potential of social media to address the current obesity epidemic as significant and call for more research in this area. We note that if unchecked the obesity epidemic will have devastating consequences for individuals, families, and the society. Furthermore, we draw attention to the fact that currently many new apps are being developed and deployed, which try to encourage physical activity, healthy diet, and other types of health behavior changes. A question that remains to be answered in general is the following: What is the long-term impact of such mobile apps on behavior change and will the behavior change affected by the app only be short term and previous behaviors reverted to after some time has passed? Some authors (Klasnja et al. 2011) believe that the key is to focus on the efficacy of the tailored behavior-change intervention strategies, that is, self-monitoring embodied on the system, and examine this. We plan to do such evaluations in our future research in order to address these questions. This chapter focused only on the design and development of the solution; yet through our design and development, we have become more convinced that the long-term behavioral implications and potential benefits will be the key to addressing the obesity epidemic.

References

AICR. (2014). What you need to know about obesity and cancer. http://www.aicr.org/learn-more-about-cancer/infographic-obesity-and-cancer.html.

AIHW. (2014). Causes of overweight and obesity. https://www.aihw.gov.au/overweight-and-obesity/causes/.

Arnaboldi, V., Passarella, A., Tesconi, M., & Gazz, D. (2011). Towards a characterization of egocentric networks in online social networks.

Boulos, M. N. K., Wheeler, S., Tavares, C., & Jones, R. (2011). How smartphones are changing the face of mobile and participatory healthcare: An overview, with example from eCAALYX. *Biomedical Engineering Online, 10*(1), 24.

Boyd, N. (2014). Self-comparison theory: Upward vs. downward social comparison. http://education-portal.com/academy/lesson/self-comparison-theory-upward-vs-downward-social-comparison.html#lesson.

Brickman, P., & Bulman, R. J. (1977). Social comparison processes: Theoretical and empirical perspectives. In J. M. Suls & R. L. Miller (Eds.), *Social comparison processes: Theoretical and empirical perspectives* (pp. 149–186). Washington, DC: Hemisphere Publishing.

Budiu, R. (2013). Mobile: Native apps, web apps, and hybrid apps. http://www.nngroup.com/articles/mobile-native-apps/.

Capita. (2013). Anytime, anyplace, anywhere…. http://www.capita.co.uk/news-and-opinion/opinion/2013/bring-your-own-device.aspx.
Carrieri, V. (2012). Social comparison and subjective well-being: Does the health of others matter? *Bulletin of Economic Research, 64*(1), 31–55.
Consolvo, S., Everitt, K., Smith, I., & Landay, J. a. (2006). Design requirements for technologies that encourage physical activity. Proceedings of the SIGCHI conference on Human Factors in computing systems—CHI '06, pp. 457–466.
De Vany, A. (2012a). Paradoxes of energy balance. http://www.artdevanyonline.com/1/post/2012/12/paradoxes-of-energy-balance.html.
De Vany, A. (2012b). Paradoxes of energy balance, Part 3: A Calorie is not a Calorie. http://www.artdevanyonline.com/1/post/2012/12/paradoxes-of-energy-balance-part-3-a-calorie-is-not-a-calorie.html.
Deforche, B. I., De Bourdeaudhuij, I. M., & Tanghe, A. P. (2006). Attitude toward physical activity in normal-weight, overweight and obese adolescents. *The Journal of Adolescent Health, 38*(5), 560–568.
Donner, E. (2013). Why do overweight people lose weight faster? http://www.livestrong.com/article/406097-why-do-overweight-people-lose-weight-faster/.
Festinger, L. (1954). A theory of social comparison processes. *Human Relations, 7*(2), 117–140.
Fisher, E., Dunn, M., & Thompson, J. K. (2002). Social comparison and body image: An investigation of body comparison processes using multidimensional scaling. *Journal of Social and Clinical Psychology, 21*(5), 566–579.
Franklin, J., Denyer, G., Steinbeck, K. S., Caterson, I. D., & Hill, A. J. (2006). Obesity and risk of low self-esteem: A statewide survey of Australian children. *Pediatrics, 118*(6), 2481–2487.
French, S., Story, M., & Perry, C. L. (1995). Self-esteem and obesity in children and adolescents: A literature review. *Obesity Research, 5,* 479–490.
Furnham, A., Badmin, N., & Sneade, I. (2002). Body image dissatisfaction: Gender differences in eating attitudes, self-esteem and reasons for exercise. *The Journal of Psychology, 136,* 581–596.
GLOBALHealthPR. (2012). GLOBALHealthPR IHSMS 2.0 Infographic.
Goethals, G. R., & Darley, J. (1977). Social comparison theory: An attributional approach. In J. M. Suls & R. L. Miller (Eds.), *Social comparison processes: Theoretical and empirical perspectives* (pp. 259–278). Washington, DC: Hemisphere Publishing.
Goethals, G. R., & Nelson, R. (1973). Similarity in the influence process: The belief-value distinction. *Journal of Personality and Social Psychology, 25,* 117–122.
Halbesleben, J. R. B., & Buckley, R. M. (2006). Social comparison and burnout: The role of relative burnout and received social support. *Anxiety, Stress, and Coping, 19*(3), 259–278.
Hevner, A. R., March, S., & Park, J. (2004). Design research in information systems research. *MIS Quarterly, 28*(1), 75–105.
Huffman, S. K. (2011). *BMI changes in Russian adults: The role of lifestyles and spousal relationships*.
Jay, M. (2012).Just say no to Facebook social comparisons! http://www.psychologytoday.com/blog/the-defining-decade/201203/just-say-no-facebook-social-comparisons.
Jetté, M., Sidney, K., & Blümchen, G. (1990). Metabolic equivalents (METS) in exercise testing, exercise prescription, and evaluation of functional capacity. *Clinical Cardiology, 13*(8), 555–565.
Jones, D. C. (2002). Social comparison and body image: Attractiveness comparisons to models and peers among adolescent girls and boys. *Sex Roles, 45,* 645–664.
Kalra, V. (2012). Generation Z. p. 12.
Kiran, V. (2013). Native vs mobile web vs hybrid applications. http://www.javacodegeeks.com/2013/12/native-vs-mobile-web-vs-hybrid-applications.html.
Klasnja, P., Consolvo, S., & Pratt, W. (2011). How to evaluate technologies for health behavior change in HCI research. Proceedings of the 29th International Conference on Human Factors in Computing Systems, ACM, pp. 3063–3072.

Kruglanski, A. W., & Mayseless, O. (1987). Motivational effects in the social comparison of opinions. *Journal of Personality and Social Psychology, 53,* 834–853.
Looper, L. (2014). How generation Z works. http://people.howstuffworks.com/culture-traditions/generation-gaps/generation-z.htm.
McDonald, K., & Thompson, J. K. (1992). Eating disturbance, body image dissatisfaction, and reasons for exercising: Gender differences and correlational findings. *The International Journal of Eating Disorders, 11,* 289–292.
McFarland, C., Buehler, R., & MacKay, L. (2001). Affective responses to social comparisons with extremely close others. *Social Cognition, 19*(5), 547–586.
Mettee, D. R., & Smith, G. (1977). Social comparison and interpersonal attraction: The case for dissimilarity. In J. Suls & R. L. Miller (Eds.), *Social comparison processes: Theoretical and empirical perspectives* (pp. 115–142). Washington, DC: Hemisphere.
Mueller, A. S., Pearson, J., Muller, C., Frank, K., & Turner, A. (2010). Sizing up peers: Adolescent girls' weight control and social comparison in the school context. *Journal of Health and Social Behavior, 51*(1), 64–78.
NHLBI. (1998). *Clinical guidelines on the identification, evaluation, and treatment of overweight and obesity in adults*. Bethesda: National Heart, Lung, and Blood Institute.
NHLBI. (2012). What Causes Overweight and Obesity? http://www.nhlbi.nih.gov/health/health-topics/topics/obe/causes.html.
O'Dell, J. (2013). Here's a chart to decide whether to build a native or web mobile app. http://venturebeat.com/2013/07/29/native-v-web-chart/.
Oliveira, R. De, & Oliver, N. (2008). TripleBeat: Enhancing exercise performance with persuasion. MobileHCI '08, 255–264.
Olson, J. M., Peter, H. C., & Zanna, M. P. (1986). *Relative deprivation and social comparison: The Ontario symposium*. Hillsdale: Erlbaum.
Palley, W. (2012). Gen Z: Digital in their DNA. April (2012).
Pappas, S. (2012). Facebook with care: Social networking site can hurt self-esteem. http://www.livescience.com/18324-facebook-depression-social-comparison.html.
Park, Y., & Chen, J. V. (2007). Acceptance and adoption of the innovative use of smartphone. *Industrial Management & Data Systems, 107*(9), 1349–1365.
Peffers, K., Tuunanen, T., Rothenberger, M. A., & Chatterjee, S. (2007). A design science research methodology for information systems research. *Journal of Management Information Systems, 24*(3), 45–77.
Pierce, J. W., & Jane, V. (1997). Cause and effect beliefs and self-esteem of overweight children. *Journal of Child Psychology and Psychiatry, 38*(6), 645–650.
Sedikides, C., & Strube, M. J. (1997). Self-evaluation: To thine own self be good, to thine own self be sure, to thine own self be true, and to thine own self be better. *Advances in Experimental Social Psychology, 29,* 209–269.
Silberstein, L. R., Striegel-Moore, R. H., Timko, C., & Rodin, J. (1988). Behavioral and psychological implications of body dissatisfaction: do men and women differ? *Sex Roles, 19,* 219–232.
Smeesters, D., Mussweiler, T., & Mandel, N. (2010). Retracted: The effects of thin and heavy media images on overweight and underweight consumers: Social comparison processes and behavioral implications. *Journal of Consumer Research, 36*(6), 930–949.
Tesser, L. (1988). Toward a self-evaluation maintenance model of social behavior. In L. Berkowitz (Ed.), *Advances in social psychology* (Vol. 21, pp. 181–227). New York: Academic.
UN. (2013). Annual population by age groups—Both sexes. http://esa.un.org/unpd/wpp/Excel-Data/EXCEL_FILES/1_Population/WPP2012_POP_F15_1_ANNUAL_POPULATION_BY_AGE_BOTH_SEXES.XLS.
VanWormer, J. J., Martinez, M. A., Martinson, C. B., et al. (2009). Self-weighing promotes weight loss for obese adults. *American Journal of Preventive Medicine, 36*(1), 70–73.
Wheeler, L. (1966). Motivation as a determinant of upward comparison. *Journal of Experimental Social Psychology Supplement, 1,* 27–31.
WHO. (2013). Obesity and overweight. http://www.who.int/mediacentre/factsheets/fs311/en/.

WHO. (2014). Childhood overweight and obesity. http://www.who.int/dietphysicalactivity/childhood/en/.

Wickramasinghe, N., Say-Yen, T., Durst, C., & Viol, J. (2013). Insights from an investigation of the design of a consumer health 2. 0 application to address the relationship between on-line social networks and health-related behaviors.

Wills, T. A. (1981). Downward comparison principles in social psychology. *Psychological Bulletin, 90,* 245–271.

Zakkas, S. (2013). HTML5 vs native vs hybrid. http://infographicsmania.com/html5-vs-native-vs-hybrid.

Farruch Kouliev was born on September 22, 1989 in Baku, Azerbaijan. In the summer of 1997, he moved to Germany and settled down in Nuremberg. He completed his bachelor's degree in information systems in October 2012 and master's degree in international information systems in October 2014 at the Friedrich-Alexander University Erlangen-Nuremberg, Germany. Currently, he is working as a software engineer at Capgemini.

Dr. Carolin Durst is an associate professor at the Chair of Information System II at the University of Erlangen-Nuremberg. She holds a Ph.D. in the field of services science, and her current research focuses on the analysis and design of sociotechnical systems in a collaborative setting. The fields of application comprise strategic management, marketing, and e-health. Her research has been published in *Communications of the AIS (CAIS), International Journal of Computer Information Systems and Industrial Management Applications,* and elsewhere, including books and conference proceedings.

Prof. Nilmini Wickramasinghe (PhD; MBA; GradDipMgtSt; BSc. Amus.A, piano;Amus.A, violin) has a well-recognized research record in the field of health care and information technology/information systems (IT/IS). Her expertise is in the strategic application and management of technology for effecting superior health-care solutions. She is currently the professor director of Health Informatics Management at Epworth HealthCare and a professor at Deakin University.

Chapter 14
An Organizing Vision Perspective for Developing and Adopting e-Health Solutions

Indrit Troshani and Nilmini Wickramasinghe

Introduction

Irrespective of its espoused benefits, investments and research in e-health lag behind those in other industries (Chiasson and Davidson 2004; Cho et al. 2008; Menon et al. 2000). Indeed, achieving e-health benefits remains both challenging and elusive (Cho et al. 2008; Ha and Lee 2008; Sohn and Lee 2007; Troshani and Wickramasinghe 2014). At least partially, these challenges are attributable to the inherent complexity of health care generally and e-health in particular including the social issues and communication patterns that characterize this environment (Davidson 2000; Kaplan 2001), the high levels of leadership and resource commitments (Garabaldi 1998), the organizational structures and cultures (Bangert and Doktor 2003), institutional changes (Schriger et al. 1997), anticipated and unanticipated health care practice changes (Massaro 1993), and inconsistent or even conflicting interests and agendas of constituent participating actors and stakeholders (Constantinides and Barrett 2006). With these challenges, health care is a complex and multidisciplinary phenomenon building on many disciplines such as medicine, biomedical engineering, computer and information science, statistics, health promotion and marketing, and management science (Anderson 1997; Chiasson and Davidson 2004; Wickramasinghe et al. 2007).

Though growing, we note that extant research in e-health remains limited particularly in a number of aspects (Anderson 1997; Chiasson and Davidson 2004; Wickramasinghe et al. 2007). Extant research offers a limited coverage of the contextual industry settings that contribute to e-health complexity. This is a limitation since such settings can improve current understanding in relation to why e-health

I. Troshani (✉)
University of Adelaide Business School, 10 Pulteney St, Adelaide, SA 5000, Australia
e-mail: indrit.troshani@adelaide.edu.au

N. Wickramasinghe
Deakin University and Epworth HealthCare, 60 Baker Ave, Kew East 3102, Australia
e-mail: n.wickramasinghe@deakin.edu.au

N. Wickramasinghe et al. (eds.), *Contemporary Consumer Health Informatics*,
Healthcare Delivery in the Information Age, DOI 10.1007/978-3-319-25973-4_14

solutions emerge the way they do and also why some solutions are more successful than others. Indeed, e-health solutions influence and are influenced by structures of interacting and dynamic industry and broader environment and societal factors (Atkinson 2000; Benbasat and Zmud 2003; Cho et al. 2008). Chiasson and Davidson (2004) argue that "accounting for industry will help researchers determine the technical and social boundaries of IT artifacts and IS theories" (p. 592). That is, e-health solutions "encapsulate[s] the structures, routines, norms, and values implicit in the rich contexts within which the artifact is embedded" (Benbasat and Zmud 2003, p. 186). Thus, the development and adoption of e-health solutions is a complex social and technological undertaking (Sohn and Lee 2007) which stems from a range of challenges including creating a new health-care culture, achieving compatibility with legacy systems, and tailoring pervasive e-health solutions to address complex expectations and needs of heterogeneous stakeholders that have different and even incompatible objectives and agendas.

This chapter makes the case for using Swanson and Ramiller's (1997) organizing vision framework for information and communication technology (ICT) innovations as an effective and compelling tool for researching the development and adoption of e-health solutions. The organizing vision framework represents a rich analytical foundation for researching the emergence of ICT innovations from an institutional perspective (Kaganer et al. 2010). By focusing on this type of solution, this chapter adds to existing literature, and it enhances current understanding concerning how (un)favorable institutional arrangements can be created for the development and adoption of e-health solutions as emerging ICT innovations.

The organizing vision of ICT innovations targets interorganizational change at the sectoral or societal level rather than at a specific organizational or individual level (Currie 2004). It captures the manner in which organizational forms, structures, and rules become institutionalized and taken for granted (Currie 2004; Zucker 1983), and how they evolve to become a socially accepted "state of affairs in which shared cognitions determine what actions are possible and what has meaning" (Zucker 1983, p. 2). As ICT innovations are becoming increasingly complex, which is, at least partially, attributed to the increasing extent of interrelatedness among organizational actors at sectoral or society levels, the organizing vision framework offers a solid conceptual basis for investigating the institutional dynamics that underpin their emergence (Kaganer et al. 2010).

In making the case for using the organizing vision framework to research the development and adoption of e-health solutions, we hope to generate insight concerning the ways in which e-health research can be extended if the contextual and social dimensions that support the complex interactions which occur in modern health-care settings are to be systematically captured (Timpka et al. 2007). We argue that such insight can be invaluable to policy-makers at both organizational and broader industry and national levels as well as to the developers of e-health solutions (Lorenzi et al. 1997; Lorenzi et al. 1998; Timpka et al. 2007). Furthermore, the discussion in this chapter may generate useful insight into issues concerning pushing new ICT into a diffusion trajectory and organizational contexts, in particular demonstrating how the use of institutional frameworks for the analysis of e-health solutions as ICT innovations, like organizing vision, can help advance institutional theory particularly for explaining phenomena in health-care contexts.

Current State of Health Care

Health-care delivery operates in a complex and dynamic environment (von Lubitz and Wickramasinghe 2006). Critical to success in this environment is the access to and transfer of pertinent information and germane knowledge in a timely fashion to assist providers and patients address treatment needs (Von Lubitz and Patricelli 2007; von Lubitz and Wickramasinghe 2006). Given the challenges of today's health-care environment (Wickramasinghe and Schaffer 2010) most notably the exponential rise in costs to a point where many countries are facing the prospect of unsustainable health-care delivery in the near future, an aging population, and the phenomenal rise of chronic diseases, it is essential that new e-health solutions that ameliorate medical problems or support a better treatment regimen subscribe to the health-care value proposition of providing superior access, quality, and value (Wickramasinghe and Schaffer 2010; Zwicker et al. 2014). Given that contemporaneous to the rise of chronic diseases has been an equally significant rise in the adoption and diffusion of mobile solutions, it would be prudent to investigate if mobile solutions might be beneficial to support health-care delivery. However, realizing that health care is indeed a conservative environment, and thus the adoption of e-health into this context would be seen as a significant ICT innovation, we draw upon the institutional information system (IS) literature regarding the development of ICT innovations to guide our argument.

We note that there is a plethora of studies that have explored and explained factors that impact on the development of ICT innovations (Fichman 2000, 2004). Using the organization as a unit of analysis, these studies culminate with rational-actor decision models which argue that organizational adopters make independent rational decisions that are driven by economic and technical efficiency objectives (Strang and Meyer 2001). While these studies constitute the "dominant paradigm of IT innovation research" (Fichman 2004), they have also been criticized on the grounds that the models that they have generated represent "overrationalized" (Kaganer et al. 2010) accounts of ICT adoption. That is, they fall short of accounting for the institutional complexities of modern organizational environments within which ICT innovations are developed and adopted (Currie and Parikh 2005). Institutional theorists are increasingly asserting that institutional arrangements are present from the beginning of the process of an innovation's adoption and diffusion (Currie 2004). However, in and of itself, "institutional theory tells us relatively little about 'institutionalization' as an unfinished process (as opposed to an achieved state)" (DiMaggio 1988, p. 12). In this vein, there is paucity of research concerning early periods of the development of innovations in particular (Garud 2001). That is, what is not well understood currently is the period of ferment (Anderson and Tushman 1990) or latency (Strang and Soule 1998) which occurs just before different development paths converge into a dominant design of ICT innovations, after which innovations emerge (Wang and Swanson 2007).

In trying to draw from this literature to assist our study, we believe that this chapter will also serve to explore how institutional arrangements are brought about and shape the nature of the collective action when heterogeneous actors engage in complex patterns of interaction as occurs in health-care contexts. Moreover, we contend that by examining these dynamics in the specific context of the design and application of e-health solutions emerging ICT innovations for a specific health-care problem, it is possible to provide rich findings to inform both IS theory and the broader health informatics literature. In addition, and of equal importance, it is also possible to provide benefits for practice and most especially patients whose lives and quality of life might be improved.

The Organizing Vision for ICT Innovations

An organizing vision is a social construction of "a focal community idea for the application of information technology in organizations" (Swanson and Ramiller 1997, p. 460). That is, organizing visions emerge as community discourse incrementally establishes, transforms, refines, and maintains shared understandings concerning the organizational applications of ICT innovations (Kaganer et al. 2010; Swanson and Ramiller 2004; Wang and Swanson 2008). By understanding the diverse mechanisms that underpin organizing vision discourse, community organizations may be better positioned to make sense of an emerging ICT innovation in which they have common interest (Firth 2001). For instance, some organizations may engage in discourse in order to understand how an emerging ICT innovation might benefit them (e.g., the innovation adopters), whereas others to understand how to better promote it (e.g., software developers or industry consortia; de Vaujany et al. 2013; Fradley et al. 2012; Kaganer et al. 2010; Klecun-Dabrowska and Cornford 2002).

The organizing vision is initiated through discourse within a community consisting of heterogeneous organizations that share interest in the emerging ICT innovation (Pawlowski et al. 2006; Ramiller and Swanson 2003; Smith et al. 2010; Wang 2001). The community and organizing vision mutually shape each other. That is, organizational actors are engaged in discourse that shapes the emerging organizing vision while opportunities are exposed which can generate interest from new participants who join the community and enrich the ongoing discourse further. In attempts to shape the organizing vision, constituent organizational actors advance interpretations and arguments into the discourse that reflect their beliefs, interests, and experiences in relation to practical aspects of commerce, processes, and outcomes concerning the adoption of the emerging ICT innovation, as well as the invention and adaptation of supporting core technology (Swanson and Ramiller 1997; Yang and Hsu 2011; Yoo et al. 2012). Given the heterogeneity of the growing numbers of constituent actors, agreements, disagreements, or even conflicts among them are possible which can make the discourse dynamic and rich, but which may also result in manifestations of low coherence and contradiction in the fabric of the emerging vision. Furthermore, the discourse is also affected by higher-level structures (Carton et al. 2007; Currie 2004; Sarpong and Maclean 2012). For instance, the cultural and linguistic resources that characterize the subculture of IS practitioners affect and are affected by the evolving interpretative framework of shared meaning that is encapsulated in the organizing vision. The reciprocity of this relationship can enhance the legitimacy of the organizing vision. Similarly, the discourse extracts interpretative meaning from existing business problematic which is central in legitimizing the relevance of the emerging organizing vision (Swanson and Ramiller 1997; Yang and Hsu 2011; Yoo et al. 2012). As the organizing vision transpires, it is engaged in a reciprocal relationship with existing core technology (Swanson and Ramiller 1997; Troshani and Lymer 2011; Wang 2001; Yang and Hsu 2011). That is, the organizing vision can interpretatively ascribe significance and meaning to available core technology or, by creating expectations, even call for new technology to be developed. Similarly, as actors, such as software developers, mobilize the organizing vision, they can also take advantage of, or be constrained by, the capabilities of existing or new technology. Finally, the organizing vision affects and is itself affected by adoption and diffusion processes of the ICT innovation (de Vaujany et al. 2013; Firth 2001; Kaganer 2007). That is, with a sound organizing vision, prospective adopters will have a compelling business case for justifying the adoption of the innovation based on its merits and the manner in which these address business needs, while growing diffusion can provide the necessary evidence for validating the soundness of the organizing vision (Pawlowski et al. 2006; Smith et al. 2010). This may mobilize organizational actors and result in bandwagon adoption impacts (Gorgeon and Swanson 2011). The key themes of the institutional production of organizing visions are summarized in Fig. 14.1.

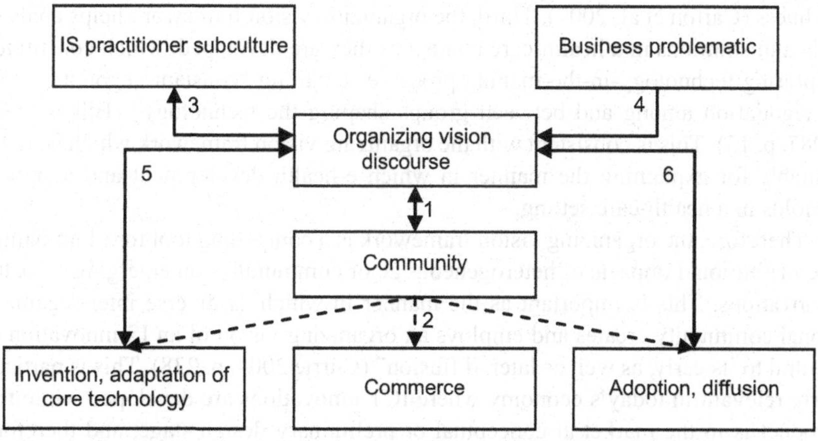

Fig. 14.1 Institutional production of organizing visions. *IS* information system (Adapted from Swanson and Ramiller 1997)

Using the Organizing Vision to Research Development and Adoption of e-Health

There is evidence that the organizing vision framework has been used previously for examining emerging ICTs, including customer relationship management (CRM; Firth 2001), telehealth (Klecun-Dabrowska and Cornford 2002), computerized physician order entry systems (Kaganer 2007; Kaganer et al. 2010), and application service provision (ASP; Currie 2004), Green IS (Fradley et al. 2012), and extensible business reporting language (XBRL; Troshani et al. 2014).

We contend that the organizing vision framework is suitable for explaining the underlying dynamics in the context of design, development, and implementation of the e-health solutions for three main reasons. First, recognizing that no ICT innovation emerges in a vacuum, this framework can improve current understanding of the institutional environment that surrounds emerging e-health innovations within health-care contexts while also capturing the dynamic, rich, and intelligible mutual shaping between the two (Carton et al. 2007). In doing so, it can highlight political, economic, and sociological impacts as part of an ongoing process that shapes the ICT adoption during its period of fermenting (Anderson and Tushman 1990; DiMaggio 1988). Given that health care is a complex industry consisting of many competing interests and often orthogonal goals between the multiple actors (Wickramasinghe and Schaffer 2010), it would appear that such a framework would be most beneficial.

Second, the organizing vision framework embodies interorganizational institutional-strategic duality, that is, it both defines an e-health solution as a socially shared meaning (i.e., institutional aspects) which is incrementally refined by active discourse among heterogeneous actors (i.e., strategic aspects; Kaganer 2007; Pawlowski et al. 2006). Furthermore, because it captures organizational changes that e-health adoption can provoke, the organizing vision framework merges interorganizational with organizational approaches thereby enhancing analysis depth and richness (Carton et al. 2007). Third, the organizing vision framework helps analyze e-health solutions in a health-care context as they are developed, which constitutes capturing technology-in-the-making processes entailing "constant negotiation and renegotiation among and between groups shaping the technology" (Bijker et al. 1987, p. 13). This is consistent with the organizing vision framework which is, thus, suitable for explaining the manner in which e-health development and adoption unfolds in a health-care setting.

Therefore, the organizing vision framework is a compelling tool for illuminating the institutional impacts of heterogeneous actor communities on emerging e-health innovations. This is important as the manner in which "a diverse inter-organizational community creates and employs an organizing vision of an IS innovation is central to its early, as well as later, diffusion" (Currie 2004, p. 238). This is particularly relevant in today's economy where ICT innovations are developed while the product is in the market at conceptual or preliminary design stage, and therefore traditional processes of rigorous design and rollout are not appropriate. Specifically, exploring the organizing vision of health can help portray the interplay of complex interests, emergent causality, reciprocalities, and organizational social interactions through which e-health solutions emerge.

By exploring the emergence of e-health solutions using the organizing vision framework, managers and policy-makers can learn that e-health entrepreneurs need to develop an organizing vision that is driven by a compelling business case that clearly stresses the manner in which actors can benefit from e-health solutions and how these can help address its existing problems. This is likely to encourage participation of individual organizations and increase the extent of their contribution in advancing the organizing vision of e-health innovations. Consequently, members in the health-care community might be in a better position to monitor the manner in which the organizing vision of e-health solutions evolves, instead of ignoring it or remaining passive. That is, by understanding how actors influence an organizing vision, organizations can better predict its evolution path and, consequently, adjust their positioning and strategies accordingly (Firth 2001). Thus, there is a significant need for these organizations to better understand why and how e-health innovations are shaped, given the idiosyncrasies of the industries to which they belong. By focusing on the emergence of e-health solutions, contribution to extant literature can be made in response to growing calls for further research in this area (Currie 2004; Kaganer et al. 2010; Wang and Swanson 2007).

Discussion and Conclusion

Taking advantage of the espoused e-health, benefits remain elusive for e-health entrepreneurs (Ha and Lee 2008; Sohn and Lee 2007). At least in part, this is attributed to the complexity of modern health-care settings where e-health applications are expected to operate (Cho et al. 2008). To improve current understanding concerning underlying contextual e-health complexity factors, this chapter presents an argument concerning how the development and adoption of e-health solutions can be addressed by using Swanson and Ramiller's (1997) organizing visions for ICT innovations as an appropriate investigative lens. Specifically, it can help specify the requirements of pervasive e-health services that are expected to operate in fluid health-care settings with fuzzy boundaries where causal and predictable behaviors can be elusive.

The organizing vision framework can help develop a deeper understanding of the critical issues, barriers, facilitators, and key success factors that underlie current modern health-care settings. We believe that as a lens for facilitating a deeper understanding of complex operations, it is particularly the most invaluable ability to (re)focus the investigative lens on the complexities of various e-health solutions at both macro- and microlevels (Gorgeon and Swanson 2011; Ramiller and Swanson 2003; Swanson and Ramiller 1997; Wang and Swanson 2007). This is particularly important in the context of consumer health informatics (CHI) given that more often than not the consumers are heterogeneous having different particular needs and wants from the data and solution. We can see this best in terms of the personally controlled electronic health record (PCEHR) solution designed in Australia (PCEHR 2015). This solution is designed to be used by all citizens and permanent residents and their respective medical professionals thereby requiring many and varied consumers to be interacting with the one system. In such a context without an organizing framework, it is most probably that such a solution will not be able to deliver to consumers what they want and how they want it and will only lead to user dissatisfaction and frustration. This is particularly problematic given the significant resources including time and money that have been invested in such projects. Thus, we close by strongly urging for more focus and care to develop e-health solutions in general and CHI solutions in particular so that they can provide consumers with what they want and how they want it.

References

Anderson, J. G. (1997). Clearing the way for physicians' use of clinical information systems. *Communications of the ACM, 40*(8), 83–90.

Anderson, P., & Tushman, M. L. (1990). Technological discontinuities and dominant designs: A cyclical model of technological change. *Administrative Science Quarterly, 35*(4), 604–633.

Atkinson, C. J. (2000). The 'soft information systems and technologies methodology' (SISTeM): Actor network contingency approach to integrated development. *European Journal of Information Systems, 9*(2), 104–123.

Bangert, D., & Doktor, R. (2003). *The role of organizational culture in the management of clinical e-health systems*. Hawaii International Conference of Systems Sciences, Computer Society Press, Big Island, Hawaii, pp. 163–171.

Benbasat, I., & Zmud, R. W. (2003). The identity crisis within the IS discipline: Defining and communicating the discipline's core properties. *MIS Quarterly, 27*(2), 83–194.

Bijker, W. E., Hughes, T. P., & Pinch, T. J. (1987). *The social construction of technological systems*. Cambridge: MIT Press.

Carton, S., De Vaujany, F.-X., & Romeyer, C. (2007). Organizing vision and local IS practices: A France–U.S. comparison. *Communications of the Association for Information Systems, 19*(11), 205–240.

Chiasson, M., & Davidson, E. (2004). Pushing the contextual envelope: Developing and diffusing IS theory for health information systems research. *Information and Organization, 14*(3), 155–188.

Cho, S., Mathiassen, L., & Nilsson, A. (2008). Contextual dynamics during health information systems implementation: An event-based actor-network approach. *European Journal of Information Systems, 17*(6), 614–630.

Constantinides, P., & Barrett, M. (2006). Negotiating ICT development and use: The case of a telemedicine system in the healthcare region of Crete. *Information and Organization, 16*(1), 27–55.

Currie, W. L. (2004). The organizing vision of application service provision: A process-oriented analysis. *Information and Organization, 14*(4), 237–267.

Currie, W. L., & Parikh, M. A. (2005). A critical analysis of IS innovations using institutional theory. Gordon B. Davis Symposium: The Future of the Information Systems Academic Discipline, Minneapolis, MN.

Davidson, E. (2000). Analyzing genre of organizational communication in clinical information systems. *Information Technology & People, 13*(3), 196–209.
de Vaujany, F.-X., Carton, S., Dominguez-Péry, C., & Vaast, E. (2013). Moving closer to the fabric of organizing visions: The case of a trade show. *Journal of Strategic Information Systems, 22*(1), 1–25.
DiMaggio, P. (1988). Interest and agency in institutional theory. In L. G. Zucker (Ed.), *Institutional patterns and organizations: Culture and environment* (pp. 3–21). Cambridge: Ballinger.
Fichman, R. G. (2000). The diffusion and assimmilation of information technology innovations. In R. W. Zmud (Ed.), *Framing the domains of IT management: Projecting the future… through the past* (pp. 105–128). Cincinnati: Pinnaflex Educational Resources.
Fichman, R. G. (2004). Going beyond the dominant paradigm for information technology innovation research. *Journal of the Association for Information Systems, 5*(8), 314–355.
Firth, D. R. (2001). The organizing vision for customer relationship management. *Americas Conference on Information Systems*, Boston, MA, pp. 834–840.
Fradley, K., Troshani, I., Rampersad, G., & De Ionno, P. (2012). *An Organizing Vision Perspective on Green IS Development*. Proceedings of the 2012 International Conference on Information Systems (ICIS2012), Orlando, Florida, 16–19 December. http://aisel.aisnet.org/cgi/viewcontent.cgi?article=1063&context=icis2012.
Garabaldi, R. (1998). Computers and the quality of care—A clinician's perspective. *New England Journal of Medicine, 338*(4), 232–238.
Garud, R. & Karnøe, P. (2001). *Path dependence and creation*. Mahwah: Lawrence Erlbaum.
Gorgeon, A., & Swanson, E. B. (2011). Web 2.0 according to wikipedia: Capturing an organising vision. *Journal of the American Society for Information Science and Technology, 62*(10), 1916–1932.
Ha, K., & Lee, J. (2008). U-health and regulatory implications in Korea. *Portland International Center for Management of Engineering and Technology (PICMET 2008 Proceedings)*, pp. 351–355, IEEE, Cape Town.
Kaganer, E. A. (2007). Institutional dynamics in IT markets: Extending the concept of organizing visions for IT innovations. Information System and Decision Sciences, Louisiana State University, Louisiana.
Kaganer, E. A., Pawlowski, S. D., & Wiley-Patton, S. (2010). Building legitimacy for IT innovations: The case of computerized physician order entry systems. *Journal of the Association for Information Systems, 11*(1), 1–33.
Kaplan, B. (2001). Evaluating informatics applications-social interactionism and call for methodological pluralism. *International Journal of Medical Informatics, 64*(1), 39–56.
Klecun-Dabrowska, E., & Cornford, T. (2002). The Organizing vision of telehealth. European Conference on Information Systems (ECIS 2002), June 6–8, Gdańsk, Poland.
Lorenzi, N. M., Riley, R. T., Blyth, A. J. C., Southon, G., & Dixon, B. J. (1997). Antecedents of the people and organizational aspects of medical informatics. *Journal of American Medical Association (JAMA), 4*(2), 79–83.
Lorenzi, N. M., Riley, R. T., Blyth, A. J. C., Southon, G., & Dixon, B. J. (1998). People and organizational aspects of medical informatics. In B. Cesnik, A. T. McCray, & J. R. Scherrer (Eds.), *MEDINFO'98 Proceedings of the Ninth World Congress on Medical Informatics* (pp. 1197–1200). IOS Press, Seoul.
Massaro, T. (1993). Introducing physician order entry at a major academic medical center: Impact on organizational culture and behavior. *Academic Medicine, 68*(1), 20–35.
Menon, N. M., Lee, B., & Eldenburg, L. (2000). Productivity of information systems in the healthcare industry. *Information Systems Research, 11*(1), 83–92.
Pawlowski, S. D., Kaganer, E. A., & Wiley-Patton, S. (2006). Building legitimacy for IT innovations: Organizing visions and discoursive strategies of legitimacy. Academy of Management Proceedings 2006.
PCEHR. (2015). www.ehealth.gov.au. Accessed 15 March 2015.

Ramiller, N. C., & Swanson, E. B. (2003). Organizing visions for information technology and the information systems executive response. *Journal of Management Information Systems, 20*(1), 13–50.
Sarpong, D., & Maclean, M. (2012). Mobilising differential visions for new product innovation. *Technovation, 32*(12), 694–702.
Schriger, D., Baraff, L., Rogers, W., & Cretin, L. (1997). Implementation of clinical guidelines using a computer charting systems. *The Journal of the American Medical Association, 278*, 1585–1590.
Smith, M. L., Noorman, M. E., & Martin, A. K. (2010). Automating the public sector and organizing accountabilities. *Communications of the Association for Information Systems, 26*, 1–16.
Sohn, M., & Lee, J. (2007). *U-health in Korea: Opportunities and challenges*. Portland International Center for Management of Engineering and Technology (PICMET 2007 Proceedings) (pp. 2791–2794), IEEE, Oregon.
Strang, D., & Meyer, M. W. (2001). In search of excellence: Fads, success stories, and adaptive emulation. *American Journal of Sociology, 107*(1), 147–182.
Strang, D., & Soule, S. A. (1998). Diffusion in organizations and social movements: From hybrid corn to poison pills. Annual Review of Sociology, J. Hagan & K. S. Cook (Eds.), Annual Reviews, Palo Alto, CA, pp. 265–290.
Swanson, E. B., & Ramiller, N. C. (1997). The organizing vision in information systems innovation. *Organization Science, 8*(5), 458–474.
Swanson, E. B., & Ramiller, N. C. (2004). Innovating mindfully with information technology. *MIS Quarterly, 28*(4), 553–583.
Timpka, T., Bång, M., Delbanco, T., & Walker, J. (2007). Information infrastructure for inter-organizational mental health services: An actor-network theory analysis of psychiatric rehabilitation. *Journal of Biomedical Informatics, 40*(4), 429–437.
Troshani, I., & Lymer, A. (June, 2011). *Institutionalizing XBRL in the UK: An organizing vision perspective*. Proceedings of the 19th European Conference on Information Systems (ECIS2011), School of Economics, Aalto University, Helsinki.
Troshani, I. & Wickramasinghe, N. (2014). *Tackling complexity in e-health with actor-network theory*. Proceedings of the 2014 47th Hawaii International Conference on System Sciences (HICSS), IEEE, Waikoloa, 6–9 January 2014, pp. 2994–3003.
Troshani, I., Parker, L. D., & Lymer, A. (2014). Institutionalising XBRL for financial reporting: Resorting to regulation. *Accounting and Business Research* (http://dx.doi.org/10.1080/00014788.2014.980772).
Von Lubitz, D., & Patricelli, F. (2007). Network-centric healthcare operations: Data warehousing and the associated telecommunications platforms. *International Journal of Services and Standards, 3*(1), 97–119.
von Lubitz, D., & Wickramasinghe, N. (2006). Healthcare and technology: The doctrine of networkcentric healthcare. *International Journal of Electronic Healthcare, 2*(4), 322–344.
Wang, P. (2001). *What drives waves in information systems: The organizing vision perspective*. Twenty-second International Conference on Information Systems, pp. 411–417. New Orleans.
Wang, P., & Swanson, E. B. (2007). Launching professional services automation: Institutional entrepreneurship for information technology innovations. *Information and Organization, 17*(1), 59–88.
Wang, P., & Swanson, E. B. (2008). Customer relationship management as advertised: Exploiting and sustaining technological momentum. *Information Technology & People, 21*(4), 323–349.
Wickramasinghe, N., & Schaffer, J. (2010). Realizing value driven e-health solutions. IBM Center for the Business of Government, Washington DC.
Wickramasinghe, N., Bali, R. K., & Tatnall, A. (2007). Using actor network theory to understand network centric healthcare operations. *International Journal of Electronic Healthcare, 3*(3), 317–328.
Yang, S. O., & Hsu, C. (2011). The organizing vision for cloud computing in Taiwan. *Journal of Electronic Commerce Research, 12*(4), 257–271.

Yoo, Y., Boland, R. J., Lyytinen, K., & Majchrzak, A. (2012). Organizing for innovation in the digitized world. *Organization Science, 23*(5), 1398–1408.

Zucker, L. G. (1983). Organizations as institutions. In S. B. Bacharach (Ed.), *Research in the sociology of organizations* (pp. 1–47). Greenwich: JAI Press.

Zwicker, R., Seitz, J., & Wickramasinghe, N. (2014). Identifying critical issues for developing successful e-health solutions. In N. Wickramasinghe, L. Al-Hakim, C. Gonzalez, & J. Tan (Eds.), *Lean thinking for healthcare* (pp. 207–224). New York: Springer.

Dr. Indrit Troshani is a senior lecturer in accounting information systems at the University of Adelaide Business School. He holds a PhD (computer science), an MSc (computer-based information systems), and a BBA (Hons). His research interests include digital business reporting (e.g., XBRL), impact of information and communication technology (ICT) on accounting, adoption, and diffusion of innovations (e.g., XBRL, Green information system/information technology (IS/IT), e-health, and mobile services). His work has been published in several journals including *Accounting and Business Research, Journal of Contemporary Accounting & Economics, Information Technology & People, Electronic Markets, Journal of Computer Information Systems, Journal of Engineering and Technology Management, European Journal of Innovation Management, and Industrial Management & Data Systems.*

Prof. Nilmini Wickramasinghe PhD, MBA, GradDipMgtSt BSc, AMusA, piano, AMusA, violin has a well-recognized research record in the field of health care and information system/information technology (IS/IT). Her expertise is in the strategic application and management of technology for effecting superior health-care solutions. She is currently the professor director of health informatics management at Epworth Health Care and a professor at Deakin University.

Chapter 15
Leveraging the Power of e-Health to Achieve Healthcare Outcomes

Indrit Troshani and Nilmini Wickramasinghe

Introduction

Information and communications technologies (ICTs) are touted to offer a huge potential to raise the quality, increase the efficiency, and decrease the costs of primary, secondary, and tertiary healthcare (Heinzelmann et al. 2005). Indeed, use of digitally enabled technologies such as ICTs to support the achievement of health goals has the potential to transform the manner in which health services are delivered (WHO 2011). Additionally, these technologies have the potential to empower patients to better understand their medical conditions and take responsibility by making informed decisions about such conditions (Raisinghani and Young 2008). In this context, e-health is emerging as an important area which can assist clinicians and patients to improve health outcomes in many ways including preventing and controlling of diseases by way of facilitating health information acquisition (Baker et al. 2003), customizing and personalizing information dissemination (Tate et al. 2006), detecting and treating diseases (Thomas et al. 2002), and encouraging the adoption of healthy lifestyles including weight control, physical activity, and quitting smoking (Tate et al. 2003). To illustrate, chronic diseases such as diabetes in addition to having a huge impact on the diabetes sufferers themselves can also be very costly to treat (AIHW 2007, 2008). Yet, pervasive diabetes monitoring solutions can offer enormous benefits which include efficient and accurate monitoring and control of glucose levels and minimizing unnecessary hospitalizations or even just doctor visits (Wickramasinghe et al. 2009). Evidence is increasingly emerging showing how these solutions can improve patients' quality of life by preventing and

---

I. Troshani (✉)
University of Adelaide Business School, 10 Pulteney St, Adelaide, SA 5000, Australia
e-mail: indrit.troshani@adelaide.edu.au

N. Wickramasinghe
Deakin University and Epworth HealthCare, 60 Baker Ave, Kew East 3102, Australia
e-mail: n.wickramasinghe@deakin.edu.au

N. Wickramasinghe et al. (eds.), *Contemporary Consumer Health Informatics*,
Healthcare Delivery in the Information Age, DOI 10.1007/978-3-319-25973-4_15

controlling disease progress and instilling preventative behaviours amongst diabetes sufferers (Koch 2006; Wickramasinghe et al. 2009).

Chiasson and Davidson (2004) argue that although there is an increasing number of contributions to e-health research, knowledge in this area remains limited and underdeveloped. Additionally, as Koch (2006) and World Health Organization (WHO 2011) argue, most modern developed healthcare systems are experiencing many challenges including (i) increasing demand for healthcare services due to increasing aging populations and changed lifestyles resulting often in chronic diseases, (ii) increasing demand for healthcare accessibility (e.g. home care), (iii) increasing need for efficiency, personalization, and quality equity in healthcare, (iv) increasing and chronic staff shortages, and (v) limited budgets. There is broad agreement in extant literature that e-health can help in addressing these challenges. It follows that knowledge and understanding of e-health developments can be useful in assisting both scholars and practitioners address these challenges since it can help understand why pervasive e-health solutions emerge and how they are shaped. Additionally, it can assist e-health scholars focus their research efforts on developing areas. Having extensively reviewed extant research, we first discuss health education, person's health information management and electronic health records (EHRs), standardization, m-health, and security and privacy. The chapter subsequently concludes with a discussion of research directions.

Health Awareness and Education

Healthcare awareness and education can have a huge impact on individual quality of life, public health, and even more widely, on national economies (Ball and Lillis 2001; Gazmararian et al. 2005; Troshani and Wickramasinghe 2013). Indeed, many organizations worldwide are using e-health technologies to address health literacy and education problems. There are a number of reasons for this. First, e-health technologies offer adaptability, cost-effectiveness, and accessibility (Eysenbach 2007). Additionally, as reported in Ball and Lillis (2001) in relation to the Deloitte & Touche and VHA Inc.'s study, two thirds of patients in the USA do not receive any literature in relation to their medical conditions, which results in patients taking matters into their own hands and look for medical information online (Ball and Lillis 2001). Second, there is evidence that health-information-seeking behaviours can lead to better health outcomes. Indeed, access to health and medical information has significantly increased in the past decade (Lustria et al. 2011) with access to health information resources, risk- and self-management tools becoming increasingly available on the Internet and used by individuals. Existing evidence suggests that consumers are becoming increasingly more proactive in the management of their healthcare with many patients conducting the research concerning their condition prior to consulting their doctors (Gauld and Williams 2009; Jones 2009). For example, a recent study found that patients who look for health information online ask more questions to doctors during their appointments and comply with doctor's recommendations better than those patients who do not look for health information online (Iverson et al. 2008). Similarly, a strong association was found to exist between using the Internet to search for health information and individual self-efficacy, problem-focused coping and social support (Kalichman et al. 2006). Indeed, documented evidence exists showing the link between self-efficacy of health education and the available of tools that support the health-related information and communication with clinicians (Lustria et al. 2011).

While numerous tools are available that can enable health consumers access health-related information online, *Web 2.0* is receiving increased attention as it offers online tools and activities that encourage interactivity and collaboration through interpersonal networking and personalization while also fostering a sense of community amongst users (Abram 2005; Troshani and Wickramasinghe 2013). There are many Web 2.0 applications that offer a huge potential for health literacy and healthcare education (Boulos and Wheeler 2007) including wikis, blogs, podcasting, Really Simple Syndication (RSS) feeds, social networking applications, and instant messaging (IM). We explain these in turn and illustrate them with examples about how they are being used in relation to health literature and education.

A *wiki* is a collaborative application that allows users to provide content while also enabling that content to be edited by anybody (Boulos et al. 2006; Troshani and Wickramasinghe 2013). In healthcare settings, wikis can be used for knowledge sharing (e.g. http://www.wikisurgery.com). Additionally, wikis offer strong localization capabilities enabling non-English posts as well. For example, DiabetesPost at http://www.diabetespost.com/ enables posts to be made in Arabic.

Blogs enable users to provide online journals or web diaries that can be easily published and updated chronologically on issues of interest or on common themes including health literacy and education (Boulos et al. 2006; Troshani and Wickramasinghe 2013). Some of the most notable health education blogs include http://drugscope.blogspot.com and http://biographyofbreastcancer.blogspot.com. As blog users are not necessarily professionals, there is a substantial risk for misinformation, although, according to Boulos et al. (2006), inherent 'collaborative intelligence' acts as a built-in quality control and assurance mechanism for blogs.

Podcasts are location- and time-independent digital files that can be downloaded automatically by free software on portable devices, such as Apple iPods/iPads or MP3/MP4 players and played by users at their leisure (Boulos and Wheeler 2007; Troshani and Wickramasinghe 2013). Notable examples of health education podcasts include http://healthliteracyoutloud.com.

RSS feeds are protocols that are used to indicate updates or additions to content to websites or blogs as per user-defined queries or requirements (Boulos and Wheeler 2007; Troshani and Wickramasinghe 2013). Typically, RSS works when users subscribe to RSS feeds using RSS aggregators that are typically supported in modern browsers. Aggregators crawl selected websites regularly and display feeds to users enabling them to conveniently and quickly overview updates on specific topics at any point in time at the selected websites (Boulos and Wheeler 2007).

Social networking applications enable forming of groups of individuals that share common interests or circumstances (Troshani and Wickramasinghe 2013).

For example, http://www.depressionnet.com.au is an Australian online community that provides comprehensive information for people living with depression. A similar social networking application is the CURE DiABETES group at http://groups.myspace.com/cureDiABETES which is run by patients and supporters in order to help and support diabetes sufferers.

IM constitutes real-time online interaction between two or more users who can share text, audio, video, and other types of files. A nurse-led web chat application enabling the public to interact with qualified nurses was well received by patients (Eminovic et al. 2004).

As patients wish to interact and exchange increasingly more information with healthcare providers, opportunities exist for using Web 2.0 tools and applications to enable or facilitate these interactions for literacy development and education purposes (Troshani and Wickramasinghe 2013). By emphasizing education, these tools empower patients to take responsibility for their conditions, thereby making them active and responsible participants in their treatment regimen (Boulos and Wheeler 2007; Boulos et al. 2006; Mackert et al. 2009; Nicholas et al. 2001).

Personal Health Information Management Through Electronic Health Records

Managing personal health information can be very challenging and is underpinned by complex and fragmented systems that include a wide array of an individual's personal health information (Pratt et al. 2006). Specifically, this information includes data concerning a patient's health history including medication regimes and treatments, medical fees, insurance and employer-related health coverage (Lustria et al. 2011). Much of this data are often stored in different often inconsistent or even incompatible systems that are distributed across many actors including doctors, clinicians, and specialists. Consequently, keeping accurate and up-to-date personal health records is of paramount importance though particularly given the current context of personal health information management (Tang et al 2006a).

EHRs represent personal health information concerning patients which is meant to support healthcare-related activities, and evidence-based medical decision support both directly or indirectly (Nelson 2009; Tang et al 2006a). This information is collected longitudinally during patient visits at any healthcare delivery setting (Raghupathi and Kesh 2009). In addition to patient demographics, EHRs also include past medical history such as medications, problems, immunizations, radiology and laboratory results, and progress notes (Raghupathi and Kesh 2009). It is anticipated that in the future, EHRs will offer rich medically relevant information in addition to text. EHRs will include still images, echocardiograms, endoscopies, and even video recordings of patient interviews or visits which will enable convenient access to expertise that is located remotely and even facilitate training of medical practitioners (Heinzelmann et al. 2005).

EHRs can offer many benefits including complete, accurate, error-free universally accessible lifetime patient health information (Raghupathi and Kesh 2009). They also offer significant productivity improvements in the healthcare industry (von Lubitz and Wickramasinghe 2006). In a healthcare setting where healthcare costs are steadily increasing while pressures are growing to satisfy unmet needs and increasing competition, the promises of EHRs to offer quality and productivity constitute the main driving forces for developing them.

There are a number of risks that need to be mitigated as EHR development progresses and design issues addressed. Although EHRs offer many benefits, healthcare professionals may find that with EHRs, they may be exchanging a set of issues with another. For example, issues experienced with traditional manual paper-based patient record systems such as lost patient charts, poor handwriting, and missing information may be exchanged with issues with data capture problems, computer crashes, programming errors, and susceptibility for viruses and other malware which are likely to affect EHRs and potentially render them useless (Glaser and Aske 2010; Goldschmidt 2005).

Another major issue with EHRs concerns the privacy and security of confidential personal medical and health information (Rao Hill and Troshani 2010; Troshani and Rao Hill 2009). For example unethical use of such information for personal gain by disgruntled or unethical employees or even legislated use of private information without an individual's prior consent constitute serious risks that need to be mitigated as EHRs are developed (Goldschmidt 2005). Thus, the question that needs further research is if the espoused benefits of EHRs will indeed outweigh their risks and development costs (Rash 2005).

Extant research shows that EHR design and development have been constrained by major challenges (Raghupathi and Kesh 2009). First, the literature suggests that existing EHRs seem to be driven by specific vendors or technologies and ignore the diverse and complex nature of modern healthcare settings and processes (Blobel 2006). For example, existing EHRs, driven by specific vendors, do not appear to comply with portability standards (Hippisley-Cox et al. 2003). Additionally, almost all exiting EHRs are based on relatively simple relational database applications which consist of patient data entry forms and report generation capabilities but lack the capacity to be interoperable in large-scale distributed environments and to inexpensively scale up to fully functional applications (Hippisley-Cox et al. 2003; Raghupathi and Kesh 2009). One possible way to address these issues is to take a holistic network-centric view to EHR design (von Lubitz and Wickramasinghe 2006).

Standardization

Standardization entails developing standards in the development and provision of pervasive e-health applications and limiting the use of other options (Choudrie et al. 2003; Damsgaard and Lyytinen 2001; King et al. 1994). Standards constitute conventions that are needed for the structure and behaviour of computing functions, formats, and processes (Engel et al. 2006). Standards play a critical role in the transmissions of electronic information, and as such, standard development, that is, standardization, is essential for the development and widespread diffusion of pervasive e-health applications. Indeed, standardization is essential as it enables the end-to-end integration of new health devices to be integrated into existing health ecosystems seamlessly (Aragüés et al. 2011). Lack of standardization can create interoperability issues adversely impacting information exchange between and among various e-health applications, that is, e-health applications can become 'information islands' and thus present difficulties to integrate with larger healthcare systems (Tang et al. 2006b).

For example, standards developed for electronic payments in the finance and banking sectors worldwide have been highly successful and have become widely diffused due to the national and international standardization approaches adopted and coordination amongst key stakeholders (WHO 2011). Similarly, governments and industry associations are collaborating by way of the Global Harmonization Task Force in order to develop standards for medical technologies (WHO 2011).

Standardization facilitates both integration and interoperability thereby enabling industry growth and development, while lack thereof can make the development of pervasive e-health applications and their integration prohibitively costly (Engel et al. 2006; Koch 2006; Lee et al. 2009). Standardization can include many aspects of e-health, ranging from terminology, text/image communications, health hardware devices, and even security and privacy (Lee et al. 2009). For example, South Korean e-health initiatives are considering the US Health Insurance Portability and Accountability Act (HIPAA) as a security standard for medical data and the International Classification of Diseases (ICD) for terminology standardization (Lee et al. 2009).

m-Health

Mobile health or simply m-health is defined as a component of e-health whereby medical practice is supported by electronic mobile devices (WHO 2011). Electronic mobile devices include mobile phones, personal digital assistants (PDAs), smart phones (e.g. iPhone), handheld computers (e.g. tablets), handheld video game devices (e.g. iPod, MP3/MP4 players) or any other wireless devices (Free et al. 2010). Use of m-health for both healthcare and public health is rapidly growing for a range of functions, which include clinical decision support systems including systems supporting collection of data for supporting clinicians and healthcare professionals (Blaya et al. 2010; Lindquist et al. 2008) and systems that support behavioural changes of patients suffering from chronic diseases (Cole-Lewis and Kershow 2010).

Mobile devices offer many key features that can make them particularly suitable and useful in healthcare settings (Free et al. 2010). First, mobile devices have wireless communication capabilities which can enable their users for ubiquitous, interactive, and continuous communication in the form of phone calls, text, and multimedia messages. Second, mobile devices are practical as they are typically small size, low weight, and are powered by rechargeable long life batteries. Third, mobile devices have sufficient processing power to manage various multimedia applications. Taken together, these features make mobile devices suitable for many types of medical interventions including those that enhance (i) management of diseases including investigation, diagnosis, treatment, and monitoring; (ii) delivery of health promotion and treatment compliance programs; and (iii) healthcare processes including setting appointments, reminders, and result notification (Free et al. 2010).

According to the International Telecommunications Union (ITU), there are over 5 billion wireless subscribers in the world, over 70 % of which reside in low- to middle-income countries (ITU 2010). The widespread accessibility and availability of mobile phones makes these devices very powerful media for reaching individuals generally (e.g. with general health promotion messages) and patients suffering from various medical conditions, in particular, by way of mobile health applications.

Evidence collected in a recent WHO study shows that there are numerous activities of m-health services that are currently being offered in member countries including health call centers, emergency toll-free telephone services, managing emergencies and disasters, mobile telemedicine, appointment reminders, community mobilization and health promotion, treatment compliance, mobile patient records, information access, patient monitoring, health surveys and data collection, surveillance, health awareness raising, and decision support systems (ITU 2010). While 83 % of WHO member states offer at least one of these m-health services, many offer four to six with the most popular m-health services being health call centers (59 %), emergency toll-free telephone services (55 %), managing emergencies and disasters (54 %), and mobile telemedicine (49 %) (WHO 2011). As might be expected, the WHO study also shows that counties in the high-income group have implemented a greater range of m-health initiatives than those in the lower-income groups while m-health call centers and healthcare help lines appear to be popular across all income groups (WHO 2011). Additionally, all income categories identified competing m- and e-health priorities was one of the greatest barriers to m-health adoption (WHO 2011).

A recent study carried out by PriceWaterhouseCoopers's Health Research Institute (HRI) presents the case for the market for m-health applications and services. For example in a recent survey they conducted, they found that 40 % of respondents are willing to pay for remote health monitoring devices and monthly service fees to send data automatically to their doctors, while based on these respondents, HRI estimates that the annual market for mobile health monitoring devices ranges between US$7.7– 43 billion (PWC 2010).

The PWC study also identifies three main business models that can be viable in the m-health market (PWC 2010). First, the operational/clinical business model enables all healthcare stakeholders including providers, payers, medical device and drug companies to use m-health applications to run their operations more efficiently. Second, the consumer products and services model provides unique value-added m-health applications to individuals. Third, the infrastructure business model offers connecting and secure infrastructures that enable m-health information and services (PWC 2010). Further research is required to evaluate the viability and effectiveness of these models in practice.

Security and Privacy

The security and privacy of patient data is of paramount importance, though achieving it is becoming increasingly challenging given the rapid evolution of modern ICT platforms, communication capabilities (e.g. use of mobile devices), and the changing user preferences (e.g. user mobility, use of shared networks) (Luxton et al. 2012). Indeed in healthcare environments where patient data can be stored in mobile devices in multiple locations, accessed by apps, and communicated wirelessly to and from various actors (e.g. patients, clinicians, health insurance providers), threats to both security and privacy become increasingly more serious both during data transmission and storage (ATA 2009).

While many standardized data encryption methods have been developed to protect patient data and securely exchange data through various types of networks in accordance with the HIPAA of 1996 requirements (CMS 2010), a number of issues exist that can threaten the security of patient data when mobile devices are used (Luxton et al. 2012). First, when Wi-Fi networks are used, it is relatively easy for third parties to monitor patient data while in transit. Although security standards protecting Wi-Fi transmissions do exist (e.g. Wi-Fi Protected Access (WPA) and Wi-Fi Protected Access II (WPA2)), their effectiveness is based on the assumption that they are set up by end users. There is no guarantee that this assumption holds particularly in home environments where end users may not be aware or have the technical know-how of operationalizing these standards. Second, while HIPAA requirements are applicable to providers to not share private patient data, these requirements do not apply to end users. End users may have many apps on their device, and the security of these apps depends on the developers' security model (Luxton et al. 2012). As there is no guarantee that apps on an end user's smartphone are HIPAA-compliant, it is possible for personal patient data to be shared with third parties (Thurm and Kane 2010).

Discussion

When we reflect on the domain of consumer health informatics, it is important in that typically consumers are everyday citizens. This includes all members of society—older individuals, disabled individuals, individuals who are less tech savvy or from lower socioeconomic backgrounds as well as Gen Y and Gen Z. A key question then becomes what are the potential risks to all users of the plethora of e-health solutions now available in the market space. Related to this question is: Are users sufficiently aware of the potential risks and benefits before they engage with a particular e-health solution, and if not, how can they best understand these risks and potential benefits. These are not simple questions and cannot be answered in a book chapter, rather they are questions that must be discussed in various forums, and key points from these discussions should serve to shape future policy and regulation so that consumers who are made up of all citizens are adequately informed, have a sound understanding, and thus can make informed and rational decisions about how and what level of e-health solutions is appropriate for their healthcare needs.

Conclusion and Future Research

The healthcare industry is under increasing pressure worldwide from many challenges including quality improvements, chronic staff shortages, and limited resources including financial and human resources. The use of ICT to enable healthcare and improve health outcomes, e-health, is touted to transform the healthcare industry and help address these challenges. Although the number of contributions in e-health research is steadily growing, knowledge in this area remains still at an embryonic stage (Chiasson and Davidson 2004). Having extensively reviewed extant research, we have discussed current e-health trends including health education, EHRs, standardization, and m-health. We believe that this discussion can assist e-health scholars hone their efforts and extend existing limited research in these areas.

For successful implementations to become a reality in the identified areas, adoption of corresponding e-health applications by both patients and healthcare providers is necessary (Raisinghani and Young 2008). In order for adoption to occur, coordinated campaigns are needed to establish public awareness and understanding concerning the value of e-health applications. These campaigns can encourage open learning and information sharing. Additionally, given the complexity of e-health applications and diversity of stakeholders that they may ultimately affect, partnerships should be fostered between the different stakeholders including vendors, patients, providers, insurers, drug and medical device companies as well as between public and private sectors (Raisinghani and Young 2008).

New research directions can extend the areas identified in the previous sections in many ways. First, controlled studies can focus on longitudinal analyses and investigations targeting the adoption of e-health applications and services in the identified areas (Cline and Haynes 2001). Second, cost/benefit evaluations can be carried out to assess whether the costs involved in developing e-health applications can be offset by espoused benefits that these applications promise to offer (Halkias et al. 2008). Third, further research needs to investigate the demographics of the patients seeking to use e-health applications, how they use them, the information they seek and its quality, and how their behaviours can be affected (Wyatt 1997). This can also help identify underserved communities, thereby addressing equity concerns. Finally, further research can also examine the manner in which public policy can assist the development of e-health applications (e.g. subsidies, training; (Cline and Haynes 2001).

References

Abram, S. (2005). Web 2.0-huh? Library 2.0, librarian 2.0. *Information Outlook, 9*(1), 44–45.

AIHW. (2007). National Indicators for Monitoring Diabetes: Report of the Diabetes Indicators Review Subcommittee of the National Diabetes Data Working Group. AIHW cat. no. CVD 38 AIHW, Canberra.

AIHW. (2008). Diabetes: Australian Facts 2008. Australian Institute of Health and Welfare, Canberra.

Aragüés, A., Escayola, J., Martínez, I., del Valle, P., Muñoz, P., Trigo, J. D., & García, J. (2011). Trends and challenges of the emerging technologies toward interoperability and standardization in e-health communications. *IEEE Communications Magazine, 49*(11), 182–188.

ATA. (2009). Practice Guidelines for Videoconferencing-Based Telemental Health. http://www.americantelemed.org/docs/default-source/standards/practice-guidelines-for-videoconferencing-based-telemental-health.pdf?sfvrsn=6. American Telemedicine Association (ATA). Accessed 17 March 2015.

Baker, L., Wagner, T. H., Singer, S., & Bundorf, M. K. (2003). Use of the Internet and e-mail for health care information: Results from a national survey. *Journal of American Medical Association (JAMA), 289*(18), 2400–2406.

Ball, M. J., & Lillis, J. (2001). E-health: Transforming the physician/patient relationship. *International Journal of Medical Informatics, 61*(1), 1–10.

Blaya, J. A., Fraser, H. S., & Holt, B. (2010). E-health technologies show promise in developing countries. *Health Affairs, 29*(2), 244–251.

Blobel, B. G. M. E. (2006). Advanced EHR architectures-promises or reality. *Methods of Information in Medicine, 45*(1), 95–101.

Boulos, M. N. K., & Wheeler, S. (2007). The emerging Web 2.0 social software: An enabling suite of sociable technologies in health and health care education. *Health Information and Libraries Journal, 24*(1), 2–23.

Boulos, M. N. K., Maramba, I., & Wheeler, S. (2006). Wikis, blogs and podcasts. A new generation of web-based tools for virtual collaborative clinical practice and education (http://www.biomedcentral.com/1472–6920/6/41). *British Medical Journal, 6*, 41.

Chiasson, M., & Davidson, E. (2004). Pushing the contextual envelope: Developing and diffusing IS theory for health information systems research. *Information and Organization, 14*(3), 155–188.

Choudrie, J., Papazafeiropoulou, A., & Lee, H. (2003). A web of stakeholders and strategies: A case of broadband diffusion in South Korea. *Journal of Information Technology, 18*, 281–290.

Cline, R. J. W., & Haynes, K. M. (2001). Consumer health information seeking on the Internet: The state of the art. *Health Education Research, 16*(6), 671–692.

CMS. (2010). Health Insurance Portability and Accountability Act of 1996 (HIPAA)—General Information. Centres for Medicare & Medicaid Services. http://www.cms.gov/Regulations-and-Guidance/HIPAA-Administrative-Simplification/HIPAAGenInfo/index.html?redirect=/HIPAAGenInfo/. Accessed 17 March 2015.

Cole-Lewis, H., & Kershow, T. (2010). Text messaging as a tool for behaviour change in disease prevention and management. *Epidemiologic Reviews, 32*(1), 56–69.

Damsgaard, J., & Lyytinen, K. (2001). The role of intermediating institutions in the diffusion of electronic data interchange (EDI): How industry associations intervened in Denmark, Finland, and Hong Kong. *The Information Society, 17*(3), 195–210.

Eminovic, N., Wyatt, J. C., Tarpey, A. M., Murray, G., & Ingrams, G. J. (2004) First evaluation of the NHS direct online clinical enquiry service: A nurse-led web chat triage service for the public (http://www.jmir.org//2/e17/). *Journal of Medical Internet Research, 6*, e17.

Engel, K., Blobel, B., & Pharow, P. (2006). Standards for enabling health informatics interoperability. In A. Hasman, R. Haux, J. Van Der Lei, E. De Clercq & F. H. R. France (Eds.), *Ubiquity: Technologies for better health in aging societies* (Studies in Health Technology and Informatics, pp. 145–150, Vol 124). Amsterdam, IOS Press.

Eysenbach, G. (2007). Credibility of health information and digital media: New perspectives and implications for youth. In B. E. Metzger & A. J. Flanagin (Eds.), *Digital media, youth, and credibility*. Cambridge, MIT Press.

Free, C., Phillips, G., Felix, L., Galli, L., Patel, V., & Edwards, P. (2010). The effectiveness of m-health technologies for improving health and health services: A systematic review protocol. *BMC Research Notes, 2*(250), 1–7.

Gauld, R., & Williams, S. (2009). Use of the internet for health information: A study of Australians and New Zealanders. *Informatics for Health and Social Care, 34*, 149–158.

Gazmararian, J., Curran, J., Parker, R., Bernhardt, J., & DeBuono, B. (2005). Public health literacy in America: An ethical imperative. *American Journal of Preventative Medicine, 28*(3), 317–322.

Glaser, J., & Aske, J. (2010). Healthcare IT trends raise bar for information security. Healthcare Financial Management, *64*, 40–44.

Goldschmidt, P. G. (2005). HIT and MIS: Implications of health information technology and medical information systems. *Communications of the ACM, 48*(10), 69–74.

Halkias, D., Harkiolakis, N., & Thurman, P. (2008). Internet use for health-related purposes among Greek consumers. *Telemedicine and e-Health, 14*(3), 255–260.

Heinzelmann, P. J., Lugn, N. E., & Kvedar, J. C. (2005). Telemedicine in the future. *Journal of Telemedicine and Telecare, 11*, 384–390.

Hippisley-Cox, J., Pringle, M., Cates, R., Wyna, A., Hammersley, V., Coupland, C., Hapwood, R., Horsfield, P., & Teasdale, S. J. (2003). The electronic patient record in primary care—regression or progression? A cross sectional study. *British Medical Journal, 326*, 1439–1443.

ITU. (2010).The World in 2010: ICT Facts and Figures (http://www.itu.int/ITU-D/material/FactsFigures2010.pdf) International Telecommunications Union (ITU), Geneva.

Iverson, S. A., Howard, K. B., & Penney, B. K. (2008). Impact of internet use on health-related behaviors and the patient-physician relationship: A survey-based study and review. *Journal of the American Osteopathic Association, 108*(12), 699–711.

Jones, S. (2009). Generations Online in 2009. http://www.faithformationlearningexchange.net/uploads/5/2/4/6/5246709/generations_online_in_2009_-_pew.pdf. Accessed 16 March 2015 Pew Research Center Publications.

Kalichman, S. C., Cherry, C., Cain, D., Pope, H., Kalichman, M., Eaton, L., Weinhardt, L., & Benotsch, E. G. (2006). Internet-based health information consumer skills intervention for people living with HIV/AIDS. *Journal of Consulting and Clinical Psychology, 74*(3), 545–554.

King, J. L., Gurbaxani, V., Kraemer, K. L., McFarlan, K. L., Raman, K. S., & Yap, C. S. (1994). Institutional factors in information technology innovation. *Information Systems Research, 5*(2), 139–169.

Koch, S. (2006). Home telehealth-current state and future trends. *International Journal of Medical Informatics, 75*, 565–576.

Lee, M., Min, S. D., Shin, H. S., Lee, B. W., & Kim, J. K. (2009). The e-health landscape: Current status and future prospects in Korea. *Telemedicine and e-Health, 15*(4), 362–369.

Lindquist, A. M., Johansson, P. E., Petersson, G. I., Saveman, B. I., & Nilsson, G. C. (2008). The use of the Personal Digital Assistant (PDA) among personnel and students in health care: A review. *Journal of Medical Internet Research, 10*(4), e31.

Lustria, M. L. A., Smith, S. A., & Hinnant, C. C. (2011). Exploring digital divides: An examination of eHealth technology use in health information seeking, communication and personal health information management in the USA. *Health Informatics Journal, 17*(3), 224–243.

Luxton, D. D., Kayl, R. A., & Mishkind, M. C. (2012). mHealth data security: The need for HIPAA-compliant standardization. *Telemedicine and e-Health, 18*(4), 284–288.

Mackert, M., Love, B., & Whitten, P. (2009). Patient education on mobile devices: An e-health intervention for low health literate audiences. *Journal of Information Science, 35*(1), 82–93.

Nelson, J. A. (2009). Personal health records. *Home Health Care Management & Practice, 21*(2), 141–142.

Nicholas, D., Huntington, P., Williams, P., & Blackburn, P. (2001). Digital health information provision and health outcomes. *Journal of Information Science, 27*(4), 265–276.

Pratt, W., Unruh, K., Civan, A., & Skeels, M. M. (2006). Personal health information management. *Communications of the ACM, 49*(1), 51–55.
PWC. (2010). Healthcare unwired: New business models delivering care anywhere. Health Research Institute and PriceWaterhouseCoopers.
Raghupathi, W., & Kesh, S. (2009). Designing electronic health records versus total digital health systems: A systemic analysis. *Systems Research and Behavioural Science, 26*(1), 63–79.
Raisinghani, M. S., & Young, E. (2008). Personal health records: Key adoption issues and implications for management. *International Journal of Electronic Healthcare, 4*(1), 67–77.
Rao Hill, S., & Troshani, I. (2010). Factors influencing the adoption of personalisation mobile services: Empirical evidence from young Australians. *International Journal of Mobile Communications, 8*(2), 150–168.
Rash, M. C. (2005). Privacy concerns hinder electronic medical records. The Business Journal of the Greater Triad Area (April 4).
Tang, P. C., Ash, J. S., Bates, B. W., Overhage, J. M., & Sands, D. Z. (2006a). Personal health records: Definitions, benefits, and strategies for overcoming barriers to adoption. *Journal of the American Medical Informatics Associations, 13*(2), 121–126.
Tang, P. C., Ash, J. S., Bates, D. W., Overhage, J. M., & Sands, D. Z. (2006b). Personal health records: Definitions, benefits, and strategies for overcoming barriers to adoption. *The Journal of the American Medical Informatics Association, 13*(2), 121–126.
Tate, D. F., Jackvony, E. H., & Wing, R. R. (2003). Effects of Internet behavioral counseling on weight loss in adults at risk for type 2 diabetes. *Journal of American Medical Association (JAMA), 289*(14), 1563–1571.
Tate, D. F., Jackvony, E. H., & Wing, R. R. (2006). A self-regulation program for maintenance of weight loss. *New England Journal of Medicine, 355*(15), 1563–1571.
Thomas, B., Stamler, L. L., Lafreniere, K. D., Out, J., & Delahunt, T. D. (2002). Using the Internet to identify women's sources of breast health education and screening. *Women Health, 36*(1), 33–48.
Thurm, S., & Kane, Y. I. (2010). Your apps are watching you. http://www.wsj.com/articles/SB10001424052748704368004576027751867039730. Accessed 17 March 2015. Wall Street Journal (December 18, 2010).
Troshani, I., & Rao Hill, S. (2009). Linking stakeholder salience with mobile services diffusion. *International Journal of Mobile Communications, 7*(3), 269–289.
Troshani, I., & Wickramasinghe, N. (2013). e-Health trends. In R. Bali, I. Troshani, S. Goldberg, & N. Wickramasinghe (Eds.), *Pervasive health knowledge management* (pp. 57–68). New York: Springer.
von Lubitz, D., & Wickramasinghe, N. (2006). Healthcare and technology: The doctrine of networkcentric healthcare. *International Journal of Electronic Healthcare, 2*(4), 322–344.
WHO (Ed.). (2011). *mHealth: New horizons for health through mobile technologies*. Geneva: WHO.
Wickramasinghe, N., Troshani, I., & Goldberg, S. (2009). Supporting diabetes self-management with pervasive wireless technology solutions. *International Journal of Healthcare Delivery Reform Initiatives, 1*(4), 17–31.
Wyatt, J. C. (1997). Commentary: Measuring quality and impact of the World Wide Web. *British Journal of Medicine, 314*, 1879–1881.

Dr. Indrit Troshani is a senior lecturer in accounting information systems at the University of Adelaide Business School. He holds a Ph.D. (computer science), an M.Sc. (computer-based information systems), and a Bachelor of Business Administration (Hons). His research interests include digital business reporting (e.g. XBRL), impact of information and communications technology (ICT) on accounting, adoption, and diffusion of innovations (e.g. XBRL, Green IS/IT, e-health, and mobile services). His work has been published in several journals including *Accounting and Business Research, Journal of Contemporary Accounting and Economics, Information Technology & People, Electronic Markets, Journal of Computer Information Systems, Journal of Engineering and Technology Management, European Journal of Innovation Management*, and *Industrial Management & Data Systems*.

Prof. Nilmini Wickramasinghe Ph.D., M.B.A., Grad.Dip.Mgt.St., B.Sc., Amus.A, piano, Amus.A, violin has a well-recognised research record in the field of healthcare and IT/IS. Her expertise is in the strategic application and management of technology for effecting superior healthcare solutions. She currently is the professor director of Health Informatics Management at Epworth HealthCare and a professor at Deakin University

Chapter 16
Remote Monitoring and Mobile Apps

Ruwini Edirisinghe, Andrew Stranieri and Nilmini Wickramasinghe

Introduction

Within consumer health informatics, one of the key driving technology enablers has been mobile solutions. These mobile solutions, whether smartphones or other sensor devices, promised to empower consumers to be better able to monitor their own health and wellbeing and thereby be better placed to engage in more meaningful and in-depth discussions with their respective clinicians. It is clear that such mobile solutions are only in their infancy in health care, and the whole area of mobile health (mHealth) care is growing exponentially. Given this, it behoves us to understand the whole domain of mobile health including remote monitoring and mobile apps, and thus, in this chapter, we proffer an appropriate taxonomy to assist us in developing a better understanding.

mHealth

The area of ubiquitous and pervasive computing as it relates to health monitoring underscores the need to be continuous and support anywhere-and-anytime monitoring, preferably in a seamless and unobtrusive fashion.

R. Edirisinghe (✉)
School of Property, Construction and Project Management, RMIT University, GPO Box 2476V, Melbourne, Australia
e-mail: ruwini.edirisinghe@rmit.edu.au

A. Stranieri
Centre for Informatics and Applied Optimization, Federation University Australia, University Drive, Mt Helen, Vic 3353, Australia
e-mail: a.stranieri@federation.edu.au

N. Wickramasinghe
Deakin University and Epworth HealthCare, 60 Baker Ave, Kew East 3102, Australia
e-mail: n.wickramasinghe@deakin.edu.au

N. Wickramasinghe et al. (eds.), *Contemporary Consumer Health Informatics*, Healthcare Delivery in the Information Age, DOI 10.1007/978-3-319-25973-4_16

As a result, with the prevalence of smartphones, mHealth emerged in the past decade. mHealth is viewed as driving force in transforming health-care delivery, making some elements of health care faster, better, more accessible, and cheaper (Levy 2012).

While a standard or a definition for mHealth is absent, we adopt the definition for "mHealth applications" provided in the American Health Information Management Association (AHIMA) guide given below:

> …the use of devices such as smartphones or tablets in the practice of medicine, and the downloading of health-related applications or 'apps'…[to] help with the flow of information over a mobile network and…improve communication, specifically between individuals and clinicians. (AHIMA Guide 2013, p. 1)

While the AHIMA guide offers a reasonable definition for mHealth applications, we argue that the above definition lacks comprehension in the following two elements:

1. The definition does not include a holistic view on the communication technology aspects of the mHealth applications. We argue that the mHealth information flow does not necessarily occur over a mobile network. Depending on the application and the adopted technology, a single mobile or networking communication technology (mobile/wireless) or hybrid communication method could be used for global connectivity in the system.
2. As Malvery and Slovensky (2014) argue, it does not include key elements of clinical purpose. The definition focuses on communication with a physician or other clinician and fails to acknowledge the important role mHealth applications play in self-care and self-management of health issues and the resulting information that is not intended to be reported to the individual's physician.

Istepanian et al. (2006) argue that mHealth redefines the original concept of telemedicine as "medicine practiced at a distance" to include the new mobility and "invisible communication technologies" to reshape the future structure of global health-care systems. Further, the definition of mHealth by Istepanian et al. (2006) is "emerging mobile communicates and network technologies for healthcare," which gives a more holistic focus to the communication aspect. They further state that convergence of future wireless communication, wireless sensor networks, and ubiquitous computing technologies will enable the proliferation of such technologies around health-care services with cost-effective, flexible, and efficient ways. Supportively, Free et al. (2010) identify mHealth as "the use of mobile computing and communication technologies in health care and public health".

Taxonomy

As the vision of pervasive computing, to be connected anywhere, anytime, on any device was accomplished, an exponential growth in mHealth systems and applications also appeared over the past decade. For example, in 2013, it was estimated that more than 40,000 mHealth apps were in use (Silow-Carroll and Smith 2013).

Similarly, an exponential growth of mHealth can be expected in the future. The market for mHealth app services is predicted to reach US$ 26 billion worldwide by 2017, according to a March 2013 report by research2guidance, a Berlin-based consulting company (in Malvery and Slovensky 2014, p. 65).

With the high growth of mobile health solutions, it is vital to introduce a taxonomy to keep track of these solutions. The purpose of the taxonomy is to present a checklist of criteria for comparison of mHealth applications. The potential users of the taxonomy are the researchers, developers, funding agencies, and users who want to compare one mHealth application with another.

This chapter presents a multidimensional taxonomy for mHealth applications and systems in a socio-technical context. The four dimensions used in the taxonomy include technological, clinical, social, and economic, and we discuss these briefly in turn.

Technology Dimension

The "technology" dimension focuses on any system/applications that is/are developed for remote monitoring of a health condition. With the rapid advancement of pervasive computing and the vision to achieve anywhere anytime connectivity on any device, a smart personal device like a smartphone with health applications, so-called mHealth applications, are becoming an essential element in day-to-day life. The mHealth applications are classified based on the mode of sensing as follows.

Clusters of Remote Monitoring (Telemonitoring) and mHealth

From the mHealth and telemonitoring points of view, the ubiquitous sensors used in the health-care industry can be of two basic types. The two clusters are the sensors inbuilt in the mobile device or the external sensors. For example, as Stanley and Osgood (2011) argue, the typical smartphones have inbuilt location (global positioning system (GPS)), activity (accelerometer), and sound (microphone) sensors. The mHealth applications developed on the smartphone to use such sensors can be visualised as telemonitoring embedded in mHealth. This is illustrated in Fig. 16.1b.

Situations where external sensors and mHealth applications jointly form a comprehensive system with or without the many other features of mHealth and telemonitoring are represented in Fig. 16.1a. These systems could have external sensors wirelessly connecting to the smartphone and or other device, with or without an mHealth application. For example, the intersection of the two sets represents an mHealth app which uses external sensors. These external sensors could be of many forms such as wearables, patches, clothing, implanted, or even a tablet that can be swallowed.

There is a tremendous number of consumer mobile apps developed in the health-care sector. It was estimated in 2013 that more than 40,000 mHealth apps were

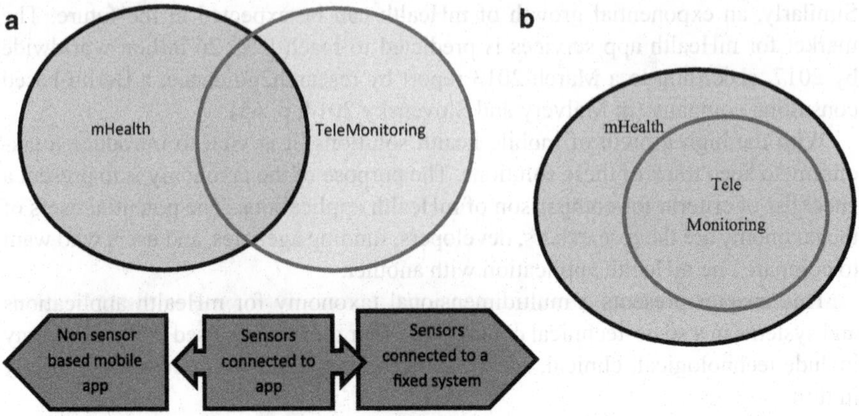

Fig. 16.1 Illustration of the two clusters of sensors

in use (Silow-Carrol and Smith 2013). The types of apps in descending order of popularity include: (1) exercise, fitness, pedometer, or heart rate (HR) monitor; (2) diet, food, and calorie counter;(3) weight; (4) menstrual or period cycles; (5) blood pressure (BP); (6) WebMD; (7) pregnancy; (8) blood sugar or diabetes; (9) medication management (tracking/alerts) (10) mood; (11) sleep; and (12) other (Malvey and Slovensky 2014, p. 5).

The technology dimension of the taxonomy is composed of a sub-dimension including: (1) context parameters sensed, (2) communication aspects, (3) scope of access and information flow, and (4) technology evaluation.

Context Parameters Captured

In ubiquitous computing paradigm, context is defined as *any information that can be used to characterise the situation of an entity* (Dey 2001). Health-care systems measure various context parameters including patient behaviours and social and environmental parameters.

- Physiological parameters: Physiological health can be monitored in patients with chronic diseases such as hypertension and diabetes. General health monitoring for wellbeing and fitness purposes is also doable. The parameters such as BP and blood glucose levels, HR, oxygenation, electrocardiogram (ECG), oxygen saturation, and respiration are measured. In addition, environmental measurements such as temperature, humidity, and visible light in the living environment are also monitored in health assessments.
- Movement-related parameter: Location information is measured to estimate motion pattern and activity recognition of elderly or physically and mentally disabled people.

- Other parameters: Activities, social parameters such as access to grocery stores or fast food restaurants, proximity of individual to each other are also considered in mHealth applications.
- Parameters inferred: These include any parameters inferred from the captured parameters above. Examples are arrhythmias and ventricular fibrillation (VF).

Architecture

The components of the system architecture include hardware (sensors and other hardware), software (operating system and processing algorithm), and the communication method(s). The communication methods are linked with the geographical boundaries and also with the clinical purpose; hence, we discuss it in detail below.

Communication Method

The sensors that measure various physiological parameters, environmental conditions, and other activities can form various communication mechanisms according to the needs such as range of communication, power consumption, and availability of the technology.

The communication aspects of a given system also depend on the capabilities of the devices in use. For example, the smartphones today have Bluetooth and Wi-Fi built in as the short-range communication method in addition to cellular communication. There are cost implications as well as available data rate and frequency of update on selection of the communication technology or the mix of technologies. We consider a holistic and generalised system, which is composed of multiple technologies.

- Body area network (BAN): The physiological sensors attached to the body and the other external sensors will be connecting to form a network of sensors using Zigbee (IEEE 802.15.4 standard) or Bluetooth. This addresses the solutions to low-power and short-range communication challenges. This sensor network data are fed to the smartphone using Bluetooth connection.
- Local area network (LAN): The smartphone then connects to the home computer or home server via Wi-Fi (IEEE 802.11 standard). In case of the absence of a smartphone, the sensor network master can directly connect to a Wi-Fi-enabled laptop/computer to transmit data.
- Global system for mobile communication (GSM): The data is transmitted through the cellular network typical in the form of short message system (SMS).
- Internet protocol (IP): The home computer connects to the cloud via Internet, and the data is transmitted to the external world.
- Alternative connectivity technologies include infrared (IR) for indoor communication and localisation and GPS for outdoor localisation.

Scope of Access and Information Flow

- BAN: This basic unit of information flow enables self-education or self-awareness for the patient. They empower patients with self-care. Ultimate benefits include saving money and time and enhancing patient satisfaction.
- LAN: This local information flow has dual purpose. One is to create a link with the external world through IP. Second is to execute complex processing of the sensor-collected sensor data such as signal and trend analysis and pattern recognition.
- Cloud: This enables sending patient monitoring information and information pertaining to treatment response to health-care providers, physicians, and other clinicians as well as hospitals. Above and beyond, this related information can be fed to the health system.

Communication method and scope of access and information flow sub-dimensions discussed above are illustrated in Fig. 16.2.

Technology Evaluation

Once the system is implemented, it is equally important to evaluate it technically as well as clinically. This technical evaluation might include quantitative system evaluation to benchmark the criteria such as error, reporting load on patients' richness of data, and qualitative user evaluation. A similar study (Berke et al. 2011) evaluates the devices that are easy to use and comfortable to wear based on a questionnaire.

Criteria to Use in Technology Evaluation

- Timely information: Health domain is inherently characterised to be a time-critical domain for decision-making. The timeliness of monitored health conditions is vital. Hence, real-time monitoring should have very little tolerance for obsolete data.
- Accuracy of system: The system should do what it intends to do with a very small error. In some critical situations such as telecardiology applications or tele-operation applications, no error is tolerable.

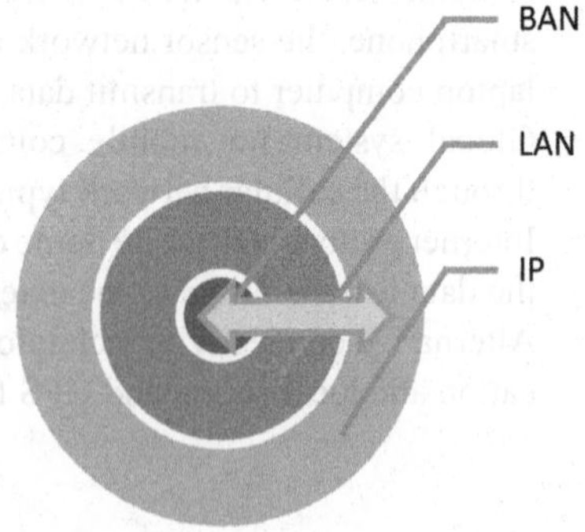

Fig. 16.2 Communication and information hierarchy

- Power management: The commercially available sensor units are generally battery powered. Hence, the limited battery life of the sensors is a limitation in any application. Energy-harvesting sensors, which are currently in the research stage, are hoped to solve this issue in the near future.
- Security: Security is a major concern when sensitive health information traverses on any network, particularity on the web. Malvery and Slovensky (2014) and Lim et al. (2010) discuss in detail the mHealth regulations and legislation and cybersecurity aspects related to mHealth.
- Privacy: The ability to protect the privacy of patients' health information is also vital as discussed by Malin et al. (2012).
- Integration with other systems: As there are a number of health systems in place, for example, the systems used by general practitioners, specialists, and hospitals, the ability of any proposed system to integrate with other systems is vital. Hence, the interoperability or compliance with Medical Information System (MIS) is an important criterion in evaluating its usefulness.
- Effectiveness (fit for purpose): It is necessary to evaluate the ability of the system to satisfy user needs. Thorough investigation and user requirement analysis prior to the implementation will result in a greater effectiveness of any mHealth system.

Clinical Dimension

The clinical aspect of the mHealth application or system is considered under clinical dimension. Clinical dimension covers three sub-dimensions: (1) clinical focus, (2) clinical purpose, and (3) clinical evaluations. These are further discussed below.

Clinical Focus

The clinical focus dimension represents whether the proposed solution is developed to focus on physical coordination or psychological coordination. The solution might be targeting both of the key segments of the health-care industry, which are primary care and chronic care management; however, regardless of the segment, the clinical focus of the system is critical for classification.

Clinical Purpose

Clinical purpose is the primary purpose of the system. Clinical purpose includes: (1) clinical diagnosis, (2) prevention, (3) providing information or monitoring, (4) self-care and awareness, (5) clinical decision support, (6) treatment and management of a medical condition, and (7) general wellbeing.

End users such as patients, health-care professionals, and caregivers use the system for various purposes. For example, patients use the system for the purpose of self-care and awareness. Health-care professionals such as doctors and nurses use for the purposes such as clinical diagnosis, prevention, treatment, and management of a medical condition. These user groups are further discussed in the section "Social Dimension" below.

Clinical Consumer Group

Despite the clinical purpose, a particular application can be developed for a target consumer group. The following are example consumer groups:

- Elderly: Providing home-assistive and other support services for elderly people living in their own home reduces the need for hospitalisation, decreases the cost of care, and improves the patients' quality of life (Norris et al. 2008).
- Disabled: Various assistive, support, and guiding services for the disabled relieve the burden on the caregivers and also improve the patients' quality of life.
- Cognitive and mental disorders: Mobile phones offer the opportunities for accessing heath information, monitoring progress, receiving personalised prompts and support, and using self-management (Judith Proudfoot 2013).
- Patients with chronic diseases: Self-monitoring and self-management of chronic diseases such as diabetes and high BP using an automated technological solution could relieve a major burden they impose on the medical systems.

Clinical Evaluations

Clinical evaluations capture whether the proposed solution has conducted clinical trials to evaluate the effectiveness of the system by monitoring the effects of health outcomes on a relative sufficient number of users. This assures that the system reliably works in a clinical setting. Clinical evaluations can be done by conducting clinical trials. Clinical trials are defined as follows.

A clinical trial is defined as a prospective research study of human subjects that is designed to answer specific questions about biomedical or behavioural interventions (vaccines; drugs; treatments; devices; or new ways of using known drugs, treatments, or devices). Clinical trials are used to determine whether new biomedical or behavioural interventions are safe, efficacious, and effective.[1]

The spectrum of the clinical evaluations could vary from rigorous trials done to no trials. Regardless of the clinical purpose whether to prevent, detect, treat, or manage various diseases or medical conditions, the clinical evaluations verify the ability of the system to perform what it is intended to. For example, the systems developed for the purpose of treatments or management of a medical condition are required to be measured with rigorous clinical trials. However, the systems developed for the purpose of general wellbeing are unlikely to be measured using clinical trials. They are measured in other ways such as technology and usability evaluations.

[1] https://docs.gatesfoundation.org/documents/clinical_trials.pdf

Social Dimension

Social dimension in the taxonomy includes the social context where the system is used and the end user of the system.

Social Context

The social context sub-dimension investigates the degree of social elements in the system. This is evaluated to see whether the system is purely for a personal diary or it goes beyond that to the level of social media health clubs, for example, or even to the level of rapidly growing social media.

Paralleling a rapidly growing online trend toward the "quantified self" and "life-logging", some individuals may choose to share this information socially, either in person or through social media sites, much like the readings on a scale in weight loss clubs. The combination of personal retrospectives and social stigma could prove sufficient to deter a person from fast-food restaurant visits if they knew that the trip would be logged and displayed for both themselves and their peers to see (Stanley and Osgood 2011).

End User

In any technological system, the end user and the end user's needs are vital. The second social sub-element of mHealth applications is to identify the end user of the system. This could be one or more of the following stakeholders:

- Patient
- Doctor
- Nurse
- Carer
- Other

User centered design (UCD) is a modern human–computer interaction (HCI) design philosophy and a multistage problem-solving process in which the needs, desires, and limitations of the end users of an interface are questioned and analysed and assumptions of user behaviour are transferred to prototypes and tested (LeRouge & Wickramasinghe 2013). Hence, it is vital to identify the end user of the system very clearly.

Usability Evaluation

Some estimate that the failure rate of software development projects is as high as 60 % due to HCI issues of poor functionality and usability and hence low uptake (LeRouge & Wickramasinghe 2013).

For several decades, HCI research and practice have focused on designing human-centred technologies, often referred to as UCD (Ritter et al. 2014). UCD is a modern HCI design philosophy and a multistage problem-solving process, in which the needs, desires, and limitations of the end users of an interface are questioned and analysed, and assumptions of user behaviour are transferred to prototypes and tested (LeRouge and Wickramasinghe 2013).

Usability is defined as the extent to which a user can fulfil a task using a tool effectively, efficiently, and with satisfaction (Shackel 2009). The level of the usability of a tool or application can be defined only in the context of its specific users and the specific tasks that are to be accomplished. Hence, designing highly usable software applications requires an in-depth understanding of the user needs.

Usability is currently one of the primary concerns of clinicians and a key factor in their decisions about adopting health information technologies for routine use (Russ et al. 2014). In this regard, several large vendors acknowledged that practices such as formal usability testing, UCD process, and routine involvement of cognitive and usability engineering experts are not common (Civan-Hartzler et al. 2010; Yen and Bakken 2014).

Economic Dimension

The focus of economic dimension is to identify the ultimate economic benefit of a proposed system. It also includes the ways to analyse the benefit flow in the workflow. Is the benefit mainly intended for the patient? Is it for the doctors or physicians? Is it for the health system or providers? The ultimate economic benefit might be even for the community. The benefit might even partially pass on to the various stakeholders. The sub-dimensions of the economic dimension are given below:

- The extent to which the mHealth application has a business case: The business case verifies that the economies of the application use are sustainable (as an initial investment or a subscription by the patient or the insurance company).
- Change management: The extent to which the app changes the current the process/method—whether it replaces the current method or adds a new component. Change management analyses the cost-benefit of the change process.
- The extent to which the app is a disruptive technology: Whether the technology transforms the way the work is done at a broader level. For example, the introduction of a blood glucose monitor for diabetes management was a disruptive technology, where the device changed the industry. The economies of benefit of the introduction of the device included the time and cost to visit the doctor for a referral for frequent blood tests.

In Fig. 16.3, we present the taxonomy discussed above with the key dimensions and sub-dimensions identified.

Discussion

Existing Solutions

To illustrate our ideas, we map some existing solutions into the proposed taxonomy. A comprehensive literature review was conducted to identify most recent mHealth-

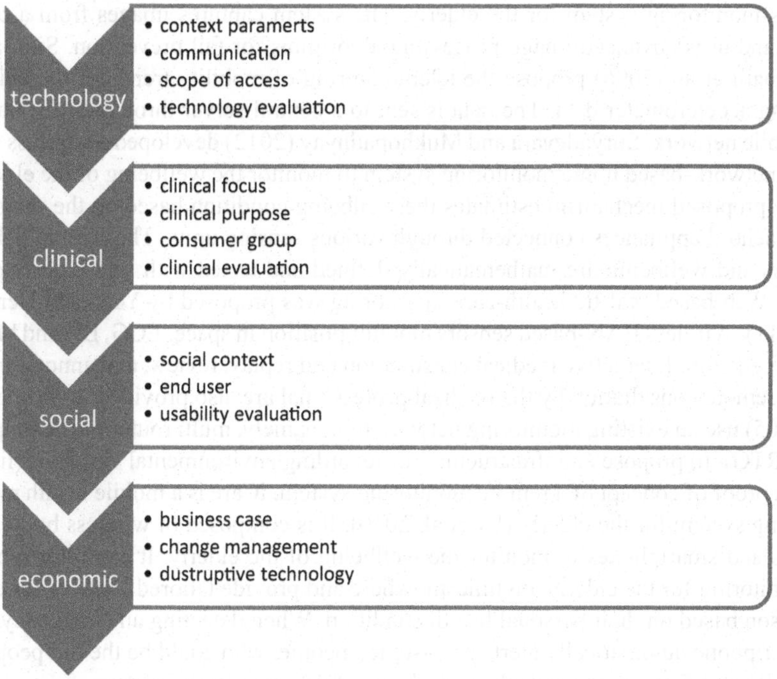

Fig. 16.3 Taxonomy for mHealth applications

related work from the year 2004. We used search terms such as "mHealth", "mobile Health", "remote health monitoring", "telemonitoring", "teleHealth", "personal health monitoring", and "telecare" in retrieving articles. The articles reviewed and are discussed below.

A tremendous number of sensor-based monitoring applications are proposed to assist the elderly in the literature (Rodrigues et al. 2014; Chan et al. 2005; Hewson et al. 2007; Scanaill et al. 2006; Suryadevara and Mukhopadhyay 2012; Yuan and Herbert 2011; Lubrin et al. 2005; Lin et al 2006 and Lv et al. 2010).

Rodrigues et al. (2014) propose a mobile health-care solution for ambient assisted living environment. Sensors attached to the body of the elderly measure ECG, BP, and temperature. The sensors forming a BAN connect to a personal computer, tablet, or smartphone through Bluetooth. The system immediately alerts both the elderly and caregivers of significant changes that might raise life-threatening situations. The accuracy and performance of the system are investigated in controlled clinical trials with three levels of surveillance (alerting). A multisensor home monitoring system (Chan et al. 2005) monitors the activities of elderly. Ten IR sensors fitted in the ceiling of the house connected to an acquisition interface, which is wired to a PC. Accuracy of the behaviour assessment is tested. Changes in activity data and correlations between in-bed restlessness and getting up variables show trends in the behaviour of elderly people (as a predictive tool in abnormal situations). The system provides information to caregivers. The system was trialled with four participants in clinical setting. Hewson et al. (2007) propose a posture- and falls-monitoring system for the elderly. The system captures images from a camera and uses advanced image-processing algorithms for fall prevention. Similarly, Scanaill et al. (2006) propose the telemonitoring of mobility trends of the elderly using accelerometer data. The data is sent to a central server through SMS via the mobile network. Suryadevara and Mukhopadhyay (2012) developed a wireless sensor network-based home monitoring system to monitor the wellbeing of the elderly. The proposed mechanism estimates the wellbeing condition based on the usage of household appliances connected through various sensing units. The normal behaviours and wellbeing are mathematically defined and tested with four elderly people. Web-based real-tie health-care monitoring was proposed by Yuan and Herbert (2011). Wireless BAN-based sensors monitor position in space, ECG, BP, and blood oxygenation. Interactive medical consultation and replay, review, and annotation of the remote consultation by the medical professional are also provided. Lubrin et al. (2005) use an existing monitoring network tool, namely, multi router traffic grapher (MRTG), to propose an infrastructure for recording environmental variables (light) as a proof of concept of a remote monitoring system. iCare is a mobile health monitoring system for the elderly (Lv et al. 2010). It is composed of wireless body sensors and smartphones to monitor the wellbeing of the elderly. It can offer remote monitoring for the elderly anytime anywhere and provide tailored services for each person based on their personal health condition. When detecting an emergency, the smartphone automatically alerts preassigned people, who could be the old people's family and friends, and calls the ambulance of the emergency centre.

Doukas et al. (2011) review the home-assistive technology developed for the elderly and disabled and highlight the social issues about acceptance and training with the technology. Raad and Yang (2009) proposed a smart home for the elderly and disabled. Medical wearable sensors such as pulse oximeter sensor and BP sensor together with a number of environmental sensors, camera, weight sensors, and motion detectors were used to form the smart home. Web interface enables integrating physicians' reports. Lyu et al. (2014) developed a robotic walking-aid system with mobility assistance and remote monitoring of the elderly and disabled. The walking accessibility robot with embedded controller uses a laser range finder, ultrasonic radar, grip sensors, and other environmental sensors. The robot can prevent collision with a navigation and adaptation speed control, and remote monitoring.

The health-care system for the elderly with dementia (Lin et al 2006) is based on radio frequency identification, GPS, global system for mobile communications, and geographic information system (GIS) to construct a stray prevention system. A service platform was implemented for indoor and outdoor monitoring, emergency rescue, and remote monitoring. Nugent et al. (2007) proposed a system of home-based assistive technologies for people with mild dementia. User requirements captured during three workshops involving people with mild dementia as well as caregivers of an ongoing project were presented with the overview of the proposed system.

Telecardiology and monitoring through implanted devices is proposed in the literature (Boriani et al. 2008; Ricci et al. 2008). Boriani et al. (2008) studied the potential for telecardiology and remote monitoring of implanted electrical devices. Ricci et al. (2008) proposed a home monitoring technology for detection and treatment of atrial fibrillation (AF). The data collected from the implanted device through the transmitter device called CardioMessenger is forwarded to the service centre through a GSM network via SMS. Web interface is provided for nurses and physicians to analyse the received data. The data is decoded, analysed, and organised at the service centre. In a follow-up study, the system is evaluated with regard to patient acceptance of and satisfaction with the home monitoring remote control system with the implanted device (Ricci et al. 2010). After 1 year, the remote control by home monitoring (HM) was evaluated. A high level of acceptance and satisfaction was detected using a five-point scale for the system, which showed a good internal reliability.

Wearable physiological remote monitoring system was developed by Pandian et al. (2008); a washable shirt, which uses an array of sensors connected to a central processing unit with firmware for continuously monitoring physiological signals. Lee and Chung (2009) developed a wireless sensor network-based wearable smart shirt for health and activity monitoring. ECG and acceleration data is transmitted via Zigbee. Similarly, Paradiso et al. (2008) developed a health monitoring system with a wearable system. ECG, HR, oxygen saturation, impedance pneumography, and activity data is transmitted via general packet radio service (GPRS; transmission control protocol (TCP)/IP) for remote access.

Agarwal and lau (2010) developed a remote monitoring system for chronic diseases (BP). The BP data collected via a mobile phone are sent to doctors via the Web so that doctors can manage the chronic condition by providing feedback to the patient remotely.

Other systems include medication support systems. Suzuki and Nakauchi (2014) conducted a month-long study with two elderly participants on a reminder system to keep recipient medication condition up to date. The system is composed of an intelligent medicine storage case, wireless sensing devices, and a database server. The medicine case recognised the presence of medicine in its storage compartments by image processing to estimate the patient's present living state (i.e. current activity) on the basis of a fuzzy inference algorithm. The sensing devices are distributed throughout the houses to collect data for living state estimation. The intelligent medicine case works with wireless sensing devices to assist a recipient in maintaining good medication compliance.

A tremendous number of health-related mobile apps are currently available. Selected examples include the studies by Mowad et al. (2014), Ketabdar and Lyra (2010), and Banos et al. (2014).

An android app developed by Mowad et al. (2014) connects with the electrical appliances and services allowing them to be remotely controlled, monitored, or accessed. Even though the health focus of this solution is limited, an arduino-based system can be connected to monitor and control the electronic house equipment from anywhere.

A mobile app to remotely monitor physical activities is developed by Ketabdar and Lyra (2010). The system uses the data retrieved from the mobile phone accelerometer sensor for monitoring physical activities of users.

Banos et al. (2014) propose a wearable health monitoring system called PhysioDroid consisting of physiological sensors and a mobile app. ECG, HR, respiration, motion (acceleration), and body temperature are measured. Two use cases are considered.

Similarly, a large number of remote monitoring systems were proposed for home health care. Some examples are Chen (2011), Berke et al. (2011), and Istrate et al. (2008).

Web-based remote human pulse monitoring system for home health care is proposed by Chen (2011). The designed arterial pulsation measurement system is recommended for assessing and pre-diagnosing the health of a human being in traditional Chinese medicine clinical practice.

Berke et al. (2011) propose mobile sensing and activity monitoring to detect changes in health. The system measures physical, social, and mental indicators. Sensors include accelerometer; a microphone (to measure the presence and style of interactions); and sensors for barometric pressure, temperature, humidity, visible light, and IR light. Concurrently conducted questionnaire survey data were well correlated with mobile sensing of sociability and activity in the study of 400 participants.

Istrate et al. (2008) propose real-time sound analysis for medical remote monitoring. The study uses everyday life sounds and distress expressions in order to participate in an alarm decision for the elderly. The speech/sound segmentation module recognised a real-time test with 9% accuracy.

Classification of Existing Solutions

The above-discussed solutions were classified using the taxonomy we proposed above. Technology and clinical and social dimensions were considered. However, none of the articles/proposed solutions discussed the economic impact of the proposed solution. Hence, the economic dimension was excluded in the classification. The sub-dimensions of technology dimension context parameters, communication, scope of access, and technology evaluation; clinical dimension-clinical focus, clinical purpose, consumer group, and clinical evaluation; and social dimension–social context, end user, and usability are considered. Table 16.1 summarises the classification of the existing solutions.

Issues Challenges and Road Ahead

The benefits of mHealth applications and systems come at a risk of their limitations and challenges. Based on our literature analysis, we find that the three key areas of limitations are:

1. Technology limitations
2. Technology adoption and user needs
3. Security

Table 16.1 Classification of existing solutions

	Technology				Clinical				Social		
	Context parameters	Communication	Scope of access	Technology evaluation	Clinical focus	Clinical purpose	Consumer group	Clinical evaluation	Social context	End user	Usability
Rodrigues et al. (2014)	ECG, blood pressure, and temperature	Bluetooth	Data store on PDA BAN	Accuracy	Physical	Self-care and awareness	Elderly	Controlled environment	N/A	Patient and caregiver	No
Hewson et al. 2007	Motion images	Camera	N/A	No	Physical	Providing information and monitoring	Elderly	No	N/A	Caregiver	No
Chan et al. (2005)	Motion	Infrared and wired	LAN	Accuracy	Physical	Providing information and monitoring	Elderly	Yes	N/A	Caregiver	N/A
Scanaill et al. 2006	Motion	Mobile network GSM	IP	No	Physical	Providing information and monitoring	Elderly	No	No	Medical personal	No
Suryadevara and Mukhopadhyay (2012)	Appliance usage data	Zigbee	LAN	Yes	Physical	Wellbeing monitoring	Elderly	No	No	N/A	No
Yuan and Herbert (2011)	Position in space, ECG, blood pressure, and blood oxygenation	Bluetooth/ Zigbee/ Wi-Fi	BAN and IP	Performance	Physical	Monitoring and remote medical consultation	At-risk patients	No	No	Patient, caregiver, and medical consultants	No
Lubrin et al. (2005)	Light		BAN, LAN, and IP	No	Physical	Proof of concept for home monitoring	Patients need monitoring	No	No	Patients and health-care professionals	
Lin et al. 2006	Location	RFID, GSM, and GPS	GSM, satellite, IP	Performance and reliability	Physical	Chronic disease patient monitoring	Elderly with dementia	No	No	Family members and caregivers	No

Table 16.1 (continued)

	Technology				Clinical				Social		
	Context parameters	Communication	Scope of access	Technology evaluation	Clinical focus	Clinical purpose	Consumer group	Clinical evaluation	Social context	End user	Usability
Lv et al. (2010)	GPS, ECG, accelerometer, blood pressure	Bluetooth, cellular, and Internet	BAN, GSM, IP	No	Physical	Patient monitoring	Elderly	No	No	Family and friends, caregiver, emergency	No
Raad and Yang (2009)	Digital IP camera, wearable pulse oximeter sensor, blood pressure sensor, environmental fall sensor/weight sensors, temperature, gas and smoke, and water sensor	N/A (wireless)	GSM, IP	No	Physical	Smart home monitoring for the elderly and disabled	Elderly and disabled	No	No	Caregivers, physicians	No
Ricci et al. (2008) Ricci et al. (2010)	Atrial and ventricular arrhythmia development or heart failure data captured from implanted device	BAN, cellular, and IP	Wireless, GSM, and Web	Yes	Physical health	Implanted device remote monitoring	Patients with pacemaker and implantable cardioverter defibrillator	Yes	No	Health-care professional	User acceptance and satisfaction evaluated
Pandian et al. (2008)	ECG, PPG, body temperature, blood pressure, GSR, and HR	BAN and GSM	Wireless, GPS	Yes	Physical	Wearable physiological monitoring	General	Yes	No	Caregivers	No
Lee and Chung (2009)	ECG and acceleration signals	LAN	Zigbee	Testing	Physical	Health and activity monitoring	Patients and fitness	No	No	Health professional	No
Paradiso et al. (2008)	ECG, HR, oxygen saturation, impedance pneumography, and activity patterns	GPRS	Web-based access	No	Physical	Health and activity monitoring	Patients and fitness	No	No	Health professional	No

Table 16.1 (continued)

	Technology				Clinical				Social		
	Context parameters	Communication	Scope of access	Technology evaluation	Clinical focus	Clinical purpose	Consumer group	Clinical evaluation	Social context	End user	Usability
Agarwal and lau (2010)	Blood pressure	N/A	LAN and Internet	N/A	Physical	Monitoring of chronic diseases remotely	Hypertension	N/A	N/A	Doctors	N/A
Lyu et al. (2014)	Image, embedded controller uses a laser range finder, ultrasonic radar, grip sensors, and other environmental sensors	Navigation aid	N/A	No	Physical	Mobility assistance and remote monitoring	Elderly and disabled	No	No	Elderly and disabled	No
Suzuki and Nakauchi (2014)	Image, activity sensing devices in house	Wireless	N/A	Accuracy	Physical	Medication support system	Elderly	Yes	No	Caregiver	No
Mowad et al. (2014)	Environmental temperature, humidity, and activity	Bluetooth and IP	BAN and Internet	No	Physical	Smart home automated control system with an android app	General	No	No	General	No
Ketabdar and Lyra (2010)	Acceleration	Mobile phone-embedded sensors	N/a	No	Physical	Monitor physical activities and assistive technology	Patients/elderly need care	No	No	Care givers	No
Banos et al. (2014)	ECG, HR, respiration, motion (acceleration), and body temperature	Bluetooth	BAN	Proof of concept	Physical	Health and wellbeing	Sports and general wellbeing	N/A	N/A	Patient	N/A
Chen (2011)	Pulse	LAN, Internet	Wi-Fi IP	Yes	Physical	Home health care	Elderly	No	No	Chinese clinical practitioner	No

Table 16.1 (continued)

	Technology				Clinical				Social		
	Context parameters	Communication	Scope of access	Technology evaluation	Clinical focus	Clinical purpose	Consumer group	Clinical evaluation	Social context	End user	Usability
Istrate et al. (2008)	Sound	Wired	Wired and SMS	Accuracy tested	Physical	Home health care	Elderly	No	No	Caregivers	No
Berke et al. 2011	Accelerometer, a microphone, sensors for barometric pressure, temperature, humidity, visible light, and infrared light	Daily data download	N/A	Yes	Physical and psychological	Health and wellbeing	General public	N/A	Social interactions monitored	N/A	Questionnaire

ECG electrocardiogram, *IP* Internet protocol, *SMS* short messaging service, *N/A* not applicable, *BAN* body area network, *LAN* local area network, *GSM* global system for mobile communication, *GPS* global positioning system, *GPRS* general packet radio service, *RFID* radio-frequency identification, *PPG* photoplethysmogram, GSR galvanic skin response, *HR* heart rate, *PDA* personal device assistance

We briefly outline each key area below.

Technology limitations: Technology limitations include the choice of the right device(s) for the right application. For example, as Boulos et al. (2011) noted, a smartphone with portability but limited internal storage, processing power, and screen size compared to a tablet or a laptop. However, the use of external cloud computing resources may prevent the needs for inbuilt processing speeds and memory requirements in the future (Kailas et al 2010). Device-related technology limitations also include the accuracy, reliability, and power supply of the sensors.

Technology adoption and user needs: It is vital to understand that the mHealth system and application users have goals and expectations around the technology, and studies should focus on clarifying those goals and exploring how technology could address these goals prior to developing the systems. For example, Dawe (2006) argues that technology adoption, particularly assistive technologies for cognitive disability, must be studied as a process, consisting of multiple stages and involving a variety of caregiver stakeholders who jointly form a caregiver network. Supportively, Spinsante (2012) studied the usability of three different systems and found that the need of a clear and intuitive graphical user interface (GUI) is expressed by the users and highlighted the need of a specific technological design suitable for the elderly or disabled, by taking into account their requirements, either physical or cognitive ones.

Security: Security has been discussed as a major challenge in mHealth application in the past (Poon et al 2006; Thilakanathan, et al. 2014). Poon et al. (2006) argue that is it essential to protect the BAN in order to ensure the security of the overall system. They also highlight the need to secure the sensitive medical information from unauthorised access, which could be hazardous to a user's life (e.g. alteration of system settings, drug dosages, or treatment procedures). They proposed a biometrics method to secure the BAN as a solution. Other issues such as loss or theft of devices which can impact the security of confidential digital health records or data held on mobile phones were also discussed in the past (Boulos et al. 2011).

Conclusions

mHealth is still only in its infancy. Scholars and practitioners alike predict that mHealth will be one if not the key driver for future health-care initiatives (gov2020). However, we believe that the move forward will also contain several challenges connected with privacy and security issues, integrity of information, the distinction between health care and wellness, and the need to have a patient-centric focus as well as support the needs of health-care providers. We do not have all the answers at this point and believe much more careful research is required. However, we do believe that a guiding framework and taxonomy is a very necessary first step in trying to understand this space and thereby design and develop appropriate solutions, policies, protocols, and guiding principles for moving forward. Thus, the proffered taxonomy is presented as a suitable framework to serve in this regard. Our next steps will include testing this taxonomy in various contexts.

References

Agarwal, S., & Chiew, T. L. (2010). Remote health monitoring using mobile phones and Web services. *Telemedicine and e-Health, 16*(5), 603–607.

AHIMA Foundation. (2013). AHIMA Guide: Mobile apps 101: A primer for consumers. http://myphr.com/Stories/NewsStory.aspx?Id=596. Accessed 02 Jan 2015.

Banos, O., Villalonga, C., Damas, M., Gloesekoetter, P., Pomares, H., & Rojas, I. (2014). PhysioDroid: Combining wearable health sensors and mobile devices for a ubiquitous, continuous, and personal monitoring. *The Scientific World Journal, 2014*, 11.

Berke, E. M., Choudhury, T., Ali, S., & Rabbi, M. (2011). Objective measurement of sociability and activity: Mobile sensing in the community. *The Annals of Family Medicine, 9*(4), 344–350.

Boriani, G., Diemberger, I., Martignani, C., Biffi, M., Valzania, C., Bertini, M., et al. (2008). Telecardiology and remote monitoring of implanted electrical devices: the potential for fresh clinical care perspectives. *Journal of General Internal Medicine, 23*(1), 73–77.

Boulos, M. N., Wheeler, S., Tavares, C., & Jones, R. (2011). How smartphones are changing the face of mobile and participatory healthcare: An overview, with example from eCAALYX. *Biomedical Engineering Online, 10*(1), 24.

Chan, M., Campo, E., & Estève, D. (2005). Assessment of activity of elderly people using a home monitoring system. *International Journal of Rehabilitation Research, 28*(1), 69–76.

Chen, C. M. (2011). Web-based remote human pulse monitoring system with intelligent data analysis for home health care. *Expert Systems with Applications, 38*(3), 2011–2019.

Civan-Hartzler, A., McDonald, D. W., Powell, C., Skeels, M. M., Mukai, M., & Pratt, W. (2010). Bringing the field into focus: User-centered design of a patient expertise locator. Proceedings of the SIGCHI Conference on Human Factors in Computing Systems (pp. 1675–1684). ACM.

Dawe, M. (2006). Desperately seeking simplicity: how young adults with cognitive disabilities and their families adopt assistive technologies. Proceedings of the SIGCHI conference on human factors in computing systems, CHI 06 (pp. 1143–1152). ACM.

Dey, A. K. (2001). Understanding and using context. *Personal and Ubiquitous Computing, 5*(1), 4–7.

Doukas, C., Metsis, V., Becker, E., Le, Z., Makedon, F., & Maglogiannis, I. (2011). Digital cities of the future: Extending@ home assistive technologies for the elderly and the disabled. *Telematics and Informatics, 28*(3), 176–190.

Hewson, D. J., Duchêne, J., Charpillet, F., Saboune, J., Michel-Pellegrino, V., Amoud, H., et al. (2007). The PARAChute project: Remote monitoring of posture and gait for fall prevention. *EURASIP Journal on Applied Signal Processing, 2007*(1), 109–109.

Free, C., Phillips, G., Felix, L., Galli, L., Patel, V., & Edwards, P. (2010). The effectiveness of M-health technologies for improving health and health services: A systematic review protocol. *BMC Research Notes, 3.1*(2010), 250.

Istepanian, R., Laxminarayan, S., & Pattichis, C. S. (2006). *M-health emerging mobile health systems*. New York: Springer.

Istrate, D., Binet, M., & Cheng, S. (2008). Real time sound analysis for medical remote monitoring. Engineering in medicine and biology society, 2008. EMBS 2008. 30th Annual International Conference of the IEEE (pp. 4640–4643). IEEE.

Kailas, A., Chong C.C., & Watanabe, F. (2010). From mobile phones to personal wellness dashboards. *IEEE Pulse, 7*(8), 57–63.

Ketabdar, H., & Lyra, M. (2010). System and methodology for using mobile phones in live remote monitoring of physical activities. Technology and Society (ISTAS), IEEE International Symposium on (pp. 350–356), 7–9 June 2010.

Lee, Y. D., & Chung, W. Y. (2009). Wireless sensor network based wearable smart shirt for ubiquitous health and activity monitoring. *Sensors and Actuators B: Chemical, 140*(2), 390–395.

LeRouge, C., & Wickramasinghe, N. (2013). A review of user-centered design for diabetes-related consumer health informatics technologies. *Journal of diabetes science and technology, 7*(4), 1039–1056.

Levy, D. (2012). Emerging mHealth: Paths for growth. https://www.pwc.com/gx/en/healthcare/mhealth/assets/pwc-emerging-mhealth-full.pdf. Accessed 7 Feb 2015.

Lim, S., Oh, T. H., Choi, Y. B., & Lakshman, T. (2010). Security issues on wireless body area network for remote healthcare monitoring. Sensor Networks, Ubiquitous, and Trustworthy Computing (SUTC), 2010 IEEE International Conference (pp. 327–332).

Lin, C. C., Chiu, M. J., Hsiao, C. C., Lee, R. G., & Tsai, Y. S. (2006). Wireless health care service system for elderly with dementia. *Information Technology in Biomedicine, IEEE Transactions, 10*(4), 696–704.

Lubrin, E., Lawrence, E., & Navarro, K. F. (2005). Wireless remote healthcare monitoring with motes. Mobile business, 2005. ICMB 2005. International Conference on (pp. 235–241). IEEE.

Lv, Z., Xia, F., Wu, G., Yao, L., & Chen, Z. (2010). iCare: A mobile health monitoring system for the elderly. Proceedings of the 2010 IEEE/ACM international conference on green computing and communications & international conference on cyber, physical and social computing (pp. 699–705). IEEE Computer Society.

Lyu, S. R., You, W. T., Chen, Y. S., Chiang, H. H., & Chen, Y. L. (2014). Development of robotic walking-aid system with mobility assistance and remote monitoring. Automation science and engineering (CASE), 2014 IEEE International Conference on (pp. 830–835). IEEE.

Malin, B. A., El Emam, K., & O'Keefe, C. M. (2012). Biomedical data privacy: problems, perspectives, and recent advances. *Journal of the American Medical Informatics Association, 20*(1), 2–6. (amiajnl-2012. mHealth, Springer US. 2014, 65–94).

Malvey, D., & Slovensky, D. J. (2014). mHealth products, markets, and trends. *mHealth* (pp. 65–94). New York: Springer.

Mowad, M. A. E. L., Fathy, A., & Hafez, A. (2014). Smart home automated control system using android application and microcontroller. *International Journal of Scientific & Engineering Research, 5*(5), 935–939.

Norris, F. H., Stevens, S. P., Pfefferbaum, B., Wyche, K. F., & Pfefferbaum, R. L. (2008). Community resilience as a metaphor, theory, set of capacities, and strategy for disaster readiness. *American journal of community psychology, 41*(1–2), 127–150.

Nugent, C., Mulvenna, M., Moelaert, F., Bergvall-Kåreborn, B., Meiland, F., Craig, D., et al. (2007). Home based assistive technologies for people with mild dementia. *Pervasive computing for quality of life enhancement* (pp. 63–69). Heidelberg: Springer.

Pandian, P. S., Mohanavelu, K., Safeer, K. P., Kotresh, T. M., Shakunthala, D. T., Gopal, P., & Padaki, V. C. (2008). Smart vest: Wearable multi-parameter remote physiological monitoring system. *Medical Engineering & Physics, 30*(4), 466–477.

Poon, C. C., Zhang, Y. T., & Bao, S. D. (2006). A novel biometrics method to secure wireless body area sensor networks for telemedicine and m-health. *Communications Magazine, IEEE, 44*(4), 73–81.

Paradiso, R., Alonso, A., Cianflone, D., Milsis, A., Vavouras, T., & Malliopoulos, C. (2008). Remote health monitoring with wearable non-invasive mobile system: The healthwear project. Engineering in medicine and biology society, 2008. EMBS 2008. 30th Annual International Conference of the IEEE (pp. 1699–1702). IEEE.

Proudfoot, J. (2013). The future is in our hands: the role of mobile phones in the prevention and management of mental disorders. *Australian and New Zealand Journal of Psychiatry, 47*(2), 111–113.

Raad, M. W., & Yang, L. T. (2009). A ubiquitous smart home for elderly. *Information Systems Frontiers, 11*(5), 529–536.

Ricci R. P., Morichelli, L., & Santini, M. (2008). Home monitoring remote control of pacemaker and ICD patients in clinical practice. Impact on medical management and health care resource utilization. *Europace, 2008*(10), 164–170.

Ricci, R. P., Morichelli, L., Quarta, L., Sassi, A., Porfili, A., Laudadio, M. T., et al. (2010). Long-term patient acceptance of and satisfaction with implanted device remote monitoring. *Europace, 12*(5), 674–679.

Ritter, F. E., Baxter, G. D., & Churchill, E. F. (2014). *Foundations for Designing User-Centered Systems*. London: Springer.

Rodrigues, D. F., Horta, E. T., Silva, B., Guedes, F. D., & Rodrigues, J. J. (2014). A mobile healthcare solution for ambient assisted living environments. e-Health networking, applications and services (Healthcom), 2014 IEEE 16th International Conference on (pp. 170–175). IEEE.

Russ, A. L., Zillich, A. J., Melton, B. L., Russell, S. A., Chen, S., Spina, J. R., Weiner M., Johnson E. G., Daggy J. K., McManus M. S., Hawsey J. M., Puleo A. G., Doebbeling B. N., & Saleem, J. J. (2014). Applying human factors principles to alert design increases efficiency and reduces prescribing errors in a scenario-based simulation. *Journal of the American Medical Informatics Association, 21*(e2), e287–e296.

Scanaill, C. N., Ahearne, B., & Lyons, G. M. (2006). Long-term telemonitoring of mobility trends of elderly people using SMS messaging. *IEEE Transactions On, Information Technology in Biomedicine 10*(2), 412–413.
Shackel, B. (2009). Usability–Context, framework, definition, design and evaluation. *Interacting with Computers, 21*(5–6), 339–346.
Silow-Carroll, S., & Smith, B. (November 2013). Clinical management apps: Creating partnerships between providers and patients. Commonwealth Fund Issue Brief. http://www.commonwealthfund.org/Publications/Issue-Briefs/2013/Nov/Clinical-Management-Apps.aspx. Accessed 7 May 2015.
Spinsante, S., Antonicelli, R., Mazzanti, I., & Gambi, E. (2012). Technological approaches to remote monitoring of elderly people in cardiology: A usability perspective. *International Journal of Telemedicine and Applications, 2012*, 3.
Stanley, K. G., & Osgood, N. D. (2011). The potential of sensor-based monitoring as a tool for health care, health promotion, and research. *The Annals of Family Medicine, 9*(4), 296–298.
Suryadevara, N. K., & Mukhopadhyay, S. C. (2012). Wireless sensor network based home monitoring system for wellness determination of elderly. *Sensors Journal, IEEE, 12*(6), 1965–1972.
Suzuki, T., & Nakauchi, Y. (2014). Field experiments of a sensor embedded medication support system. *SICE Journal of Control, Measurement, and System Integration, 7*(5), 263–272.
Thilakanathan, D., Chen, S., Nepal, S., Calvo, R., & Alem, L. (2014). A platform for secure monitoring and sharing of generic health data in the Cloud. *Future Generation Computer Systems, 35*, 102–113.
Yen, P. Y., Sousa, K. H., & Bakken, S. (2014). Examining construct and predictive validity of the Health-IT usability evaluation scale: Confirmatory factor analysis and structural equation modeling results. *Journal of the American Medical Informatics Association, 21*(e2), e241–e248.
Yuan, B., & Herbert, J. (March 2011). Web-based real-time remote monitoring for pervasive healthcare. Pervasive Computing and Communications Workshops (PERCOM Workshops), 2011 IEEE International Conference on (pp. 625–629). IEEE.

Dr. Ruwini Edirisinghe is a vice chancellor's research fellow at RMIT University. Ruwini received her Ph.D. in information technology from Monash University in 2009. Ruwini is a member of the Institute of Electrical and Electronics Engineers (IEEE) and a committee member of IEEE Victorian Women in Engineering group. Among the awards she holds is the Endeavour Postdoctoral Research Fellowship.

Assoc. Prof. Andrew Stranieri is a researcher in the Centre for Informatics and Applied Optimization at Federation University Australia. His research in health informatics spans data mining in health, complementary and alternative medicine informatics, telemedicine, and intelligent decision support systems. He is the author of over 150 peer-reviewed journal and conference articles and has published two books.

Prof. Nilmini Wickramasinghe Ph.D., M.B.A., Grad.Dip.Mgt.St., B.Sc., Amus.A, piano, Amus.A, violin has a well-recognised research record in the field of healthcare and IT/IS. Her expertise is in the strategic application and management of technology for effecting superior healthcare solutions. She currently is the professor director of Health Informatics Management at Epworth HealthCare and a professor at Deakin University.

Chapter 17
Mobile Nursing

Jianqiu Kou and Nilmini Wickramasinghe

Introduction

Health-care delivery today is facing many challenges such as escalating costs, pressure to provide high-quality care, increase in life expectancy and an aging population, higher patient expectations, and shortages of clinical staff (Wickramasinghe and Schaffer 2010). Thus, delivering more efficient, safe, and high-quality clinical treatments is a priority (Pearce and Haikerwal 2010; Porter and Teisberg 2006; Wickramasinghe and Schaffer 2010). To address this, many have turned to technology solutions; however, it is also noted that this has led to an apparent rise in harmful medical errors (Kohn et al. 2000). Hence, a critical problem now is how to reduce these medical errors and yet improve the efficiency of clinical treatments. The use of information and communication technology (ICT) within health care has already shown its significance in improving the effectiveness and outcome of health-care delivery (Shekelle et al. 2006). We contend that it should also be possible to use such technology solutions to reduce harmful medical errors.

To achieve safe and high-quality health-care service, closed-loop medication administration is an efficient solution (Franklin et al. 2007). With regard to medical errors, medication administration is one key area where problems always occur (Kohn et al. 2000). There are various steps in the medication administration process from the physicians prescribing the order to the medication being administered by nurses (Garg et al. 2005; Members of Emerge et al. 2009), in which closed-loop medication administration records, traces, and captures every step throughout the process, whereby the users can identify and avoid potential medical errors with the aid of automated check and reminder features embedded in the system (Franklin et al. 2007).

J. Kou (✉)
Deakin University Australia, 60 Baker Ave, Kew East 3102, Australia
e-mail: kjq1102@hotmail.com

N. Wickramasinghe
Deakin University and Epworth HealthCare, 60 Baker Ave, Kew East 3102, Australia

N. Wickramasinghe et al. (eds.), *Contemporary Consumer Health Informatics*,
Healthcare Delivery in the Information Age, DOI 10.1007/978-3-319-25973-4_17

In the medication administration loop, nurses play an important role as they are critical in managing the patient's journey (Richardson and Storr 2010). According to O'Shea (1999), although the medication order is prescribed by the physicians and dispensed by the pharmacists, medication errors are constantly reoccurring issues in nursing practice because the rest of the processes such as preparing, checking, and giving medications as well as monitoring the effectiveness or the adverse reaction are all the responsibilities of nurses; and these are more likely to lead to medical errors. As a consequence, we suggest that a mobile nursing system brings great opportunity to the closed-loop medication administration process. In particular, mobile nursing systems can smooth the workflow through providing all the related information anywhere anytime and recording every step in a timely and accurate fashion. Although there is some research about closed-loop medication administration (Franklin et al. 2007; Lenderink and Egberts 2004), most just focus on computerized prescriber order entry (CPOE) systems or electronic medical record (EMR) systems (Franklin et al. 2007; Sensmeier 2009; Whiting and Gale 2008) and seldom, if at all, try to explore the achievement through a mobile nursing information system.

Research Questions

The objective of this exploratory research is to design and implement a mobile nursing system with the purpose of achieving closed-loop medication administration throughout the life cycle of medication orders. The main research question is:

How can a mobile nursing system be used to achieve closed-loop medication administration?

Literature Review

The relevant extant literature for this study focuses on three main aspects. The first part is medical error and closed-loop medication administration. The second part focuses on the continuum of nursing care and mobile nursing system. Finally, the third part presents examples of technology tools to be utilized in mobile nursing systems such as clinical decision support.

Medical Error and Information Technology

Medical error is defined as "an act of omission or commission in planning or execution that contributes or could contribute to an unintended result" (Grober and Bohnen 2005). The harm caused by medical error is huge and can be classified into two sections: (1) the direct physical hurt caused to the patients and (2) the indirect

Table 17.1 Steps, error rates, and information technology (IT) systems in medication management (Agrawal 2009)

Stage	Error rate %	Intercept rate %	True error rate %	Relevant IT systems
Prescription	39	48	22	CPOE with decision support
Transcription	12	33	11	Automated transcription
Dispensing	11	34	10	Robots, automated dispensing cabinets
Administration	38	2	51	Bar coding, electronic medication administration

financial burden on the entire society, that is, the increased costs in order to deal with the medical errors (Kumar and Steinebach 2008). According to the literature, there are a great number of serious injuries or deaths of patients occurring concurrently with significantly increased costs caused by medical errors every year all around the world. The famous "To Err Is Human" report shows that there are around 44,000–98,000 patients died every year in hospitals because of preventable medical errors, and the total costs were about US$17 billion to US$29 billion annually in America (Kohn et al. 2000). Furthermore, the most serious problem is that there is no evidence for obvious improvement after several years. There are still more than 100,000 patients died due to medical errors in America (Union 2010), and the annual cost for USA caused by measurable medical errors was US$17.1 billion in 2008 (Van Den Bos et al. 2011). Therefore, the issue of how to reduce medical errors is critical to both the clinical practitioners and patients.

In recent years, the use of information technology to reduce medical errors has become an attractive field with more and more successful evidences (Bates and Gawande 2003). In order to reduce medical errors, the process of medication management should be evaluated and checked. The process includes prescription by the physicians, transcription by the nurses, dispensing by the pharmacists, and the administration by the nurses. As summarized in Table 17.1 (Agrawal 2009), the error rate, the intercept rate, and the true error rate are dissimilar, and there are some kinds of information systems contributed to reduce medical errors in different stages.

Because the error rates at every stage differ and due to the diverse degrees of intervention by information systems toward medication management, the contributions to the reduction of medical errors are different. As shown in Fig. 17.1, the CPOE system with some decision support reduced the ordering errors by 55 %; 67 % of the dispensing errors were eliminated by the pharmacy bar code identification system; and the reduction of administration errors by 51 % and the elimination of all transcription errors were achieved through the bar code electronic medication administration records (EMAR) system (Poon et al. 2010).

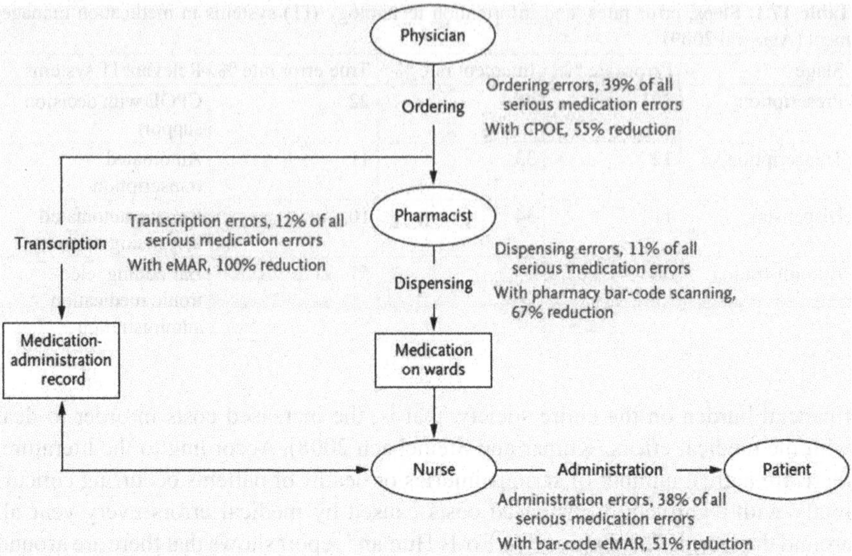

Fig. 17.1 The effect of information technology (IT) at key stages in the process of medication use (Poon et al. 2010)

Closed-Loop Medication Administration

The major target of medication administration is to achieve the five rights: The right drug with the right dosage is taken by the right patient through the right route just at the right time (Members of Emerge et al. 2009). Since medication administration contains several steps and involves many departments and various kinds of clinical staff such as doctors, nurses and pharmacists, it is one of the most sophisticated processes in hospitals. The occurrence of potential medical errors will definitely increase if there is no integrated coordination management through the whole process as all the clinical staff carry out their individual tasks at different times and different places, which will result in many information gaps, process gaps, and management gaps (Kelly and Rucker 2006). Therefore, it is vital that the medication administration management should present integrated, accurate, and timely information to all the related clinical staff so that they can identify all the potential gaps and take actions to bridge the gaps so as to prevent potential medical errors. Another critical factor of a successful medication administration system is making the whole process to be recorded timely so that the wrong points can be traced and identified afterward for future improvement in the case of medical error occurrence.

Closed-loop medication administration is a solution of the best practice for medication management in hospitals. Closed-loop medication administration ensures that the medicine and the patients are verified through every stage, and every step is recorded and can be traced (Lenderink and Egberts 2004). The first important point of closed-loop medication administration is verification using appropriate technology. For example, the right medicine is confirmed by scanning the bar code on the medicine, and the right patient is ensured through scanning the wristband with bar code printed. The other key characteristic is documentation in suitable format of all the related information including the time, dose, route, patient, and responsible nurse, which makes the whole medication process to be retrievable. Traditionally, only the process of prescribing by physicians is recorded, whereas the following procedures are not recorded and cannot be traced. But when a closed-loop medication administration is attained, all the information from different entries is recorded and shared at every step of the process. Therefore, the possibility of medication errors is minimized, and an error alert will be raised rapidly in case of unmatched information is identified by the system.

Continuum of Nursing Care

Nurses act as the most important roles in the whole patient-care process in hospitals, including the medication administration process (Spears 2005). The job of nurses is always unpredictable; they are involved in almost all medication management processes and need to communicate with all the other clinical staff. Moreover, nurses stay with the patients during most of their working period, and they are more likely to identify any tiny potential harm toward patients due to medical errors and thereby prevent them from the beginning. It is reported that there is close correlation between long periods of high-quality care by registered nursing staff and the low ratio of some kinds of medical errors (Needleman et al. 2002). In other words, most of the medical errors could be recognized, handled, and prohibited by nurses. On the other hand, the job of nurses through the whole medication process is very difficult to monitor. They have many kinds of tasks, some of which are very trivial, and they need to do them in different places. Consequently, much more attention should be paid to the processes conducted by nurses when designing and implementing closed-loop medication administration.

Three domains come together to make up the nursing continuum (Haggerty et al. 2003): information continuity, which means obtaining past and concurrent patient situation to give an appropriate therapy; management continuity that refers to reliable and coherent management responsible for patients' varying requirements; and relational continuum that means a continuing therapeutic relationship between a patient and all the care providers (Haggerty et al. 2003). From the perspective of nurses, the continuum of care means having adequate professional knowledge of the treatment, access to patient information over time, and seamless cooperation with other care providers (Haggerty et al. 2003). The lack of knowledge; the inefficient and insufficient information transfer; inadequate and ambiguous communication among various clinical professionals, between patients and clinicians, and among fragmented systems are all interrupting factors to the continuum of nursing care (Sparbel and Anderson 2000). Therefore, the continuum of nursing care should be ensured when designing nursing information systems to promote patient safety (Cook et al. 2000)—this concept will be incorporated into this study.

Mobile Nursing Information System

Nurses need to conduct their responsibilities anytime anywhere through the whole medication process. Although information systems are demonstrated to have the ability to reduce medical errors and increase patient safety, they impose higher documentation workload on the daily job of nurses in order to achieve a closed-loop and traceable system (Ammenwerth et al. 2011). Mobile nursing system is a wonderful tool for nurses to conduct their daily job as the system can provide a quick and easy way for them to check the information whenever they need it and record what they do just at the point of care with the utilization of wireless technology (Wickramasinghe and Goldberg 2009). Therefore, nurses can have more time to take care of the patients rather than spend lots of time on recording their jobs using the computers in the office after finishing clinical treatments. What is more important is that nurses can treat the patients in a safer manner as the mobile nursing system can make the verification simpler and more accurate using bar code verification technology (Johansson et al. 2010). From this point of view, a mobile nursing system does not just transfer what is displayed and presented on the screen of computers to a personal digital assistant (PDA) or a tablet PC, but it can both improve the quality and efficiency of health care and reduce medical errors with the combination of some emerging technology.

Clinical Decision Support Systems

Clinical decision support systems (CDSS) refer to the kind of information systems that can provide suggestions or reminders at the point of care to improve health-care service quality (Berner 2007). There are many types of CDSS: some are stand-alone systems, while some are embedded in the existing information systems such as the CPOE or EMAR system. There are many examples which illustrate that with the help of CDSS providing drug information and preventive care reminders at the time when physicians make medication decisions, the performance of clinicians is improved (Blackmore et al. 2011; Garg et al. 2005). It is assumed that the characteristics of CDDSs including automatic supply of decision support embedded in clinical workflow, offering recommendations, presenting decision support just at the point of care, and computer-based automated support will improve patient care considerably when implementing clinical information systems (Kawamoto et al. 2005). However, there is very little evidence for applying CDSS to mobile nursing information systems. In this study, we are interested to enhance the mobile nursing information system with CDSS as we believe that doing so could improve the quality of health-care outcome with less medical errors and empower the tablet PC to be a smarter secretary for nurses.

Research Design and Methodology

In this research, a mobile nursing system will be designed using a user-centered design approach to achieve a user friendly system, and then a mixed-methods approach that consist of qualitative and quantitative methods will be adopted to explore the research questions.

User-Centered Design

The dynamic complexity of the nursing care process in hospitals determines that the traditional waterfall lifecycle processes in software design are not appropriate for the design of a mobile nursing system (Konstantinidis et al. 2012). For that reason, a user-centered design methodology would be adopted in this research as this method focuses on the needs of users and can achieve an efficient system in the context of health care; moreover, there are some successful examples from the literature (Holzinger et al. 2011; Turner et al. 2013). A user-centered design has six key principles, which are illustrated in Table 17.2 (DIS 2009).

According to these main principles, the system design will be based on careful observation and cooperation with nurses to fully understand the workflow of nurses and thus to obtain a mobile nursing system that satisfies the requirements of users. In addition to this, the convenience and security from the perspective of patients will also be considered at the same time since the main aim is to provide efficient and safe service to the patients. Because of the sophistication of nursing care, the requirement and design processes will be iterative until achieving the satisfaction of end users. Furthermore, in order to achieve truly closed-loop medication administration, all the processes of all kinds of drugs would be examined thoroughly in light of the prescribed orders. In addition to that, more attention would be paid to the user interface design since good user experience of such a system installed in a tablet PC with a small 6-in. screen is really challenging. The buy-in of nurses will only be achieved if the system navigation is easy and clear, and the working process is simplified.

Table 17.2 Key principles of a user-centered design

The design is based upon an explicit understanding of users, tasks, and environment
Users are involved throughout design and development
The design is driven and refined by user-centered evaluation
The process is iterative
The design addresses the whole user experience
The design team includes multidisciplinary skills and perspectives

Case Study

Qualitative research is an interpretive research strategy for gathering and analyzing nonquantitative data of some kinds of social phenomena and trying to explain "how things work in particular contexts" (Mason 2002). The main research question is how a mobile nursing system can be used to achieve closed-loop medication administration. Therefore, in order to explore in depth, qualitative methods are appropriated to be utilized. Since closed-loop medication administration is a complicated management issue and mobile nursing system is rather a new information system, exemplar case study is a suitable research method for this kind of sophisticated problem. Case study is defined as follows: "Case studies are analyses of persons, events, decisions, periods, projects, policies, institutions, or other systems that are studied holistically by one or more methods" (Thomas 2011). In this research, a single-exemplar case study is appropriate since the case could represent, illustrate, and examine existing theories and could be used as a prelude to future research (Yin 2003). Moreover, since a case study provides a further study of all the relationships among various associated parts and how they affect the researched social phenomenon, the research results will present an in-depth and comprehensive depiction (Sturman 1999).

A single-case study of designing and implementing a mobile nursing system with the purpose of completing closed-loop medication administration in a large hospital located in China will be conducted to investigate the research question. The case site is the largest hospital in Jiangsu Province, which contains around 3000 inpatient beds and treats more than 10,000 outpatients per day and around 100,000 inpatients every year. Consequently, the situation there is very complicated, and therefore the solution would be reliable to be spread since various kinds of problems would be encountered and solved in this single case. As shown in Fig. 17.2, in the data collection phase, semi-structured interviews, focus group interviews, and site observation will be utilized to achieve primary qualitative data, and secondary data will be acquired through reading related files and archives.

Structured Questionnaire

Quantitative research strategy collects quantifiable numerical data and analyzes them in an arithmetical or statistical manner to test some hypotheses or theories (Johnson and Christensen 2008). In order to find the most important points in designing and implementing such a mobile nursing system and the significance level of various benefits and problems of the system, quantitative research methods will also play an important role. As illustrated in Fig. 17.2, a structured questionnaire will be conducted to provide some quantitative data in the data collection stage, and an arithmetic analysis will be used in the data analysis phase to evaluate the impact factors and the effect of such a mobile nursing system.

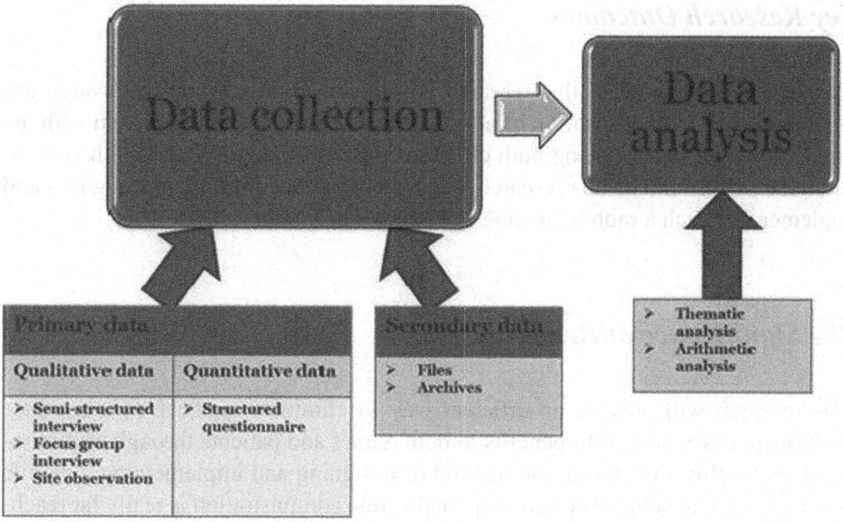

Fig. 17.2 Data collection and data analysis phases

Discussion

This proposed solution of a mobile nursing information system to support closed-loop medication administration has many key aspects as will now be discussed in turn.

Contribution to Knowledge

Medical error is a critical and intractable crisis all around the world because of the direct physical injury and indirect financial problem. Closed-loop medication administration is demonstrated to be able to reduce medical errors through the intervention and documentation in the whole medication management process. Although there is much research on closed-loop medication administration, rarely has it been approached with the focus on a mobile nursing system. For that reason, this research identifies the main aspects when designing and implementing closed-loop medication administration through mobile nursing system and therefore makes closed-loop medication administration and patient safety knowledge to be more integrated in the academic field. Moreover, the findings of this research will contribute to the pursuit of high quality and efficient health-care delivery in practice. In addition to this, the results of this research will also provide some ideas when supplying decision support with the information derived using big data technology in the future.

Key Research Outcomes

The expected outcome of this research is to achieve closed-loop medication administration with the utilization of a well-designed mobile nursing system with the final completed system being both effective and diffusible to other health-care institutions. At the end of this research, some recommendations about designing and implementing such a mobile nursing system will be given.

The Significance of Research

This research will provide an efficient way to eliminate medical errors, reduce health-care costs, and bring benefits to both nurses and patients through streamlining the workflow. Moreover, the method of designing and implementing a mobile nursing system to achieve closed-loop medication administration is really far reaching as there are more and more health-care institutions using or planning to use mobile nursing system. As a result, how to design and implement such an efficient mobile nursing system is very significant. This research will just present a meaningful attempt to accomplish this goal.

Apart from mobile technology, big data is also an emerging field and has the possibility to bring obvious benefits to health-care delivery. It is well known that there are huge amounts of data behind all kinds of clinical information systems, and how to make them useful is a critical problem. From this point of view, the result of this research can disclose some information points, which can derive from the existing big data and provide more intelligent decision support to the clinicians.

Conclusions

At this stage, preliminary in-depth analyses which have included a needs analysis and a feasibility analysis clearly indicate the likely and far-reaching benefits of the proposed mobile nursing information system. Next steps include the design and building of the system and then the testing. There are still some limitations to this research: (1) Being a single-case study, the findings may not be appropriate to all health-care institutions, and hence we recommend caution when trying to design and develop a similar mobile nursing information system for a different health-care context. (2) As the presented language of the mobile nursing system is Mandarin (as the case is in China), translation will be needed before promoting the specific solution to health-care contexts in other countries. In spite of these limitations, we are confident that there is a future for mobile nursing information systems and close by calling for more research into the area.

References

Agrawal, A. (2009). Medication errors: Prevention using information technology systems. *British Journal of Clinical Pharmacology, 67*(6), 681–686. doi:10.1111/j.1365–2125.2009.03427.x.

Ammenwerth, E., Rauchegger, F., Ehlers, F., Hirsch, B., & Schaubmayr, C. (2011). Effect of a nursing information system on the quality of information processing in nursing: An evaluation study using the HIS-monitor instrument. *International Journal of Medical Informatics, 80*(1), 25–38. doi:10.1016/j.ijmedinf.2010.10.010.

Bates, D. W., & Gawande, A. A. (2003). Improving safety with information technology. *New England Journal of Medicine, 348*(25), 2526–2534. doi:10.1056/NEJMsa020847.

Berner, E. S. (2007). *Clinical decision support systems theory and practice* (2nd ed.). New York: Springer.

Blackmore, C. C., Mecklenburg, R. S., & Kaplan, G. S. (2011). Effectiveness of clinical decision support in controlling inappropriate imaging. *Journal of the American College of Radiology, 8*(1), 19–25. doi:http://dx.doi.org/10.1016/j.jacr.2010.07.009.

Cook, R. I., Render, M., & Woods, D. D. (2000). Gaps in the continuity of care and progress on patient safety. *British Medical Journal, 320*(7237), 791–794.

DIS, I. (2009). 9241–210: 2010. Ergonomics of human system interaction-Part 210: Human-centred design for interactive systems. International Organization for Standardization (ISO), Switzerland.

Franklin, B. D., O'Grady, K., Donyai, P., Jacklin, A., & Barber, N. (2007). The impact of a closed-loop electronic prescribing and administration system on prescribing errors, administration errors and staff time: A before-and-after study. *Quality and Safety in Health Care, 16*(4), 279–284. doi:10.1136/qshc.2006.019497.

Garg, A. X., Adhikari, N. K., McDonald, H., Rosas-Arellano, M. P., Devereaux, P. J., Beyene, J., et al. (2005). Effects of computerized clinical decision support systems on practitioner performance and patient outcomes: A systematic review. *Journal of the American Medical Association, 293*(10), 1223–1238. doi:10.1001/jama.293.10.1223.

Grober, E. D., & Bohnen, J. M. (2005). Defining medical error. *Canadian Journal of Surgery, 48*(1), 39–44.

Haggerty, J. L., Reid, R. J., Freeman, G. K., Starfield, B. H., Adair, C. E., & McKendry, R. (2003). Continuity of care: A multidisciplinary review. *British Medical Journal, 327*(7425), 1219–1221. doi:10.1136/bmj.327.7425.1219.

Holzinger, A., Kosec, P., Schwantzer, G., Debevc, M., Hofmann-Wellenhof, R., & Fruhauf, J. (2011). Design and development of a mobile computer application to reengineer workflows in the hospital and the methodology to evaluate its effectiveness. *Journal of Biomedical Informatics, 44*(6), 968–977. doi:10.1016/j.jbi.2011.07.003.

Johansson, P. E., Petersson, G. I., & Nilsson, G. C. (2010). Personal digital assistant with a barcode reader—a medical decision support system for nurses in home care. *International Journal of Medical Informatics, 79*(4), 232–242. doi:10.1016/j.ijmedinf.2010.01.004.

Johnson, B., & Christensen, L. (2008). *Educational research: Quantitative, qualitative, and mixed approaches*. Thousand Oaks: Sage.

Kawamoto, K., Houlihan, C. A., Balas, E. A., & Lobach, D. F. (2005). Improving clinical practice using clinical decision support systems: A systematic review of trials to identify features critical to success. *British Medical Journal, 330*(7494), 765. doi:10.1136/bmj.38398.500764.8F.

Kelly, W. N., & Rucker, T. D. (2006). Compelling features of a safe medication-use system. *American Journal of Health System Pharmacy, 63*(15), 1461–1468. doi:10.2146/ajhp050343.

Kohn, L. T., Corrigan, J. M., & Donaldson, M. S. (2000). *To err is human: Building a safer health system* (Vol. 627). Washington, D.C.: National Academies Press.

Konstantinidis, G., Anastassopoulos, G. C., Karakos, A. S., Anagnostou, E., & Danielides, V. (2012). A user-centered, object-oriented methodology for developing health information systems: A Clinical Information System (CIS) example. *Journal of Medical System, 36*(2), 437–450. doi:10.1007/s10916-010-9488-x.

Kumar, S., & Steinebach, M. (2008). Eliminating US hospital medical errors. *International Journal of Health Care Quality Assurance, 21*(5), 444–471.

Lenderink, B., & Egberts, T. G. (2004). Closing the loop of the medication use process using electronic medication administration registration. *Pharmacy World and Science, 26*(4), 185–190. doi:10.1023/B:PHAR.0000035843.42226.e0.

Mason, J. (2002). *Qualitative researching*. Thousand Oaks: Sage.

Members of Emerge, E. M. E. R. G., Agrawal, A., Aronson, J. K., Britten, N., Ferner, R. E., de Smet, P. A., et al. (2009). Medication errors: Problems and recommendations from a consensus meeting. *British Journal of Clinical Pharmacology, 67*(6), 592–598. doi:10.1111/j.1365-2125.2009.03414.x.

Needleman, J., Buerhaus, P., Mattke, S., Stewart, M., & Zelevinsky, K. (2002). Nurse-staffing levels and the quality of care in hospitals. *New England Journal of Medicine, 346*(22), 1715–1722. doi:10.1056/NEJMsa012247.

O'Shea, E. (1999). Factors contributing to medication errors: A literature review. *Journal of Clinical Nursing, 8*(5), 496–504.

Pearce, C., & Haikerwal, M. C. (2010). E-health in Australia: Time to plunge into the 21st century. *Medical Journal of Australia, 193*(7), 397–398.

Poon, E. G., Keohane, C. A., Yoon, C. S., Ditmore, M., Bane, A., Levtzion-Korach, O., et al. (2010). Effect of bar-code technology on the safety of medication administration. *New England Journal of Medicine, 362*(18), 1698–1707. doi:10.1056/NEJMsa0907115.

Porter, M. E., & Teisberg, E. O. (2006). *Redefining health care*. Boston: Harvard Business Press.

Richardson, A., & Storr, J. (2010). Patient safety: A literative review on the impact of nursing empowerment, leadership and collaboration. *International Nursing Review, 57*(1), 12–21.

Sensmeier, J. (2009). Close the loop on med errors. *Nursing Management, 40*(11PS), 2–3.

Shekelle, P. G., Morton, S. C., & Keeler, E. B. (2006). Costs and benefits of health information technology. *Evidence Report Technology Assessment (Full Rep)*, (132), 1–71.

Sparbel, K. J., & Anderson, M. A. (2000). Integrated literature review of continuity of care: Part 1, Conceptual issues. *Journal of Nursing Scholarship, 32*(1), 17–24.

Spears, P. (2005). Managing patient care error: Nurse leaders' perspectives. *Journal of Nursing Administration, 35*(5), 223–224.

Sturman, A. (1999). Case study methods. In J. P. Keeves & G. Lakomski (Eds.), *Issues in educational research* (pp. 103–112). Kidlington: Pergamon.

Thomas, G. (2011). A typology for the case study in social science following a review of definition, discourse, and structure. *Qualitative Inquiry, 17*(6), 511–521. doi:10.1177/1077800411409884.

Turner, A. M., Reeder, B., & Ramey, J. (2013). Scenarios, personas and user stories: User-centered evidence-based design representations of communicable disease investigations. *Journal of Biomedical Informatics, 46*(4), 575–584. doi:10.1016/j.jbi.2013.04.006.

Union, C. (2010). To err is human—to delay is deadly. May 2009. www.safepatientproject.org/safepatientproject.org/pdf/safepatientproject.org-ToDelayIsDeadly.pdf. Accessed 1 Feb.

Van Den Bos, J., Rustagi, K., Gray, T., Halford, M., Ziemkiewicz, E., & Shreve, J. (2011). The $17.1 billion problem: The annual cost of measurable medical errors. *Health Affairs (Millwood), 30*(4), 596–603.

Whiting, S. O., & Gale, A. (2008). Computerized physician order entry usage in North America: The doctor is in. *Healthcare Quaterly, 11*(3), 94–97.

Wickramasinghe, N., & Goldberg, S. (2009). M-Health: A new paradigm for mobilizing healthcare delivery. *Medical informatics: Concepts, methodologies, tools, and applications* (pp. 1773–1787). Hershey: IGI Global.

Wickramasinghe, N., & Schaffer, J. (2010). Realizing value driven e-health solutions. Report for IBM. Washington, D.C.

Yin, R. K. (2003). *Case study research: Design and methods* (Vol. 5). Thousand Oaks: Sage.

Jianqiu Kou is a Ph.D. student of Deakin University Australia and she has 15 years of work experience in the field of construction and management of information systems in health-care institutions. Her main research interests lie in the application of information technology in the area of health care.

Nilmini Wickramasinghe PhD; MBA; GradDipMgtSt; BSc. Amus.A, piano; Amus.A, violin has a well-recognised research record in the field of healthcare and IT/IS. Her expertise is in the strategic application and management of technology for effecting superior healthcare solutions. She is currently the professor director of Health Informatics Management at Epworth HealthCare and a professor at Deakin University.

Chapter 18
An Ontology of Consumer Health Informatics

Arkalgud Ramaprasad and Thant Syn

Introduction

The concept of consumer health informatics (CHI) is about two decades old. Some of the earliest users of the term are Ferguson (1995), Jimison and Sher (1995), and Taylor et al. (1996). CHI has garnered much attention in recent years as its application has come to permeate the health-care industry. Its growth is partly driven by the self-empowerment of consumers of health care due to the advances in information technology, and partly by the health-care systems' need to empower its consumers (Jimison and Sher 1995) in the evolving health-care environment. Advances in information technology such as the widespread availability of the Internet, accessibility of health-care information, and ease of communication between the stakeholders in health care is reshaping the provider–consumer relationship (Bader and Braude 1998; Brennan 1999; Committee on Enhancing the Internet for Health Applications 2000; Hewitt-Taylor and Bond 2012). Consumers in health care are shifting from being passive recipients of care to active participants and proactive partners in care. Simultaneously, the increasing expectations of health-care systems are driving the providers of and other stakeholders (hospitals, insurers, pharmacists, etc.) in health care to encourage and facilitate the participation and partnership of the consumers using CHI (Brennan 1999).

Amidst this increasing interest in CHI, a clear definition of the concept and its domain is absent (Flaherty et al. 2015). Researchers and practitioners have focused selectively on different parts of the whole, neglecting the "big picture"—a theme analogous to the story of the five blind men and the elephant (Börner et al. 2003;

A. Ramaprasad (✉)
University of Illinois at Chicago, 601 S Morgan Street (MC 294), Chicago, IL 60607, USA
e-mail: prasad@uic.edu

T. Syn
Division of International Business and Technology Studies, A. R. Sanchez,
Jr. School of Business, Texas A&M International University,
5201 University Boulevard, Laredo, TX 78041, USA
e-mail: thant.syn@tamiu.edu

N. Wickramasinghe et al. (eds.), *Contemporary Consumer Health Informatics*,
Healthcare Delivery in the Information Age, DOI 10.1007/978-3-319-25973-4_18

Ramaprasad and Papagari 2009). This selectivity has resulted in fragmentation of the research and development agenda; the sum of the parts simply falls short of making the whole. There is a need to articulate and make the combinatorial complexity of CHI visible to facilitate both the effective design and evaluation of CHI systems (Ramaprasad and Syn 2013a). As Flaherty et al. (2015, p. 92) suggest: "Without a clear definition it will be difficult to develop core competencies for the training of consumer health informatics professionals. CHI professionals can help the public (consumer) with accessing health information via Internet-based technologies (e.g., health websites, applications). This is vitally important at the present time, as the Internet has brought about a huge array of health information that is frequently, but not always accurately, accessed by the population." We seek to address these concerns using an ontology to visually represent the complexity of CHI systemically and systematically.

We will start with the analysis of 23 key definitions of CHI presented by Flaherty et al. (2015) and then logically deconstruct the concept using an ontology. We will then describe how the ontology can be used to define the domain of CHI, and how the ontology can be extended, reduced, refined, and coarsened to adapt to the evolving technology and environment for health care. Last, we will delineate how the ontology can be used to develop a systematic roadmap for research and practice in CHI.

Definitions of CHI

"Consumer health informatics (CHI) is an emerging field that utilizes technology to provide health information to enhance health-care decision making by the public" (Flaherty et al. 2015, p. 91). It is "an important subfield of health informatics, addresses the needs of health consumers and medical and public health practitioners in order to bolster healthcare" (Flaherty et al. 2015, p. 91). It "is the field devoted to informatics from multiple consumer or patient views. These include patient-focused informatics, health literacy and consumer education. The focus is on information structures and processes that empower consumers to manage their own health—for example, health information literacy, consumer-friendly language, personal health records, and Internet-based strategies and resources. The shift in this view of informatics analyzes consumers' needs for information, studies and implements methods for making information accessible to consumers, and models and integrates consumers' preferences into health information systems. Consumer informatics stands at the crossroads of other disciplines, such as nursing informatics, public health, health promotion, health education, library science, and communication science" (American Medical Informatics Association 2015).

Flaherty et al. (2015) present a systematic review of 23 definitions of CHI derived from an exhaustive search of the literature in the domain. Based on latent semantic analysis (LSA) of these definitions, they suggest "that the subject matter among the 23 definitions is quite similar" (p. 107). Three definitions with the highest LSA scores are quoted below. They presumably encapsulate the core sense of all the 23 definitions:

> Consumer health informatics is defined as "any electronic tool, technology or electronic application that is: (1) primarily designed to interact with health information users or consumers (anyone who seeks or uses healthcare information for nonprofessional work), (2) interacts directly with the consumer who provides personal health information to the CHI system and receives personalized health information from the tool application or system, and (3) is one in which the data, information, recommendations, or other benefits provided to the consumer, may be used in coordination with a healthcare professional but is not dependent on a healthcare professional" (Gibbons et al. 2011, p. 72). We note that Flaherty et al. (2015) paraphrase this definition.

> CHI generally encompasses two areas: the use of Internet technology to connect to online services for health care information, such as that contained in medical journals and professional publications; and systems and software provided by clinicians to patients to help in the diagnosis and treatment of specific conditions and diseases. (Anonymous 1998, p. 51)

> Consumer health informatics is the branch of medical informatics that analyses consumers' needs for information; studies and implements methods of making information accessible to consumers; and models and integrates consumers' preferences into medical information systems. Consumer informatics stands at the cross-roads of other disciplines, such as nursing informatics, public health, health promotion, health education, library science and communication science, and is perhaps the most challenging and rapidly expanding field in medical informatics. (Eysenbach 2000, p. 1713)

Flaherty et al. (2015) also summarize the most frequently used words in the CHI definitions. Their table is shown in Fig. 18.1. In a sense, these words represent the domain of CHI as expressed in the 23 definitions (Table 18.1).

In the following section, we logically deconstruct the CHI construct using an ontology. In doing so, we draw upon the extent definitions reviewed and analyzed by Flaherty et al. (2015), and at the same time extend and refine the connotation of CHI. The ontology, we will argue, is a systematic and systemic representation of the CHI domain.

An Ontology of CHI

An ontology represents the conceptualization of a domain (Gruber 2008); it organizes the terminologies and taxonomies of the domain. It is an "explicit specification of a conceptualization," (Gruber 1995, p. 908) and can be used to systematize the description of a complex system (Cimino 2006). "Our acceptance of an ontology is … similar in principle to our acceptance of a scientific theory, say a system of physics; we adopt, at least insofar as we are reasonable, the simplest conceptual scheme into which the disordered fragments of raw experience can be fitted and arranged." (Quine 1961, p. 16). Using an ontology, we hope to make the metaphorical "elephant" visible.

An ontology of CHI is shown in Fig. 18.1. Three illustrative components of CHI derived from the ontology are listed below the ontology, each with an example. A

Informatics								Health			
Structure		**Function**		**Semiotics**		**Consumer**		**Outcome**		**Focus**	
Devices	[to]	Acquire	[health]	Data	[by/to]	Patients	[to manage the]	Cost	[of]	Wellness	[care]
Software		Store		Record		Caretakers		Quality		Preventive	
Networks		Retrieve		Knowledge		Families		Safety		Maintenance	
People		Process				Citizens		Parity		Illness	
Policies		Interpret				Communities		Timeliness		Chronic	
Procedures		Translate								Episodic	
		Distribute									
		Protect									

Total number of components = 6*8*3*5*5*4 = 14,400

Illustrative components:

Devices to acquire health data by patients to manage the cost of wellness $_{\text{preventive}}$ care.

Example: Devices for patients to monitor blood pressure periodically without visiting the doctor.

Software to retrieve health record by caretakers to manage the safety of illness $_{\text{chronic}}$ care.

Example: Software which allows caretakers to check drug dosage and schedule for chronically ill patients.

Procedures to distribute health knowledge to citizens to manage timeliness of illness $_{\text{episodic}}$ care.

Example: Procedures to distribute knowledge about measles infection in California, USA.

Fig. 18.1 Ontology of consumer health informatics (CHI)

glossary of all the terms is given in Appendix 1. We will discuss the construction of the ontology, its dimensions, taxonomies, elements, and the components encapsulated within.

Table 18.1 Most frequently used words in CHI definitions. (Flaherty et al. 2015, p. 106)

Health	48	Designed	4
Informatics	28	Defined	4
Information	26	Communication	4
Consumer	25	Tools	3
Consumers	12	Telecommunication	3
Medical	10	Technologies	3
Care	10	Studies	3
Systems	7	Science	3
Computer	7	Models	3
Technology	5	Management	3
Patients	5	Making	3
Health care	5	Electronic	3
Support	4	Development	3
Public	4	Delivery	3
Patient	4	Decisions	3
Needs	4	Better	3
Internet	4		

Construction of the Ontology

Our method of constructing the CHI ontology is explained by Ramaprasad and Syn (2013a, 2013b). It was iterative amongst the authors of the paper (two information systems professors) and by the authors with the extent literature. The challenge was to construct an ontology which is logical, parsimonious, and complete. It had to be logical in the deconstruction of the domain, parsimonious yet complete in the representation of the domain. It had to be a closed description of the CHI domain.

The challenge was also to adapt the information system terminology to CHI. This was done by iterating with the literature and creating a glossary of terms (Appendix 1). In this context, we should note that the ontology presented is one of many possible ontologies of the CHI domain. A complex domain like CHI can be studied from many points of view, each with its own ontology. It is a "wicked" (Churchman 1967) problem with many potential formulations. Each ontology can be seen as a lens through which one may study the domain—ours is one of many possible lenses.

Dimensions of the Ontology

The ontology deconstructs the domain of CHI into three dimensions: Consumer, Health, and Informatics (Note: Words which refer to the dimensions and sub-dimensions of the ontology are capitalized. We will also capitalize references to elements of a dimension—its categories and subcategories.) The dimensions are represented by columns or a combination of columns in Fig. 18.1. Health is represented by two columns—Outcome and Focus; Consumer by a single column; and Informatics by three columns—Structure, Function, and Semiotics. Thus:

$$\text{Consumer Health Informatics} = \text{Consumer} + \text{Health} + \text{Informatics}$$

It can be further parsed as:

$$\text{Consumer Health Informatics} = \text{Consumer} + \left(\text{Health}_{\text{Outcome}} + \text{Health}_{\text{Focus}}\right) + \left(\text{Informatics}_{\text{Structure}} + \text{Informatics}_{\text{Function}} + \text{Informatics}_{\text{Semiotics}}\right)$$

Note: Subcategories are shown as subscripts.

The definitions of CHI discussed earlier include these dimensions latently; we have explicated them in the ontology. On the other hand, not all the definitions include all the dimensions and sub-dimensions of the ontology. Very few of them, for example, specifically allude to $\text{Health}_{\text{Outcome}}$. It is a significant omission; ultimately the efficacy (Gibbons et al. 2011) of CHI will be based on the $\text{Health}_{\text{Outcomes}}$ engendered by its use, not just its use. In the same vein, the definitions bundle the Structure, Function, and Semiotics sub-dimensions of Informatics and label it as information system or information technology. Their disaggregation can provide a more refined understanding of the dynamics of CHI and its efficacy.

Each dimension is articulated by a one- or two-level taxonomy of elements. These taxonomies can be extended by adding more elements, reduced by deleting elements, refined by adding more levels, and coarsened by aggregating existing levels. The elements and the number of levels in the taxonomy define the scale and granularity of the dimension. In the following sections, we will discuss each dimension in slightly greater detail.

Health

The objective of CHI is to improve the consumers' health. The Health dimension is represented by the two right columns in the ontology—its Focus and its Outcome. Today, the focus of Health is both Wellness and Illness care. Wellness care, in turn, consists of Preventive care and Maintenance care; Illness care consists of Chronic care and Episodic care.

The Outcomes are the desired results of health care sought through the meaningful use of CHI for the management of health-care information. Extending the concept of meaningful use of health-care information systems (Centers for Medicare & Medicaid Services; Ramaprasad et al. 2014), the ontology enumerates the management of Cost, Quality, Safety, Parity, and Timeliness of health care as the desired outcomes.

Thus, the Health dimension of the ontology encapsulates 20 (5 × 4) objectives. They are to manage the Cost/Quality/Safety/Parity/Timeliness of $\text{Wellness}_{\text{Preventive}}$/$\text{Wellness}_{\text{Maintenance}}$/$\text{Illness}_{\text{Chronic}}$/$\text{Illness}_{\text{Episodic}}$ care. These 20 represent the domain of CHI's objectives. A particular CHI may address only a subset of these—for example, to manage: (1) the cost of $\text{wellness}_{\text{preventive}}$ care, and (2) the timeliness of $\text{illness}_{\text{episodic}}$ care. The choice of objectives will drive the design of the CHI. The ontology provides a systematic basis to consider the full range of objectives.

The CHI requirements for each Focus, Outcome, and combinations of Focuses, Outcomes, and Focus × Outcome are different in many ways and similar in others. For example, while in many cases wellness- and illness-care may be distinct, they can also be very strongly coupled in other cases. It is necessary to systematically differentiate these requirements and systemically integrate them to develop an efficacious CHI. The panoramic view provided by the ontology will help do so, and help minimize design bias due to a selective focus.

Consumer

The Consumer dimension is represented by the third column from the right by a single-level taxonomy. It includes Patients, Caretakers, Families, Citizens, and Communities. The first three generally fall under the ambit of personal health care, the last two of public health care. CHIs can be used for both types of care. Extending the two examples above, the design of a CHI may be for (1) communities to manage the cost of wellness$_{preventive}$ care—as with vaccinations, and (2) caretakers to manage the timeliness of illness$_{episodic}$ care—as with illnesses of the elderly.

The Consumers of CHI may be independent entities as listed in the taxonomy, or interacting entities which can be derived by crossing the taxonomy with itself. Thus, a CHI may be used by a Patient, a Caretaker, and a Family independently but also in collaboration with each other (and with the provider of health care). In the latter case, the CHI may have to serve as a collaboration (Brennan 1999) tool too. A well-formed taxonomy of Consumers, as initially presented in the ontology, can help specify each entity's requirements individually and their requirement for collaboration collectively.

Informatics

The ontology deconstructs Informatics into three sub-dimensions: Structure, Function, and Semiotics. The Structure defines the physical and organizational objects (nouns) constituting the information system; the Function defines the actions (verbs) of the system; and the Semiotics the information objects managed by the system. The structural/functional deconstruction is widely used in analysis of physical, biological, and logical systems. The explicit identification of the Semiotics dimension recognizes the centrality of management of the morphology, syntax, semantics, and pragmatics of information (Ramaprasad and Rai 1996) in CHI.

CHI—Structure

The taxonomy of elements is based on the common body of knowledge in information systems (e.g., Rainer and Cegielski 2012). The structure of an information system is commonly described in terms of Hardware, Software, Networks, data, Processes, People, and Policies. To limit the redundancy of elements, we have excluded data from the taxonomy because of its articulation in a separate Semiotics dimension. In keeping with the current developments, we have changed Hardware to Devices.

The technological elements of Structure (Devices, Software, and Networks) have to work symbiotically with the non-technological elements (Processes, People, and Policies) for the CHI to be effective. However, very often, the technological elements become the dominant focus of design to the exclusion of the non-technological elements. The potential of a smartphone (Device) in CHI may, for example, be severely limited by a provider's access policies and processes. The design has to address the sociotechnical challenges (Ancker et al. 2014). The design of CHI using a smartphone, for example, has to encompass the design of associated Policies and Processes to be effective. The Functions (discussed next) of the Structure elements have to be systematically differentiated and systemically integrated.

CHI—Function

We started with the commonly used taxonomy of information system Functions: acquire, store, retrieve, process, and distribute. These functions are relevant to CHI but need to be extended to fit the focus of CHI in research and practice. Hence, we modified the taxonomy of Functions to include: Acquire, Store, Retrieve, Process, Interpret, Translate, Distribute, and Protect. The modified taxonomy overlaps with but also extends the common taxonomy.

The elements of Function are in an approximate ordinal order. Each element follows the preceding one generally, except Protect, which may occur in each Function. The full set of Functions is essential for an effective CHI, although the emphasis on each may vary. A CHI designed for dissemination of public-health information about vaccinations may emphasize Translate and Distribute more than the other Functions with little emphasis on Protection. On the other hand, a CHI designed for patients' access to doctors' notes (Vodicka et al. 2013) may incorporate the full spectrum of Functions, with particular emphasis on privacy Protection.

The Structure × Function interaction is a critical part of CHI design. For example, while Devices' capability to Acquire information is increasing rapidly due to technological advances, their capability to Interpret and Translate information is still limited. People (e.g., nurses or help desks), perhaps in combination with Devices, may be critical to effective Interpretation and Translation in a CHI. The Functions and the Structure × Function interaction have to be systematically differentiated and systemically integrated in a CHI.

CHI—Semiotics

Here we use the variant of the traditional taxonomy of data, information, and knowledge. We substitute information with Record and keep Data and Knowledge. These correspond to the morphological, syntactic, and semantic levels (Ramaprasad and Rai 1996) of semiotics. It must be noted that there is no element corresponding to the pragmatic level.

The three elements of Semiotics are ordinal—Record is derived from Data, and Knowledge is derived from Record. The CHI Structure and Function has to be designed for the Semiotics to be effective.

Further extending the two examples above, the design of a CHI may be for (1) policies to acquire data by communities to manage the cost of wellness$_{\text{preventive}}$ care, and (2) devices to distribute information by caretakers to manage the timeliness of illness$_{\text{episodic}}$ care. There are 14,398 other similar components encapsulated in the ontology.

Components of CHI

The dimensions (and sub-dimensions) of the ontology are arranged left to right with adjacent words/phrases with a purpose. The concatenation of an element from each dimension with the adjacent words/phrases creates a natural English sentence illustrating a potential component of CHI. The concatenation has been demonstrated with the two examples carried through the discussion of the dimensions of the ontology as well as the three illustrative components with examples listed below the ontology.

At the most detailed level, the ontology encapsulates 14,400 potential components of CHI. The components and fragments (of these components) define the domain of CHI. It would be laborious and voluminous to enumerate all the components. The ontology provides a convenient and concise "big picture" of CHI. It helps visualize its combinatorial complexity and make the "elephant" visible.

It may be possible to instantiate a component in many different ways. Consider the second example above: devices to distribute information by caretakers to manage the timeliness of illness$_{\text{episodic}}$ care. Instantiations may vary in terms of the devices used (computer, smartphone, or telephone), information distributed (change in blood sugar, blood pressure, or diet), caretakers (spouse, child, or nurse), timeliness (immediate or delayed), and illness episode (pneumonia or fever) addressed. The same logic can be extended to the other example.

A particular CHI system may instantiate only a small number of components encapsulated in the ontology. Further, some components may be instantiated frequently and some infrequently. We will call those frequently instantiated as "bright" spots, those infrequently instantiated as "light" spots, and those uninstantiated as "blind/blank" spots. A component may be "bright" because of its relative value to the field and/or ease of study/implementation; it may be "light" due to its lack of value and/or difficulty for study/implementation; it may be "blind" if it has been overlooked; or it may be "blank" due to infeasibility of study. By mapping the state-of-the-research and the state-of-the-practice onto the ontology, one can discover the "bright," "light," and "blind/blank" spots in each, thereby demonstrating deficiencies existing both between and among research and practice. Further, since the possible explanations for the luminosity of a component is equivocal, one must dig deeper to find the underlying cause. An important "bright" spot would be functional but an easy one would be dysfunctional. Similarly, an unimportant "light" spot may be acceptable but a difficult, highly valued "light" spot may be unacceptable. Last, a "blind" spot has to be investigated deeper lest it be important, and a "blank" spot clearly demarcated so as not to waste one's effort. In the next section, we will discuss how the ontology can be used as a lens to study the topography of CHI research and practice (Ramaprasad and Syn 2014).

Discussion—Ontology of CHI as a Lens

The ontology of CHI presented in this chapter makes visible the combinatorial complexity of an emerging topic in health care. Our attempt seeks to include, refine, and extend the previous definitions and conceptualizations (Flaherty et al. 2015).

The ontology is logically constructed but grounded in the theory and practice of the domain. The dimensions are logically specified and not empirically generated.

They are deduced from the definition of the domain. In contrast to our method, an ontology may be induced from the corpus of a domain. There are a number of automated ontology extraction tools based on linguistic extraction techniques such as part-of-speech (POS) tagging and natural language processing (NLP) (Alani et al. 2003). Based on the nouns and verbs in the corpus, the techniques can help develop comprehensive and detailed (with reference to the corpus) OWL-based ontologies (W3C 2013), thesauruses of hierarchically arranged terms, and other ISO-based ontology exchange standards (Ahmad and Gillam 2005). The automated tools are designed for standardizing terminologies (Burton-Jones et al. 2005; Evermann and Fang 2010; Staab et al. 2004), as for example, in medicine, but not to deduce semantically meaningful logical components of a domain as we seek to do. The automated tools cannot yet formulate an ontology which is (a) parsimonious as the one we propose, and (b) organized such that the domain components can be concatenated to form natural language sentences.

The logical construction of the ontology minimizes the errors of omission and commission. For example, inclusion of the Outcome dimension compels the research designer to explicitly pose the question of how a CHI might affect Cost, Quality, Safety, Parity, or Timeliness of care. Without consideration for outcomes (error of omission), CHI systems are unlikely to advance the field. Indeed, the ontology can help specify the precise outcomes it can achieve, instead of broadly specifying that it can improve health care (error of commission).

Finally, the ontology is a multidisciplinary lens. The Structure and Function dimensions are drawn from the information systems literature and refined for health care; the Semiotics dimension draws from the knowledge management literature and adapted to health care; the Focus dimension is from the health-care policy literature; and the Outcome dimension from the health-care information technology literature. The ontology compels the user to analyze the CHI problem and synthesize solutions by drawing upon these disciplines.

Conclusion

The proposed ontology of CHI can advance the state-of-the-research and the state-of-the-practice in the domain. It can be used to systematically identify the "bright," "light," and "blind/blank" spots in the two states and between the two states. Such mapping will reveal opportunities for research and development. In the past 20+ years, the connotation of CHI has shifted from the use of personal computers and CD-ROMs (Jimison and Sher 1995) to the use of social media (Ho 2011; Prybutok et al. 2014) such as Facebook (Zhang et al. 2013) and Twitter (Lee et al. 2014) on smartphones. While the instantiations of the elements, subcomponents, and components of a CHI have changed significantly during the period, the ontology itself had been virtually unchanged. The changes are likely to continue, perhaps at an accelerated pace, in the future. In this context, the ontology can serve as a foundational framework to map the changes in and the trajectory of CHI. It can be used to develop a road map for CHI.

Appendix 1

Glossary
Informatics: The science of managing information
Structure: The objects (nouns) for managing information
Devices: The hardware for managing information—computers, smartphones, etc.
Software: The programs/apps for managing information—to record data, to search, etc.
Networks: The connections to transfer information—Bluetooth, Wi-Fi, Internet, etc.
People: The people involved in managing the information—providers, help aides, etc.
Policies: The policies of the stakeholders guiding the management of information—HIPAA, security, etc.
Procedures: The protocols and processes for managing the information—sign-in, access, log-off, etc.
Function: The processes (verbs) for managing information
Acquire: To measure, elicit, obtain information—blood sugar level, advice, suggestion, etc.
Store: To record information—record prescription, advice, etc.
Retrieve: To recover information—recover prescription, advice, etc.
Process: To manipulate the information—computing the BMI, cancer risk, etc.
Interpret: To articulate the meaning of the information—the meaning of a person's BMI, cancer risk, etc.
Translate: To translate the meaning of information into action—recommendations for managing BMI, cancer risk, etc.
Distribute: To distribute the information to the consumers—distributing measles vaccination information, medication schedule, etc.
Protect: To manage the confidentiality, integrity, and availability of information—per HIPAA guidelines, state privacy guidelines, etc.
Semiotics: The levels of information management
Data: Management of information at the morphological level—raw numerical measurements, text, etc.
Record: Management of information at the syntactic level—data organized into a health record, report, etc.
Knowledge: Management of information at the semantic level—meaning of health record, research report, etc.
Consumer: The consumers of health information
Patients: The recipients of health care—adults, children, mothers, etc.
Caretakers: Those taking care of patients—nurses, family members, social workers, etc.
Families: Families, as a group, receiving health care or assisting in providing care—families of children with disability, etc.
Citizens: Citizens at large—entitled to or requiring health care
Communities: Communities of patients—with similar conditions, needs, ethnicity, etc.
Health: The care for the health of the consumers—individual patients, families, public at large, etc.
Outcome: The focal attributes of health care—low cost, high quality, optimal timeliness, etc.
Cost: The cost of health care—primarily financial, but also physical, psychological, etc.
Quality: The quality of health care—adherence to guidelines, mortality rates, etc.
Safety: The safety of health care—the safety of drugs, treatment, care, etc.

Glossary
Parity: The parity of health care—geographical (urban, rural), socioeconomic, gender, etc.
Timeliness: the timeliness of health care—the time to access/deliver care based on the condition, etc.
Focus: Assurance of wellness and the elimination/management of illness of the consumer
Wellness: Care to assure an acceptable, normal state of being of the consumer
Preventive: Care to assure wellness through prevention of illness—vaccination, cleanliness, sanitation, etc.
Maintenance: Care to maintain wellness through healthy habits—exercise, sleep, etc.
Illness: Care to restore normalcy—through drugs, surgery, therapy, etc.
Chronic: Care of persistent illness—diabetes, blood pressure, etc.
Episodic: Care of transient illness—fever, chicken pox, etc.

HIPAA Health Insurance Portability and Accountability Act, *BMI* body mass index

References

Ahmad, K., & Gillam, L. (2005). Automatic ontology extraction from unstructured texts. In R. Meersman & Z. Tari (Eds.), *On the move to meaningful internet systems 2005: Coopis, Doa, and Odbase* (pp. 1330–1346). Berlin: Springer.

Alani, H., Kim, S., Millard, D. E., Weal, M. J., Hall, W., Lewis, P. H., & Shadbolt, N. R. (2003). Automatic ontology-based knowledge extraction from web documents. *Intelligent Systems, IEEE, 18*(1), 14–21.

American Medical Informatics Association. (2015). Consumer health informatics. www.amia.org/applications-informatics/consumer-health-informatics. Accessed 4 April 2015.

Ancker, J. S., Miller, M. C., Patel, V., & Kaushal, R. (2014). Sociotechnical challenges to developing technologies for patient access to health information exchange data. *Journal of the American Medical Informatics Association, 21*(4), 664–670.

Anonymous. (1998). Online services facilitate self-care practice, p. 51.

Bader, S. A., & Braude, R. M. (1998). "Patient informatics": Creating new partnerships in medical decision making. *Academic Medicine, 73*(4), 408–411.

Börner, K., Chen, C., & Boyack, K. W. (2003). Visualizing knowledge domains. *Annual Review of Information Science and Technology, 37*(1), 179–255.

Brennan, P. (1999). Health informatics and community health: Support for patients as collaborators in care. *Methods of Information in Medicine, 38*(4/5), 274–278.

Burton-Jones, A., Storey, V. C., Sugumaran, V., & Ahluwalia, P. (2005). A semiotic metrics suite for assessing the quality of ontologies. *Data & Knowledge Engineering, 55*(1), 84–102.

Centers for Medicare & Medicaid Services. Meaningful use. https://www.cms.gov/Regulations-and-Guidance/Legislation/EHRIncentivePrograms/Meaningful_Use.html. Accessed 23 Nov 2012.

Churchman, C. W. (1967). Wicked problems. *Management Science, 14*(4), B141.

Cimino, J. J. (2006). In defense of the desiderata. *Journal of Biomedical Informatics, 39*(3), 299–306.

Committee on Enhancing the Internet for Health Applications. (2000). *Networking health: Prescriptions for the internet* (p. 388). Washington, D.C.: National Academy Press.

Evermann, J., & Fang, J. (2010). Evaluating ontologies: Towards a cognitive measure of quality. *Information Systems, 35*(4), 391–403.

Eysenbach, G. (2000). Recent advances: Consumer health informatics. *BMJ: British Medical Journal, 320*(7251), 1713.

Ferguson, T. (1995). Consumer health informatics. *The Healthcare Forum Journal, 38*(1), 28–31.

Flaherty, D., Hoffman-Goetz, L., & Arocha, J. F. (2015). What is consumer health informatics? A systematic review of published definitions. *Informatics for Health and Social Care, 40*(2), 91–112.

Gibbons, M. C., Wilson, R. F., Samal, L., Lehmann, C. U., Dickersin, K., Lehmann, H. P., Aboumatar, H., Finkelstein, J., Shelton, E., & Sharma, R. (2011). Consumer health informatics: Results of a systematic evidence review and evidence based recommendations. *Translational Behavioral Medicine, 1*(1), 72–82.

Gruber, T. R. (1995). Toward principles for the design of ontologies used for knowledge sharing. *International Journal Human-Computer Studies, 43*(5–6), 907–928.

Gruber, T. R. (2008). Ontology. In L. Liu & M. T. Ozsu (Eds.) *Encyclopedia of database systems*. New York: Springer-Verlag.

Hewitt-Taylor, J., & Bond, C. S. (2012). What e-patients want from the doctor-patient relationship: Content analysis of posts on discussion boards. *Journal of Medical Internet Research, 14*(6), e155.

Ho, J. (2011). Functional themes across blogs, wikis and social networking sites relating to pregnancy. *Electronic Journal of Health Informatics, 6*(2), e17.

Jimison, H. B., & Sher, P. P. (1995). Consumer health informatics: Health information technology for consumers. *Journal of the American Society for Information Science, 46*(10), 783–790.

Lee, J. L., DeCamp, M., Dredze, M., Chisolm, M. S., & Berger, Z. D. (2014). What are health-related users tweeting? A qualitative content analysis of health-related users and their messages on twitter. *Journal of Medical Internet Research, 16*(10), e237.

Prybutok, G. L., Koh, C., & Prybutok, V. R. (2014). A content relevance model for social media health information. *CIN—Computers Informatics Nursing, 32*(4), 189–200.

Quine, W. V. O. (1961). *From a logical point of view* (2nd revised ed.). Boston: Harvard University Press.

Rainer, R.K., and Cegielski, C. G. (2012). Introduction to information systems: Supporting and transforming business. (4th ed.). Hoboken, NJ: Wiley.

Ramaprasad, A., & Papagari, S. S. (2009). Ontological design. Proceedings of DESRIST 2009. Malvern, PA.

Ramaprasad, A., & Rai, A. (1996). Envisioning management of information. *Omega-International Journal of Management Science, 24*(2), 179–193.

Ramaprasad, A., & Syn, T. (2013a). Design thinking and evaluation using an ontology. Proceedings of the European Design Science Symposium (EDSS) 2013. Dublin, Ireland.

Ramaprasad, A., & Syn, T. (2013b). Ontological meta-analysis and synthesis. Proceedings of the Nineteenth Americas Conference on Information Systems. Chicago, IL, USA.

Ramaprasad, A., & Syn, T. (2014). Ontological topography: Mapping the bright, light, blind/blank spots in healthcare knowledge. Proceedings of big data analysis in healthcare 2014. Singapore.

Ramaprasad, A., Syn, T., & Thirumalai, M. (2014). An ontological map for meaningful use of healthcare information systems (Muhis). In M. Bienkiewicz, C. Verdier, G. Plantier, T. Schultz, A. Fred, & H. Gamboa (Eds.), Proceedings of HEALTHINF 2014—International Conference on Health Informatics. Angers, France: SCITEPRESS.

Staab, S., Gómez-Pérez, A., Daelemana, W., Reinberger, M. L., & Noy, N. F. (2004). Why evaluate ontology technologies? Because it works! *Intelligent Systems, IEEE, 19*(4), 74–81.

Taylor, P. T., Motley, C. M., Heyl, N. F., Ricks, R. L., Fruitman, M. P., Loschiavo, J. F., Higginbotham, C. L., Brown, T. D., Vigil, Y. J., & Sikich, J. P. (1996). *Consumer health informatics: Emerging issues*. Washington, D.C.: Accounting and Information Management Division, United States General Accounting Office.

Vodicka, E., Mejilla, R., Leveille, S. G., Ralston, J. D., Darer, J. D., Delbanco, T., Walker, J., & Elmore, J. G. (2013). Online access to doctors' notes: Patient concerns about privacy. *Journal of Medical Internet Research, 15*(9), e208.

W3C. (2013). OWL 2 Web Ontology Language Document Overview. Second Edition. http://www.w3.org/TR/2012/REC-owl2-overview-20121211/. Accessed 2 May 2013.

Zhang, Y., He, D., & Sang, Y. (2013). Facebook as a platform for health information and communication: A case study of a diabetes group. *Journal of Medical Systems, 37*(3), 9942.

Dr. Arkalgud Ramaprasad is professor emeritus of Information and Decision Sciences at the University of Illinois at Chicago (UIC). His current research focus is on the application of ontological analysis and design for envisioning and realizing large, complex systems—especially higher education systems and health-care information systems. He has a Ph.D. from the University of Pittsburgh, Pittsburgh, PA, 1980; M.B.A. from the Indian Institute of Management, Ahmedabad, India, 1972; and B.E. (Electrical), from the University of Mysore, Karnataka, India, 1970.

Thant Syn is an assistant professor of Management Information Systems at the Texas A&M International University. He received his Ph.D. from the Florida International University, M.B.A. from the International University of Japan, and B.E. (Aeronautics) from the Yangon Technological University. His current research focuses on ontology development and application.

Chapter 19
The Acceptance of Nursing Information Systems: An Analysis Using UTAUT

Lemai Nguyen, Peter Haddad, Hoda Moghimi, Imran Muhammad, Kimberley Coleman, Bernice Redley, Mari Botti and Nilmini Wickramasinghe

Introduction

Nurses are the largest group of health-care professionals in hospitals providing 24-h care to patients. Hence, nurses are pivotal in coordinating and communicating patient care information in the complex network of health-care professionals, services, and other care processes. Yet, despite nurses' central role in health-care delivery, information communication technologies (ICTs) have historically rarely been designed around nurses' operational needs. This could explain the poor integration of technologies into nursing work processes and consequent rejection by many nursing professionals (Rogers et al. 2013; Stevenson et al. 2010). The complex nature of acute care

L. Nguyen (✉)
Department of Information Systems and Business Analytics, Deakin University, Deakin Business School, 70 Elgar Rd, Burwood, VIC 3125, Australia
e-mail: lemai.nguyen@deakin.edu.au

P. Haddad · H. Moghimi · I. Muhammad
Epworth HealthCare, 185-187 Hoddle st., Richmond, VIC 3121, Australia
e-mail: peter.e.haddad@gmail.com

H. Moghimi
e-mail: moghimi87@gmail.com

I. Muhammad
e-mail: drimran.work@gmail.com

K. Coleman
Deakin-Epworth Centre for Clinical Nursing Research, 185-187 Hoddle st., Richmond, VIC 3121, Australia
e-mail: kimberley.coleman@epworth.org.au

B. Redley
Deakin University and Monash Health Partnership, Centre for Nursing Research, 221 Burwood Highway, Burwood, VIC 3125, Australia
e-mail: Bernice.redley@deakin.edu.au

N. Wickramasinghe et al. (eds.), *Contemporary Consumer Health Informatics*, Healthcare Delivery in the Information Age, DOI 10.1007/978-3-319-25973-4_19

delivery in hospitals and the frequently interrupted patterns of nursing work suggest that nurses require flexible intelligent systems that can support and adapt to their variable workflow patterns. This study was designed to explore nurses' initial reactions to a new integrated point-of-care solution for acute health-care contexts. The following reports on the first stage of a longitudinal project to use an innovative approach involving nurses in the development and refinement of this solution: from conceptualization to implementation. In this project, unified theory of acceptance and use of technology (UTAUT) was used to evaluate acceptance (Venkatesh et al. 2003).

Background

Given the advances of ICT solutions, it is reasonable to assume that it should be possible to design and develop suitable solutions to support nursing workflows in acute care contexts. It is essential that the design of such systems demonstrate high fidelity to nursing work and usability within real clinical work settings to increase the likelihood that they will be adopted by the expected end users, that is, nurses.

Information Technology Solutions and Nursing Practice

The complexities associated with the coordination, communication, and delivery of health care at the point of care present particular challenges for the design of information technology (IT) systems. In an Australia-wide qualitative study that examined nurses' experiences of already established computerized patient information systems (CPIS), Darbyshire (2004) found that nurses often considered that these established systems made no "clinical sense" and were perceived to waste time. Overriding of the system, duplication of documentation, and a reversion to familiar systems such as paper recording have all been reported as work-around strategies used to continue delivery of safe and reliable clinical communication and care in the face of technological solutions that do not meet clinicians' needs (Alaszewski 2005; Dowding et al. 2009; Lau et al. 2010; Viitanen et al. 2011).

Creating an ongoing collaborative process whereby nursing and IT industries both actively contribute to the development and sequential implementation of an intelligent tool for nursing work within health-care settings is proposed as a feasible, viable, and crucial solution.

M. Botti
Deakin-Epworth Centre for Clinical Nursing Research, 221 Burwood Highway, Burwood, VIC 3125, Australia
e-mail: marib@deakin.edu.au

N. Wickramasinghe
Deakin University and Epworth HealthCare, 60 Baker Ave, Kew East 3102, Australia
e-mail: nilmini.work@gmail.com

Building Intelligent Systems Suited to Support Nursing Care

An intelligent system specifically designed for the discipline of nursing that can adequately and appropriately meet the requirements of nursing in terms of design and flexibility is challenging. Jennings et al. (2009) recommends that intelligent systems need to be designed to meet full epidemiological clinical and research needs of the clinical nurse. This idea is supported by suggestions that intelligent systems for nursing should encompass a set of standard elements directly related to the routine of everyday nursing practice (Yu et al. 2009; Yun-Ke et al. 2009). There is evidence that intelligent systems often address some of the needs of nursing care delivery, but fall short of supporting the full scope of nurses' work in complex clinical settings: that is, the system doesn't "think" like a nurse "thinks" (Yun-Ke et al. 2009).

Over more than 98 hours of nurses' workflow patterns, Cornell et al. (2010a) observed that nurses often made important decisions about care delivery quickly and decisively; their workflow was often sporadic and chaotic in nature, incorporating a complex mix of patient and environmental data and clinical experience. They also discovered that the workflow patterns of nurses changed little after the introduction of technology. Indeed, the technology added an extra task (Cornell et al. 2010b).

Disparities between the clinical work of nursing and the effectiveness of intelligent systems in supporting that work are commonly reported. Issues such as responsiveness, reliability, and ease of use are often cited problems (Alaszewski 2005; Garg et al. 2005; Kawamoto et al. 2005; Yun-Ke et al. 2009). In addition, difficulties with security, maintenance, and confidentiality of patient records (Garg et al. 2005; Holden 2010; Viitanen et al. 2011; Weber et al. 2009) are often seen as barriers to the assimilation of a nursing information system into acute clinical contexts.

In pursuing the goal of a fully integrated e-health system in health care, it is useful for IT solutions to focus on nursing care as a central part of the communication and care processes that occur in acute care settings. The IT solution then needs to be sufficiently robust and flexible to be easily integrated into the multidisciplinary nature of care so that it is accepted as the "preferred" method of planning and documenting care across the health-care team (Oroviogoicoechea 2008). In the past, many IT applications have focused on aspects of nursing care delivery such as health records, medication administration, and decision-making, but few have managed to successfully integrate all of these processes into one all-encompassing system (Kowitlawakul 2011; Weber 2007). With a focus on patient-centered care, the notion of care being integrated across multidisciplinary teams has emerged as an important consideration that impacts patient safety and quality of care. Nurses are consistently the core of multidisciplinary health-care teams.

Understanding and applying a theory that is closely aligned to nursing practice and reflects the relativity of clinical application is essential to the success or failure of IT solutions (Turley 1996). Determinants such as interactional workability, relational integration, and skill set workability are clear factors in the success or failure of an intelligent nursing care system. This approach is based on the premise that if acceptance by nurses is obtained in the first instance, a "relative flow on" effect could lead to a wider acceptance by other members of the multidisciplinary health-care team.

Technology Acceptance

User adoption is a central theme in much of the information systems (IS) literature (see for example Rogers 2003; Venkatesh et al. 2003; Venkatesh et al. 2012). This is primarily due to the fact that user adoption is used as a proxy for trying to determine a priori if a system will be successful or not. Given the amount of time and financial resources invested in so many IS/IT projects, not to mention the impact these systems have on critical service and business functions and the expectation that these projects will deliver significant benefits, it is understandable that user acceptance is an important early consideration.

Health care is now witnessing many initiatives to embrace IS/IT, including but not limited to diverse projects focused at designing and implementing various types of electronic medical records (EMRs), numerous e-health initiatives as well as the application of Web 2.0 in the form of personally controlled health-care records and patient portals. More recently, we are also observing the introduction of personal monitoring, mobile, and wireless devices. It is of particular importance in the health-care domain that such implementations are successful, first and foremost because ultimately a patient's well-being may be at stake. In addition, health care in general is experiencing challenges regarding provision of cost-effective and high-quality services and treatments; hence, situations such as costly implementations of less than successful IS/IT solutions can have widespread detrimental effects.

To date, within the IS field, several models have been developed to examine the critical issue of user acceptance including theory of reasoned action (TRA), technology acceptance model (TAM/TAM2), theory of planned behavior (TPB), combined TAM and TPB, motivational model (MM), model of PC utilization (MPCU), social cognitive theory (SCT), and innovation and diffusion theory (IDT). However, as noted by Venkatesh et al. (2003), due to a need "…to integrate the fragmented theory and research on individual acceptance of information technology that captures the essential elements of eight previously established models," they developed UTAUT, which we used as a conceptual model for our research.

Succinctly stated, UTAUT proposes that four constructs; namely, performance expectancy (i.e., by using the technology, will this have a positive impact on performance/outcome?), effort expectancy (i.e., will using this technology require much effort on the user's part?), social influence (i.e., is using this technology a socially acceptable activity?), and facilitating conditions (i.e., other benefits or positives that make using this technology positive) act as determinants of behavioral intentions and usage behaviors. In addition, there are four key moderator variables including: gender, age, experience, and voluntariness of use (Venkatesh et al. 2003).

Given that our interest was to examine what drives nurses to adopt a novel technology in acute care contexts, it was important to look closely at the role of nurses as it related to technology adoption and the workflow of activities and tasks they must perform.

Consequently, we focused on the following research question: "Based on various UTAUT dimensions, what are initial reactions of nurses to the proposed solution?" We contend that by answering this question it is possible to then better understand nurses' requirements and improve their acceptance of new ICT solutions.

Research Approach

To answer the posed research question, a mixed method design was adopted for a clinical trial to critically examine nurses' use of a novel information system called SW in acute care contexts (both surgical and medical wards), within a single hospital service in Melbourne, Australia. The following describes the key aspects of the research setting, data collection, and data analysis.

Research Setting

SW is a new ICT solution to support nursing work. It is a sophisticated, multifunctional technology designed to support nurses in documentation of the delivery of patient care by decreasing time spent by nurses on administrative tasks to allow direct patient care, create an electronic record of patient care delivery, reduce errors, and provide a positive enhancement to nurses' work experience.

SW was tested with nurses working in two acute care wards (medical and surgical) using a three-stage project across two hospital sites of a large Victorian public health service over an 8-week period in 2013. Temporary implementation of the SW system at 4 beds in each ward was used to evaluate fidelity of the system to nursing work as well as usability and acceptability of the SW system to nurses. The test wards included a 25-bed general surgical ward with 32 regular nursing staff at Site A and a 32-bed general medical and neurology ward with 50 regular nursing staff at Site B. In stage 1, over a 2-week period, the SW system was installed and nurses were recruited and introduced to the system prior to implementation. Baseline workflow data were also collected during stage 1. In stage 2, SW was partially integrated into nursing care processes; during this stage, all nurses were invited to familiarize themselves with the SW system and they began to adopt it into care processes for patients in the selected beds. During this stage, issues of concern related to usability and risk were identified and subsequently modified by the developers prior to stage 3. The duration of this stage was 3 weeks. In stage 3, the SW system was used exclusively for documentation of nursing care delivery for selected patients by a small number of nurse "super users." An UTAUT-based survey was distributed during stage 1. The primary research objective was to capture initial reactions to the system by the nurses participating in the trial.

Data Collection

The UTAUT-based survey reported in this chapter was conducted during the clinical trial. The surveys collected demographic data, responses to UTAUT items, and additional questions related to the training, support, and implementation of the SW system. This chapter reports findings related to nurses' responses to 26 items addressing the five UTAUT constructs and four key moderator variables using a 7-point Likert scale (from 1 being totally disagree to 7 being totally agree). The items included:

- Performance expectancy (PE), $n=8$
- Effort expectancy (EE), $n=4$
- Social influence (SI), $n=5$
- Facilitating conditions (FC), $n=4$
- Behavioral intentions (BI), $n=5$. As the system was in a testing stage, only intention rather than actual use was included.

Overall contextual variables included:

- Gender
- Age
- Experience
- VU voluntariness, $n=3$

A brief descriptive analysis of these variables is included below with the results for the interest of readers. The intention here was not to validate the UTAUT model nor predict the nurses' behavioral intention but to describe and examine the constructs PE, EE, SI, FC and explore the impact of these constructs on BI.

Response rates are presented in Table 19.1:

Data Analysis

The survey data were entered into an Excel 2010 file. Duplicate and invalid records were removed prior to analysis leaving 38 complete responses. Data were then cleaned and imported into SPSS v22 and Excel for statistical analysis and data visualization. The following statistical analyses were conducted:

- Descriptive analysis techniques were employed for each individual survey construct, particularly PE, EE, SI, FC, and BI.
- Reliability analysis was conducted using Cronbach's alpha to examine the internal consistency of the items included in the scale for each UTAUT construct.
- Calculation of a composite score was used to summarize items with strong correlation with each other. Pearson Correlation was used to examine the strength of relationships between BI and each of the UTAUT constructs (PE, EE, SI, and FC). The intention of this chapter was not to predict BI, hence a regression analysis was not included in analyses. As a result of reliability analysis, FC3 was re-

Table 19.1 Response rates to UTAUT-based surveys

Administered	Responses	Response rate
50	43 (valid: 38)	86%

moved from the FC construct. This approach to data analysis using the UTAUT framework has been followed in previous studies (Heselmans et al. 2012; Wills et al. 2008) in the context of health care.

Findings

Gender, Age, Computer Skills, and Perceived Voluntariness of Use

Most (95 %) of the nurse respondents were female; only 2 out of the 38 respondents (5 %) were male. The mean age was 38 (95 % confidence interval for mean: 34.25–41.75, range: 23–58, median = 41.5, interquartile range (IQR): 27.75–42.25). Examination of the age distribution revealed large clusters: 38.2 % (n = 13) were younger than 30 and 29.4 % (n = 10) were aged between 41 and 45 years.

Most nurse participants rated their computer skills as average (52.6 %, n = 20) and above average (26.3 %, n = 10), and over half rated themselves as being comfortable or very comfortable with computers (52.6 %, n = 20; Figs. 19.1 and 19.2).

Five of the voluntariness of use (VU) items refer to nurses' perceptions about whether the SW system should be compulsory or not (VU1), and if they should be required (VU2) or expected (VU3) to use it (Table 19.2).

Please see Table 19.2 for IQR and Fig. 19.2 for the data shapes. The distribution of the responses to these items is slightly to moderately positively skewed, indicating that nurses tended to disagree with the suggestion that the SW system should not be compulsory.

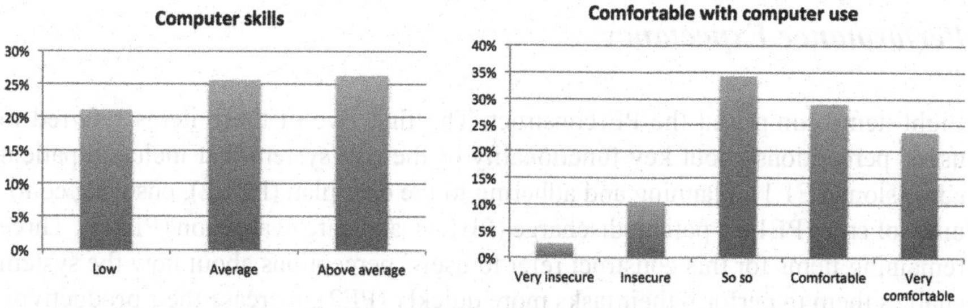

Fig. 19.1 Computer skills and comfortable with computer use

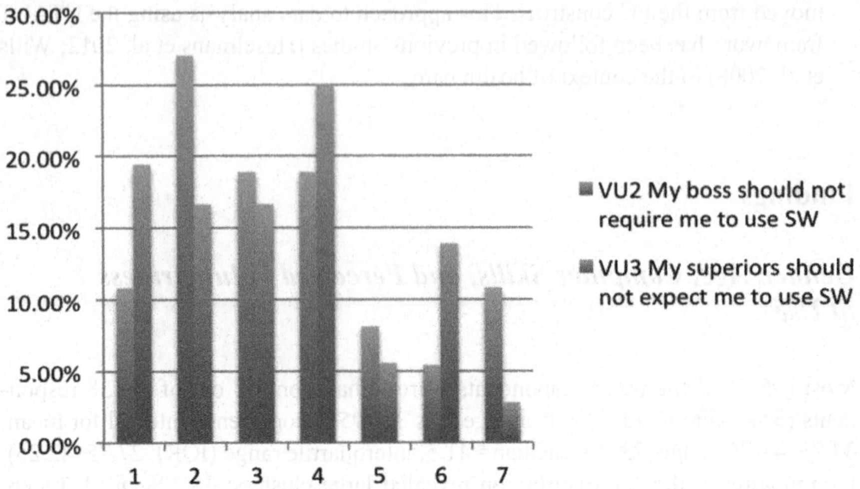

Fig. 19.2 Voluntariness of use (VU)

Table 19.2 Descriptive statistics summary—Voluntariness of Use (VU)

	N	Mean	Median	IQR	Min	Max	Mode
VU1 Although it might be helpful, using SW should certainly not be compulsory in my job	37	3.84	4	2–5	1	7	2
VU2 My boss should not require me to use SW	37	3.46	3	2–4.75	1	7	2
VU3 My superiors should not expect me to use SW	36	3.33	3	2–4	1	7	4

IQR interquartile range, *VU* voluntariness of use

Performance Expectancy

Eight items comprised the PE construct. The first five of these items referred to users' perceptions about key functionality of the SW system that included patient admission (PE1.1), planning and adhering to the care plan (PE1.2), ensuring continuity of care (PE1.3), patient discharge (PE1.4), and care evaluation (PE1.5). Three remaining items for this construct refer to users' perceptions about how the system enables them to perform their tasks more quickly (PE2), increase their productivity (PE3), and provide a chance for career advancement (PE4).

Overall, all medians were between 4 (neutral) and 5 (slightly agree), see Table 19.3 for the IQR for each of the items. Examination of the distribution of responses shows that approximately one quarter of responses were neutral across all the PE items, except for PE1.1 where fewer (18.4%, $n=7$) responding nurses

Table 19.3 Descriptive statistics summary—performance expectancy (PE)

	N	Mean	Median	IQR	Min	Max	Mode
PE1.1 I would find SW useful for my job for patient admission	38	4.63	5	4–6	1	7	5
PE1.2 useful for planning and adhering to the care plan	38	4.29	4	3.25–6	1	7	4
PE1.3 useful for ensuring continuity of care	37	4.35	4	3.25–5	1	7	5
PE1.4 useful for patient discharge	36	4.64	5	3.25–6	1	7	6
PE1.5 useful for care evaluation	36	4.39	4	3.25–6	1	7	4
PE2 Using SW would enable me to accomplish tasks more quickly	38	4.26	4	3–6	1	7	4
PE3 Using SW will increase my productivity	38	4.24	4	3–6	1	7	4
PE4 If I use SW, I will increase my chances for career advancement	38	4.47	5	4–5.75	1	7	Bimodal: 4, 5

IQR interquartile range, *PE* performance expectancy

were neutral. Overall, nurses' responses to the PE items suggest they were slightly positive in their perceptions about the usefulness of the system (see Figs. 19.3 and 19.4). A small number of nurses disagreed with the system's usefulness across almost all the PE items. A notable proportion of the respondents reported extreme negative views in response to the items that "using SW would enable me to accomplish tasks more quickly (PE2; 15.8 %, $n=6$) and improve my productivity" (PE3; 18.4 %, $n=7$; see Table 19.3 and Fig. 19.4 for examples).

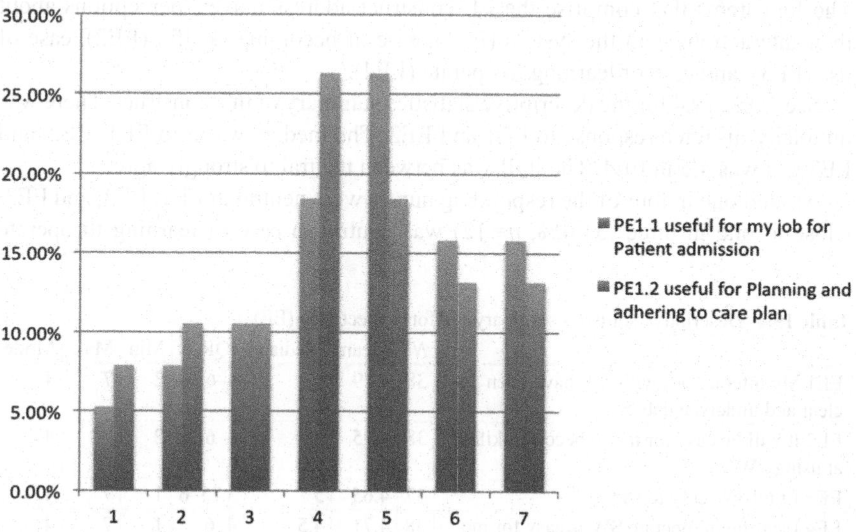

Fig. 19.3 PE1.1 and PE1.2

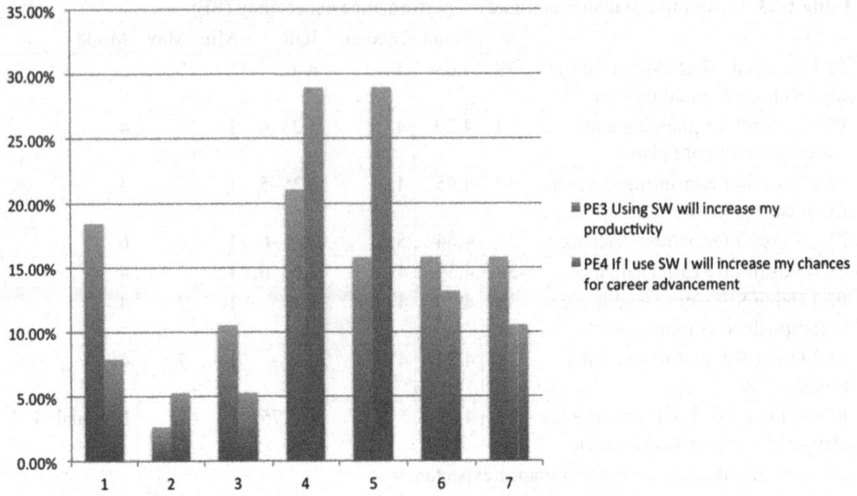

Fig. 19.4 PE3 and PE4

Summary
Overall responses suggest nurses were generally positive about the PE construct.

Effort Expectancy

The four items that comprise the EE construct address nurses' perceptions about their interactions with the system (EE1), ease of becoming skillful (EE2), ease of use (EE3), and ease of learning to operate (EE4).

See Table 19.4 for the descriptive statistics summary of this construct. There was no totally disagree response to EE1 and EE2. The median was 5 in EE1, EE2, and EE3 and was 4.5 in EE4. The IQR was between neutral to strongly agree.

Around one in four of the responding nurses were neutral in EE1, EE2, and EE3. Close to one in three (31.6%, $n=12$) was neutral in ease of learning to operate

Table 19.4 Descriptive statistics summary—effort expectancy (EE)

	N	Mean	Median	IQR	Min	Max	Mode
EE1 My interactions with SW have been clear and understandable	38	4.79	5	4–6	2	7	4
EE2 It will be easy for me to become skillful at using SW	38	4.95	5	4–6	2	7	4
EE3 I find SW easy to use	37	4.65	5	3.75–6	1	7	4
EE4 Learning to operate SW is easy for me	38	4.71	4.5	4–6	1	7	4

IQR interquartile range, *EE* effort expectancy

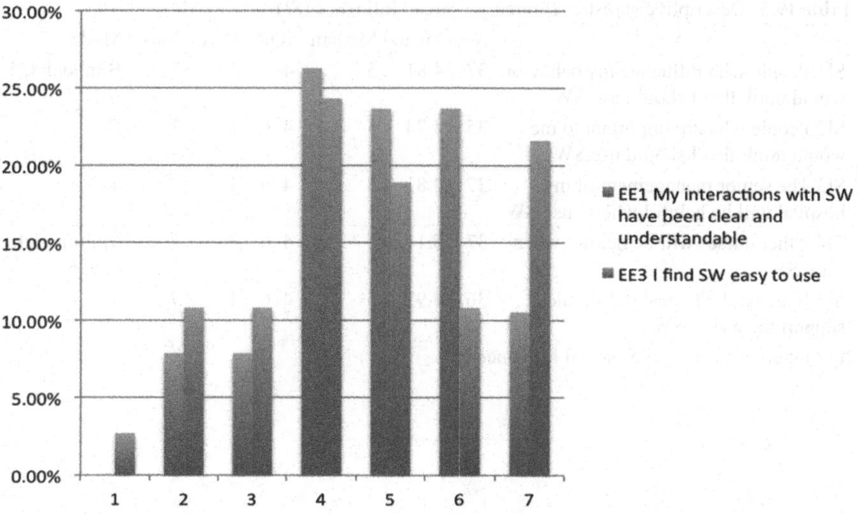

Fig. 19.5 EE1 and EE3

(EE4). Most skeptical is EE3, easy to use, as almost one in four (cumulative 24.3 %, $n=9$) disagreed to some degree (Fig. 19.5).

Summary
Most of the responses regarding EE were positive, suggesting they perceived the SW system easy to learn, while few were skeptical about how easy it would be to learn to use.

Social Influence

The five SI items referred to perceived influences on nurses to use SW by other people (SI1), by people important to them (SI2), nurses' perceived helpfulness of senior management (SI3), perceived helpfulness of other nurses (SI4), and hospital support for the use of the SW system (SI5). Overall, responses to these items were positive indicating SIs were present.

Examination of distributions reveal that the responses were centered around neutral and "slightly/moderately agree" (median: 5, IQR: 4–6). Responses to SI4 were most positive, suggesting nurses highly valued help from other nurses. A clear minority of responses were negative (Table 19.5).

Summary
Nurses were generally positive about SI and the helpfulness of other nurses (SI4) was most positively perceived by the respondents (Fig. 19.6).

Table 19.5 Descriptive statistics summary—social influence (SI)

	N	Mean	Median	IQR	Min	Max	Mode
SI1 People who influence my behavior would think that I should use SW	37	4.81	5	4–6	1	7	Bimodal:4, 5
SI2 People who are important to me would think that I should use SW	35	4.74	5	4–6	1	7	5
SI3 The senior management of my hospital will be helpful when I use SW	37	4.81	5	4–6	1	7	4
SI4 Other nurses will be helpful when I use SW	37	5.11	5	4–6	3	7	Multimodal: 4, 5, 6
SI5 In general, the hospital should support the use of SW	36	4.92	5	4–6	1	7	4

IQR interquartile range, *SI* social influence

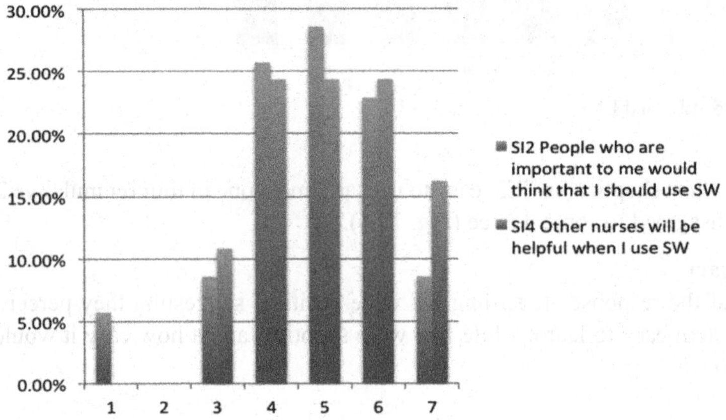

Fig. 19.6 SI2 and SI4

Facilitating Conditions

The four items used to examine facilitating conditions (FC) examined nurses' perception about resources (FC1) and knowledge (FC2) necessary to use SW, whether SW is compatible with other systems (FC3), and the availability of assistance (FC4).

Examination of the distribution shows that a clear minority of responses to FC1, FC2, and FC4 items were positive (see Table 19.6 and Fig. 19.7). Responses about the system's compatibility with other systems in their hospital (FC3) was less positive (see mean, median, and IQR of this item in Table 19.6).

Summary

Nurses were generally positive about their knowledge, resources, and assistance to use the SW system. However, some were slightly skeptical that the system would be compatible with other systems in their hospital.

Table 19.6 Descriptive statistics summary—facilitating conditions (FC)

	N	Mean	Median	IQR	Min	Max	Mode
FC1 I have the resources necessary to use SW	37	5.22	6	4.5–6	2	7	6
FC2 I have the knowledge necessary to use SW	38	5.11	5	4–6	3	7	4
FC3 SW is compatible with other systems I use in my hospital	37	3.59	4	2–5	1	7	4
FC4 Someone is available for assistance with the system difficulties	38	5.82	6	5–7	3	7	7

IQR interquartile range, *FC* facilitating conditions

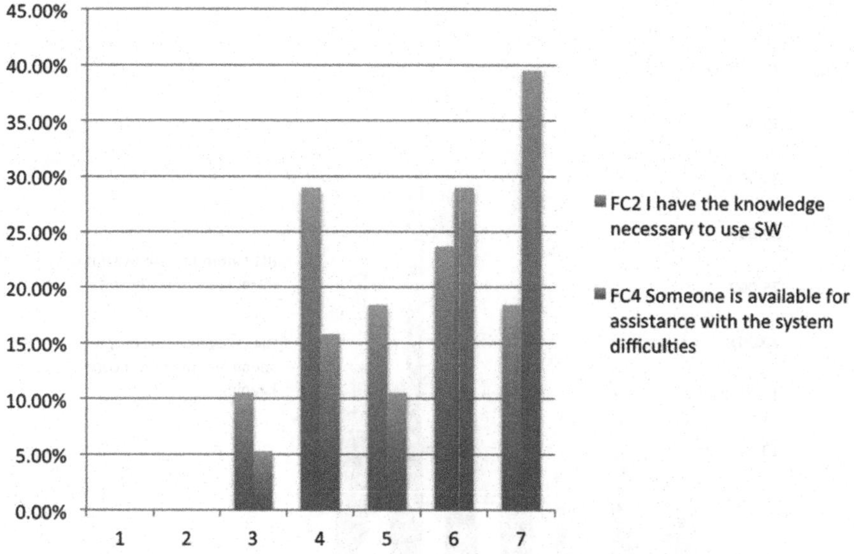

Fig. 19.7 FC2 and FC4

Behavioral Intentions

The five items that comprise the construct behavioral intentions (BI) refer to nurses' intentions (BI1), prediction (BI2), planning (BI3) to use SW when it is introduced as well as perception about whether SW will help them reduce record-keeping time (BI4) and spend more time with patients (BI5) (Table 19.7, Fig. 19.8).

Distribution of responses to BI1, BI2, and BI3 were skewed toward positive answers (5, 6, and 7). All their medians and modes were 6– showing half of the responses moderately or strongly agreed, and the most frequent responses were "moderately agree". In comparison to BI1, BI2, and BI3, the responding nurses were found to be slightly less positive in regard to BI4 and BI5. Medians and modes were 5– "slightly agree".

Table 19.7 Descriptive statistics summary—behavioral intentions (BI)

	N	Mean	Median	IQR	Min	Max	Mode
BI1 I intend to use SW if it is introduced to my hospital	38	5.45	6	5–7	1	7	6
BI2 I predict I would use SW in my hospital	38	5.34	6	5–7	1	7	6
BI3 I plan to use SW if it is introduced in my hospital	38	5.39	6	5–7	1	7	6
BI4 Using SW enables me to spend less time on record keeping	37	4.38	5	3–7	1	7	5
BI5 Using SW allows me to spend more time with my patients	37	4.11	5	2–7	1	7	5

IQR interquartile range, *BI* behavioral intentions

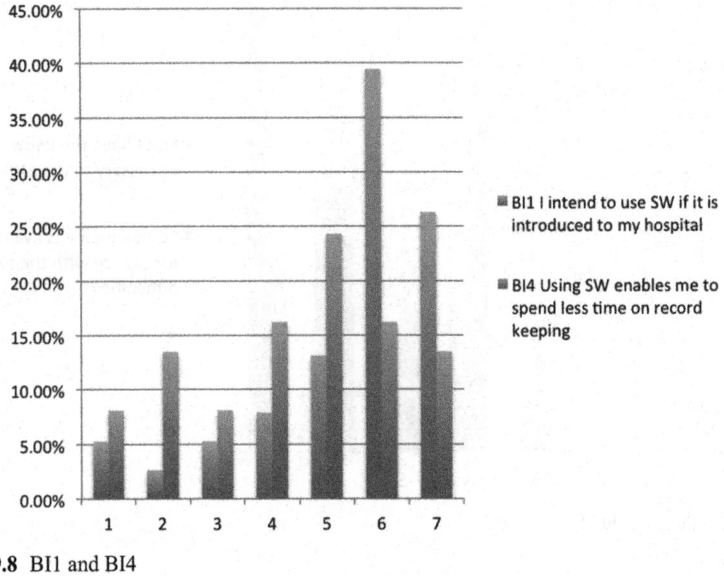

Fig. 19.8 BI1 and BI4

Summary
Overall, the responding nurses were moderately positive that they intend, predict, and plan to use the SW system when it is introduced to the hospital, whereas they were less positive in perceiving that the system would reduce their documentation time and enable them to have more time with patients.

Reliability of the Subscale Constructs

Despite the small sample, the Cronbach's alpha coefficient was greater than 0.8 (over the acceptable level .07) indicating a high level of internal consistency between items within each construct (Table 19.8).

Table 19.8 Reliability statistics

	Cronbach's alpha	Cronbach's alpha based on standardized items	No. of items
PE	0.969	0.970	8
EE	0.972	0.974	4
SI	0.859	0.859	5
FC	0.813	0.816	3
BI	0.943	0.946	5

PE performance expectancy, *EE* effort expectancy, *SI* social influence, *FC* facilitating conditions, *BI* behavioral intentions

Table 19.9 Correlation matrix

		PE	EE	SI	FC
BI	Pearson correlation	*0.772*[a]	*0.751*[a]	*0.613*[a]	*0.600*[a]
	Sig. (2-tailed)	*0.000*	*0.000*	*0.000*	*0.000*
	N	38	38	38	38

[a] Correlation is significant at the 0.01 level (2-tailed)
Bootstrap results are based on 1000 bootstrap samples
PE performance expectancy, *EE* effort expectancy, *SI* social influence, *FC* facilitating conditions, *BI* behavioral intentions

Correlations Between the Constructs (PE, EE, SI, and FC) and BI

Correlations between the construct subscales were examined revealing moderately positive and significant correlations between each of the constructs (PE, EE, SI, and FC[1]) and BI (Table 19.9).

Hypotheses under examination include:

- H1: There is no significant correlation between PE and BI.
- H2: There is no significant correlation between EE and BI.
- H3: There is no significant correlation between SI and BI.
- H4: There is no significant correlation between FC and BI.

All p-value <0.01; hence we can reject all the above hypotheses (that there is no significant correlation between each of the construct PE, EE, SI, and FC and BI). Hence, at the 0.01 significant level, there is statistical evidence for positive correlation between each of the constructs and BI.

While the above analysis suggests a positive correlation between each of the constructs and BI, this analysis does not predict the nurses' BI based on the UTAUT constructs nor did it test the moderators (Fig. 19.9).

[1] FC* was calculated without FC3.

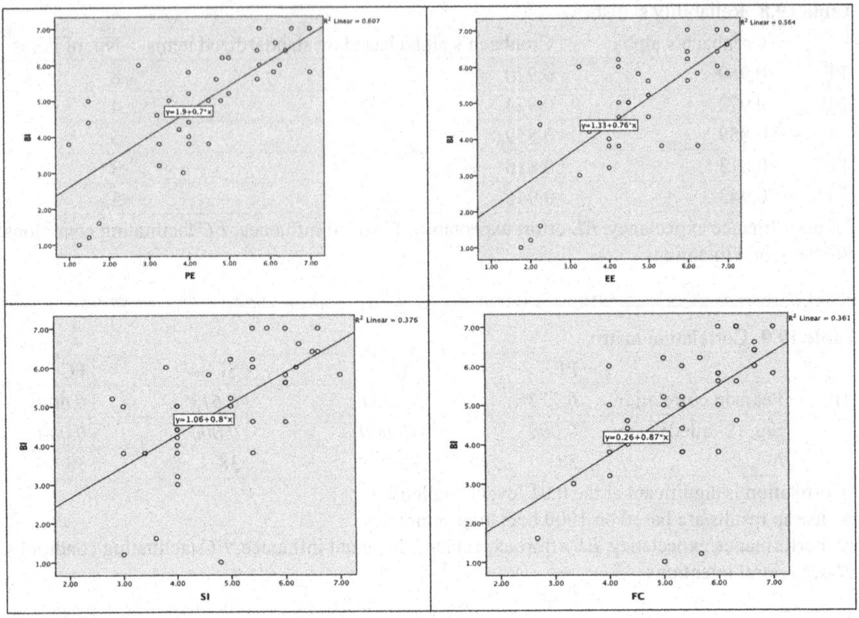

Fig. 19.9 Scatter plots

Discussion and Conclusion

Nurses' initial reactions to a novel technology, SW, were examined through the UTAUT lens. Overall, the nurses had slightly positive perceptions about PE, EE, and SI and moderately positive perception toward FC. These findings indicate that nurses intend, predict, and plan to use the SW system when it is introduced to the hospital. They reported slightly positive perceptions that the SW would reduce their documentation time and enable them to spend more time with patients.

The findings confirm positive correlations between each of the constructs (PE, EE, SI, FC) and BI as described in UTAUT (Venkatesh et al. 2003). The findings also support the use of the UTAUT tool to explore and plan nurse user requirements and evaluate their acceptance of innovative technology solutions and feedback to design. A subsequent analysis is underway to test whether age, gender, VU, and years of experience moderate the relationships between each of the independent variables (PE, EE, SI, FC) and the dependent variable BI.

The findings suggested redesigning the solution and developing an implementation plan to fit in with the dynamic and complex nursing care. Firstly, while nurses were found to be moderately positive in their intention to use the proposed system, they were less positive in perceiving the system's usability. This suggests the importance of improving the system's usability. Secondly, nurses perceived more strongly about peer support (other nurses being helpful—SI4) and were slightly/moderately positive with SI/FC respectively. This suggests the importance of peer support, training, and technical support during implementation and training.

Our study appears to indicate, then, that while the participating nurses expressed a generally positive view to the use of the SW technology in their nursing context, this may not translate directly into strong acceptance of the specific solution. Clearly, this was not the finding we were expecting; however, on closer examination, we note this is reflective of the general trend in practice with health care and technology use (Lau et al. 2010; Mills et al. 2013). Currently, we are witnessing a plethora of IS/IT solutions being adopted into health-care organizations, but these solutions all show poor user acceptance and oftentimes even have to be terminated (e.g., most notably the NHS Connecting for Health project). To address this issue, we recommend follow-up analyses and studies that include a mixed method approach and use qualitative techniques to assist in the uncovering of why acceptance might be low.

There are three key limitations in this study worthy of consideration. First, this was not an empirical validation of UTAUT (Venkatesh et al. 2003). Second, due to the complex nature of acute care wards and patient safety requirements, only a small number of nurses participated in the software trial. All these resulted in a small sample size of the acceptance surveys. Third, survey research by nature does not reveal a deep understanding of how and why behind the findings. A good response rate indicates a good level of interest in the participating nurses.

This chapter contributes to theory in a very important way. It suggests that conceptual models such as UTAUT need further extension of IS theory to facilitate a deeper understanding of the complex and dynamic nature of health care and the how and why of acceptance of specific solutions despite appearance of a general acceptance that IS/IT. For practice, the message is even stronger: user needs and requirements must be carefully considered when developing IS/IT solutions for health-care contexts. More research into how to better meet the demands of a multiple heterogeneous user system such as the dynamic and complex health-care environment is definitely needed.

References

Alaszewski, A. (2005). Risk, safety and organizational change in health care? *Health, Risk & Safety, 7*(4), 315–318.

Cornell, P., Herrin-Griffith, D., Keim, C., Petschonek, S., Sanders, A. M., D'Mello, S., Golden, T. W., & Shepherd, G. (2010a). Transforming nursing workflow, part 1: The chaotic nature of nurse activities. *Journal of Nursing Administration, 40*(9), 366–373. doi:310.1097/NNA.1090b1013e3181ee4261.

Cornell, P., Riordan, M., & Herrin-Griffith, D. (2010b). Transforming nursing workflow, part 2: The impact of technology on nurse activities. *Journal of Nursing Administration, 40*(10), 432–439. doi:410.1097/NNA.1090b1013e3181f1092eb1093f.

Darbyshire, P. (2004). 'Rage against the machine?': Nurses' and midwives' experiences of using computerized patient information systems for clinical information. *Journal of Clinical Nursing, 13*(1), 17–25.

Dowding, D., Mitchell, N., Randell, R., Foster, R., Lattimer, V., & Thompson, C. (2009). Nurses' use of computerised clinical decision support systems: A case site analysis. *Journal of Clinical Nursing, 18*(8), 1159–1167. doi:10.1111/j.1365-2702.2008.02607.x.

Garg, A. X., Adhikari, N. K. J., McDonald, H., Rosas-Arellano, M. P., Devereaux, P. J., Beyene, J., Sam, J., & Haynes, R. B. (2005). Effects of computerized clinical decision support systems on practitioner performance and patient outcomes: A systematic review. *Journal of the American Medical Association, 293*(10), 1223–1238.

Heselmans, A., Aertgeerts, B. P. D., Geens, S., Van de Velde, S., & Ramaekers, D. (2012). Family physicians' perceptions and use of electronic clinical decision support during the first year of implementation. *Journal of Medical Systems, 36*(6), 3677–3684. doi:10.1007/s10916-012-9841-3.

Holden, R. J. (2010). Physicians beliefs about using EMR and CPOE: In pursuit of a contextualized understanding of health IT use behavior. *International Journal of Medical Informatics, 79*(2), 71–80. doi:10.1016/j.ijmedinf.2009.12.003.

Jennings, J. M., Stover, J. A., Bair-Merritt, M. H., Fichtenber, C., Munoz, M. G., Maziad, R., Ketemepi, S. J., & Zenilman, J. (2009). Identifying challenges to the integration of computer-Based surveillance information systems in large city health department: A case study. *Public Health Reports, 124*(2), 39–48.

Kawamoto, K., Houlihan, C. A., Balas, E. A., & Lobach, D. F. (2005). Improving clinical practice using clinical decision support systems: A systematic review of trials to identify features critical to success. *BMJ, 330*(7494), 765. doi:10.1136/bmj.38398.500764.8F.

Kowitlawakul, Y. (2011). The technology acceptance model: Predicting nurses' intention to use telemedicine technology (eICU). *Computers Informatics Nursing, 29*(7), 411–418. doi:410.1097/NCN.1090b1013e3181f1099dd1094a.

Lau, F., Kuziemsky, C., Price, M., & Gardner, J. (2010). A review on systematic reviews of health information system studies. *Journal of the American Medical Informatics Association, 17*(6), 637–645. doi:10.1136/jamia.2010.004838.

Mills, J., Chamberlain-Salaun, J., Henry, R., Sando, J., & Summers, G. (2013). Nurses in Australian acute care settings: Experiences with and outcomes of e-health. An integrative review. *International Journal of Management & Information Technology, 2*(2), 1–8.

Rogers, E. (2003). *Diffusion of innovations* (5th ed.). New York: Free Press.

Rogers, M. L., Sockolow, P. S., Bowles, K. H., Hand, K. E., & George, J. (2013). Use of a human factors approach to uncover informatics needs of nurses in documentation of care. *International Journal of Medical Informatics, 82*(11), 1068–1074.

Stevenson, J., Nilsson, G., Petersson, G., & Johanssson, P. (2010). Nurses' experience of using electronic patient records in everyday practice in acute/inpatient ward settings: A literature review. *Health Informatics Journal, 16*(1), 63–72.

Turley, J. P. (1996). Toward a model for nursing informatics. *Journal of Nursing Scholarship, 28*(4), 309–313.

Venkatesh, V., Morris, M. G., Gordon, B. D., & Davis, F. D. (2003). User acceptance of information technology: Toward a unified view. *MIS Quarterly, 27*(3), 425–478.

Venkatesh, V., Thong, J. Y. L., & Xin, X. (2012). Consumer acceptance and use of information technology: Extending the unified theory of acceptance and use of technology. *MIS Quarterly, 36*(1), 157–178.

Viitanen, J., Hypponen, H., Laaveri, T., Vanska, J., Reponen, J., & Winblad, I. (2011). National questionnaire study on clinical ICT systems proofs: Physicians suffer from poor usability. *International Journal of Medical Informatics, 80*(10), 708–725.

Weber, S. (2007). A qualitative analysis of how advanced practice nurses use clinical decision support systems. *Journal of the American Academy of Nurse Practitioners, 19*(12), 652–667. doi:10.1111/j.1745-7599.2007.00266.x.

Weber, S., Crago, E. A., Sherwood, P. R., & Smith, T. (2009). Practitioner approaches to the integration of clinical decision support system technology in critical care. *Journal of Nursing Administration, 39*(11), 465–469. doi:10.1097/NNA.0b013e3181bd5fc2.

Wills, M. J., El-Gayar, O. F., & Bennett, D. (2008). Examining health care professionals' acceptance of electronic medical records using UTAUT. *Issues in Information Systems, 9*(2), 396–401.

Yu, P., Li, H., & Gagnon, M.-P. (2009). Health IT acceptance factors in long-term care facilities: A cross-sectional survey. *International Journal of Medical Informatics, 78*(4), 219–229. doi:10.1016/j.ijmedinf.2008.07.006.

Yun-Ke, C., Khoo, C., Nourbakhsh, A., & Gan, A. (26–27 Sept 2009). *Requirement analysis for a nursing decision support system*. Paper presented at the Science and Technology for Humanity (TIC-STH), 2009 IEEE Toronto International Conference.

Prof. Nilmini Wickramasinghe Ph.D.; MBA; Grad.Dip.Mgt.St; B.Sc. Amus.A, piano; Amus.A, violin has a well-recognized research record in the field of health care and IT/IS. Her expertise is in the strategic application and management of technology for effecting superior health-care solutions. She currently is the professor director of Health Informatics Management at Epworth HealthCare and a professor at Deakin University.

Prof. Mari Botti was appointed the Epworth Deakin Chair of Nursing in 2004, and has held academic appointments for over 20 years. Professor Botti coordinates the Bachelor of Nursing (Honours) program, is chair of the Deakin University Human Research and Ethics Committee, and a member of the Epworth Human Research and Ethics Committee. She also leads the Epworth Deakin Centr for Clinical Nursing Research.

Her specific research and clinical interests are in postoperative pain management, investigation of models of care that encourage patient engagement in their care, safety and wellbeing, and the use of data to improve quality and safety in health care.

Dr. Hoda Moghimi is a data analyst professional with experience in different industries over the past 10 years, working closely with various participants to address their analytical requirements and issues as well as developing new prototypes. Her major research and technology interests include data analytics, predictive modeling, and data visualization. She also has over 30 peer-reviewed scholarly publications in informatics contexts.

Imran Muhammad (PhD Business Information Systems, Masters in Business (ERP Systems), Masters in Business Information Systems) is a research fellow at Royal Melbourne Institute of Technology (RMIT University), Australia. His primary research interests are in the area of business information systems, especially in the area of health-care information systems management and electronic health records (EHR). He has more than 10 years of teaching and research experience in different areas of business information systems, health informatics, and management.

Peter Haddad is working towards his PhD from Deakin University, Australia. He is involved in different research projects that concentrate on IS/IT in health care. Mr Haddad comes from an engineering management background and has over 12 years' experience in this area, both in academic and professional contexts.

Lemai Nguyen (PhD) is a senior lecturer in the Department of Information Systems and Business Analytics, Deakin Business School, Deakin University. Lemai is currently an honorary research affiliate at Epworth HealthCare. In health informatics, Lemai conducts research in implementing and evaluating nursing information systems and their impacts on various aspects of care delivery. She also conducts research in electronic health records implementation evaluation, health-care analytics, and information needs and information behaviors of clinicians, patients, and their carers. Lemai publishes widely in many high quality international scholarly journals, conferences, and books. She is the section editor of the *Australasian Journal of Information Systems* (AJIS).

Dr. Bernice Redley is an associate professor in the School of Nursing and Midwifery at Deakin University research partnership with Monash Health. Her research interests include health-care quality and patient safety in complex health-care settings, inter-professional teamwork, and communication, using health informatics to support nursing practice and health service evaluation.

Chapter 20
Using e-Mental Health Services for the Benefit of Consumers in Saudi Arabia

Bader Binhadyan, Konrad Peszynski and Nilmini Wickramasinghe

Introduction

The fast developments of the Internet and mobile technologies during the past two decades have enabled health-care providers globally to adapt these technologies in order to facilitate better service delivery (Eysenbach 2001). Recently, the mental health sector is realising the benefit of using technologies, due to the fact that such technologies have the promise to improve mental health services especially by enabling early intervention and treatment for many people with mental illnesses (Christensen et al. 2002).

The mental health sector in Saudi Arabia started to get some attention from the Saudi authorities and mental health providers to develop a strategic plan to facilitate this sector and improve the mental health services quality in Saudi (Al-Habeeb and Qureshi 2010; Koenig et al. 2014). However, although Saudi Arabia has invested billions of dollars to improve the quality and the delivery of e-health in the past 10 years (Altuwaijri 2010), less focus has been given to e-mental health. This is a key void and one this chapter sets out to address.

The emphasis of this research in progress design will be on examining e-mental health services and how these services benefit the consumers in Saudi Arabia. It also

B. Binhadyan (✉)
Ministry of Education, Saudi Arabia & School of Business IT and Logistics, RMIT University, GPO Box 2476V, 3001 Melbourne, VIC, Australia
e-mail: binhadyan@gmail.com

K. Peszynski
School of Business IT and Logistics, RMIT University, GPO Box 2476V, Melbourne, VIC 3001, Australia
e-mail: konrad.peszynski@rmit.edu.au

N. Wickramasinghe
Deakin University and Epworth HealthCare, 60 Baker Ave, Kew East 3102, Australia
e-mail: n.wickramasinghe@deakin.edu.au

N. Wickramasinghe et al. (eds.), *Contemporary Consumer Health Informatics*, Healthcare Delivery in the Information Age, DOI 10.1007/978-3-319-25973-4_20

explores how e-mental health can facilitate the mental health services and improve the barriers that affect the mental health services and delivery in that country. Australian e-mental health services programme was chosen to be the case study to assist with the investigation. The research question guiding this study is: How e-mental health services can be implemented for the benefit of Saudi Arabia consumers?

Literature Review

In this section, a brief background of mental health sector in Saudi and e-health development in Saudi Arabia is provided, followed by a definition of e-mental health and the use of technology in mental health services in general, and in Australia in particular.

Background

Technology in health care has the potential to assist developed and developing countries to solve many issues they are facing, such as creating easy access to information and services, coping with changing population health patterns and satisfaction and safety of stakeholders and specific population groups. Health care is becoming technology-driven (Moumtzoglou 2011) with the possibility of superior health-care delivery with the adoption of e-business in the form of e-health (Eysenbach 2001).

e-Health covers a broad area in health care (Eysenbach 2001). e-Mental health is one of the areas that e-health covers. e-Mental health is a relatively new area of e-health and hence, few, if any, policies or strategic directions currently exist.

Even though the use of technologies in mental health care is relatively new, there is a positive trend towards using technologies among different age groups, for different mental illness preventions and treatments (Ben-Zeev et al. 2012; Proudfoot et al. 2010; Whittaker et al. 2012). Technology has the potential to improve efficiency, accessibility and the opportunities for early intervention and treatment for young adults (Anthony et al. 2010; Christensen et al. 2002).

Technological tools and methods, such as Internet-based interventions and mobile-based application or short message services (SMS) therapy are used for the treatment of people with mental illnesses such as depression and anxiety (Anthony et al. 2010; Christensen and Petrie 2013b; Whittaker et al. 2012). They can also target young adults seeking mental health attention (Christensen et al. 2002).

Recently, the mental health sector is getting a massive transformation and new policies and acts have been applied by the Saudi authorities to improve the mental health services and deliveries (Koenig et al. 2014; Qureshi et al. 2013).

Saudi Mental Health Sector

Recently, the mental health sector has started to gain some attention from the Saudi authorities; in 2006 national mental health policy was developed and special mental health programmes in general medical systems were established. The following year the Saudi Arabian Mental and Social Health Atlas was introduced, which aimed to establish a well-developed plan that would improve the quality of mental health services, mental health promotion/education and improve the mental literacy (Al-Habeeb and Qureshi 2010). Almalki et al. (2011) argue that the Saudi government has recently introduced a Mental Health Act which focus on the following objectives: (1) improving accessibility, (2) less restrictive level of care, (3) improving the accreditation of professionals and facilities, (4) ensuring better mental health policy and procedure enforcement, and (5) protecting patients and their family members' rights.

Between the years 2006 and 2012, the Ministry of Health (MoH) reported that the total number of outpatients seeking mental health services at public hospitals increased by 59.40% (from 310,848 to 495,484 cases), and the total number of inpatients increased by 12.90% (MoH 2011, 2012). MoH (2012) used the International Classification of Diseases (ICD-10) to identify disease groups and reported that in 2012:

- 48.93% of the total number of mental health outpatients and inpatients were women.
- 53.19% were between the age of 15–40.
- 35% suffered from depression.
- 36% suffered from anxiety.

In addition, Islam plays a momentous part in Saudi's culture by shaping the social protocols, traditions, practices of society and responsibilities (Al-Saggaf 2004; Aldraehim et al. 2012). Therefore, Saudi health system is strongly grounded in religion and culture, which needs to be taken into consideration when examining and treating patients and planning health services (Koenig et al. 2014).

e-Health of Saudi Arabia

"Saudi Arabia offers a picture of spectacular progress in health care …. Although many nations have seen sizable growth in their health care systems, probably no other nation of large geographic expanse and population has, in comparable time, achieved so much on a broad national scale, with a relatively high level of care made available to virtually all segments of the population" (Gallagher 2002, p. 182).

In the past decade, the Saudi Arabian government made the development of health-care systems a high priority and has invested billions of dollars to improve the delivery and quality of health services. For example, the MoH has allocated just over US$1 billion to develop and improve e-health programmes for public sector between 2008–2011 (Qurban and Austria 2008). Because of these huge investments and the high level of care and attention, the Saudi population's health services has improved significantly (Almalki et al. 2011).

Due to a number of challenges that the Saudi Arabian health sector is facing, such as vast growth, vast geography and emergence of lifestyle diseases (Ministry of Health Portal 2011), MoH quickly started to adapt and implement the e-health concept. e-Health focus and strategies in Saudi Arabia concentrate on patient-centric care (Fig. 20.1) by building a significant nationwide e-health network that will allow more than 3500 e-health-care facilities to use a single patient record by 2020 (Ministry of Health Portal 2011; Nuviun Digital Health 2014).

The national e-health program of Saudi Arabia aims to achieve the following:

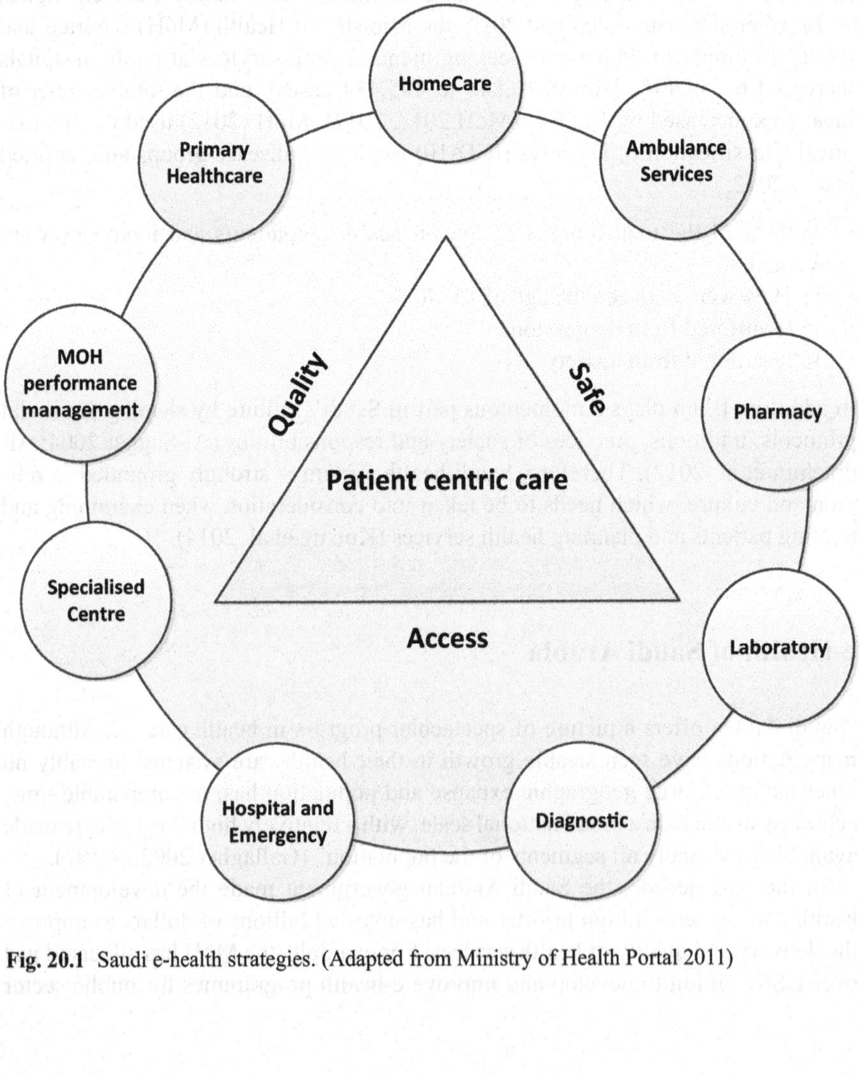

Fig. 20.1 Saudi e-health strategies. (Adapted from Ministry of Health Portal 2011)

- Interoperable electronic health record (iEHR) for every patient
- Patient health information will be available to clinicians in all health-care services
- Deliver an efficient system to transfer patients between health-care services
- Offer electronic services to all health-care facilities

The national e-health project plan will cover the mental health sector in 4–6 years with no further details of mental health program or the role of IS/IT in mental health (Ministry of Health Portal 2011) even though the Saudi King, King Abdullah bin Abdul-Aziz Al Saud, has given his order to allocate over US$4 billion to establish 22 health projects, which includes three health centres for children's growth and behaviour disorders (Ministry News 2013).

The need of e-mental that will facilitate mental health sector in Saudi Arabia is timely and important. e-Mental health services are showing significant outcomes to improve the barriers that are affecting the traditional mental health services.

e-Mental Health

e-Mental health is defined as providing treatment and/or support to people with mental disorders through sensible technologies such as telephone, mobile phone, computer and online applications which can range from the provision of information, peer support services, virtual applications and games to real-time interaction with trained clinicians (Australian Government 2012). The e-mental health services have the abilities to improve accessibility, reduce costs, flexibility and better consumer interactivity and engagement (Lal and Adair 2014).

e-Mental health services can assist in overcoming issues that are preventing people from accessing mental health services and creating barriers to treatment. This includes lack of access of mental health services due to location, time or perhaps financial matters (Booth et al. 2004); stigma incurred by seeing a therapist (Burns et al. 2010; Christensen and Hickie 2010) and therapist time and efficacy (Jorm et al. 2013; Jorm et al. 2007).

Technologies such as social media, SMS, emails, website, chat or instant messaging (IM) can be used to better the delivery of interventions and treatment options for people with mental illnesses such as depression and anxiety (Anthony et al. 2010; Christensen and Petrie 2013b; Whittaker et al. 2012). They can also be used to target young adults seeking mental health attention better than traditional methods (Christensen et al. 2002).

However, Lal and Adair (2014) argue that there are a number of disadvantages of e-mental health services, such as lack of quality control, they are limited only to people with low to moderate mental illness as well as the services available are limited to people who are familiar with using technology.

One of the countries that is considered a leader in e-mental health services is Australia.

Table 20.1 Australian mental health services types

Number	Mental health services type	Example
1	Health promotion, wellness promotion and psycho-education	Beyondblue www.beyondblue.org.au
2	Prevention and early intervention	Kids helpline www.kidshelp.com.au MoodGYM moodgym.anu.edu.au
3	Crisis intervention and suicide prevention	Lifeline www.lifeline.org.au
4	Treatment	myCompass www.mycompass.org.au/
5	Recovery and mutual peer support	BlueBoard www.blueboard.anu.edu.au

e-Mental Health in Australia

In the past decade, Australia has become one of the leading countries in providing e-mental health services along with Sweden and the Netherlands; also lately 50% of the publications in e-mental health are from Australian resources (Christensen and Petrie 2013a). Majority of e-mental health programs in Australia are targeting young people who suffer depression, anxiety and suicidal thoughts (Australian Government 2012). There are five types of e-mental health services in Australia as shown in Table 20.1.

Method and Research Design

e-Mental health in Saudi Arabia has not been explored before, and it does not have defined characteristics; an exploratory qualitative research method is the most suitable method and a single case study is used (Yin 2009). At this stage of the research, the answer to the research question of "How can e-mental health services be implemented to facilitate the current mental health in Saudi Arabia?" will be examined and explored.

Case Study

Creswell (2013) argue that case study as a tool of investigation is found in many fields which allow the research to develop in-depth analysis of a field. According to Stake (1995), there are three types of case study research: intrinsic, instrumental and collective case studies. To gain more insight and knowledge into this research topic, an instrumental case study has been chosen.

In general, case study methodology is not strictly planned but the researchers will be guided by what they will see in the field, given a planned field study with specific steps with data collection and analyses (Fidel 1984). This will enable the researcher to deal with unexpected results. This research has employed the case study framework that was developed by Eisenhardt (1989). It includes eight steps as follow:

Getting Started

In this step, after reviewing and outlining the literature, the research question will be developed and defined. A priori constructs will be examined for further measuring. At this stage of the research, the research question is developed and the related literatures are articulated.

Selecting the Case Study

Australian mental health services programme is chosen as the single case study that will be examined against the Saudi's mental health sector.

Crafting the Instruments and Protocols

Observation is the main method adopted to collect data for this research. Observation is a fundamental and highly important method in all qualitative inquiry (Yin 2009). Observing and examining Australian mental health services will be the most stable method at this stage of the research. Tools, such as NVivo and MS Visio, will be used to facilitate this stage of the research to explore the relationships and identify differences in both contexts. Some of the aspects that will be observed and taken into consideration include the culture and how the role of e-mental health will be different in a Saudi Arabian context.

Entering the Field

In this stage, the data will be collected. Data collection and analysis overlap and research can go back and forth until the main theory emerges.

Data Analysis

The case study approach allows the researcher to move back and forth from data collection and analysis, and it will continue until the main theory starts to develop. The data is analysed by using within-case analysis (Yin 2009). The data collected will be inspected for common characteristics that represent categories or themes (Boyatzis 1998). For instance, the important data or information collected will be divided into categories that will later involve a group of subcategories after more in-depth analysis occurs.

Hypotheses Formulation

In this step, the relationship between the core categories/themes will be validated and refined. Most likely in this stage, all findings will be considered and the overall theory can be shaped and tested. The relationships and findings will be verified among the unique and specific constructs and aspects identified, for instance the hypotheses benefits that patients, mental health professional and the Saudi government will gain from the e-mental health will discussed later in this chapter.

Enfolding Literature

In this level, the findings will be compared with similar and conflicting literature.

Recommendation

Based on the outcomes of the data analysis and findings and the literature, a recommendation will be proposed.

Discussion

This research aims to investigate how an IS/IT solution that is designed to facilitate mental health services delivery in an Australia context can be applied to a Saudi Arabian context. This will be done through observing and analysing the status of current mental health service delivery in Saudi Arabia and examining the cultural similarity and differences between Saudi Arabia and Australia. Kavanagh, Andrews, Scharr, Helpline and Spence (2014) argue that the availability of the e-mental health services will allow the patients and their family members to overcome already known barriers to treatment such as stigma associated with visiting practitioners' clinics, geographical location, social aspects and isolation, as well as the high cost and transport difficulties. e-Mental health services will provide convenient and flexible services and easy access anywhere and anytime with a high level of confidentiality. Confidentiality can be seen in providing the choice of the patient to remain anonymous.

Moreover, people experiencing multiple mental health conditions can access multiple treatments in one location (Kavanagh et al. 2014). e-Mental health services can help mental professionals by reducing the over load on their clinic, which on the other hand will increase the clinic availability for people with high or complex mental health conditions (Lal and Adair 2014). Mental health professionals can find it easy to access education tools and support resources and improve their clinic's integration with primary health-care services (Kavanagh et al. 2014).

From a government's perspective, e-mental health will reduce the cost of e-mental health delivery and services, and provide better service policy by targeting groups that are not benefiting from the traditional services or delivery (Kavanagh et al. 2014). e-Mental health has the ability to provide real-time data collections and better population information management to provide high-quality future planning and developments.

Conclusion

The outcome of this research will not only assist consumers to get better mental health care, but will also assist health-care providers to deliver better services with lower cost to help consumers with their general happiness, mental health and well-being. Technology will help the mental health sector in Saudi to provide better treatment and services for people with mental illness in Saudi Arabia.

By 2020, Saudi Arabia aims to develop a nationwide e-health program that will cover all services and facilities of health care which will allow these services and facilities to use one single patient record; therefore, we believe our study will serve to match this development by calling from research in this area. This research will also contribute to e-mental health practice in Australia as well as theory regarding e-health and e-mental health.

References

Al-Habeeb, A., & Qureshi, N. (2010). Mental and social health atlas I in Saudi Arabia. *EMHJ, 16*(5), 570–577.

Al-Saggaf, Y. (2004). The effect of online community on offline community in Saudi Arabia. *The Electronic Journal of Information Systems in Developing Countries, 16*, 1–16.

Aldraehim, M. S., Edwards, S. L., Watson, J. A., & Chan, T. (2012). Cultural impact on e-service use in Saudi Arabia: The role of nepotism. *International Journal for Infonomics (IJI), 5*(3/4), 655–662.

Almalki, M., Fitzgerald, G., & Clark, M. (2011). Health care system in Saudi Arabia: an overview. *Eastern Mediterranean Health Journal, 17*(10), 784–793.

Altuwaijri, M. (2010). Supporting the Saudi e-health initiative: The Master of Health Informatics programme at KSAU-HS. *Eastern Mediterranean Health Journal, 16*(1), 119–124.

Anthony, K., Nagel, D. M., & Goss, S. (2010). *The use of technology in mental health: Applications, ethics and practice*. Springfield: Charles C Thomas Pub Limited.

Australian Government. (2012). E-mental health strategy for Australia.http://www.health.gov.au/internet/main/publishing.nsf/Content/7C7B0BFEB985D0EBCA257BF0001BB0A6/$File/emstrat.pdf.

Ben-Zeev, D., Davis, K. E., Kaiser, S., Krzsos, I., & Drake, R. E. (2012). Mobile technologies among people with serious mental illness: Opportunities for future services. *Administration and Policy in Mental Health and Mental Health Services Research, 40*, 340–343.

Booth, M. L., Bernard, D., Quine, S., Kang, M. S., Usherwood, T., Alperstein, G., & Bennett, D. L. (2004). Access to health care among Australian adolescents young people's perspectives and their sociodemographic distribution. *Journal of Adolescent Health, 34*(1), 97–103.

Boyatzis, R. E. (1998). *Transforming qualitative information: Thematic analysis and code development*: Thousand Oaks: Sage.

Burns, J. M., Davenport, T. A., Durkin, L. A., Luscombe, G. M., & Hickie, I. B. (2010). The internet as a setting for mental health service utilisation by young people. *Medical Journal of Australia, 192*(11), S22.

Christensen, H., Griffiths, K. M., & Evans, K. (2002). *e-Mental health in Australia: Implications of the internet and related technologies for policy*. Canberra: Commonwealth Department of Health and Ageing Canberra.

Christensen, H., & Hickie, I. B. (2010). E-mental health: A new era in delivery of mental health services. *Medical Journal of Australia, 192*(11), S2.

Christensen, H., & Petrie, K. (2013a). Information technology as the key to accelerating advances in mental health care. *Australian and New Zealand Journal of Psychiatry, 47*(2), 114–116.

Christensen, H., & Petrie, K. (2013b). State of the e-mental health field in Australia: Where are we now? *Australian and New Zealand Journal of Psychiatry, 47*(2), 117–120.

Creswell, J. W. (2013). *Research design: Qualitative, quantitative, and mixed methods approaches* (4th ed.). London: Sage Publications, Incorporated.

Eisenhardt, K. M. (1989). Building theories from case study research. *Academy of management review, 14*(4), 532–550.

Eysenbach, G. (2001). What is e-health? *Journal of Medical Internet research, 3*(2), E20.

Fidel, R. (1984). The case study method: A case study. *Library and Information Science Research, 6*(3), 273–288.

Gallagher, E. B. (2002). Modernization and health reform in Saudi Arabia, Chapter 4. In A. C. Twaddle (Eds.), *Health care reform around the world* (pp. 181–197). London: Auburn House.

Jorm, A. F., Morgan, A. J., & Malhi, G. S. (2013). The future of e-mental health. *Australian and New Zealand Journal of Psychiatry, 47*(2), 104–106.

Jorm, A. F., Wright, A., & Morgan, A. J. (2007). Where to seek help for a mental disorder? *The Medical Journal of Australia, 187*(10), 556–560.

Kavanagh, D., Andrews, G., Scharr, S., Helpline, K., & Spence, S. (2014). E-Mental health services in Australia 2014: Current and future. The e-Mental Health Alliance.

Koenig, H. G., Al Zaben, F., Sehlo, M. G., Khalifa, D. A., Al Ahwal, M. S., Qureshi, N. A., & Al-Habeeb, A. A. (2014). Mental health care in Saudi Arabia: Past, present and future. *Open Journal of Psychiatry, 4*(02), 113.

Lal, S., & Adair, C. E. (2014). E-mental health: A rapid review of the literature. *Psychiatric Services, 65*(1), 24–32.

Ministry News. (2013). King Abdullah approves of allocating SR 15 billion to establish 22 health projects. http://www.moh.gov.sa/en/Ministry/MediaCenter/News/Pages/News-2013-04-24-003.aspx. Accessed 15 July 2014.

Ministry of Health Portal. (2011). National e-health strategy. http://www.moh.gov.sa/en/Ministry/nehs/Pages/Overview-of-eHealth.aspx. Accessed 12 July 2014.

MoH. (2011). Statistical Book for the Year 1432. http://www.moh.gov.sa. http://www.moh.gov.sa/en/Ministry/Statistics/book/Documents/1431.rar.

MoH. (2012). Statistical Book for the Year 1433. http://www.moh.gov.sa. http://www.moh.gov.sa/en/Ministry/Statistics/book/Documents/1433.pdf.

Moumtzoglou, A. (2011). E-Health: A Bridge to People-Centered Health Care. In A. Moumtzoglou & A. Kastania (Eds.), *E-Health Systems Quality and Reliability:* Models and Standards (pp. 47–63). Hershey, PA: . doi:10.4018/978-1-61692-843-8.ch005.

Nuviun Digital Health. (2014). Saudi Arabia is building a massive nationwide ehealth network. http://nuviun.com/content/blog/saudi-Arabia-eHealth. Accessed 14 July 2014.

Proudfoot, J., Parker, G., Pavlovic, D. H., Manicavasagar, V., Adler, E., & Whitton, A. (2010). Community attitudes to the appropriation of mobile phones for monitoring and managing depression, anxiety, and stress. *Journal of Medical Internet Research, 12*(5), e64.

Qurban, M., & Austria, R. (2008). Public Perception on E-Health Services: Implications of Preliminary Findings of the King Fahd Military Medical Complex for Military Hospitals in the Kingdom of Saudi Arabia. Paper presented at the European and Mediterranean Conference on Information Systems (EMCIS), Dubai.

Qureshi, N. A., Al-Habeeb, A. A., & Koenig, H. G. (2013). Mental health system in Saudi Arabia: An overview. *Neuropsychiatric Disease and Treatment, 9*, 1121.

Stake, R. E. (1995). The art of case study research.

Whittaker, R., Merry, S., Stasiak, K., McDowell, H., Doherty, I., Shepherd, M., Dorey, E., Parag, V., Ameratunga, S., & Rodgers, A. (2012). MEMO—A mobile phone depression prevention intervention for adolescents: Development process and postprogram findings on acceptability from a randomized controlled trial. *Journal of Medical Internet Research, 14*(1), e13.

Yin, R. K. (2009). *Case study research: Design and methods* (Vol. 5). Thousand Oaks: Sage.

Bader Binhadyan (Dip.Comp.Prog., B.I.T., M.B.I.S. (Prof.) Ph.D. candidate) has worked and studied in Australia, the Middle East and North America, which helped him to get insight into different cultures and crafted his ability to introduce new ideas. He has interests in psychology, and technology has influenced his research interests.

Dr. Konrad Peszynski His specific research interests include supply chain management and associated technologies, eBusiness, eProcurement and the social aspects of information.

His Ph.D. titled "Power and Politics in a System Implementation" was awarded in 2006 at Deakin University (Victoria, Australia). His Ph.D. had a strong focus on the social issues surrounding systems implementation. The study aimed to identify the role of power and politics in systems implementation.

Since joining Royal Melbourne Institute of Technology (RMIT), Konrad has been involved in the School of Business IT and Logistics and teaches the Masters of Strategic Procurement, Masters of Logistics and Supply Chain Management, Masters of Business (Information Technology) and the Masters of Commerce.

Prof. Nilmini Wickramasinghe (Ph.D.; M.B.A.; Grad.Dip.Mgt.St.; B.Sc.; Amus.A, piano; Amus.A, violin) has a well-recognised research record in the field of health care and information systems and information technology (IT/IS). Her expertise is in the strategic application and management of technology for effecting superior health-care solutions. She currently is professor director of Health Informatics Management at Epworth HealthCare and a professor at Deakin University.

Chapter 21
Data Accuracy in mHealth

Zaid Zekiria Sako, Vass Karpathiou and Nilmini Wickramasinghe

Introduction

Reports from the World Health Organization indicate that noncommunicable diseases are the leading cause of deaths worldwide, where the number of deaths from 2012 are projected to increase from 38 million to 52 million by 2030 (World Health Organization 2015). According to the World Health Organization, noncommunicable diseases are chronic diseases such as cardiovascular diseases, cancers, respiratory diseases, and diabetes. Chronic diseases, change in demographics, increasing costs of medical services, ongoing quality, and safety issues in healthcare are all major health-care challenges that must be dealt with (Armstrong et al. 2007).

These health-care challenges mean finding newer, effective, and innovative ways of battling chronic diseases which ultimately decrease the pressure on health-care systems. The number of mobile phone subscriptions as per the 2014 statistics released by the International Telecommunication Union is estimated to be 6.9 billion worldwide (International Telecommunication Union 2015). This presents an opportunity for mobile phone devices to be used for the management of health and as an intervention in the rising number of chronic diseases, as half of smartphone owners frequently browse for health information online and monitor their health using mobile health (mHealth) applications (Fox and Duggan 2012). As such, the new role for mobile phones is mHealth. The definition of mHealth is the use of portable devices such as smartphones and tablets to improve health (Hamel et al. 2014).

Z. Z. Sako (✉)
60 Baker Ave, Kew East, VIC 3102, Australia
e-mail: zsako@hotmail.com

N. Wickramasinghe
Deakin University and Epworth HealthCare, 60 Baker Ave, Kew East 3102, Australia
e-mail: n.wickramasinghe@deakin.edu.au

V. Karpathiou
School of Business IT and Logistics, Building 80 Level 7, 445 Swanston Street,
Melbourne, VIC 3000, Australia
e-mail: VASS.KARPATHIOU@rmit.edu.au

N. Wickramasinghe et al. (eds.), *Contemporary Consumer Health Informatics*,
Healthcare Delivery in the Information Age, DOI 10.1007/978-3-319-25973-4_21

mHealth has enabled people to play an active role in managing their health rather than being the passive object when seeking treatment during traditional methods (Niilo et al. 2006). The advances in sensor technology such as heart rate, respiratory and blood pressure sensors, along with mobile phone devices, have allowed patients to self-monitor their health before conditions deteriorate and risk being readmitted to hospital (Tarassenko and Clifton 2011).

Individuals can self-monitor the status of their health using any form of mHealth as presented in Table 21.1, which allows for different uses and applications.

While smartphones have a new role to play in the effective management of health and diseases, the technology must be clear of medical errors. Medical error has been defined as a preventable adverse outcome that results from improper medical management (a mistake of commission) rather than from the progression of an illness resulting from lack of care (a mistake of omission) (Van Den Bos et al. 2011). Errors in the medical field belong to a number of domains such as development and use of technologies, ergonomics, administration, management, politics, and economics (Vincent 2010).

A common root cause is human error, where errors are of omission (forgetting to do something) and commission (intentionally doing something that is not meant to be done) (BCS, The Chartered Institute for IT 2012). The Institute of Medicine

Table 21.1 Classification of devices and sensors. (Adapted from Ade 2012)

Form	Description	Examples
Traditional	Medical devices connected to a mobile phone via Bluetooth and which use the phone as a data gateway	Blood pressure monitors, precision weight scales, spirometers
Implantable	Implantable medical devices embedded just below the surface of the skin and which use a small transmitter to send data to a gateway attached to the patient or located in their vicinity. Implantable devices are typically used to monitor disease conditions such as chronic diabetes where constant monitoring 24 h a day is required	GlySens—wireless-enabled glucometer
Wearable	Body sensors and wearable devices contain one or more small, embedded sensors capable of monitoring different physiological and physical parameters	BodyMedia Armband and monitoring system
Ingestible	Small micro-transmitters in chemical agents, which react with the contents of the stomach to generate small electrical signals which are then transmitted via a data hub to a medical station	Proteus ingestible sensor and monitoring system
Mobile peripherals	Devices that can be plugged directly into a mobile phone and which turn the mobile phone into a new medical instrument	AgaMetrix device manufactured by Sanofi Aventis and which is used to monitor diabetes
Mobile apps	Applications that are developed to replicate functionality that is normally provided by a dedicated medical device	iPhone Stethoscope app that records a heart rhythm and plays back a cardiogram

Report “To Err Is Human” estimates that approximately 98,000 people die each year in hospitals due to preventable medical errors (Institute of Medicine 2015). Similarly, 50 % of individuals with chronic diseases have experienced a medication error, while another 30 % with no chronic diseases suffered from the same error (Nuovo 2010).

Medical errors have progressed from human to technological errors. Jenicek (2010) defines technology errors in medicine as errors that relate to data and information recording, processing, and retrieval caused by information technology and its uses (information technology inadequacy and failure). The use of mobile phone technology for managing health has its own set of challenges and complexities, such as accuracy, integrity, privacy, security, and confidentiality. These challenges are of concern to both medical professionals and the Food and Drug Administration (FDA; Wired 2015). Thus, to prevent the spread of medical errors and eliminate risks associated with it, mHealth solutions must be error free.

While the primary concern for mHealth solution is delivering high-quality care through cost-effective technology for better patient outcomes, there are other key areas which are part of the health-care system that can add to the negative effect of inaccurate data and the misleading information. These key areas are:

- Financial and sustainability matters: According to The Data Warehousing Institute, poor data quality has endured businesses a large deficit of around US$600 billion a year with no comparison of cost for health data (Linda 2012).
- Legal: In an overview of the Health Insurance Portability and Accountability Act (HIPAA) privacy laws, personal health information (PHI) must be accurate, complete, up-to-date, and be protected by security safeguards (Cheng and Hung 2008).
- Regulator: As data must be transmitted in a timely manner for it to conform to integrity and for the treatment to be effective and relevant, quality of service and the liability in delayed transmission of health data across operators’ networks in a timely manner must be established, as some aspects of health data communication is still not covered in operators’ licenses (Ade 2012).
- Research and emerging technologies: Big data and emerging technologies, such as Watson, require accurate data as their primary function is to provide insights through different sources of data that help drive decision-making and create competitive advantages.
- Quality: If the mHealth systems cannot be trusted to deliver a high level of quality, it will then remain underutilized, be bypassed or used as a measure of last resort (Akter et al. 2013).

To overcome these challenges and benefit from such promising technology, techniques such as machine learning, which applies probabilistic reasoning after the analysis of data, can help deliver robust and accurate solutions. The effective solution will eventually build on data accuracy and information integrity, which are two fundamental components of mHealth solution that ultimately lead patients to decision-making and affect the quality of health care.

Background

This section will explore and define the key areas of machine learning algorithms, data accuracy, and information integrity as they relate to the specific context of mHealth.

Machine Learning Algorithm

mHealth is a great opportunity and convenient way of tackling diseases and illnesses from both child diseases to chronic diseases (Curioso and Mechael 2010). Smarter technology has been battling chronic diseases by using mobile phones and other devices that have multiple intrinsic sensors, as well as data connectivity that provide around-the-clock support (Haddad et al. 2012). This technology is fast growing and can help solve complex problems and diagnosis of diseases (Lev-Ram 2012). The ability to solve complex problems and perform diagnosis is due to the new generation of smartphones having more advanced computing and communication (Internet access, geo locations) capabilities compared to older versions of mobile phones, where they performed simple tasks and had limited capabilities (Boulos et al. 2011).

As a result of using smartphones for health management, this has enabled smarter use of data as we shift from curing to anticipating and preventing diseases before they occur through real-time data analysis (Kumar et al. 2013). Figure 21.1

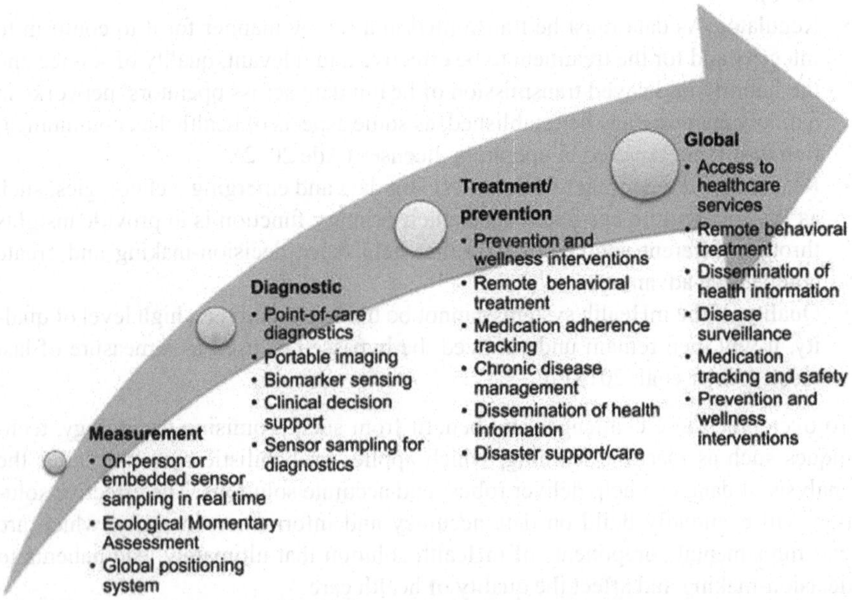

Fig. 21.1 Continuum of mHealth tools. (Adapted from Kumar et al. 2013)

illustrates how mHealth can collect large amount of data as more opportunities emerge for mHealth to be used as tools, such as measurement (GPS locations, sensor readings), diagnosis, treatment and prevention, and access to global health-care services. Despite the opportunities and benefits mHealth brings, the risk of medical errors occurring, such as those found while seeking treatment inside the hospital, can exist and therefore must be constrained. Varshney (2009) describes common medical errors as those found during investigation, diagnosis, treatment, communication, and office administration errors.

Eliminating errors in mHealth can be achieved by learning about the collected data and applying analysis techniques to find new insights that help facilitate a better understanding of how the technology works. A common method is using machine learning algorithms. Machine learning is a knowledge extraction method used when there is great amount of data, and it is achieved through well-designed models or algorithms that can predict for new and unseen data (Lambin et al. 2013). The machine learning algorithms learn and improve the outcomes through experience and observations (Oquendo et al. 2012).

Table 21.2 illustrates the different algorithms used in mHealth developments that accurately detect the symptoms of a disease, perform diagnosis, and monitor patients. These machine learning algorithms are usually trained using available datasets from an existing solution or collected through other means, from which accuracy of the data is then examined through the results produced by the algorithms.

The concept of machine learning is learning that improves with experience at some task. That is (Bell 2014):

- Improve over task, T
- With respect to performance measure, P
- Based on experience, E

Machine learning algorithms can play a pivotal role in acquiring accurate data through pre-trained algorithms that can be deployed in mHealth solutions. The

Table 21.2 Role of machine learning in mobile health

Machine learning algorithm	Applications	Uses	Source
Artificial neural networks	Diabetes	Diagnosing diabetes using neural networks on small mobile devices	Karan et al. 2012
Support vector machines, sparse multinomial logistic regression (SMLR), Naïve Bayes, decision trees, k-nearest neighbor	Fall detection	Fall classification by machine learning using mobile phones	Albert et al. 2012
Bayesian network	Heart rate	Real-time robust heart rate estimation based on Bayesian framework and grid filters	Radoslav and Pavel 2012
Classifiers	Autism	Use of machine learning to shorten observation-based screening and diagnosis of autism	Wall et al. 2012

support vector machine (SVM) algorithm was deployed in a blood pressure measurement application on an android tablet that detected the patient's arm and ensured stability, in order to acquire accurate reading of the data performed by the cuffs (Murthy and Kotz 2014). In a fall detection scenario, recorded data were used from a database which contained 95 instances of recorded falls, from which four types of machine learning algorithms were then applied to accurately detect a fall (Sannino et al. 2014)..

Machine learning techniques can close the "gap" of incomplete or inaccurate data through reasoning capabilities that they have (Martha and Bart 2006). In the medical field, trained algorithms can be used to overcome uncertainties in medical diagnosis and provide crisp results. A simple method is the use of fuzzy logic algorithms. Fuzzy logic is a method that renders precise what is imprecise and is excellent in handling ambiguous, fuzzy data, and imprecise information prevalent in medical diagnosis (Djam and Kimbi 2011). This method along with other machine learning algorithms, such as artificial neural networks or association rules, can be applied at the stage of data collection where values captured are of exact or approximate reflection of the patient's current condition.

The role of machine learning in detecting inaccurate data through reasoning could prove crucial in enhancing the quality of data collection stage of mHealth as the accuracy aspect of data is a major challenge itself. Removing inaccuracy and assuring high-data quality would mean a plethora of solutions that can be developed to help manage diseases and lower the premature rate of deaths, as well as reduce health-care costs. This makes data accuracy a critical part of the overall design of mHealth solution that must be present at all time.

Data Accuracy

The term data itself can be defined as information in the form of facts or figures obtained from experiments or surveys, used as a basis for making calculations or drawing conclusion, as defined by Dumas (2013). According to the World Health Organization, accuracy of data is an element of data quality that is intended to achieve desirable objectives using legitimate means, and its accuracy is the original source of the data (World Health Organization 2014). In mHealth, the collected data is simply the patient describing their symptoms, side effects, and providing other information when suffering from an illness (Estrin and Sim 2010). The quality of the data helps evaluate health, assess effectiveness of interventions, monitor trends, inform health policy, and set priorities (van Velthoven et al. 2013).

Accuracy of the data provided through mHealth solution helps convey a better picture of ones' health status. When data lacks accuracy, currency, or certainty, it can have catastrophic results (Sadiq 2013). For mHealth solution to be effective and safe, the data collected from mHealth devices, wearables, and applications must be accurate and secure (Mottl 2014). Data accuracy is a foundational feature or dimension that contributes to data quality (Gregori and Berchialla 2012), and it is still a major part of mHealth developments, as some of the traditional ways of assessing the patients provide inaccurate data (Lin 2013).

The common standard for data collection in the medical field is the Gold Standard, which is direct observation of patients at the clinic (Eisele et al. 2013). This standard is missing in mHealth solutions as there is no direct observation from the medical professionals when data is collected. The common method of data collection in mHealth is through data entry by users or collected automatically if it is a sensor-based solution. This step can prove crucial, and if not addressed appropriately, this innovative mHealth technology can build on existing health-care challenges and contribute significantly to health problems.

Figure 21.2 is an illustration of how observation through mHealth differs from the traditional direct observation and the risk of not conveying the full picture of patients' health status.

The issue of data inaccuracy can be classified into four categories. These categories are initial data entry, data decay, moving and restructuring, and using data (Olson 2003).

1. *Initial data entry*: Mistakes, data entry processes, deliberate, system errors
2. *Data decay*: Accuracy of data when originally created over time
3. *Moving and restructuring*: Extract, cleansing, transformation, loading, integration
4. *Using*: Faulty reporting, lack of understanding

In addition to the four categories described above, intentional and unintentional wrong data entry and speed of data collection that are misleading can result in misallocating resources or interventions when needed for the patients (Patnaik, Brunskill and Thies 2009). Inaccurate readings, insufficient amount of data, movement and physical activities also contribute to inaccurate data provided through the mHealth devices (Mena et al. 2013). Another factor that affects the quality of data is security breaches, where unauthorized modification or alteration is made to patients' data that compromise their confidentiality and privacy (Mena et al. 2013).

Concerns associated with data accuracy and validity are persistent and can become a risk to patients' safety (Linda 2012). For data to be accurate, it must always

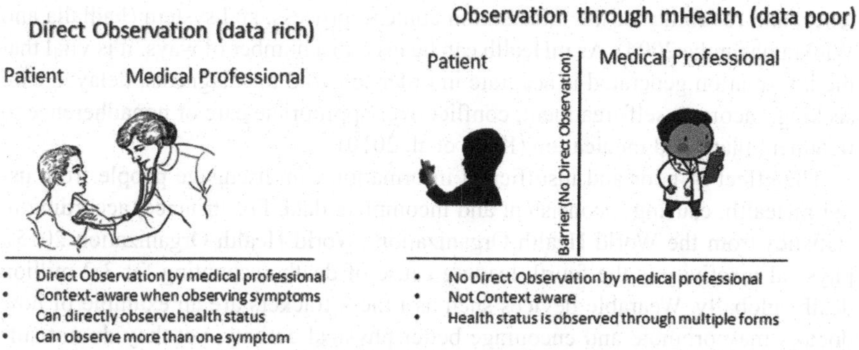
Direct Observation (data rich)
Patient
Medical Professional
Observation through mHealth (data poor)
Patient
Barrier (No Direct Observation)
Medical Professional
• Direct Observation by medical professional
• Context-aware when observing symptoms
• Can directly observe health status
• Can observe more than one symptom
• No Direct Observation by medical professional
• Not Context aware
• Health status is observed through multiple forms

Fig. 21.2 Direct observation compared to observation through mHealth consist of completeness, consistency, currency, relevance, and accuracy (Närman et al. 2011). In mHealth, these elements of data quality can be compromised as data goes through five different stages. These are: (1) collection, (2) transmission, (3) analysis, (4) storage, and (5) presentation (Klonoff 2013).

To increase the accuracy, often a single-value data does not sufficiently convey the whole health status of a patient. WE-CARE system is an mHealth solution for the detection of cardiovascular diseases, in which seven electrocardiogram (ECG) leads are used to guarantee that data is accurate (Anpeng et al. 2014). In direct observation, when the medical professional performs blood pressure reading (collecting data), there is usually other observations made to help evaluate the patients. In an mHealth solution, a single reading of blood pressure does not convey the full picture and is often measured against thresholds (high and low limits) which trigger an alarm.

Acquiring context-aware rich data from which rules and knowledge can be inferred from is enabling mHealth techniques to mimic real-life scenarios and provide resourceful feedback. An example of obtaining context-aware data is demonstrated in a study where a Microsoft Sensecam camera analyzed photos of food for dietary analysis to help athletes and sporting people calculate calories, energy intake and prepare for events (O'Loughlin et al. 2013).

The accuracy of the data contributes to data integrity that has been defined as maintaining and assuring the accuracy and consistency of data over its entire life cycle (Cucoranu et al. 2013). Therefore, data accuracy and consistency are critical to increasing data integrity as it goes through the five stages. The information produced based on the set of data must not only be of high quality but also conform to integrity expectation of the user.

Information Integrity

Information at the very basic level is raw data that is processed and transformed into information from which knowledge is then extracted (Dumas 2013). Thus, information integrity is about having the right properties of information including sensitivity in which information is used, as well as encompassing accuracy, consistency, and reliability of the information content, process, and system (Fadlalla and Wickramasinghe 2004). As mHealth can be used in a number of ways, it is vital that the information generated is accurate in order to avoid misdiagnosis, delayed care seeking, incorrect self-treatment, conflict over appropriate care or nonadherence to treatment plans and medication (Kahn et al. 2010).

The effect of poor and insufficient information can disengage people from using mHealth, causing inconsistent and incomplete data. For instance, according to statistics from the World Health Organization (World Health Organization 2015), physical inactivity is the fourth leading cause of death accounting for 3.2 million deaths globally. Wearable devices such as fitness trackers are an example of how doctors may promote and encourage better physical activity, yet they do not sufficiently satisfy the patient with the information provided and therefore can deter people from exercising (Product Design & Development 2015).

As important as it is to have accurate and valid data, it is equally important to have information integrity. The integrity of information produced as a result of shift in the dynamics of technology has been getting more focus as the interaction experience has changed (Cunningham 2012). The shift from clinician care towards patient-centered model is encouraging patients to actively self-manage and make decisions concerning their health (David et al. 2011). Smartphones have allowed people access to health information (Boulos et al. 2011), and to harness the power of mHealth in order to benefit from it, the technology must be error free and provide rich health information.

Errors in health-care systems due to data loss, incorrect data entry, displayed or transmitted data can lead to loss of information integrity (Bowman 2013). Thus, when patients are treated inside the hospital, their details and information are checked prior to being provided with the treatment to ensure that there are no medical errors.

During the data collection stage, if the data is inaccurate, it continues through the data transformation cycle (as per Fig. 21.3) till it reaches the medical professional where they apply their reasoning based on the data provided, from which a recommended set of actions or treatment is then suggested. This can be a disastrous way of recommending treatment if there are no pre-checks or control behind the reasoning, specifically when there are no tools or guidance used to provide the treatment.

To overcome the challenge of correctly treating patients using mHealth and ensure information integrity, data governance, information workflow management, internal controls, confidentiality, and data privacy processes must exist (Flowerday and Solms 2008). These processes along with information technology can improve the quality of care by decreasing medical errors due to inaccurate and untimely information (Mahmood et al. 2012). Using a semantic tool when processing the data and transforming it into information can prove crucial in detecting errors when inaccurate information is generated, thus stopping it from being turned into actions and preventing medical errors.

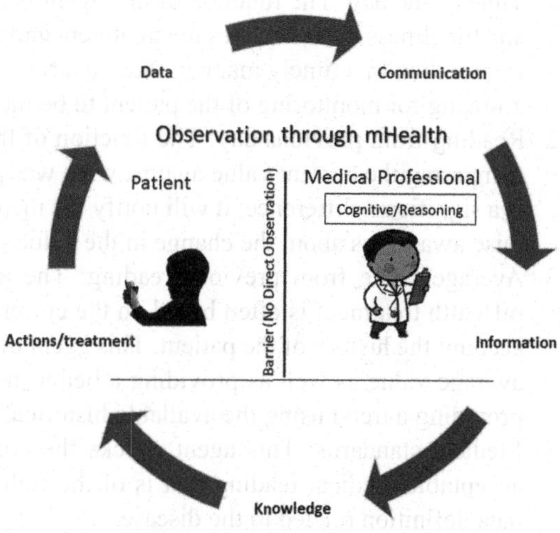

Fig. 21.3 Transformation of data into knowledge in order to provide right treatment

The Omaha System (latest 2005 edition) is a semantic tool that is used in a number of domains including medical diagnosis, which involves the aggregation and analysis of clinical data and better information management (The Omaha System 2015). This comprehensive guide can enhance the quality of mHealth solution and control the quality of information, as wrong information can potentially have significant repercussions resulting in misleading information fed through to all the stakeholders involved in an mHealth transaction.

Research Question

The following will investigate data accuracy and information integrity in the context of mHealth solutions in health care by first answering the research question:

How can machine learning be applied in mHealth solutions to provide data accuracy and information integrity?

Conceptual Model

To help address the accuracy problem in mHealth, the conceptual model (see Fig. 21.5) addresses data inaccuracy and allows medical professionals to detect errors in data through the use of multiple agents. This conceptual model not only detects data inaccuracy, but also positions the data to be checked from the same perspective as would a medical professional during direct observation of the patients.

The four agents described in the conceptual model can perform smart functions which help detect and assess the accuracy of the value that is received from a patient during the use of mHealth.

1. Time of the day: The function of this agent is to check for data decay, currency, and timeliness, which makes the treatment and actions to be relevant and provide information in a timely manner, thus ensuring no delay in seeking treatment and allowing for monitoring of the patient to be more relevant.
2. Reading from previous day: The function of this agent is to detect mistakes by comparing the current value against what was provided previously. Where there is a significant difference, it will notify the medical professional of such event to raise awareness about the change in the value.
3. Average value from previous reading: The advice given to a patient during mHealth treatment is often based on the current value and does not take into an account the history of the patient. This agent performs calculations that finds the average value as well as providing a better insight of the patient's behavior by providing a trend using the available historical data.
4. Medical standards: This agent checks the current value against the standard, acceptable medical reading that is of the right range and conforms to medical data definition related to the disease.

The objective of these four initial collective agents is to address data integrity elements and contextualize the data to help bring the gold direct observation standard that is often used when a medical professional examines the patient at a medical clinic. Having performed all these checks, the medical professional who provides the treatment based on the data can now have more context around the data that helps remove any biased opinion or uncertainty.

Once the data is of high accuracy and integrity, the Omaha System (as illustrated in Fig. 21.4) can be implemented as a guide to classify the problem (disease) and list down the signs and symptoms that must be observed in order for the designated intervention method to be relevant and effective. The ratings of the outcomes from the intervention method will provide knowledge and feedback to both the patient and the medical professional.

Using the four agents along with the exhaustive Omaha System semantic tool for mHealth solutions will not only enable accurate data to be collected but also cover the big picture of how a patient should be treated and provide an understanding of how the disease is progressing.

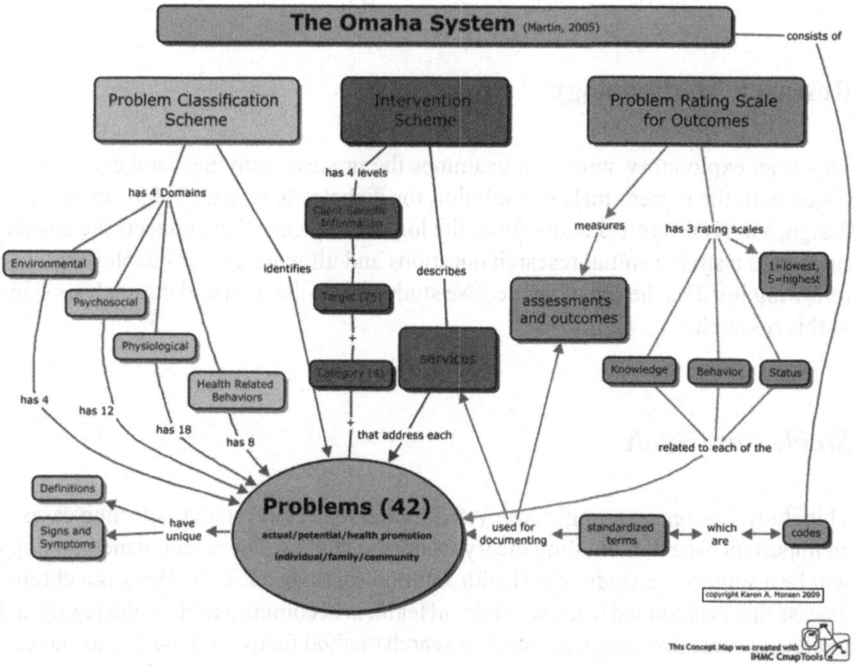

Fig. 21.4 The Omaha System 2005 version. (Adapted from The Omaha System Chart 2015)

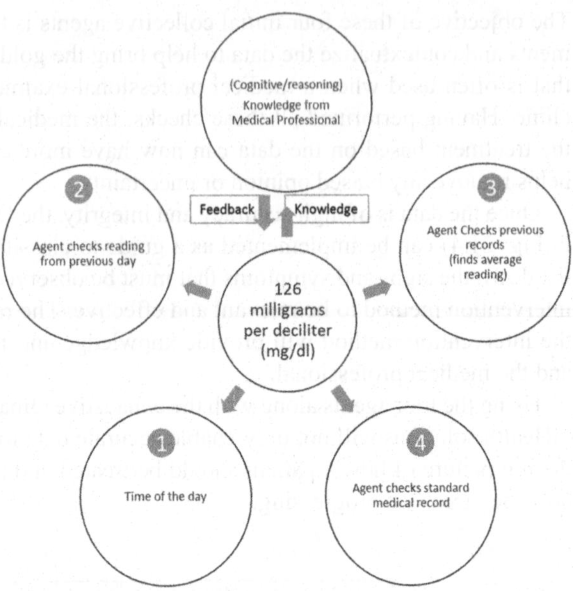

Fig. 21.5 Conceptual model consisting of agents that contextualize data

Research Methodology

This is an exploratory study that examines the process, activities, and events associated with the current mHealth solution for diabetes (Creswell 2003). In research design, Yin (2003) refers to design as the logical sequence that connects the empirical data to a study's initial research questions and ultimately to its conclusions. The following justifies the use of single case study, data collection and the analysis stage of this research.

Single Case Study

This study focuses on a single case. As Gummesson (1991) stated, selecting cases is an important aspect of building theory from case studies. The research methodology will be a single case study of mHealth solution for diabetes, as diabetes is a chronic disease that is predicted to grow, while mHealth is becoming a tool for managing and treating chronic diseases. Case study research method focuses on the circumstances, dynamics, and complexity of a single case study as they are explored in depth using detailed observations or information from records as explained by Bowling (2009). For health-care organizations and health-related studies, case study is an appropriate method to investigate and explore the complexities and issues (Caronna 2010).

Data Collection

For the purpose of this research, secondary, de-identified data will be used, that is, data used for research purposes and do not identify or represent a person (McGraw 2012). Secondary data can include a number of empirical forms, such as those that are generated from systemic reviews, documentary analysis, as well as those generated from large-scale datasets (Smith 2008). It can also provide further interpretation other than the one originally intended for (Singleton 1988).

Data Triangulation

The datasets used for the purpose of this research will be drawn from a single source at different times to check the accuracy and support the analysis of the data (Flick et al. 2004).

Data Sampling

Convenience sampling will be used for this research, as secondary data from an existing mHealth solution is available for research purposes (Abbott and McKinney 2013). Convenience sampling is simply when people are available to participate in a research or can be conveniently be recruited (Gideon 2012).

Data Analysis Techniques

For the data analysis phase of this research design, archival and hermeneutic analysis techniques will be used in this research (Creswell 2003). Archival records are those of computer files and records (Yin 2009). Archives can contain official sources such as government papers, organizational records, medical records, personal collection, and other contextual materials (Corti 2004).

The hermeneutic analysis approach will be applied using the following phenomenological method which involves (Taylor et al. 2013):

1. Turning to the nature of the lived experience
2. Investigating experience as we live it, rather than as we conceptualize it
3. Reflecting on the essential themes, which characterize the phenomenon
4. Describe the phenomenon through the art of writing and rewriting
5. Maintaining a string and oriented relation to the phenomenon
6. Balancing the research context by considering the parts and the whole

Organize and Prepare Data

For the data to be ready for data analysis stage, it is reviewed for any missing values and format to ensure it is ready for analysis.

Detailed Analysis (Steps)

Analyze the data by applying code to each of the data integrity elements and categorize it using nVivo software, along with small write-ups regarding the quality of the data to perform within case data analysis (Eisenhardt 1989).

Steps

1. Collect 6 months of de-identified raw data that has been transmitted over for processing.
2. Create 4 different data sets and label them from 1 to 4.
3. Obtain the same data after processing.
4. Plot the data both raw and processed (field vs. values) using graphs.
5. Compare the results against:
   - *Accuracy*: Origin of the data when it was transmitted and values (range, low value, high value). Check if any correction has been made after processing.
   - *Reliability*: Consistency of the values over time.
   - *Currency*: Time stamps of the process and the values produced as a result.
   - *Timeliness*: Verify values and check for consistency.
   - *Completeness*: Fields and the values entered correctly.
   - *Readable*: Format of the values and content created.
   - *Relevancy*: What information is produced and how relevant are they.
6. Match the right machine learning algorithm that best describes step 5 and simulate it using any machine learning tool (i.e., Weka tool).
7. Compare machine learning output against the processed data.
8. Use the Omaha System as a guide for producing the information, and find the correlation between the processed data and the Information generated from the Omaha System.

Coding Process

Code the data using qualitative content analysis technique by identifying themes and patterns (thematic analysis) based on the data element and timeline of the data (Wahyuni 2012).

Discussion and Conclusions

This chapter serves to present a research in progress study that focuses on trying to optimize data assets in an mHealth context. In particular, it focuses on critical considerations regarding data accuracy and information integrity. Further, it has provided the conceptual model and described the research design to be followed. While still at an early stage, the research should provide important implications for theory and practice pertaining to achieving more accurate data in mHealth solutions.

From the perspective of practice, the research should provide an exhaustive examination into why data accuracy is of paramount importance to not just the delivery of high-quality health services through mHealth technology, but also the ripple effect it has on other key stakeholders and areas associated with it.

From the perspective of theory, the study will assist in developing a new area of knowledge that establishes methods of bringing a Gold Standard direct observation to mHealth using machine learning as a step to validate the accuracy of the data and extending the data collection method to include more than a single based value that helps convey one's health status.

As mHealth grows and the domain of consumer health informatics matures, we will see more and more mobile solutions being embraced to support health and wellness. Central to the success of these solutions is that they provide accurate data and information to consumers who in turn make decisions with far-reaching implications based on the data and information received. The findings from this study will clearly be significant in ensuring optimal value from such mHealth solution.

With the key areas for implications being highlighted earlier, the limitations faced in this research must also be highlighted. This research focuses on one mHealth solution that utilizes data entry process for data collection. The data collection methods in mHealth vary from one solution to another, as some incorporate automatic data capturing through sensors or image analysis, in which the data is then sent for analysis based on the design of the solution. However, although the data capturing methods differ, data entry process is still a common method that is used in mHealth, and the consequent need for accurate and integritous data will always be important.

A key challenge for this research that requires mentioning is the use of secondary data. Using secondary data does not allow this research to observe the patients nor their behavior during the use of the mHealth solution, specifically when the patient enters the data. Thus, this research does not take into consideration the human factors that can affect the accuracy of the data. Despite this difficulty, this is a major challenge in mHealth as there is no direct observation of the patient or their behavior when the data is collected. Using the secondary data will help establish methods that can overcome this challenge and ensure data accuracy in mHealth.

References

Abbott, M. L., & McKinney, J. (2013). *Understanding and applying research design.* Hoboken: Wiley.

Ade, B. (2012). *Mobile healthcare: Challenges and opportunities mobile technology consumption: Opportunities and challenges* (pp. 77–98). Hershey: IGI Global.

Akter, S., Ray, P., & D'Ambra, J. (2013). Continuance of mHealth services at the bottom of the pyramid: The roles of service quality and trust. *The International Journal on Networked Business, 23*(1), 29–47. doi:10.1007/s12525-012-0091-5.

Albert, M. V., Kording, K., Herrmann, M., & Jayaraman, A. (2012). Fall classification by machine learning using mobile phones. *PLoS ONE, 7*(5), e36556. doi:10.1371/journal.pone.0036556.

Anpeng, H., Chao, C., Kaigui, B., Xiaohui, D., Min, C., Hongqiao, G., & Linzhen, X. (2014). WE-CARE: An intelligent mobile telecardiology system to enable mHealth applications. *IEEE Journal of Biomedical and Health Informatics, 18*(2), 693–702. doi:10.1109/JBHI.2013.2279136.

Armstrong, B. K., Gillespie, J. A., Leeder, S. R., Rubin, G. L., & Russell, L. M. (2007). Challenges in health and health care for Australia. *Medical Journal of Australia, 187*(9), 485–489.

Bell, J. (2014). *Machine Learning: Hands-on for developers and technical professionals*. Indianapolis: Wiley.

Boulos, M. N. K., Wheeler, S., Tavares, C., & Jones, R. (2011). How smartphones are changing the face of mobile and participatory healthcare: An overview, with example from eCAALYX. *BioMedical Engineering OnLine, 10*, 24–24. doi:10.1186/1475-925X-10-24.

Bowling, A. (2009). *Research methods in health: Investigating health and health services* (3rd ed.). Maidenhead: McGraw-Hill Education.

Bowman, S. (2013). Impact of electronic health record systems on information integrity: Quality and safety implications. *Perspectives in Health Information Management, 10*, 1–1c.

Caronna, C. A. (2010). Why use qualitative methods to study health care organizations? Insights from multi-level case studies. In I. Bourgeault, R. Dingwall, & D. V. Raymond (Eds.), *The SAGE handbook qualitative methods health research.* London: Sage.

Cheng, V., & Hung, P. (2008). *An overview of the HIPAA-compliant privacy access control model.*

Corti, L. (2004). *Archival research. The SAGE encyclopedia of social science research methods.* Thousand Oaks: Sage.

Creswell, J. W. (2003). *Research design: Qualitative, quantitative, and mixed method approaches* (2nd ed.). Thousand Oaks: Sage.

Cucoranu, I. C., Parwani, A. V., West, A. J., Romero-Lauro, G., Nauman, K., Carter, A. B., & Pantanowitz, L. (2013). Privacy and security of patient data in the pathology laboratory. *Journal of Pathology Informatics, 4*, 4. doi:10.4103/2153-3539.108542.

Cunningham, P. (2012). It's most important role: Ensuring information integrity. *Information Management, 46*(3), 20–22, 24, 47.

Curioso, W. H., & Mechael, P. N. (2010). Enhancing 'M-health' with south-to-south collaborations. *Health Affairs (Project Hope), 29*(2), 264. doi:10.1377/hlthaff.2009.1057.

David, W., Sara, U., & Erin, J. (2011). *Personal health information in the age of ubiquitous health clinical technologies: Concepts, methodologies, tools and applications* (pp. 50–72). Hershey: IGI Global.

Djam, X., & Kimbi, Y. (2011). Fuzzy expert system for the management of hypertension. *The Pacific Journal of Science and Technology, 12*(1), 390–402.

Dumas, M. B. (2013). *Diving into the bitstream: Information technology meets society in a digital world.* New York: Routledge.

Eisele, T. P., Silumbe, K., Yukich, J., Hamainza, B., Keating, J., Bennett, A., & Miller, J. M. (2013). Measuring coverage in MNCH: Accuracy of measuring diagnosis and treatment of childhood malaria from household surveys in Zambia. *PLoS Medicine, 10*(5), e1001417. doi:10.1371/journal.pmed.1001417.

Eisenhardt, K. M. (1989). Building theories from case study research. *Academy of Management. The Academy of Management Review, 14*(4), 532.

Estrin, D., & Sim, I. (2010). Health care delivery. Open mHealth architecture: An engine for health care innovation. *Science, 330*(6005), 759–760. doi:10.1126/science.1196187.

Fadlalla, A., & Wickramasinghe, N. (2004). An integrative framework for HIPAA-compliant I*IQ healthcare information systems. *International Journal of Health Care Quality Assurance Incorporating Leadership in Health Services, 17*(2–3), 65–74.

Flick, U., Kardorff, E. v., & Steinke, I. (2004). *A companion to qualitative research*. London: Sage.

Flowerday, S., & Solms, R. V. (2008). What constitutes information integrity? *South African Journal of Information Management, 10*(2), 2–11.

Fox, S., & Duggan, M. (2012). Mobile health 2012. *Washington, DC: Pew Internet & American Life Project.*

Gideon, L. (2012). *Handbook of survey methodology for the social sciences*. New York: Springer.

Gregori, D., & Berchialla, P. (2012). Quality of electronic medical records. In F. W. Faltin, R. S. Kenett, & F. Ruggeri (Eds.), *Statistical methods in healthcare* (pp. 456–480). Wiley.

Gummesson, E. (1991). *Qualitative methods in management research* (Rev. ed.). London: Sage.

Haddad, D., Selsky, J., Hoffman, J. E., Kravitz, R. L., Estrin, D. E., & Sim, I. (2012). Making sense of mobile health data: An open architecture to improve individual- and population-level health. *Journal of Medical Internet Research, 14*(4), 10–10.

Hamel, M. B., Cortez, N. G., Cohen, I. G., & Kesselheim, A. S. (2014). FDA regulation of mobile health technologies. *The New England Journal of Medicine, 371*(4), 372–379.

Institute of Medicine. (2015). To err is human. http://www.iom.edu/~/media/Files/Report%20 Files/1999/To-Err-is-Human/To%20Err%20is%20Human%201999%20%20report%20brief.pdf. Accessed 1 May 2015.

International Telecommunication Union. ICT Facts and Figs. (2015). http://www.itu.int/en/ITU-D/Statistics/Documents/statistics/2015/ITU_Key_2005–2015_ICT_data.xls. Accessed 16 July 2015.

BCS, The Chartered Institute for IT. (2012). *Health informatics: Improving patient care*. Swindon: British Informatics Society Limited.

Jenicek, M. (2010). *Medical error and harm understanding, prevention, and control*. Hoboken: Taylor and Francis.

Kahn, J. G., Yang, J. S., & Kahn, J. S. (2010). 'Mobile' health needs and opportunities in developing countries. *Health Affairs, 29*(2), 252–258.

Karan, O., Bayraktar, C., Gümüşkaya, H., & Karlık, B. (2012). Diagnosing diabetes using neural networks on small mobile devices. *Expert Systems with Applications, 39*(1), 54–60. doi:10.1016/j.eswa.2011.06.046.

Klonoff, D. C. (2013). The current status of mHealth for diabetes: will it be the next big thing? *Journal of Diabetes Science and Technology, 7*(3), 749–758.

Kumar, S., Nilsen, W. J., Abernethy, A., Atienza, A., Patrick, K., Pavel, M., & Swendeman, D. (2013). Mobile health technology evaluation: The mHealth evidence workshop. *American Journal of Preventive Medicine, 45*(2), 228–236. doi:10.1016/j.amepre.2013.03.017.

Lambin, P., Roelofs, E., Reymen, B., Velazquez, E. R., Buijsen, J., Zegers, C. M., & Dekker, A. (2013). 'Rapid Learning health care in oncology'—an approach towards decision support systems enabling customised radiotherapy. *Radiotherapy and Oncology, 109*(1), 159–164. doi:10.1016/j.radonc.2013.07.007.

Lev-Ram, M. (2012). The supercomputer will see you now. *Fortune, 166*(9), 50.

Lin, J. Y. (2013). Mobile health tracking of sleep bruxism for clinical, research, and personal reflection.

Linda, L. K. (2012). Information integrity: A high risk, high cost vulnerability; proper information goverance includes paying attention to some key building blocks (GOVERNANCE). *Health Data Management, 20*(4), 44.

Mahmood, N., Burney, A., Abbas, Z., & Rizwan, K. (2012). Data and Knowledge management in designing healthcare information systems. *Growth, 9*(10), 11.

Martha, E. P., & Bart, P. (2006). Computer science tools and techniques. In A. Mihailidis, E. B. Jakob, & D. Wan (Eds.), *Pervasive computing in healthcare* (pp. 21–45). Florida: CRC Press.

McGraw, D. (2012). Building public trust in uses of Health Insurance Portability and Accountability Act de-identified data. *Journal of the American Medical Informatics Association, 20*(1), 29. doi:10.1136/amiajnl-2012-000936.

Mena, L. J., Felix, V. G., Ostos, R., Gonzalez, J. A., Cervantes, A., Ochoa, A., & Maestre, G. E. (2013). Mobile personal health system for ambulatory blood pressure monitoring. *Computational and Mathematical Methods in Medicine, 2013*, 13. doi:10.1155/2013/598196.
Mottl, J. (2014). The imperative of safety in mHealth and why it can't be ignored.
Murthy, R., & Kotz, D. (2014). *Assessing blood-pressure measurement in tablet-based mHealth apps*. Paper presented at the COMSNETS.
Närman, P., Holm, H., Johnson, P., König, J., Chenine, M., & Ekstedt, M. (2011). Data accuracy assessment using enterprise architecture. *Enterprise Information Systems, 5*(1), 37–58. doi:10.1080/17517575.2010.507878.
Niilo, S., Ilkka, K., & Elina, M. (2006). Mobile and personal health and wellness management systems. A. Mihailidis, J. E. Bardram, & D. Wan (Eds.), *Pervasive computing in healthcare* (pp. 105–134). CRC Press.
Nuovo, J. (2010). *Chronic disease management*. Dordrecht: Springer.
O'Loughlin, G., Cullen, S. J., McGoldrick, A., O'Connor, S., Blain, R., O'Malley, S., & Warrington, G. D. (2013). Using a wearable camera to increase the accuracy of dietary analysis. *American Journal of Preventive Medicine, 44*(3), 297–301. doi:10.1016/j.amepre.2012.11.007.
Olson, J. E. (2003). Sources of inaccurate data. In J. E. Olson (Ed.), *Data quality* (pp. 43–64). San Francisco: Morgan Kaufmann.
Oquendo, M. A., Baca-Garcia, E., Artes-Rodriguez, A., Perez-Cruz, F., Galfalvy, H. C., Blasco-Fontecilla, H., & Duan, N. (2012). Machine Learning and data mining: strategies for hypothesis generation. *Molecular Psychiatry, 17*, 956+.
Patnaik, S., Brunskill, E., & Thies, W. (2009, 17–19 April 2009). *Evaluating the accuracy of data collection on mobile phones: A study of forms, SMS, and voice*. Paper presented at the Information and Communication Technologies and Development (ICTD), 2009 International Conference on.
Product Design & Development. (2015). Challenges for doctors using fitness trackers & apps. http://www.pddnet.com/news/2015/02/challengesdoctorsusingfitnesstrackersapps. Accessed 24 Feb 2015.
Radoslav, B., & Pavel, S. (2012). *Real-time robust heart rate estimation based on Bayesian framework and grid filters medical applications of intelligent data analysis: Research advancements* (pp. 67–90). Hershey: IGI Global.
Sadiq, S. E. (2013). *Handbook of data quality research and practice*. Berlin: Springer.
Sannino, G., De Falco, I., & De Pietro, G. (2014). *A general-purpose mHealth system relying on knowledge acquisition through artificial intelligence ambient intelligence-software and applications* (pp. 107–115). Springer.
Singleton, J. F. (1988). Secondary data analysis. *Journal of Physical Education, Recreation and Dance, 59*(4), 38.
Smith, E. (2008). *Using secondary data in educational and social research*. Maidenhead: McGraw-Hill. Education.
Tarassenko, L., & Clifton, D. A. (2011). Semiconductor wireless technology for chronic disease management. *Electronics Letters, 47*(26), S30–S32. doi:10.1049/el.2011.2679.
Taylor, B. J., Francis, K., & Hegney, D. (2013). *Qualitative research in the health sciences methodologies, methods and processes*. London: Routledge.
The Omaha System. (2005). Chart. http://cmapspublic3.ihmc.us/rid=1290438215218_1896624281_17913/2010-11-22%20Omaha%20System%20for%20NSFr.cmap. Accessed 10 June 2015.
The Omaha System. (2015). http://www.omahasystem.org/. Accessed 17 June 2015.
Van Den Bos, J., Rustagi, K., Gray, T., Halford, M., Ziemkiewicz, E., & Shreve, J. (2011). The $17.1 billion problem: The annual cost of measurable medical errors. *Health Affairs, 30*(4), 596–603.
van Velthoven, M. H., Car, J., Zhang, Y., & Marušić, A. (2013). mHealth series: New ideas for mHealth data collection implementation in low- and middle-income countries. *Journal of Global Health, 3*(2), 020101. doi:10.7189/jogh.03.020101.
Varshney, U. (2009). *Pervasive healthcare computing*. Dordrecht: Springer.
Vincent, C. (2010). Putting medical error in context *medical error and harm* (pp. 1–14). New York: Productivity Press.
Wahyuni, D. (2012). *The research design maze: Understanding paradigms, cases, methods and methodologies*. Institute of Certified Management Accountants.

Wall, D. P., Kosmicki, J., DeLuca, T. F., Harstad, E., & Fusaro, V. A. (2012). Use of machine learning to shorten observation-based screening and diagnosis of autism. *Translational Psychiatry, 2*(4), e100. doi:10.1038/tp.2012.10.

WIRED. (2015). These medical apps have doctors and the FDA worried, http://www.wired.com/2014/07/medical_apps/. Accessed 5 May 2015.

World Health Organization. (2014). Improving data quality. http://www.wpro.who.int/publications/docs/Improving_Data_Quality.pdf. Accessed 26 August 2014.

World Health Organization. (2015). Global Status Report on noncommunicable diseases 2014. http://apps.who.int/iris/bitstream/10665/148114/1/9789241564854eng.pdf?ua=1. Accessed 27 April 2015.

Yin, R. K. (2003). *Case study research: Design and methods* (3rd ed.). Thousand Oaks: Sage.

Yin, R. K. (2009). *Case study research: Design and methods* (4th ed.). California: Sage.

Zaid Zekiria Sako graduated in Bachelor of Business (business information systems) from RMIT University and is currently a storage specialist at IBM. His research interests are around mHealth technologies, innovative wearable devices and artificial intelligence.

Vass Karpathiou has a varied experience in academia, business, technology and engineering spanning over 30 years. His interests are developing business technology solutions with a social engagement outcome and value. His current research is focusing on health-care value in the interaction of business, technology, and medicine.

Prof. Nilmini Wickramasinghe Ph.D.; M.B.A.; Grad.Dip.Mgt.St.; B.Sc.; Amus.A, piano; Amus.A, violin has a well-recognized research record in the field of healthcare and IT/IS. Her expertise is in the strategic application and management of technology for effecting superior health-care solutions. She currently is the professor director of Health Informatics Management at Epworth HealthCare and a professor at Deakin University.

Chapter 22
Intelligent Home Risk-Based Monitoring Solutions Enable Post Acute Care Surveillance

Hoda Moghimi, Jonathan L. Schaffer and Nilmini Wickramasinghe

Introduction

A key challenge for healthcare delivery in Organisation for Economic Co-operation and Development (OECD) countries is the projected significant increases in people aged 65 years and over. In particular, Australia will experience an increase of 16.4 % by 2015 while Canada will experience an increase of 16 %, the UK an increase of 17.9 % and the USA an increase of 14.3 % in the same time period (Australian Bureau of Statistics 2010). Such increase in the respective ageing populations will have significant and far reaching implications for healthcare delivery, labour force participation, housing and demand for skilled labour (Australian Bureau of Statistics 2010). Given the impending economic impact of providing healthcare services to this projected increase of seniors, it behoves us to look at possible technology solutions that serve to provide effective and efficient healthcare delivery as well as meet other key considerations highly desired by seniors such as remaining in their own home.

More recently, studies are showing a rapid growth in the number of seniors now using computers in the USA and other developed countries, and this growth is projected to increase (Jimison et al. 2006). In particular, there appears to be a growth in the potential for health-monitoring technologies (Clifford and Clifton 2012). The key aim of such technologies is the maintenance of a seniors' autonomy through understanding how he or she can manage his or her individual health problem, and

H. Moghimi (✉)
15 Pentlowe Ave., Templestowe Lower, Manningham, VIC 3107, Australia
e-mail: moghimi87@gmail.com

J. L. Schaffer
Cleveland Clinic, 9500 Euclid Avenue, Desk A-41, Cleveland, 44195 OH, USA
e-mail: schaffj@ccf.org

N. Wickramasinghe
Deakin University and Epworth HealthCare 60 Baker Ave, Kew East 3102, Australia
e-mail: n.wickramasinghe@deakin.edu.au

N. Wickramasinghe et al. (eds.), *Contemporary Consumer Health Informatics,*
Healthcare Delivery in the Information Age, DOI 10.1007/978-3-319-25973-4_22

what necessary actions should be taken and when (Ludwig et al. 2012). Another important factor concerning home health-based technologies is concerned with reducing the national cost of seniors' treatments by keeping them more at home (Aanesen et al. 2011). Projections by the Congressional Budget Office for Social Security, Medicare and Medicaid transfers as a percentage of gross domestic product (GDP) show the share of output spent on seniors' care programs in the USA rising from 7.6 % in 2000 to 13.9 % in 2030 to 21.1 % in 2075 (Zhang et al. 2009; Falls 2008). Despite the increased number of home-monitoring technologies in age-care contexts, there are several challenges that have to be met before integrating such services into the practice as a real-life application (Ludwig et al. 2012). Some of the major relevant challenges are reliability of the technology due to the lack of prototypes and clinical trials (Karunanithi 2007; Bui and Fonarow 2012), poor technical design and development to address interdisciplinary workflow in the care process (Demiris et al. 2001; Wai et al. 2013), and the other main challenge is using information in a different way rather than adapting the existing healthcare process and health information systems (Essén and Conrick 2008).

Hence, continuing research is still needed to better understand how these monitoring technology solutions can be beneficial for older adults through enhancing adoption of home-monitoring technologies more pervasive in real-world settings (Boise et al. 2013; Larizza et al. 2013). We contend that until there is an overarching framework to guide the use of such monitoring technologies at best incremental, progress will be made. Thus, this research in progress looks at the benefits of applying the intelligence continuum (Wickramasinghe and Schaffer 2006) to explore the benefits, barriers and components of designing and developing home-monitoring technologies in the specific context of postsurgery risks and complications, after discharge, in the case of hip and knee replacements in seniors. Given the number of total knee and or total hip replacements projected to be performed on seniors will increase over sixfold between 2010 and 2030 in the USA (Kurtz et al. 2007), this appears to be a prudent and pressing case context. It is expected that the proffered model will assist in:

- Reducing the number of unplanned readmissions in hospitals
- Improving postoperative quality by continuous monitoring of risk factors at home
- Reducing rehabilitation costs by developing/expanding home care and thereby reducing the burden on already stretched rehabilitation care facilities
- Reducing hospital postoperative costs

In addition, the solution will serve to comply with meaningful use of technology. The research question guiding this study is: *How can home-monitoring technologies be developed to aid in the detection of postoperative complications and risk factors after discharge from total knee and/or total hip arthroplasty in senior citizens?* In this exploratory research, a qualitative approach using an exemplar data site as a single case study is adopted to answer the research question.

Background

The following section provides details on key bodies of literature that taken together serve to underscore the importance of understanding the role of home health monitoring technologies in the context of senior citizens.

Home-Monitoring Technologies in the Context of Seniors

In recent years, there has been an increase in studies focussing on home health monitoring to identify seniors' changes in their health and behaviour, in home settings in order to try to enable seniors to stay at home for longer (Boise et al. 2013). Outcomes of previous studies show that older adults have generally expressed willingness to adopt in-home monitoring technologies and also share monitoring data with physicians and family members (Demiris and Hensel 2008; Andersson et al. 2002; Melenhorst et al. 2004; Courtney et al. 2008; Steele et al. 2009; Wild 2010; Bowman et al. 2013; Larizza et al. 2013).

Specifically, Boise's et al. (2013) identified that the most important values of monitoring identified by older adults included achieving the goal of independent living, in responding to emergencies, and in tracking of specific medical parameters (Boise et al. 2013). Services provided through these technologies for elderly people are categorised into six major groups (Ludwig et al. 2012): handling adverse conditions, assessing state of health, consultation/education, motivation/feedback, service ordering and social inclusion. Further, the literature shows that the most common application of disease monitoring is focused on medical conditions that are highly prevalent amongst the aged (Ludwig et al. 2012), particularly in cardiovascular disease (Antonicelli et al. 2008; Birati et al. 2008; Stratakisf et al. 2006; Kielblock et al. 2007), in the respiratory systems (Lamothe et al. 2006; Horton 2008; Gale and Sultan 2013; Gellis et al. 2012) and diabetes mellitus (Dang et al. 2006, 2007; Barnett et al. 2006). For example, one of these monitoring applications is "Health Buddy" device to monitor the results of a coronary artery bypass graft (CABG; Barnason et al. 2006). The daily answers of the seniors concerning these symptoms are uploaded to a website and reviewed by nurses, combined with educating and motivating messages (Barnason et al. 2006). To date though, technology solutions providing continuous monitoring of specific factors taking a process centric perspective are not evident in the literature nor are their studies that present systematic enabling frameworks being used to facilitate a macro level understanding of the key issues. These voids will be the focus of the current study.

The Importance of Home-Monitoring Solutions in Seniors After Hip and Knee Replacements

Hip and knee replacements are the procedures performed frequently to relieve pain and improve function in patients with advanced hip and knee joint destruction (Davidson et al. 2008) . The Australian Orthopaedic Association National Joint Replacement Registry (AOANJRR; Davidson et al. 2008) categorizes hip replacements as either primary or revision procedures.

By 2030, the number of total hip replacement (THR) and total knee replacement (TKR) performed annually in the USA is projected to exceed 500,000 (Kurtz et al. 2007). Age is the most important patient factor affecting the outcome of both knee replacement (Losina et al. 2012) and hip replacement (Wetters et al. 2013). Most patients undergoing knee replacement are elderly; the mean age during surgery is close to 70 years (Smith et al. 2011). Also, in terms of THR, 40 % increased risk for complications after the surgery is noted for every decade above the age of 65 years (Keener et al. 2003). Numerous studies state that monitoring post operation risk factors (Wetters et al. 2013), estimating the quality of life (Arenaza 2009; Bruyère et al. 2012) and planning relevant wellness services (Wagenmakers et al. 2011; Stevens et al. 2012) may impact morbidity rates after THR and TKR.

Postsurgical indications for THR and TKR are guided by pain, functional impairment, physical examination and radiographic (Philippon et al. 2009). However, an initial course of conservative therapy should always be monitored and attempted with analgesia, activity modification, ambulatory aids and weight loss (Hunter and Lo 2008). Also, regular postoperative assessment of patient and implant outcomes is necessary to monitor long-term patient satisfaction, results of surgical techniques and patient perceptions (Carr et al. 2012; Westby and Backman 2010; Dorr et al. 2010). Another important risk factor that should be monitored after the surgery is infection. Most infections occur within 2 years of the initial surgery (Urquhart et al. 2010), such as prosthetic joint infections (Jämsen et al. 2010; Senneville et al. 2011). Patient risk factors for deep postoperative infection include previous surgery of the joint, rheumatoid arthritis, corticosteroid therapy, diabetes mellitus, poor nutritional state, obesity and advanced age (Senneville et al. 2011; Lau et al. 2010; Wright 2013).

In general, total hip and total knee replacement surgeries are successful and are performed frequently, especially for people experiencing pain associated with degenerative joints (Katz et al. 2004). However, types of partial hip and knee replacements are complex and involve many postoperative risk factors. Since, these risk factors can attribute to a decrease in the patient's quality of life (Dijkman et al. 2008), the continuous assessment and regular monitoring are of significant importance for post hip and knee replacements. Additionally, hip and knee implants are undergoing a rapid rate of innovation and improved technology with unknown outcomes that should be monitored effectively (Wickramasinghe et al. 2009). As long term and continuous monitoring of these risk factors in hospitals is costly and and time consuming, a home-montioring solution is proposed to monitor the postoperative risk factors efficiently in real time.

Current and Proposed Orthopaedic Care Process

Decision-making regarding the treatment and surgery for patients under hip and knee replacements is especially multifaceted and complex, including for example the clinical condition of the patients, their age, activity and mobility levels and size (Karlson et al. 2003). The decision to undertake treatments with either drugs, or surgery or a combination of both depends on a large number of factors (Roy and Brunton 2008). The decision-making process in the context of THR and TKR can be divided into six broad phases (Fig. 22.1). In phase 1 and phase 2, awareness programmes and outpatient clinic vary in different hospitals. In phase 3 or preoperation phase, the surgeon having received much information about the patient and their medical conditions, needs to make a decision relating to whether surgery is the best medical option. Once patients and surgeons have agreed to proceed, in phase 4, ad hoc decisions pertaining to the unique situations that may arise during the surgery must be addressed. Then, in the postoperating phase, or phase 5, decision-making is primarily done at two levels:

a. Assessing relevant clinical factors to ensure a sustained successful result for the patient during aftercare and beyond
b. Developing an initial plan for postoperative treatment through rehab programs.

Research Method

Qualitative inquiry can improve the description and explanation of complex, real-world phenomena pertinent to health services research (Bradley et al. 2007). Hence, in this research a qualitative approach using an exemplar data site as a single case study is adapted to address research objectives and to answer the research question. This study is exploratory in nature to explore main components, barriers, issues and requirement to design and develop a home-monitoring technology in senior citizens

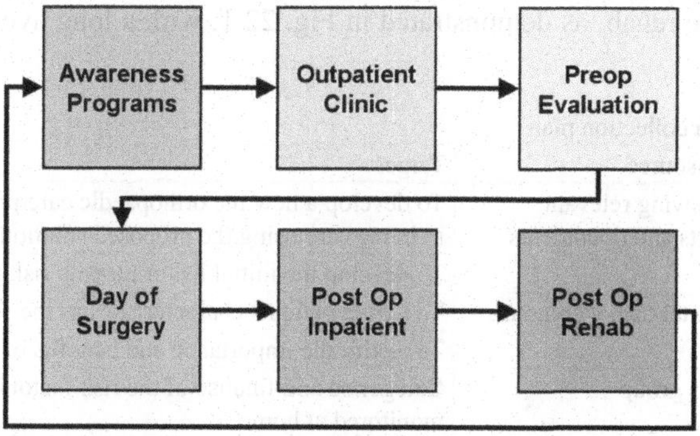

Fig. 22.1 Orthopaedic continuum of care. (Adapted from Wickramasinghe et al. 2009)

to detect postoperative complications and risk factors in the case of hip and knee replacements. As the case study methodology is a mature method to investigate contemporary phenomena in their context (Runeson and Höst 2009), in this research we applied the single case study approach referred to general definitions of the term case study according to Robson (2002), Yin (2009) and Benbasat et al. (1987).

During the design time of a case study, ethical considerations must be made (Singer and Vinson 2002). Hence, the research study will subscribe to the necessary ethics requirements. Qualitative data will be collected mainly through data sources such as a focus group of orthopaedic surgeons, hospital data warehouse as well as reviewing relevant reports and documents in the study site. Five orthopaedic surgeons in the hospital are identified as an expert group of orthopaedic clinicians who perform THA/total knee arthroplasty (TKA). Table 22.1 presents the data collection plan.

The use of thematic analysis will apply in the analysis of data in this research as it provides a structured way of understanding how to develop thematic codes and sense themes (Boyatzis 1998).

Preliminary Findings

Patients' characteristics of the study population is presented in Table 22.2, who are seniors admitted for hip and knee replacement operations between 2004 and 2012. As shown in the table, during this period totally 4645 patients (60+) had hip replacement and 4790 had knee replacement operation.

Research results from this exploratory pilot study by the date is collected, from phase 1 and 2, by reviewing relevant reports and documents as well as reviewing data inside of the hospital data warehouse. Initial results present better gaining insights into early identification of postoperative risks after discharge through regular monitoring of patients clinical conditions at home.

Table 22.3 presents possible risk factors for monitoring at home, through the proposed technology, after discharge.

Table 22.4 presents the economic benefits of the proposed solution. As the table shows, in 2012 all the patients who had undertaken hip and knee replacement were admitted to the rehab, as demonstrated in Fig. 22.1, with a long average length of

Table 22.1 Data collection plan

Steps	Data source	Target
1st step	Reviewing relevant reports and documents	To develop a new the orthopaedic care process included in home care using the proposed solution
		To develop the initial list of post-op risk factors
2nd step	Hospital data warehouse	To define patients characteristics as the solution users
		To justify the importance and benefits of the solution
3rd step	Focus group	Categorise and finalise of the risk factors that should be monitored at home
		Categorise of the solution services

Table 22.2 Patients' characteristics in the hospital between 2004 and 2012

Total hip replacement		Total knee replacement	
Female—age group	No. of admitted patients	Female—age group	No. of admitted patients
061–070	1058	061–070	1293
071–080	1053	071–080	1107
081–090	590	081–090	458
091–100	48	091–100	13
Total	*2749*	*Total*	*2871*
Male	*No. of admitted patients*	*Male*	*No. of admitted patients*
061–070	869	061–070	958
071–080	727	071–080	698
081–090	291	081–090	254
091–100	9	091–100	9
Total	*1896*	*Total*	*1919*

Table 22.3 Possible risk factors to be monitored by the proposed technology at home after discharge

Possible risk factors that should be monitored at home	Description
BMI	Patient with higher BMI's has worse postoperative functional score. Hence, it should be monitored regular and long term (Wylde et al. 2011; Lash et al. 2013)
Loss of motion	One of the most common postoperative complications is the loss of range of motion, particularly after TKR
Instability	Knee prosthesis instability is cited as the third most frequent cause of failure of total knee arthroplasty. It has been reported that 10–22% of the revision surgeries after TKA are due to instability (Vince et al. 2006; Parratte and Pagnano 2008; Song et al. 2013)
Infection	Urinary tract infection (Herwaldt et al. 2013; Ollivere et al. 2013; Richards et al. 2012)
Postoperative hyperglycaemia	Diabetes is an established risk factor for complications following total joint arthroplasty (Malinzak et al. 2009; Cohn et al. 2012; Jämsen et al. 2012)
Hypertension	Hypertension should also be monitored regularly after discharge because it effects the transfusion rates (Russo et al. 2012; Ahmed et al. 2011)
Depression	The prevalence of depressive and anxiety symptoms is relatively high in patients after THR or TKR compared with the prevalence in other chronic diseases (Vissers et al. 2012; Pinto et al. 2013; Duivenvoorden et al. 2013). Hence it is important to monitor and score it

BMI body mass index, *TKR* total knee replacement, *TKA* total knee arthroplasty, *THR* total hip replacement

stay while a considerable number of patients were in low or moderate risk that could be discharged to be monitored at home through a home-based monitoring technology.

Table 22.4 Number of patients (60+) admitted in rehab in 2012 and length of stay in rehab

	Number of patients	Ave length of stay in rehab
Admitted in OR for THR or TKR	30	
Admitted in rehab	30	207
Female	20	147
Total hip replacement	10	77
Total knee replacement	10	70
Male	10	60
Total hip replacement	3	24
Total knee replacement	7	36

THR total hip replacement, *TKR* total knee replacement, *OR* operating room

Table 22.5 Number of identified patients (60+) at the study site, between 2004 and 2012, who readmitted within 7 days or 28 days after hip and knee surgeries

Row labels	Is readmission within 7 days	Is readmission within 28 days
Hip	32	96
Female	24	66
Male	8	30
Knee	6	26
Female	3	13
Male	3	13
Grand total	38	120

Moreover, through home-based risk monitoring technology, number of unplanned readmission in the hospital can be reduced significantly as most of these readmissions are accrued due to the postoperative risk factors, captured in this study (Table 22.5).

These risk factors are explored through reviewing the hospital reports and relevant literatures in the first phase of data collection. However, these risk factors should be validated by clinical experts' focus group in the third phase of data collection.

In addition, it is likely that there will be economic benefits of the proposed solution. For example, in 2012 all the patients who had hip and knee replacements were admitted to rehab with a long average length of stay while a considerable number of patients were in low or moderate risk that could be discharged to be monitored at home through a home-based monitoring technology, as proposed in Fig. 22.2. However, through home-based risk monitoring technology, the number of unplanned readmission in the hospital can be reduced significantly as most of these readmissions are accrued due to the postoperative risk factors, captured in this study (Table 22.3).

Discussion

Grandpapa, a 73-year old-man with a long history of congestive heart failure, diabetes type 2 and severe right knee medial arthrosis has a knee replacement. He is doing well on postoperative day #2 with good adherence to the exercise regimen. He is ready for discharge to home and has been provided with a prescription-based home monitoring solution that includes a heart rate monitor, smart medication container, event monitor, dual accelerometer system that measure his knee range of motion and activity patterns, a scale and a glucometer to measure his glucose level. Each of these Bluetooth-based monitoring systems communicates with his base station, an autonomous system that has been programmed with his specific medical regimen and communicates the data to his medical care team. Once home, he and his spouse plug the unit into an electrical outlet and the system autonomously connects to either his pre-existing home network or establishes a new local network if needed. Each of the monitoring devices sends its data through this base station to his care providers in an encrypted secure communication. Feedback and regimen changes can be sent to the patient as needed. The system, having his regiment preprogrammed also provides alerts and reminders to him and his family to ensure compliance with his medication and activity regimen. He recuperates and within 6 weeks is more active and healthier than he was before the surgery. This is the objective of such intelligent solutions.

Conclusion

This research in progress has far reaching implications especially in light of the challenges facing many healthcare systems of an ageing population coupled with escalating healthcare costs and increases in chronic diseases as well as workforce shortage issues. It is the thesis of this work that intelligent technology solutions hold the key to addressing this apparently intractable situation. To begin to delve further into this, the current study starts to identify how we might harness the strengths from information system/information technology (IS/IT) and incorporate them into the healthcare delivery processes so that we might realise benefits for patients, clinicians and other stakeholders in healthcare and ultimately society.

References

Aanesen, M., Lotherington, A. T., & Olsen, F. (2011). Smarter elder care? A cost-effectiveness analysis of implementing technology in elder care. *Health Informatics Journal, 17,* 161–172.
Ahmed, A. A., Mooar, P. A., Kleiner, M., Torg, J. S., & Miyamoto, C. T. (2011). Hypertensive patients show delayed wound healing following total hip arthroplasty. *PloS ONE, 6,* e23224.

Andersson, N.-B., Hanson, E., Magnusson, L., & Nolan, M. (2002). Views of family carers and older people of information technology. *British Journal of Nursing, 11,* 827–831.

Antonicelli, R., Testarmata, P., Spazzafumo, L., Gagliardi, C., Bilo, G., Valentini, M., Olivieri, F., & Parati, G. (2008). Impact of telemonitoring at home on the management of elderly patients with congestive heart failure. *Journal of Telemedicine and Telecare, 14,* 300–305.

Arenaza, J. C. (2009). Predictors of health-related quality-of-life change after total hip arthroplasty. *Clinical Orthopaedics and Related Research®, 467,* 2886–2894.

Australian Bureau of Statistics. (2010). *Population by age and sex, Australian States and Territories.* http://www.abs.gov.au/Ausstats/abs@.nsf/mf/3201.0. Accessed 22 Oct 2013.

Barnason, S., Zimmerman, L., Nieveen, J., & Hertzog, M. (2006). Impact of a telehealth intervention to augment home health care on functional and recovery outcomes of elderly patients undergoing coronary artery bypass grafting. *Heart & Lung: The Journal of Acute and Critical Care, 35,* 225–233.

Barnett, T. E., Chumbler, N. R., Vogel, W. B., Beyth, R. J., Qin, H., & Kobb, R. (2006). The effectiveness of a care coordination home telehealth program for veterans with diabetes mellitus: A 2-year follow-up. *American Journal of Managed Care, 12,* 467.

Benbasat, I., Goldstein, D. K., & Mead, M. (1987). The case research strategy in studies of information systems. *MIS Quarterly, 11*(3) 369–386.

Birati, E. Y., Malov, N., Kogan, Y., Yanay, Y., Tamari, M., Elizur, M., Steinberg, D. M., Golovner, M., & Roth, A. (2008). Vigilance, awareness and a phone line: 20 years of expediting CPR for enhancing survival after out-of-hospital cardiac arrest: The 'SHL'-Telemedicine experience in Israel. *Resuscitation, 79,* 438–443.

Boise, L., Wild, K., Mattek, N., Ruhl, M., Dodge, H. H., & Kaye, J. (2013). Willingness of older adults to share data and privacy concerns after exposure to unobtrusive in-home monitoring. *Gerontechnology: International Journal on the Fundamental Aspects of Technology to Serve the Ageing Society, 11,* 428.

Bowman, S., Hooker, K., Steggell, C. D., & Brandt, J. (2013). Perceptions of communication and monitoring technologies among older rural women: Problem or panacea? *Journal of Housing For the Elderly, 27,* 48–60.

Boyatzis, R. E. (1998). *Transforming qualitative information: Thematic analysis and code development.* Thousand Oaks: Sage.

Bradley, E. H., Curry, L. A., & Devers, K. J. (2007). Qualitative data analysis for health services research: Developing taxonomy, themes, and theory. *Health Services Research, 42,* 1758–1772.

Bruyère, O., Ethgen, O., Neuprez, A., Zégels, B., Gillet, P., Huskin, J.-P., & Reginster, J.-Y. (2012). Health-related quality of life after total knee or hip replacement for osteoarthritis: A 7-year prospective study. *Archives of Orthopaedic and Trauma Surgery, 132,* 1583–1587.

Bui, A. L., & Fonarow, G. C. (2012). Home monitoring for heart failure management. *Journal of the American College of Cardiology, 59,* 97–104.

Carr, A. J., Robertsson, O., Graves, S., Price, A. J., Arden, N. K., Judge, A., & Beard, D. J. (2012). Knee replacement. *Lancet, 379,* 1331–1340.

Clifford, G. D., & Clifton, D. (2012). Wireless technology in disease management and medicine. *Annual Review of Medicine, 63,* 479–492.

Cohn, D. M., Hermanides, J., DeVries, J. H., Kamphuisen, P.-W., Kuhls, S., Homering, M., Hoekstra, J. B., Lensing, A., & Büller, H. R. (2012). Stress-induced hyperglycaemia and venous thromboembolism following total hip or total knee arthroplasty: Analysis from the RECORD trials. *Thrombosis and Haemostasis, 107,* 225.

Courtney, K. L., Demiris, G., Rantz, M., & Skubic, M. (2008). Needing smart home technologies: The perspectives of older adults in continuing care retirement communities. *Informatics in Primary Care, 16,* 195–201.

Dang, S., Ma, F., Nedd, N., Aguilar, E. J., & Roos, B. A. (2006). Differential resource utilization benefits with internet-based care coordination in elderly veterans with chronic diseases associated with high resource utilization. *Telemedicine Journal & e-Health, 12,* 14–23.

Dang, S., Ma, F., Nedd, N., Florez, H., Aguilar, E., & Roos, B. A. (2007). Care coordination and telemedicine improves glycaemic control in ethnically diverse veterans with diabetes. *Journal of Telemedicine and Telecare, 13,* 263–267.

Davidson, D., Steiger, R. D., Ryan, P., Griffith, L., Mcdermott, B., Pratt, N., Miller, L., & Stanford, T. (2008). *Hip and knee arthroplasty. Annual report*. Adelaide: Data Management & Analysis Centre and University of Adelaide.

Demiris, G., & Hensel, B. (2008). Technologies for an aging society: A systematic review of "smart home" applications. *Yearbook of Medical Informatics, 47,* 33–40.

Demiris, G., Finkelstein, S. M., & Speedie, S. M. (2001). Considerations for the design of a Web-based clinical monitoring and educational system for elderly patients. *Journal of the American Medical Informatics Association, 8,* 468–472.

Dijkman, B. A., Kooistra, B. A., Ferguson, T. B., & Bhandari, M. A. C. (2008). Decision making open reduction/internal fixation versus arthroplasty for femoral neck fractures. *Techniques in Orthopaedics, 23,* 288–295.

Dorr, L. D., Thomas, D. J., Zhu, J., Dastane, M., Chao, L., & Long, W. T. (2010). Outpatient total hip arthroplasty. *The Journal of Arthroplasty, 25,* 501–506.

Duivenvoorden, T., Vissers, M. M., Verhaar, J. A. N., Busschbach, J. J. V., Gosens, T., Bloem, R. M., & Reijman, M. (2013). Anxiety and depressive symptoms before and after total hip and knee arthroplasty: A prospective multicentre study. *Osteoarthritis and Cartilage, 21*(12), 1834–1840.

Essén, A., & Conrick, M. (2008). New e-service development in the homecare sector: Beyond implementing a radical technology. *International Journal of Medical Informatics, 77,* 679–688.

Falls, C. E. (2008). Palliative healthcare: Cost reduction and quality enhancement using end-of-life survey methodology. *Journal of Gerontological Social work, 51,* 53–76.

Gale, N., & Sultan, H. 2013. Telehealth as 'peace of mind': Embodiment, emotions and the home as the primary health space for people with chronic obstructive pulmonary disorder. *Health & Place, 21,* 140–147.

Gellis, Z. D., Kenaley, B., McGinty, J., Bardelli, E., Davitt, J., & Ten Have, T. (2012). Outcomes of a telehealth intervention for homebound older adults with heart or chronic respiratory failure: A randomized controlled trial. *The Gerontologist, 52,* 541–552.

Herwaldt, L., Bailin, S., Johannsson, B., Noiseux, N., Haleem, A., & Johnson, S. (2013). P198: Antimicrobial treatment for urinary tract infection (UTI) among patients having total hip (THA) or total knee arthroplasty (TKA). *Antimicrobial Resistance and Infection Control, 2,* P198.

Horton, K. (2008). The use of telecare for people with chronic obstructive pulmonary disease: Implications for management. *Journal of Nursing Management, 16,* 173–180.

Hunter, D. J., & Lo, G. H. (2008). The management of osteoarthritis: An overview and call to appropriate conservative treatment. *Rheumatic Disease Clinics of North America, 34,* 689–712.

Jämsen, E., Varonen, M., Huhtala, H., Lehto, M. U., Lumio, J., Konttinen, Y. T., & Moilanen, T. (2010). Incidence of prosthetic joint infections after primary knee arthroplasty. *The Journal of Arthroplasty, 25,* 87–92.

Jämsen, E., Nevalainen, P., Eskelinen, A., Huotari, K., Kalliovalkama, J., & Moilanen, T. (2012). Obesity, diabetes, and preoperative hyperglycemia as predictors of periprosthetic joint infection: A single-center analysis of 7181 primary hip and knee replacements for osteoarthritis. *The Journal of Bone & Joint Surgery, 94,* e101, 1–9.

Jimison, H., Jessey, N., Mckanna, J., Zitzelberger, T., & Kaye, J. Monitoring computer interactions to detect early cognitive impairment in elders. Distributed Diagnosis and Home Healthcare, 2006. D2H2. 1st Transdisciplinary Conference on, 2006. IEEE, 75–78.

Karlson, E. W., Mandl, L. A., Aweh, G. N., Sangha, O., Liang, M. H., & Grodstein, F. (2003). Total hip replacement due to osteoarthritis: The importance of age, obesity, and other modifiable risk factors. *The American Journal of Medicine, 114,* 93–98.

Karunanithi, M. (2007). Monitoring technology for the elderly patient. *Expert Review of Medical Devices, 4,* 267–277.

Katz, J. N., Barrett, J., Mahomed, N. N., Baron, J. A., Wright, R. J., & Losina, E. (2004). Association between hospital and surgeon procedure volume and the outcomes of total knee replacement. *The Journal of Bone and Joint Surgery (American), 86,* 1909–1916.

Keener, J. D., Callaghan, J. J., Goetz, D. D., Pederson, D. R., Sullivan, P. M., & Johnston, R. C. (2003). Twenty-five-year results after Charnley total hip arthroplasty in patients less than fifty years old: A concise follow-up of a previous report*. *The Journal of Bone & Joint Surgery, 85,* 1066–1072.

Kielblock, B., Ch, F., Kottmair, S., Hudler, T., Siegmund-Schultze, E., & Middeke, M. 2007. Impact of telemetric management on overall treatment costs and mortality rate among patients with chronic heart failure. *Deutsche medizinische Wochenschrift (1946)*, 132, 417–422.

Kurtz, S., Ong, K., Lau, E., Mowat, F., & Halpern, M. (2007). Projections of primary and revision hip and knee arthroplasty in the United States from 2005 to 2030. *The Journal of Bone & Joint Surgery, 89,* 780–785.

Lamothe, L., Fortin, J.-P., Labbe, F., Gagnon, M.-P., & Messikh, D. (2006). Impacts of telehomecare on patients, providers, and organizations. *Telemedicine Journal & E-Health, 12,* 363–369.

Larizza, M. F., Zukerman, I., Bohnert, F., Busija, L., Bentley, S. A., Russell, R. A., & Rees, G. (2013). In-home monitoring of older adults with vision impairment: Exploring patients', caregivers' and professionals' views. *Journal of the American Medical Informatics Association, 21*(1), 56–63.

Lash, H., Hooper, G., Hooper, N., & Frampton, C. (2013). Should a patients BMI status be used to restrict access to total hip and knee arthroplasty? Functional outcomes of arthroplasty relative to BMI-single centre retrospective review. *The Open Orthopaedics Journal, 7,* 594.

Lau, E., Bozic, K. J., Berry, D., & Parvizi, J. (2010). Prosthetic joint infection risk after TKA in the Medicare population. *Clinical Orthopaedics and Related Research®, 468,* 52–56.

Losina, E., Thornhill, T. S., Rome, B. N., Wright, J., & Katz, J. N. (2012). The dramatic increase in total knee replacement utilization rates in the United States cannot be fully explained by growth in population size and the obesity epidemic. *The Journal of Bone & Joint Surgery, 94,* 201–207.

Ludwig, W., Wolf, K.-H., Duwenkamp, C., Gusew, N., Hellrung, N., Marschollek, M., Wagner, M., & HAUX, R. (2012). Health-enabling technologies for the elderly-an overview of services based on a literature review. *Computer Methods and Programs in Biomedicine, 106,* 70–78.

Malinzak, R. A., Ritter, M. A., Berend, M. E., Meding, J. B., Olberding, E. M., & Davis, K. E. (2009). Morbidly obese, diabetic, younger, and unilateral joint arthroplasty patients have elevated total joint arthroplasty infection rates. *The Journal of Arthroplasty, 24,* 84–88.

Melenhorst, A.-S., Fisk, A. D., Mynatt, E. D., & Rogers, W. A. (2004) Potential intrusiveness of aware home technology: Perceptions of older adults. *Proceedings of the Human Factors and Ergonomics Society Annual Meeting, 48*(2), 266–270 (Sage).

Ollivere, B., Kurien, T., Morris, C., Forward, D., & Moran, C. (2013). Post-operative urinary tract infection results in higher rates deep infection in patients with proximal femoral fractures. *Bone & Joint Journal Orthopaedic Proceedings Supplement, 95,* 133–133.

Parratte, S., & Pagnano, M. W. (2008). Instability after total knee arthroplasty. *The Journal of Bone & Joint Surgery, 90,* 184–194.

Philippon, M., Briggs, K., Yen, Y.-M., & Kuppersmith, D. (2009). Outcomes following hip arthroscopy for femoroacetabular impingement with associated chondrolabral dysfunction: Minimum two-year follow-up. *Journal of Bone & Joint Surgery, British Volume, 91,* 16–23.

Pinto, P. R., Mcintyre, T., Ferrero, R., Almeida, A., & Araújo-Soares, V. (2013). Predictors of acute postsurgical pain and anxiety following primary total hip and knee arthroplasty. *The Journal of Pain, 14*(5), 502–515.

Richards, C., Garbuz, D., & Masri, B. (2012). Diagnosis of infection after total knee arthroplasty. *The Knee Joint*. New York: Springer.

Roy, C. B., & Brunton, S. (2008). Managing multiple cardiovascular risk factors. *The Journal of Family Practice, 57,* 13–20.

Runeson, P., & Höst, M. (2009). Guidelines for conducting and reporting case study research in software engineering. *Empirical Software Engineering, 14,* 131–164.

Russo, R. R., Dasa, V., Duarte, R., Beakley, B., Mishra, M., & Thompson, H. (2012). Post-operative hypertension after total knee arthroplasty and the effects on transfusion rates. *PloS ONE, 7,* e50967.

Senneville, E., Joulie, D., Legout, L., Valette, M., Dezèque, H., Beltrand, E., Roselé, B., D'Escrivan, T., Loïez, C., & Caillaux, M. (2011). Outcome and predictors of treatment failure in total hip/knee prosthetic joint infections due to *Staphylococcus aureus*. *Clinical Infectious Diseases, 53,* 334–340.

Singer, J., & Vinson, N. G. (2002). Ethical issues in empirical studies of software engineering. *IEEE Transactions on Software Engineering, 28*(12), 1171–1180.

Smith, T. O., Blake, V., & Hing, C. B. (2011). Minimally invasive versus conventional exposure for total hip arthroplasty: A systematic review and meta-analysis of clinical and radiological outcomes. *International Orthopaedics, 35,* 173–184.

Song, S. J., Detch, R. C., Maloney, W. J., Goodman, S. B., & Huddleston, J. I. III (2013). Causes of instability after total knee arthroplasty. *The Journal of Arthroplasty, 29*(2), 360–364.

Steele, R., Lo, A., Secombe, C., & Wong, Y. K. (2009). Elderly persons' perception and acceptance of using wireless sensor networks to assist healthcare. *International Journal of Medical Informatics, 78,* 788–801.

Stevens, M., Reininga, I. H., Bulstra, S. K., Wagenmakers, R., & Van Den Akker-Scheek, I. (2012). Physical activity participation among patients after total hip and knee arthroplasty. *Clinics in Geriatric Medicine, 28,* 509–520.

Stratakisf, M., Fontanellig, R., Guerrig, D., Salvettish, O., Tsiknakisi, M., Chiarugii, F., Gambergerj, D., & Valentinik, M. 2006. HEARTFAID: A knowledge based platform of services for supporting medical-clinical management of heart failure within elderly population. *Medical and Care Compunetics 3, 121,* 108.

Urquhart, D. M., Hanna, F. S., Brennan, S. L., Wluka, A. E., Leder, K., Cameron, P. A., Graves, S. E., & Cicuttini, F. M. (2010). Inciden
ce and risk factors for deep surgical site infection after primary total hip arthroplasty: A systematic review. *The Journal of Arthroplasty, 25,* 1216–1222. e3.

Vince, K. G., Abdeen, A., & Sugimori, T. (2006). The unstable total knee arthroplasty: Causes and cures. *The Journal of Arthroplasty, 21,* 44–49.

Vissers, M., Duivenvoorden, T., Verhaar, J., Busschbach, J., Gosens, T., Pilot, P., Bierma-Zeinstra, S., & Reijman, M. (2012). Depressive and anxiety symptoms before and after total hip and knee arthroplasty. *Recovery After Total Hip or Knee Arthroplasty Physical and Mental Functioning, 109.*

Wagenmakers, R., Stevens, M., Groothoff, J. W., Zijlstra, W., Bulstra, S. K., van Beveren, J., van Raaij, J. J., & van den Akker-Scheek, I. (2011). Physical activity behavior of patients 1 year after primary total hip arthroplasty: A prospective multicenter cohort study. *Physical Therapy, 91,* 373–380.

Wai, A. A. P., Kenneth, L. J. H., Yen, A. L. V., Phua, C., Tiberghien, T., Aloulou, H., Yan, L., Zhang, X., Biswas, J., & Yap, P. (2013). Challenges, experiences and lessons learned from deploying patient monitoring and assistance system at Dementia Care Hostel. *Inclusive society: Health and wellbeing in the community, and care at home*. Berlin: Springer.

Westby, M. D., & Backman, C. L. (2010). Patient and health professional views on rehabilitation practices and outcomes followi ng total hip and knee arthroplasty for osteoarthritis: A focus group study. *BMC Health Services Research, 10,* 119.

Wetters, N. G., Murray, T. G., Moric, M., Sporer, S. M., Paprosky, W. G., & Della Valle, C. J. (2013). Risk factors for dislocation after revision total hip arthroplasty. *Clinical Orthopaedics and Related Research®, 471,* 410–416.

Wickramasinghe, N., & Schaffer, J. L. (2006). Creating knowledge-driven healthcare processes with the intelligence continuum. *International Journal of Electronic Healthcare, 2,* 164–174.

Wickramasinghe, N., Bali, R., Gibbons, C., Choi, J. H. J. & Schaffer, J. L. (2009). A systematic approach: Optimization of healthcare operations with knowledge management. *Journal of Healthcare Information Management, 23*(3), 44–50. http://www.himss.org/ASP/publications_jhim_issue.asp?issue=6/27/2009.

Wild, K. (2010). Unobtrusive in-home monitoring of cognitive and physical health: Reactions and perceptions of older adults. *Gerontechnology, 9,* 124–125.

Wright, W. F. (2013). *Essentials of clinical infectious diseases.* New York: Gasch Printing.

Wylde, V., Hewlett, S., Learmonth, I. D., & Dieppe, P. (2011). Persistent pain after joint replacement: Prevalence, sensory qualities, and postoperative determinants. *Pain, 152,* 566–572.

Yin, R. K. 2009. *Case study research: Design and methods*. thousand Oaks: Sage.

Zhang, B., Wright, A. A., Huskamp, H. A., Nilsson, M. E., Maciejewski, M. L., Earle, C. C., Block, S. D., Maciejewski, P. K., & Prigerson, H. G. (2009). Health care costs in the last week of life: Associations with end-of-life conversations. *Archives of Internal Medicine, 169,* 480.

Dr. Hoda Moghimi is a data analyst professional with experience in different industries over the past 10 years, working closely with various participants to address their analytical requirements and issues as well as developing new prototypes. Her major research and technology interests are including data analytics, predictive modelling and data visualisation. She also has over 30 peer-reviewed scholarly publications in informatics contexts.

Dr. Jonathan L. Schaffer is a managing director in the Information Technology Division at Cleveland Clinic, where he leads the eClevelandClinic effort to connect the participants in the care process. An active board certified joint replacement surgeon, he is also the program director for the advanced operative technology group in the orthopaedic and rheumatologic research centre. Prior to the Cleveland Clinic, Dr. Schaffer was the CEO of Harmonie Group, Inc, a corporate spin off from the informatics lab at Brigham and Women's Hospital and Harvard Medical School. He has participated in many healthcare software development projects from clinical applications to supply chain management systems and has been a founder of or consultant to four healthcare technology companies. He is also active with the medical industry and venture community having participated in a number of medically related start-ups.

Prof. Nilmini Wickramasinghe PhD, MBA, GradDipMgtSt, BSc. Amus.A, piano, Amus.A violin has a well-recognised research record in the field of healthcare and IT/IS. Her expertise is in the strategic application and management of technology for effecting superior healthcare solutions. She, currently, is the Epworth Chair in health information management and a professor at Deakin University.

Chapter 23
Investigating Parents' Attitude Towards Using Intelligent Solutions in Care Process: The Case of Paediatric Congenital Heart Disease

Hoda Moghimi and Nilmini Wickramasinghe

Introduction

Although developing web-based health communication technologies and decision support solutions are increasing rapidly (Gentles et al. 2010), designing these systems in the highly complex and dynamic domain of clinical contexts is a serious challenge for solution providers (Blumenthal and Glaser 2007; Musen et al. 2014). Design of communication channels, decision criteria, alerts, reminders and other types of intervention requires detailed analysis of numerous factors that affect their accuracy, specificity, clarity, clinical relevance and, in turn, the ability of clinicians to take timely and appropriate actions in response (Horsky et al. 2012). Hence, developers need to adopt design practices that include user-centred, iterative design and common standards based on human–computer interaction (HCI) research methods rooted in ethnography and cognitive science (Trafton et al. 2010; Yen and Bakken 2011).

Previous studies have already presented multiple innovations associated with electronic health record systems, developed to support evidence-based medicine practice (Brunette et al. 2011). These studies mainly highlighted a new construct, based on the technology acceptance model, to explain end users' acceptance of this technology through a lens of continuous behavioural adaptation and change (Johnson et al. 2014). Literature review shows that end-users of these technologies are clinical staffs, health providers, administrators and executives in healthcare organisations (Musen et al. 2014, Jones et al. 2014) and there are just a few studies focusing on parents' and patients' attitude in terms of using new intelligent solutions (de Graaf et al. 2014; Mitchell et al. 2014).

H. Moghimi (✉)
Epworth HealthCare, 89 Bridge Rd, Richmond, VIC 3121, Australia
e-mail: moghimi87@gmail.com

N. Wickramasinghe
Deakin University and Epworth HealthCare, 60 Baker Ave, Kew East 3102, Australia
e-mail: n.wickramasinghe@deakin.edu.au

N. Wickramasinghe et al. (eds.), *Contemporary Consumer Health Informatics*,
Healthcare Delivery in the Information Age, DOI 10.1007/978-3-319-25973-4_23

Hence, due to the important role of patients' parents in paediatric diseases to facilitate care process, the aim of this study is investigating parent's attitude to use an intelligent decision support solution during the care process as well as to enhance their intention to be involved in the SDM process. Also, the possible role of knowledge sharing through the intelligent solutions in order to improve their home care management and their children's post operation quality of life is discussed. This study is exploratory in nature and endeavours to explore the parents' point of views and their needs in order to design and develop an intelligent web-based solution to be applied to healthcare contexts, in particular of congenital heart disease (CHD) for children. Data collection was through performing a paper-based survey with the patients' parents in the study site admitted between 2006 and 2013.

Background

CHD is a common health problem affecting many children around the world. The term 'congenital heart disease' refers to 'disorders of heart or central blood vessels present at birth' (Larrazabal et al. 2007). 'CHD is one of the biggest killers of infants less than one year old' (AIHW 2009) and the risk of death remains significantly high for these patients throughout their life, with over 40% unable to reach the age of five. Unfortunately, surgery is not considered a final cure, as it can result in a considerably high rate of complications, and the coexistence of certain other diseases such as diabetes or various types of cancer needs to be considered. Along with the direct adverse impact on the patients and their families, CHD also carries significant societal and economic implications. Furthermore, infants born with complex CHD are not only at risk of serious heart-related complications, but also of developing a deadly bowel disease, regardless of the type of surgical intervention they receive for their heart (Hospital 2010).

While considering CHD surgery, it is not only important to consider immediate medical results but also the ongoing risk of increased probability of sudden death, exercise intolerance, neurodevelopment and psychological problems as well as long-term impacts on the family unit as a whole. This multifaceted consideration is important because:

- The risk of late sudden death for patients surviving the operation for common CHD is 25–100 times greater than an age-matched control population (Silka et al. 1998).
- Exercise intolerance is significantly increased in many survivors of the surgery.
- More than 50% of patients after surgery demonstrate abnormalities in neurodevelopment testing.
- Between 1-in-8 and 1-in-3 survivors exhibit post-traumatic stress disorder (PTSD) and a similar percentage display signs of PTSD symptoms (Ben-Amitay et al. 2006).

- Children with complex CHD are rated by their parents and their teachers as being more withdrawn, experiencing more social problems and engaged in fewer physical activities.
- Fewer parents have attachment relationships with their CHD-affected infants compared to those of healthy infants (Goldberg and Rock 1992), and parents of children with CHD are found to be overprotective, overindulgent and inconsistent in disciplining their children.
- Families of children with CHD experience more financial strain and greater familial/social stress compared to control groups (Casey et al. 1996). As can be seen, the decisions relating to treatment strategies for children suffering from CHD are both complex and high risk.

In CHD patients, infants with hypoplastic left heart syndrome (HLHS) are amongst the most challenging subgroups of cardiac patients to care for and manage. This challenge may begin at birth, it may begin earlier in those with a prenatal diagnosis, and the period of greatest acute risk often continues until the time of stage II palliation, when the patient is between 4 and 6 months. Infants with HLHS often respond poorly to seemingly minor external stresses, or to subtle changes in their medical management. These events can lead to significant morbidity and mortality.

Shared Decision-Making in Healthcare

The literature informs the reader that shared decision-making (SDM) is recognised as the active participation of both clinicians and families in clinical treatment decisions, the exchange of clinical information, discussion of treatment preferences, and the joint determination of a treatment plan (Makoul and Clayman 2006; Barry and Edgman-Levitan 2012; Légaré et al. 2011; Charles et al. 1997). A physician may sometimes make a decision unilaterally, obtaining the patient's consent without offering the patient a choice out of all options; this is not an actual SDM but it is still information exchange between patients or their family with practitioners to improve the care process (Whitney et al. 2003). SDM has been conceptualised in several different ways, and usually involves a process in which an individual is informed of the seriousness of the illness; the benefits, harms, alternatives and uncertainty of preventive or treatment options; weighs his or her options and participates in the decision-making process with the clinician in a shared role (Head et al. 2011; Pentz et al. 2012; Sheridan et al. 2004).

The benefit of sharing the decision-making process is that it allows doctors to clarify with patients or their families' an understanding of key facts and relevant values, highlight the unique circumstances that might alter the decision for any individual and add a considered clinical perspective on the decision (Sheridan et al. 2004). Several of these functions may not be necessary when decision aids are available, particularly if patients or their families are known to be health literate and the decision aid allows for deliberation on values and preferences (Kennedy et al.

2002). Instead, independent decision-making by the doctor in a supporting role may sometimes be appropriate and improve patients or their families' self-efficacy for following through with a decision (Kiesler and Auerbach 2006a).

Typically, cases using SDM are of major importance and high uncertainty in which patients' values, and hence SDM, are highly relevant. Continuing life support, for example, for patients in a persistent vegetative state, surgery for localised breast cancer or care or termination of care for severely burned persons are in this category (Whitney et al. 2004). To date, SDM studies are developed in different domains of healthcare and this is presented in Table 2.

Although SDM is supported in many disease management domains, some concerns and issues still remain with respect to adopting SDM solutions, these concerns including a perception among some medical practitioners that the ultimate responsibility for treatment should remain under their authority (Schauer et al. 2007; Edwards and Elwyn 2009). Client capacity to participate in decisions (O'Brien et al. 2011), identifying the SDM components (Sheridan et al. 2004; van der Weijden et al. 2011) and SDM user acceptance (Scholl et al. 2011) are the main issues to promote this type of CDSS in the healthcare context.

SDM also has some limitations—for example, SDM is appropriate for situations in which two or more medically reasonable choices exist (O'Connor et al. 2009), regardless of whether the degree of risk is high or low (Whitney et al. 2003). Therefore, SDM is not appropriate in these cases while patients or their families would still like to have participation in the care process. Hence, more studies are needed to deepen the understanding of interactions between patient decision aid use and the patterns of patient–practitioner communication. The format of delivery of patient decision aids, such as web-based patient decision aids, also needs further consideration (O'Connor et al. 2009; Cousin et al. 2012; Parsons et al. 2012; Flight et al. 2012).

Research on SDM has been undertaken (Deegan and Drake 2006; Barry and Edgman-Levitan 2012), but much more research is needed in this area of clinical support. Future work might also explore other intervention components or component content that might make SDM interventions more effective in promoting shared decisions (Sheridan et al. 2004).

User-Centred Design

According to Hauge et al. (2007) study, two elements of clinical decision support applications are critical to the applications success, independent of the implementation environment, as follows (Haug et al. 2007):

1. The mechanism by which the systems acquire the data used in their decision algorithms
2. The interface through which they interact with clinicians/users to report their results

User-centred design (UCD) is well recognised as an effective human factor engineering strategy to design ease of use into the total customer experience with products and information technology (IT) that has been applied specifically to healthcare IT systems (Vredenburg et al. 2002).

The shift from 'system-centred' to 'user-centred' design has increased the effectiveness of software systems (Díaz et al. 2008). This is because of the iterative nature of UCD that means all stages of the process can be revisited to make a more efficient development process which results in a product that is less likely to require major redesign after the final evaluation process is completed (De Matos et al. 2013). Hence, in this study, users' perspectives in order to enhance the clinical decision support system (CDSS) usability and acceptability are a critical component.

Summary and Significance of Study Based on the Literature

Overall, considering the study aims and goals to improve the surgical decision efficiency by detecting risk factors, more than 500 relevant publications in total in the period from 2003 to 2013 were reviewed while almost 350 publications were focused on information systems and health informatics. Approximately 150 reviewed papers were related to healthcare. Through the initial literature review in healthcare contexts, the following issues and challenges have been identified and demonstrate the importance of designing and developing such a computer-based decision support solution.

- Lack of communication facilitators to share decisions between clinicians, and between clinicians and patients or their families, in order to support clinical decisions by understanding the treatment risk factors and anticipated outcomes (Bates et al. 2003).
- Lack of some specific Socio-technical components of people, process, technology and environment in healthcare to make a successful implementation of a new technology to address data importance and accuracy issues (Kuhn et al. 2006; Candelieri et al. 2009; Gosain and Kumar 2009; Srinivas et al. 2010; Peter and Somasundaram 2012; Bernabe et al. 2012; Yoo et al 2012; Padhy et al. 2012; Amin et al. 2013).

Methodology and Research Design

This study is exploratory in nature and is designed to achieve the research aim of reducing the burden of surgery on cardiac patients, their parents and society. The strategic benefits of this research are well aligned with the research main objectives of exploring parents' attitude to use an intelligent solution in order to empower them by improving SDM and information exchange between paediatric families and health professionals and also to assess their interest in using such a solution. To address the research objectives, this study is designed to answer this question:

- How can an intelligent decision support solution be beneficial to patients' parents in the case of paediatric CHD?

Throughout this research, a qualitative approach using an exemplar data site as a case study is adopted and the approach incorporates well established qualitative data collection techniques (Boyatzis 1998; Glesne and Peshkin 1992; Yin 1994; Yin 2003). The data collection techniques will assist in collecting requirements and capturing the main components to develop the solution in healthcare contexts (Mantzana et al. 2007).

At the time of designing a case study, ethical considerations must be made (Singer and Vinson 2002). The research study is to be strictly confined to ethical research processes and it has to be approved by the Human Research Ethics Committee (HREC) of the case study site, as a low-risk study.

An open-ended survey is administrated to collect data. The survey questionnaire is mailed to participants in a package including a consent form and the study information statement. The study participants are parents of CHD patients who were admitted in the research site, between 2006 and early 2012. Although 115 participants were captured at the first stage of the study, 27 patients were diseased by the data collection time. Hence, I mailed our open-ended questionnaire and consent form to the 88 patients' parents not only in Victoria, but around Australia.

Results

Patients' parents described their point of view related to the surgical decision-making process by completing the questionnaire. The questionnaire sought parent's attitude to understanding the surgical risk factors and their intention to be involved in the surgical decision-making process. The questionnaire asked parents about their children's quality of life after surgery, the possible role of knowledge sharing and the importance of the solution in improving their home care management and their children's quality of life (Table 1).

In the USA, low-income adults experience substantial health and healthcare inequities when compared with higher income individuals (Berenson et al. 2012). In consideration of this fact, the first set of questions in the questionnaire asked parents to state their household income. The aim of ascertaining participant's income was to examine any relation between parents' income and their level of receiving and understanding clinical information. The participant's interest in using an intelligent application during their child care process was also investigated by the first set of questions. Results from the questionnaire pertaining to parents' income are shown in below table (Table 2):

- Parents' level of understanding about the surgery outcomes and risks

Table 1 Units of analysis and reference for questionnaire

No	Questionnaire code	Category of questionnaires	Number of received questionnaires and consent forms
1–35	P1,..., P35	Non-clinical, questionnaire	35

Table 2 Parents' total annual household income

Income	Questionnaire code	% response
Less than $40k	P11, P18, P21, P31	11
$40–60k	P1, P2, P12, P13, P25, P29, P33, P34	23
$60–80k	P7, P10, P14, P15, P16, P17, P23, P27, P28, P30, P32, P35	34
$80–120k	P3, P4, P5, P19, P20, P22, P26	20
More than $120k	P6, P8, P9, P24	11

The next set of questions in the questionnaire is designed to seek information with respect to the level of understanding of parents in understanding surgical risk factors and expected outcomes. Most parents stated that:

> ...Surgeons and cardiologists described the surgery process and possible outcomes very well and our level of understanding was high....P3, P4, P5, P8, P9, P12, P18, P19, P21, P32, P33, P35, Parents

> The internet was fantastic. It provided a lot of information that was simple to read and understand. There was a lot of negative feedback on his condition by the 1st cardiologist. We saw evidence of this, as did the sonographer who did the 2nd scan. The cardiologist did not even have the latest information and we received a lot of pressure to 'let nature take its course'. It was not until we went to Melbourne and the specialist was able to put our worries at ease. Our cardiologist we have now is fantastic and informative....
> P13, Parents

However, some parents had a medium level of understanding and one of them had no interest to know about surgical risk factors and possible outcomes.

> ...We had a basic knowledge of the risk factors which were explained in great detail. However, we think our level of understanding was medium because of lots of clinical terms....
> P31, Parents

> ...It was not too easy for us to understand what's going on, although Sam's cardiologist tried to describe all conditions in details....
> P29, Parents

> ...During that time we were very disappointed and confused. My wife was really depressed. So, we had no interest to hear about the surgery risks. We were trying to think positive and be hopeful....
> P14, Parents

- Parents' attitude towards the surgery decision-making process

In the next set of questions in the questionnaire, parents were asked about details of their decision-making process before agreeing to surgery for their child. The aim of this set of questions was to elucidate how understanding the surgical risk factors may affect the parents' decision to agree to surgical procedures for their child.

All parents answered that they accepted undertaking surgery without consideration of surgery risks and outcomes.

> …doesn't matter how many risks is involved. We accepted to do the surgery even when the chance of treatment was 1 % because it was the only way to keep him alive….
> P08, Parents

- Parents' intention to use the solution

In the other part of the questionnaire parents were asked about their intention to use such a real-time decision support solution to seek information about the surgical risks and outcomes prior to undertaking surgery. Most parents had an intention to use the solution (Table 3).

Parents' positive point of view to use the solution is expressed in the following comments:

> …I preferred to get more information to predict my kid's status because often I'm surprising about his reactions….
> P04, Parents

> …I preferred to receive more information also after surgeries when we are taking care him at home….
> P05, Parents

> …Because of my background that is clinical I was familiar with the surgery risks however, I'm always seeking new information and knowledge in this area….
> P06, Parents

> …Overall we got enough information but at some key moments there were situations where doctors failed to communicate with us. So, this solution might be helpful in these serious conditions….
> P08, Parents

> …We received lots of information during all surgeries but in the gap between surgeries we didn't any source of information to ask about any new condition or any sudden changes….
> P09, Parents

> …I would like to know more about similar patients who are growing up with the same problems….
> P11, Parents

Table 3 Parents' intention

Parents intention	
70 %	Positive
10 %	Negative
20 %	No Idea

…Enough information but I wish it was explained in more simple terms through this application as it was a lot to take on board given the circumstances….
P12, Parents

A total of 20 % parents were ignorant with respect to using a computer-based clinical application and 10 % did not like to use any clinical application to know more about their child's health, surgery risks or the surgery outcomes.

…I prefer to discuss with doctors directly rather than rely on the application or receive information via a computer based system….
P26, Parents

…I'm not good in using computer….
P31, Parents

…I don't like to know too much or in details about clinical procedures or conditions….
P14, Parents

- Patients' quality of life after the surgery

In this set of questions parents were asked about their child's quality of life after undergoing the surgical procedure. The aim of this question was comparing the anticipated surgical outcomes with the actual surgical outcomes to support the importance of the solution in predicting the surgical results before doing the surgery. Although most of parents were informed about the expected surgical outcomes, the parents would like to receive detailed information as they are aware of the current status of their child's health condition. They ascertained their child's quality of life after surgery and remarked as followed:

…Excellent. Issac is incredibly sensitive and aware of life and everyone in his life. He is a very happy little boy.
P02, Parents

Good. He is a healthy happy boy but less active than his 2 years age.
P04, Parents

Mental health issues 18 months post surgery. We still see a psychologist regularly. It was out of our expectation.
P03, Parents

Good. Oscar's physical health is now great, however he still suffers severe mental health problems as a result of a lengthy a complicated hospitalization 18 months ago. Although we were informed about these possible outcomes we were still surprised on some occasions.
P05, Parents

Excellent. He is doing very well in the school. Better than our expectation.
P06, Parents

Not really good. But it is not because of the surgery. He is affected by some physical problems because of staying in the hospital for a long time.
P08, Parents

Slightly, less than normal. I am already informed than he might have some physical or neurological issues but I didn't know what it means exactly. So, it was out of my expectations.
P10, Parents

Mildly limited. Breathlessness/fatigue only real issues (they are still quite mild at this stage). Gross …. Development, particularly leg strength as tight issue, as is stamina.
P12, Parents

She has a smaller frame and it is very difficult for her to put on weight. She is approximately 16 kg at 6.5 years old. She has a 6000 points appetite. However, she burns a lot of energy for daily tasks. The biggest concern I have is her mental development. She has a very poor memory, struggles to retain information, comprehend new info, and gives up very quickly.
P16, Parents

She has delayed physical and mental development but I wasn't surprised because of my information about these possible limitations for CHD patients. However, I don't consider them too much reducing her quality of life. She is a happy girl and enjoys all aspects of her childhood just like any other children.
P19, Parents

I must say, when we had spoken to by that 1st cardiologist, we didn't think he would be this good! Thanks goodness for medical staff with correct up to date information!
P20, Parents

He does get short of breath; he also suffers from frequent bouts of croup due to an airway stricture from repeated intubations…We didn't know about these special possible conditions.
P23, Parents

Less than normal. Shortage of breath, blueness around the lips & limitation in physical activities are his main problems
P28, Parents

Sam had a stroke as a result of the surgery but has no residual effects. Stroke was not discussed before the surgery. He had so many complications that can occur in the post-surgery but still surgery was Sam's best option.
P32, Parents

- Social impact on the family life

The last set of questions were related to the social impact of CHD and surgical intervention on parents' family life and seeks to find out how an intelligent decision support solution can improve these sorts of issues. Table 4, shows that 65% of parents considered that their child's CHD had a negative impact on their family and social life.

Negative impact. My husband has suffered chronic depression.
P01, Parents

Negative impact. Unpredictable health conditions; school and work absences; hospital visits' inpatient/outpatient and organizing the other 2 children are some of my problems.
P04, Parents

Table 4 Social impact of CHD on parents' family life

Social impact on the family life	
26%	Positive
65%	Negative
9%	Both

> The answer to this question depends on the day you ask it. Initially it had a negative impact, nowadays mostly positive. A really difficult question to answer honestly.
> P10, Parents

> Negative impact. Moved house due to living in a remote area & having less access to the hospital. Also I had to reduce my work hours significantly due to my sons' recurrent hospitalizations.
> P14, Parents

> Negative—mainly financial (travelling from country NSW to Melbourne for check-ups/ surgeries). Emotional—Father can get quite down about condition.
> P19, Parents

> Positive impact. Numerous lengthy procedures, hospitalizations plus frequent medical appointments plus ongoing mental health issues associated with hospitalization are challenging, however I feel blessed every day for all that I have, especially my heart kid.
> P03, Parents

> Positive impact. It has brought us closer together. We don't worry about trivial things anymore. So overall we are loss stressed.
> P07, Parents

> Positive impact. We have made some new friends, my job has changed to support and help families with heart problems and I love doing it to be more appreciate of life.
> P09, Parents

> Positive impact. We have learnt to be more grateful and appreciate what we have.
> P21, Parents

Discussion

Results show parents positive attitude towards using the intelligent solution and also that they would like to contribute more to the surgical decision-making process. This is based on the fact that the parents and family prefer to receive more information during the surgical decision-making process rather than just signing the consent form before surgery. Hence the parents' intention towards the surgical decision-making process is one of the findings in this study. Information transferred between patients' parents and clinicians. Also, based on the study findings, the importance of designing appropriate functions and components to facilitate transferring information between patients' parents and clinicians is very high.

Most of the parents in the research case had a positive attitude towards using a real-time intelligent decision support solution, also during the surgical decision-making process, especially, in the research case, parents would like to use the solution to improve knowledge sharing between clinicians and parents rather than using the intelligent solution to assist them to make a decision whether to perform the surgery or not. This is because all parents stated that there had no choice except to do the surgery.

In fact, the parent's description of how they view their role (i.e. during the treatment process) is a reflection of the expert's suggestions concerning the care of their sick baby rather than sharing in the decision-making process.

Studies examining parents' participation in clinical decision-making have usually focused on the choice of treatment (Kiesler and Auerbach 2006b; Say et al. 2006). However, this study's findings show there is no opportunity for patients' parents to discuss one or more decisions with regard to the clinical treatment of their children. Due to the nature of CHD, the only possible curative treatment is the surgery. Hence, parental decision-making is not meaningful in the research case study.

The study has identified that there is no decision sharing or parental decision-making process in children with CHD as there is no decision alternative for parents other than surgery. Hence, this study recommends a knowledge sharing process, rather than a decision sharing process between clinicians and parents in the CHD surgical decision-making process, particularly post surgery. The study defines this recommendation as an important component of designing such a real-time intelligent decision support solution in the research case study.

In summary, the findings related to practice include:

1. The importance of knowledge sharing between clinicians as well as between clinicians and patients through an on-line application;
2. The clinicians' involvement during systems development;
3. The acceptability and capability of the system and high demand of outcome predictions to improve decision efficiency.

This study highlighted the role of parent's income and the quality of their social life with respect to their intention to understand and monitor post-operative risk factors. In the case of CHD, post-operative home care is very important to assist in avoiding any side effects or sudden death. Hence, such a solution can be effective to monitor parent's quality of social life and their income to provide them with training or special services in order to assist them to improve their knowledge and information towards post-operative home care.

The logical next step of this research is to design and develop an appropriate prototype of the solution in order to identify and address issues associated with usability and acceptability of the solution for use in paediatric cardiac surgery.

UCD guidelines can be applied in the design and development of the decision support solution in order to explore the explicit understanding the of users' tasks and environments with the users' multidisciplinary skills and perspectives.

The exploration of clinicians' perspectives and patients'/parents' perspectives informs the design phase about their collective attitudes towards the solution potential as an enabler to applying intelligent solutions in the healthcare context.

This exploratory research also reveals various social-technical concerns about the potential impacts of the solution on clinical knowledge sharing, critical thinking and complex decision-making processes.

The study findings emphasise the significant role of patients' parents in the design of healthcare solutions, the parents being 'information receivers', a component of the system users. In this study, 'information receivers' are patients/patients' parents who need to receive understandable information pertaining to different treatment processes. The parent's point of view is important to improve the capability and acceptability of the designed solution, and is due to patient/parents empowerment role in the care process.

Small number of participants was the biggest limitation in this study. Collecting data through parents as a group of participants was the other challenge in this study, as there were found to be highly emotional events for parents as a group of participants, and this may have compromised this group's ability to recollect what happened during the surgical and recovery processes.

Conclusion

Overall, this study confirmed that paediatric primary care parents, even those with lower income and low level of technology understanding are interested to use a computer-based intelligent application to improve their contribution in a care process. They are mainly interested to have knowledge sharing, real-time communication and information exchange with healthcare professional as well as with the other patients' parents around the world who are in the same situation.

This study is an important first step in understanding acceptability of a web-based solution in the Australian population. However, more specific information would be necessary for designing technologies and applications in order to respond to their requirements, collected in this study.

References

(AIHW), A. I. O. H. A. W. (2009). Impact of falling cardiovascular disease death rates: Deaths delayed and years of life extended. (Online). http://www.aihw.gov.au/publications/aus/bulletin70. Accessed 20 May 2010.

Amin, S. U., Agarwal, K., & Beg, R. (2013). Data mining in clinical decision support systems for diagnosis, prediction and treatment of heart disease. *International Journal of Advanced Research in Computer Engineering & Technology (IJARCET), 2*(1), 218–223.

Barry, M. J., & Edgman-Levitan, S. (2012). Shared decision making—the pinnacle of patient-centered care. *New England Journal of Medicine, 366,* 780–781.

Bates, D. W., Kuperman, G. J., Wang, S., Gandhi, T., Kittler, A., Volk, L., Spurr, C., Khorasani, R., Tanasijevic, M., & Middleton, B. (2003). Ten commandments for effective clinical decision support: Making the practice of evidence-based medicine a reality. *Journal of the American Medical Informatics Association, 10,* 523–530.

Ben-Amitay, G., Korov, I., Reiss, A., Toren, P., Yoran-Hagesh, R., Kotler, M., & Mozes, T. (2006). Is elective surgery traumatic for children and their parents? *Journal Pediatrics and Child Health, 42,* 618–624.

Berenson, J., Doty, M. M., Abrams, M. K., & Shih, A. (2012). Achieving better quality of care for low-income populations: The roles of health insurance and the medical home in reducing health inequities. *Issue Brief (The Commonweath Fund), 11,* 1–18.

Bernabe, R. D., Thiel, G. J. v., Raaijmakers, J. A., & Delden, J. J. v. (2012). Decision theory and the evaluation of risks and benefits of clinical trials. *Drug Discovery Today.*

Blumenthal, D., & Glaser, J. P. (2007). Information technology comes to medicine. *The New England Journal of Medicine, 356,* 2527–2534.

Boyatzis, R. E. (1998). *Transforming qualitative information: Thematic analysis and code development.* USA: Sage.

Brunette, M. F., Ferron, J. C., Mchugo, G. J., Davis, K. E., Devitt, T. S., Wilkness, S. M., & Drake, R. E. (2011). An electronic decision support system to motivate people with severe mental illnesses to quit smoking. *Psyciatric Services, 62*(4), 360–366.

Casey, F. A., Sykes, D. H., Craig, B. G., Power, R., & Mulholland, H. C. (1996). Behavioral adjustment of children with surgically palliated complex congenital heart disease. *Pediatric Psychology, 21,* 335–352.

Candelieri, A., Conforti, D., Sciacqua, A., & Perticone, F. (2009). *Knowledge discovery approaches for early detection of decompensation conditions in heart failure patients.* Paper presented at the Ninth International Conference on Intelligent Systems Design and Applications.

Charles, C., Gafni, A., & Whelan, T. (1997). Shared decision-making in the medical encounter: What does it mean?(or it takes at least two to tango). *Social Science & Medicine, 44*(5), 681–692.

Cousin, G., Schmid Mast, M., Roter, D. L., & Hall, J. A. (2012). Concordance between physician communication style and patient attitudes predicts patient satisfaction. *Patient Education and Counseling, 87,* 193–197.

De Matos, P., Cham, J. A., Cao, H., Alcántara, R., Rowland, F., Lopez, R., & Steinbeck, C. (2013). The enzyme portal: A case study in applying user-centred design methods in bioinformatics. *BMC Bioinformatics, 14,* 103.

De Graaf, M., Totté, J. E., Van Os-Medendorp, H., Van Renselaar, W., Breugem, C. C., & Pasmans, S. G. (2014). Treatment of infantile hemangioma in regional hospitals with ehealth support: Evaluation of feasibility and acceptance by parents and doctors. *JMIR Research Protocols, 3,*(5), e52.

Deegan, P., & Drake, R. (2006). Shared decision making and medication management in the recovery process. *Psychiatric Services, 57,* 1636–1639.

Díaz, A., García, A., & Gervás, P. (2008). User-centred versus system-centred evaluation of a personalization system. *Information Processing & Management, 44,* 1293–1307.

Edwards, A., & Elwyn, G. (2009). *Shared decision-making in health care: Achieving evidence-based patient choice.* USA: Oxford University Press.

Flight, I. H., Wilson, C. J., Zajac, I. T., Hart, E., & Mcgillivray, J. A. (2012). Decision support and the effectiveness of web-based delivery and information tailoring for bowel cancer screening: an exploratory study. *JMIR Research Protocols, 1,* e12.

Gentles, S. J., Lokker, C., & Mckibbon, K. A. (2010). Health information technology to facilitate communication involving health care providers, caregivers, and pediatric patients: A scoping review. *Journal of Medical Internet Research, 12*(2), e22.

Glesne, C., & Peshkin, A. (1992). *Becoming qualitative researchers: An introduction.* New York: Longman White Plains.

Goldberg, A. L., & Rock, K. L. (1992). Proteolysis, proteasomes and antigen presentation (Online). http://www.nature.com/doifinder/. Accessed 10 May 2010.

Gosain, A., & Kumar, A. (2009). *Analysis of health care data using different data mining techniques*. Paper presented at the International Conference on Intelligent Agent & Multi-Agent Systems, 2009. IAMA 2009. Chennai.

Haug, P. J., Gardner, R. M., Evans, R. S., Rocha, B. H., & Rocha, R. A. (2007). Clinical decision support at intermountain healthcare. In E. Berner (Ed.), *Clinical decision support systems: Theory and Practice* (pp. 159–189). Springer.

Head, S. J., Bogers, A. J. J. C., Serruys, P. W., Takkenberg, J. J. M., & Kappetein, A. P. (2011). A crucial factor in shared decision making: The team approach. *Lancet, 377,* 1836.

Horsky, J., Schiff, G. D., Johnston, D., Mercincavage, L., Bell, D., & Middleton, B. (2012). Interface design principles for usable decision support: A targeted review of best practices for clinical prescribing interventions. *Journal of Biomedical Informatics, 45,* 1202–1216.

Hospital, N. C. S. (2010). Infants born with complex congenital heart disease also at risk for life-threatening gastrointestinal diseases (Online). http://www.news-medical.net/news/. Accessed 29 May 2010.

Johnson, M. P., Zheng, K., & Padman, R. (2014). Modeling the longitudinality of user acceptance of technology with an evidence-adaptive clinical decision support system. *Decision Support Systems, 57,* 444–453.

Jones, S. S., Rudin, R. S., Perry, T., & Shekelle, P. G. (2014). Health information technology: An updated systematic review with a focus on meaningful use. *Annals of Internal Medicine, 160,* 48–54.

Kennedy, A. D. M., Sculpher, M. J., Coulter, A., Dwyer, N., Rees, M., Abrams, K. R., Horsley, S., Cowley, D., Kidson, C., & Kirwin, C. (2002). Effects of decision aids for menorrhagia on treatment choices, health outcomes, and costs. *JAMA: The Journal of the American Medical Association, 288,* 2701–2708.

Kiesler, D. J., & Auerbach, S. M. (2006a). Optimal matches of patient preferences for information, decision-making and interpersonal behavior: Evidence, models and interventions. *Patient Education and Counseling, 61*(3), 319–314.

Kiesler, D. J., & Auerbach, S. M. (2006b). Optimal matches of patient preferences for information, decision-making and interpersonal behavior: Evidence, models and interventions. *Patient Education and Counseling, 61,* 319–341.

Kuhn, K., Wurst, S., Bott, O., & Giuse, D. (2006). Expanding the scope of health information systems. *IMIa Yearbook of Medical Informatics Methods of Information in Medicine, 45(suppl 1), S43–S52.*

Larrazabal, L. A., Jenkins, K. J., Gauvreau, K., Vida, V. L., Benavidez, O. J., Gaitán, G. A., Garcia, F., & Castañeda, A. R. 2007. Improvement in congenital heart surgery in a developing country: The Guatemalan experience. *Circulation, 116,* 1872–1877.

Légaré, F., Stacey, D., Pouliot, S., Gauvin, F. P., Desroches, S., Kryworuchko, J., Dunn, S., Elwyn, G., Frosch, D., & Gagnon, M. P. (2011). Interprofessionalism and shared decision-making in primary care: A stepwise approach towards a new model. *Journal of Interprofessional Care, 25,* 18–25.

Makoul, G., & Clayman, M. L. (2006). An integrative model of shared decision making in medical encounters. *Patient Education and Counseling, 60,* 301.

Mantzana, V., Themistocleous, M., Irani, Z., & Morabito, V. (2007). Identifying healthcare actors involved in the adoption of information systems. *European Journal of Information Systems, 16*(1), 91–102.

Mitchell, S. J., Godoy, L., Shabazz, K., & Horn, I. B. (2014). Internet and mobile technology use among urban African American parents: Survey study of a clinical population. *Journal of Medical Internet Research, 16*(1), e9.

Musen, M. A., Middleton, B., & Greenes, R. A. (2014). Clinical decision-support systems. In E. H. Shrotliffe & J. J. Cimmino (Ed.), *Biomedical informaitcs* (pp. 643-674). London: Springer.

O'Brien, M. S., Crickard, E. L., Rapp, C., Holmes, C., & Mcdonald, T. (2011). Critical issues for psychiatric medication shared decision making with youth and families. *Families in Society, 93,* 310–316.

O'Connor, A., Bennett, C., Stacey, D., Barry, M., Col, N., Eden, K., Entwistle, V., Fiset, V., Holmes-Rovner, M., & Khangura, S. (2009). Decision aids for people facing health treatment or screening decisions (Review). The Cochrane Collaboration published in the Cochrane Library, 3. http://onlinelibrary.wiley.com/doi/10.1002/14651858.CD001431.pub2/full. Accessed Dec 2014.
Padhy, N., Mishra, P., & Panigrahi, R. (2012). The survey of data mining applications and feature scope. *International Journal of Computer Science, Engineering & Information Technology, 2*(3).
Parsons, S., Harding, G., Breen, A., Foster, N., Pincus, T., Vogel, S., & Underwood, M. (2012). Will shared decision making between patients with chronic musculoskeletal pain and physiotherapists, osteopaths and chiropractors improve patient care? *Family Practice, 29,* 203–212.
Pentz, R. D., Pelletier, W., Alderfer, M. A., Stegenga, K., Fairclough, D. L., & Hinds, P. S. (2012). Shared decision-making in pediatric allogeneic blood and marrow transplantation: What if there is no decision to make? *The Oncologist, 17*(6), 881–885.
Peter, T., & Somasundaram, K. (2012). *An empirical study on prediction of heart disease using classification data mining techniques.* Paper presented at the Advances in Engineering, Science and Management (ICAESM), 2012 International Conference on.
Say, R., Murtagh, M., & Thomson, R. (2006). Patients' preference for involvement in medical decision making: A narrative review. *Patient Education and Counseling, 60,* 102–114.
Schauer, C., Everett, A., Del Vecchio, P., & Anderson, L. (2007). Promoting the value and practice of shared decision-making in mental health care. *Psychiatric Rehabilitation Journal, 31,* 54–61.
Scholl, I., Loon, M. K., Sepucha, K., Elwyn, G., Légaré, F., Härter, M., & Dirmaier, J. (2011). Measurement of shared decision making—a review of instruments. Zeitschrift für Evidenz. *Fortbildung und Qualität im Gesundheitswesen, 105,* 313–324.
Sheridan, S. L., Harris, R. P., & Woolf, S. H. (2004). Shared decision making about screening and chemoprevention. *American Journal of Preventive Medicine, 26,* 56–66.
Srinivas, K., Rani, B. K., & Govrdha, A. (2010). Applications of data mining techniques in healthcare and prediction of heart attacks. *International Journal on Computer Science & Engineering, 2*(2).
Silka, J., Hardy, G., Menashe, D., & Morris, D. (1998). A population-based prospective evaluation of risk of sudden cardiac death after operation for common congenital heart defects pediatric cardiology and medical informatics and clinical outcomes. USA Published by the American College of Cardiology Foundation.
Singer, J., & Vinson, N. (2002). Ethical issues in empirical studies of software engineering. *IEEE Transactions on Software Engineering, 28*(12), 1171–1180.
Trafton, J. A., Martins, S. B., Michel, M. C., Wang, D., Tu, S. W., Clark, D. J., Elliott, J., Vucic, B., Balt, S., & clark, M. E. (2010). Research article Designing an automated clinical decision support system to match clinical practice guidelines for opioid therapy for chronic pain.
Van Der Weijden, T., Van Veenendaal, H., Drenthen, T., Versluijs, M., Stalmeier, P., Loon, M. K., Stiggelbout, A., & Timmermans, D. (2011). Shared decision making in the Netherlands, is the time ripe for nationwide, structural implementation? Zeitschrift für Evidenz. *Fortbildung und Qualität im Gesundheitswesen, 105,* 283–288.
Vredenburg, K., Mao, J. Y., Smith, P. W., & Carey, T. (2002). A survey of user-centered design practice. In Proceedings of the SIGCHI conference on Human factors in computing systems (pp. 471–478). ACM.
Whitney, S. N., Mcguire, A. L., & McCullough, L. B. (2003). A typology of shared decision making, informed consent, and simple consent. *Annals of Internal Medicine, 140,* 54–59.
Whitney, S. N., Mcguire, A. L., & McCullough, L. B. (2004). A typology of shared decision making, informed consent, and simple consent. *Annals of Internal Medicine, 40,* 54–61.
Yen, P.-Y., & Bakken, S. (2011). Review of health information technology usability study methodologies. *Journal of the American Medical Informatics Association, 19*(3), 413–422 (amiajnl-2010–000020).
Yin, R. K. (1994). *Case study research: Design and methods.* CA: Thousand Oaks.
Yin, R. K. (2003). *Case study research: Design and methods.* CA: Sage.
Yoo,Y., Boland, R., Lyytinen, K., & Majchrzak, A. (2012). Organizing for innovation in the digitized world. *Organization Science, 23*(5), 1398–1408.

Dr. Hoda Moghimi is a data analyst professional with experience in different industries over the past 10 years, working closely with various participants to address their analytical requirements and issues as well as developing new prototypes. Her major research and technology interests include data analytics, predictive modelling and data visualisation. She also has over 30 peer-reviewed scholarly publications in Informatics contexts.

Prof. Nilmini Wickramasinghe (Ph.D., M.B.A., Grad.Dip.Mgt.St., B.Sc. Amus.A, piano, Amus.A, violin) has a well-recognised research record in the field of healthcare and IT/IS. Her expertise is in the strategic application and management of technology for effecting superior healthcare solutions. She currently is the Epworth Chair in Health Information Management and a professor at Deakin University.

Chapter 24
Managing Gestational Diabetes Mellitus (GDM) with Mobile Web-Based Reporting of Glucose Readings

Nilmini Wickramasinghe and Steve Goldberg

Introduction

The need for improvement in the delivery of healthcare is paramount. Today, much of the literature pertaining to healthcare continually discusses the many severe challenges such as exponentially increasing costs, pressures to provide appropriate quality and access as well as incorporating best practice and recent new findings at the point of care (Wickramasinghe and Schaffer 2010). Government agencies and the private sector are alarmed with rising costs and the decline in quality, access and availability of care. In addition, we are now witnessing the increased role of chronic diseases as a major cause of death and morbidity, replacing communicable diseases, which only serves to further stress the resources of an already strained healthcare delivery system.

Without a question, then, there is a clear need for short- and long-term solutions to this current crisis in the delivery of care. Such a search for a solution has led to the growing focus on technology, especially telemedicine and remote care, as a useful alternative to the prevailing models of inpatient care. The utilization of information communication technologies (ICTs) seems particularly attractive given its allure in the support and enablement of a cost-effective model of care for patients with chronic diseases. Moreover, mobile phone penetration has been exponentially increasing over the last decade, with most individuals now having at least one mobile device (Business Insider Australia 2013). However, the implementation of new ICT infrastructures needs to consider the users and the management of the information that can be captured and shared by such systems.

N. Wickramasinghe (✉)
Deakin University and Epworth HealthCare,
60 Baker Ave, Kew East 3102, Australia
e-mail: n.wickramasinghe@deakin.edu.au

S. Goldberg
Inet International Inc., 131 Glen Crescent, Thornhill, ON L4J 4W4, Canada
e-mail: sgoldberg@inet-international.com

N. Wickramasinghe et al. (eds.), *Contemporary Consumer Health Informatics*,
Healthcare Delivery in the Information Age, DOI 10.1007/978-3-319-25973-4_24

This chapter sets out to describe a unique research in progress that focuses on a specific issue to address this current dilemma: the use of smartphones to effect better information access and sharing between patients and clinicians and, thus, improved control of a chronic illness. The study is conducted with the focus on gestational diabetes in an Australian healthcare context.

Prevalence of Diabetes

Today, chronic diseases have replaced infectious diseases as the top global cause of deaths and morbidity (Zuvekas and Cohen 2007; Zimmet 2000). Noncommunicable diseases—such as cardiovascular disorders and strokes, respiratory illnesses such as asthma, arthritis and diabetes—now account for more deaths, and for a disproportionate burden on healthcare budgets of governments, compared with infectious diseases such as tuberculosis, human immunodeficiency virus/acquired immunodeficiency syndrome (HIV/AIDS) and malaria. This trend is magnified by the demographic realities of this century. Aging of the population and increased longevity of major segments of the population are key contributors to the emerging picture of a crisis in the delivery of health services. More patients afflicted by chronic diseases will continue to be a burden on an already drained healthcare delivery system (Windrum 2008; Wickramasinghe and Geisler 2008). Diabetes, the leading chronic disease, has been described by the World Health Organization (WHO) as the silent epidemic (Windrum 2008; WHO 2012; Wild et al. 2004).

Chen et al. (2012) indicate that over the last three decades, the number of people with diabetes mellitus worldwide has more than doubled. Their comment is based on data collected up to 2011 and reinforces the concern of other research that identified the continued global prevalence of diabetes mellitus. The 2012 update of the International Diabetes Federation Annual Report (IDF 2012) indicates that 8.3 % of the global adult population live with diabetes, and of these, 50 % are undiagnosed; usually type 2 (non-insulin-dependent) diabetics. The federation predicts that by 2030, the prevalence of diabetes will have risen to 9.9 % of the global adult population (IDF 2012).

Uncontrolled diabetes can lead to other very unpleasant complications, and thus there is a broader medical impact of diabetes, which includes comorbidities and higher risks of contracting other diseases (WHO 2012). One of the measures of diabetic control and management is the haemoglobin A1c (or HbA1c) blood test, which is used to indicate the average blood sugar control over a period of time, generally 3-month intervals (WHO 2013). Stratton et al. (2000) indicated that a 1 % decrease in the results of the A1c test can lead to substantial decreases in the risk of associated conditions. The results of Stratton et al.'s (2000) study suggests that this could be a 43 % decrease in the risk of peripheral vascular disease, 37 % decrease in microvascular disease and 14 % decrease in myocardial infarction (heart attack). This reinforces the importance of controlling diabetes as tighter control leads to less complications and therefore to less impact on the medical infrastructure.

Where tighter control is explicitly required is in the management of gestational diabetes mellitus (GDM; Hoffman et al. 1998). Diabetes Australia estimates that 3–8 % of pregnant women will develop GDM (Diabetes Australia 2012). Unmanaged GDM has many problematic concerns including the impact of the mother passing high levels of glucose to the baby, which may then lead to several complications at birth and beyond for both mother and baby. Tight control and management of GDM is therefore necessary, and a team of medical practitioners, diabetic nurses and dieticians are needed to assist the mother to manage her blood sugar during the pregnancy. Getahun et al. (2008) note that there is an increased prevalence of GDM in women aged between 25 and 34 years.

The Management of Diabetes

Diabetes is a chronic disease, and therefore, by definition, there is no cure for it. This makes the adoption of various management strategies paramount in the successful care of diabetic patients (Britt et al. 2007; AIHW 2008; AIHW 2007).

The management of diabetes is typically based on a mixture of self-management protocols linked with the support of a dedicated medical care team (Victorian Government 2007). An essential element of self-management relies on regular testing of blood glucose using a glucometer or blood glucose monitor. These monitors provide a point-in-time reading of blood sugar, which then informs the diabetic of the need for insulin (if Type 1) or activity/exercise (if Type 2). The preferred range of readings for Type 1/2 diabetic is between 4 and 8 mmol/L (Hoffman et al. 1998).

GDM requires tight control of blood sugar levels, with a preferred range of readings between 4 and 6 mmol/L (Hoffman et al. 1998; Siri and Thomas 1999; Diabetes Australia 2012). The management of GDM is conducted over a shorter period of time (that of the pregnancy), and thus a tighter management of sugar levels is required. The need for such control draws into question the information that a diabetic may need when self-managing their condition.

In 2008, Hedtke posed the question as to whether it would be possible for wireless technology could enable new diabetes management tools? (Hedtke 2008). The question was raised in relation to the ways that mobile phone technology could assist in the recording and management of blood glucose. More specifically, can mobile communication and data sharing be integrated with the process of glucose reading? Hedtke (2008) suggested that mobile technology and glucose monitoring technology could be integrated in three ways. The first is 'user integration', where the technology is not physically integrated but rather the information is by having the user rekey data from a glucose monitor into a mobile phone application. The second is 'cable/Bluetooth integration', where the glucose monitor and phone are connected through a direct (physical) cable or through a close-vicinity network (Bluetooth or infrared communication). And the third approach is 'physical integration', where the glucose monitor is built into or attached to the mobile phone.

This paper extends the notion of integration by reporting on the development of a pilot solution to support GDM which has been adapted from a technology solution developed in North America. The study has demonstrated proof of concept but has also uncovered other important aspects. Blood glucose monitors and even smartphone apps tend to act as recording devices. Any information is transferred to medical practitioners as a 'batch' data transfer, usually at the time of medical visit. This study, however, proposes that diabetes control may be more easily managed if there is integration of the captured mobile data with the e-health systems employed by key medical staff in real time.

Specifically, this exploratory study is examining usability and fidelity issues focussing on the following questions:

1. Can the mobile phone 'integrate' glucose monitoring as real-time data for the effective management of GDM?
2. How do patients and clinicians find the use of such a mobile solution for GDM management?

The focus is on GDM as this short-term form of diabetes may benefit from immediate feedback that an integrated information and communication process can provide. Moreover, the patient population with GDM is highly motivated and generally technology savvy and desirous to have better strategies to effectively and efficiently monitor their blood sugar levels.

The Information and Support Model

A comprehensive review of the literature around the development of technology solutions to assist in diabetes care was performed by Le Rouge and Wickramasinghe (2013). They found that an integral key success criteria is the incorporation of a user-centred design approach (Le Rouge and Wickramasinghe 2013). It is precisely this, a subscription to a user-centred paradigm, that has guided the development of the mobile Web-based solution developed by Inet International Inc. (2013) This mobile solution is Web-based and has been developed over several years (Goldberg 2002a, b, c, d; Wickramasinghe and Goldberg 2004; Wickramasinghe et al. 2010).

The development of this mobile solution and information-sharing model aims to assist in the information management processes needed for the self-care and self-management of diabetes. Often a system-based development focuses on the technology and how it can be adopted and integrated. This project, however, explores the potential of mobile development from the perspective of the patient and the clinical team; hence the user-centred nature of the project. However, the project team is also drawing on principles of information need and information management that stem from the understanding of library science. Thus, the project will examine whether increased access to information and feedback can assist in patient self-care. Chronic illnesses, such as GDM, rely on the ability of the patient to self-monitor their daily condition. Blood glucose readings form the basis for this process. However, such self-monitoring also needs to draw on the 'knowledge base' of the clinical professionals. This is usually done during clinical visits where the blood readings over a period of time are accessed and discussed. If aspects of the 'knowledge base' can be accessible on a daily basis, then there is a potential that this information can alter the patient behaviour earlier and lead to and maintain tighter control of the diabetic condition. The blood monitoring processes provide patients with information about their glucose readings at any given time. However, the information solution proposed in this study adds to this a layer of knowledge access that is not readily available for individual readings. That is, the 'real-time' nature of the information sharing between patient and the clinical team means that feedback can be accessed on readings that are out of the norm.

Winter et al. (2001) suggest that 'Information management in hospitals is the sum of all management activities in a hospital that transpose the potential contribution of information processing to fulfill the strategic hospital goals into hospital's success'. The existing information management of patient glucose readings would be based on the record of HbA1c results of tests ordered by the clinical team. The daily glucose readings of the patient will be reviewed at clinical appointments, but they may not be recorded and stored unless the data is batch uploaded from the monitor and then stored against the patient record. However, such information management processes would generally not be conducted, and rather the daily readings may be reviewed only during the patient/clinician discussion. The model being tested in this research captures and stores the daily glucose readings and makes them accessible to the clinical team. These readings can be displayed graphically, and the patterns of daily reading can be easily monitored. This information can then complement other patient tests, such as the HbA1c data. Thus, the project has the potential to offer an information management process that improves access to the daily glucose readings of a patient. This information can then assist in identification of trends in daily care that can support the information decisions associated with HbA1c data. However, as Winter (2001) suggests, this then needs to form part of the overall information management practice and systems employed by a hospital. This study can also examine how the clinical team use, monitor and exploit the additional information processes that the project's mobile solution can provide.

Figures 24.1 and 24.2 depict the respective Web-based model and how the solution actually works. In particular, Fig. 24.1 highlights the key inputs (people process, protection and platform) all essential considerations for a solution of this type that impacts a clinical environment of care. In addition, the dynamic nature of healthcare is captured by ensuring on-going updating and integration of new research findings, and the sustainability of the solution is achieved through the broad base of financing options. Lastly, the model supports the necessary delivery framework and the interaction of patient and clinician, with the clinician being the lead on all projects and the patient being the empowered consumer of the data and information.

From Fig. 24.2 we see how the solution works: The patient must take their blood sugar reading, then enter it into the mobile solution and submit it. Once the solution is received by the designated clinician, it is processed and reviewed by the clinician in conjunction with all other relevant medical data before a recommendation is then sent back to the patient. To the right of Fig. 24.2, it is possible to see a typical screenshot showing the four readings normally taken for GDM patients, that is, be-

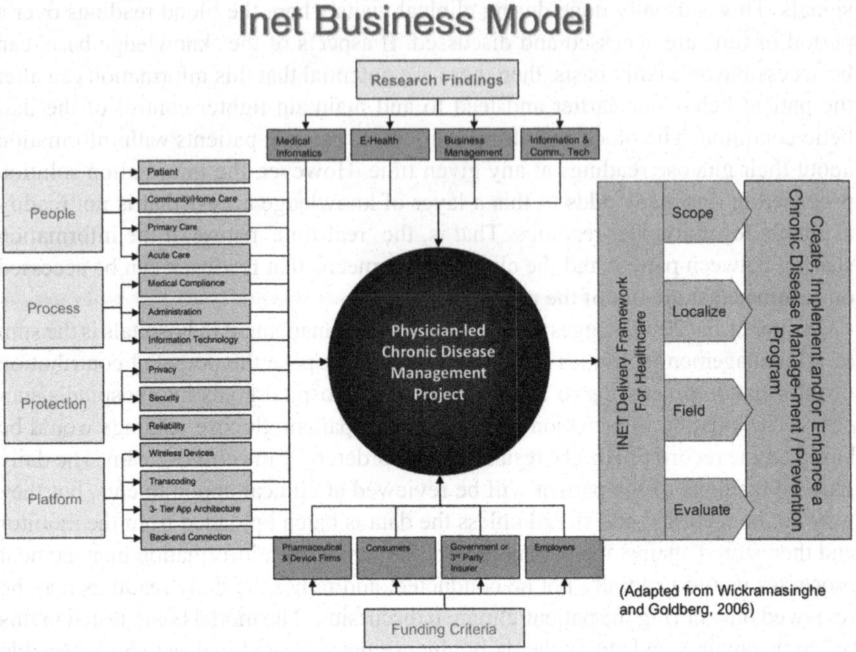

Fig. 24.1 Web-based model

Fig. 24.2 Solution in a nutshell

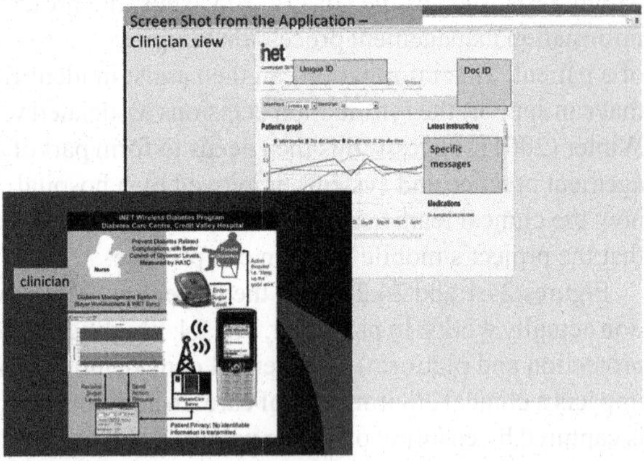

fore breakfast, 2 h after breakfast, 2 h after lunch and 2 h after dinner. Patients can also write messages about their food consumption and exercises to the right, and the clinician can review all these aspects on receipt.

The process means that there is continued information sharing between patient and clinician. While not unique in the management of glucose readings, the graphic representations assist clinicians in identifying trends associated with glucose management. The ability to add further information to the digital record (e.g. food intake or increased exercise) can assist the clinician in interpreting what may be impacting these trends or changes in the glucose readings. What is different to current glucose recording processes is the ability of the clinician to send feedback to the patient if there are concerns with the readings. Usually, such feedback is provided during a patient's physical visit with the clinical team; however, this mobile-based solution provides the opportunity for ongoing or 'real-time' feedback if required. As suggested above, this assists in the communication dialogue between patient and clinical team and has the potential to, therefore, change the information exchange and knowledge sharing between the two parties. In a review of literature associated with GDM, Devsam (2013; p. 70) suggests that 'Women reported feeling "shocked", "upset", "panicked", "scared", "numbed", "depressed", "fearful", "terrified", "disappointed", "surprised", "horribly sad", "anxious" and "worried" when first diagnosed with GDM'. Devsam et al. (2013) then indicate that when information about the condition was presented, 'Women expressed they felt unprepared and unable to assimilate this knowledge because everything was new and uncertain to them'. While this initial shock may still be evident for the participants in this study, the mobile data collection and information management processes proposed in this pilot may assist in alleviating the information uncertainty that Devsam (2013) has identified.

Carolan (2013) indicates that 'In terms of support from health professionals, the women's experiences differed quite substantially, and information and support were rated from excellent to poor. When the woman felt she had sufficient information at her disposal to self-manage her condition, then she generally was satisfied'. The near-real-time information exchange that is made possible by this pilot study may assist in reinforcing women's need for adequate information access during the management of their GDM. An outcome of the study may be perceived improved support for the participants as they will engage in a potential two-way dialogue through the mobile model being tested.

Methodology

A quasi-experimental approach was adopted (Britt et al. 2007; Coronato and De Pietro 2010), employing a two-period crossover clinical trial strategy (Hills and Armitage 1979; Rigby 2003; Senn 2002)[1] over a 10-week duration. Specifically, two groups were used. The first group experienced 'standard care' protocols and treatments, and the second group was introduced to the 'technology solution'. Patients were offered the opportunity to participate in the trial once a diagnosis of gestational diabetes had been made based on a glucose tolerance test administered between 26 and 28 weeks of pregnancy. Enrolment in the study was done by the endocrinologist under the supervision of the consultant obstetricians and was totally optional. At the time of enrolment, all pertinent information regarding the study was shared with patients, including the crossover strategy employed. Following enrolment in the study, patients were randomly allocated to either the 'technology

[1] Several references indicate that crossover is especially beneficial when trials focus on alleviating a condition and not necessarily effecting a cure especially in the case of chronic diseases (e.g. [12–14]), and we believe that for this context it is the preferred strategy to acquire the richest possible data and findings from this pilot.

solution' or 'standard care' arms of the study. All patients were then educated in the technique of blood glucose monitoring (BSLs) by a diabetic educator as per standard clinical practice. They were also then educated in the use of 'technology-based' or 'traditional' recording techniques for BSLs. Decisions regarding the need for insulin or other medical therapy were always made at the discretion of the clinician and based on current treatment guidelines and standard care. At the time of enrolment into the study, patients were asked to complete a short questionnaire, exploring demographic details, their familiarity with technology in general and their understanding of gestational diabetes. Five weeks into the study, crossover occurred; thus, patients initially in the 'standard care' arm now entered the 'technology solution' arm and vice versa. Once again, the diabetic educator provided the necessary education regarding the use of 'technology-based' or 'traditional' recording techniques for BSLs. Also at this time, a short questionnaire was administered to patients regarding their experiences during the first 5 weeks. At the completion of the study, patients again completed a questionnaire, this time also evaluating their experiences with the respective techniques. In addition, data were collected on patient outcomes, including use of insulin, frequency of 'out of target range' BSLs, compliance with monitoring (number of readings actually completed) and baby birth weight and delivery outcomes. At the completion of the study, the clinicians involved (diabetic educator, endocrinologist, obstetricians) also completed a questionnaire evaluating their experiences, in particular their opinions of the technology relative to standard techniques. All participants participated in a debriefing session at the conclusion of the study.

Established qualitative techniques have been employed to analyse the collected data (Kvale 1996; Boyatzis 1998; Yin 1994). Specifically, from the qualitative data, thematic analysis was performed in accordance with standard approaches described by Kvale (1996) and Boyatzis (1998).

Anticipated Benefits and Potential Outcomes

The study aims to determine if this approach to diabetic information management can assist in maintaining a tighter control of GDM. It is hoped that the mobile solution may provide a more enticing way to maintain information associated with glucose reading logs. While glucose monitors have a memory of readings, there are still some who maintain a written journal as an approach to information capturing for their glucose readings. The mobile phone (as a personal information device) may add an enticement for a more frequent recording of glucose readings. The feeding back of this information to the clinical team may also provide reassurance to the patient that their management is being monitored and that the information that they collate is being accessed regularly.

Initial Results

It is noted that the sample size (seven participants) in this pilot is small; thus, while not statistically significant, we have established proof of concept and demonstrated the benefit of a real-time smartphone solution to facilitate the self-management and monitoring of GDM patients. Most notably, all patients preferred the technology solution to the standard care, and those patients who start with the technology solution found the change to the standard care disappointing. 'Can't I just stay with the smartphone? [Patient 1]' was what one patient said, and this sentiment was repeated by all the others who had the technology solution for the first 5 weeks. In addition, the clinical care team (obstetricians, diabetic educator and endocrinologist) also preferred the technology solution over the standard care approach. The questionnaires and debrief sessions also generated many useful and innovative suggestions for additional features such as an interactive food diary. In keeping with a user-centred design approach, these suggestions will now be incorporated into the technology solution for the next larger-scale trial.

Discussion and Conclusion

This paper serves to report on a research in progress that focusses on the application of a smart technology solution to assist in the enablement of self-management and patient empowerment for sufferers of GDM. The technology solution itself has been designed and developed following a user-centred design approach, and this pilot trial represented the first of its type in an Australian healthcare context. The directional data obtained to date has served to establish proof of concept and that patients and clinicians alike for similar and different reasons prefer the solution to standard care approaches. Clearly, future studies will serve to provide statistically significant results to support this and confirm hypotheses that this study will generate.

The study also serves to uncover some important implications from an information management perspective. In particular, it would appear that presenting patients with pertinent information in an easy-to-understand form (i.e. a graph of blood sugar results) anytime anywhere has the result of facilitating better and appropriate behaviour modification towards control of blood sugar. We know that pregnant women represent a group in the population that is highly motivated to follow suggested beneficial behaviour modifications for the benefit of their unborn child, but our study shows that the way the information is presented as well as the time and regularity appears to be effective in facilitating the rapid adoption of appropriate and prudent behaviour modification for their own and baby's better health and wellbeing.

In conclusion, we believe that solutions of this type that try to incorporate leading-edge technology possibilities to support better patient care represent a key imperative for the future of healthcare delivery, especially in regard to superior chronic disease management in today's challenging healthcare environment.

Acknowledgments This study was made possible through funding from Epworth HealthCare, ATN-DAAD and a Schoeller Senior Fellowship awarded to Professor Nilmini Wickramasinghe. During the course of the longitudinal study, several individuals assisted, and the authors thank Drs. Len Kliman and Steve Cole for their support as well as research assistants (RAs) Hoda Moghimi and Imran Muhammed for their contributions and Say Yen Teoh and Paul Mercieca.

References

AIHW. (2007). *National indicators for monitoring diabetes: Report of the diabetes indicators review subcommittee of the National Diabetes Data Working Group. AIHW cat. no. CVD 38.* Canberra: AIHW.

AIHW. (2008). *Diabetes: Australian facts 2008.* Canberra: AIHW.

Boyatzis, R. E. (1998). *Transforming qualitative information: Thematic analysis and code development.* Thousand Oaks: Sage.

Britt, H., Miller, G. C., Charles, J., Pan, Y., Valenti, L., & Henderson, J. (2007). *General practice activity in Australia 2005–06. Cat. no. GEP 16.* Canberra: AIHW.

Business Insider Australia. (2013). Chart: Global mobile phone penetration NEwars 100 % percent [Online]. http://www.businessinsider.com.au/mobile-penetration-nears-100-percent-2013-7. Accessed 30 July 2013.

Carolan, M. (2013). Women's experiences of gestational diabetes self-management: A qualitative study. *Midwifery, 29*, 637–645.

Chen, L., Magliano, D., & Zimmet, P. (2012). The worldwide epidemiology of type 2 diabetes mellitus - present and future perspectives. *Nat Rev Endcrinol. 8*, 228–236.

Coronato, A., & De Pietro, G. (2010). An investigation into the use of pervasive wireless technologies to support diabetes healthcare. In: N. Wickramasinghe, I. Troshani, & S. Goldberg (Eds.), *Pervasive and smart technologies for healthcare: Ubiquitous methodologies and tools.* Hershey: Medical Information Science Reference.

Devsam, B. U., Bogossian, F. E., & Peacock, A. S. (2013). An interpretive review of women's experiences of gestational diabetes mellitus: Proposing a framework to enhance midwifery assessment. *Women and Birth, 26*, e69–e76.

Diabetes Australia. (2012). Gestational diabetes [Online]. http://www.diabetesaustralia.com.au/living-with-diabetes/gestational-diabetes/. Accessed 29 April 2013.

Getahun, D., Nath, C., Ananth, C. V., Chavez, M. R., & Smulian, J. C. (2008). Gestational diabetes in the United States: Temporal trends 1989 through 2004. *American Journal of Obstetrics and Gynecology, 198*, 525.e1–5.

Goldberg, S. (2002a). *Building the evidence for a standardized mobile internet (wireless) environment internal INET documentation.* Ontario: INET.

Goldberg, S. (2002b). *HTA presentation rendering component summary. Internal INET documentation 2002.* Ontario: INET.

Goldberg, S. (2002c). *HTA quality assurance component summary. Internal INET documentation 2002.* Ontario: INET.

Goldberg, S. (2002d). *Wireless POC device component summary. Internal INET documentation 2002.* Ontario: INET.

Hedtke, P. A. (2008). Can wireless technology enable new diabetes management tools? *Journal of Diabetes Science and Technology, 2*, 127–130.

Hills, M., & Armitage, P. (1979). The two-period cross-over clinical trial. *British Journal of Clinical Pharmacology, 58*, 7–20.

Hoffman, L., Nolan, C., Wilson, J., Oats, J., & Simmons, D. (1998). Gestational diabetes mellitus—management guidelines. *Medical Journal of Australia (MJA), 169*, 93–97.

IDF. (2012). Annual Report. http://www.idf.org/idf-annual-report-2012. Accessed Dec 2014.

Inet International Inc. (2013). http://www.indet-interantioanl.com. Accessed 30 July 2013.

Kvale, S. (1996). *Interviews: An introduction to qualitative research interviewing.* London: Sage.

Le Rouge, C., & Wickramasinghe, N. (2013). A review of user-centered design for diabetes-related consumer health informatics technologies. *Journal of Diabetes Science and Technology, 7*, 1039–1056.

Rigby, A. (2003). Cross-over trials in clinical research. *Journal of the Royal Statistical Society, 52*, 417–418.
Senn, S. (2002). *Cross-over trials in clinical research*. New York: Wiley.
Siri, L., & Thomas, A. (1999). Gestational diabetes mellitus. *Journal of Medicine, 341*, 1749–1756.
Stratton, I. M., Adler, A. I., Neil, H. A. W., Matthews, D. R., Manley, S. E., Cull, C. A., Hadden, D., Turner, R. C., & Holman, R. R. (2000). Association of glycaemia with macrovascular and microvascular complications of type 2 diabetes (UKPDS 35): Prospective observational study. *BMJ, 321*, 405–412.
Victorian Government. (2007). *Diabetes prevention and management: A strategic framework for Victoria 2007–2010*. Melbourne: Victorian Government, Department of Human Services.
WHO. (2012). World health statistics 2012 report [Online]. http://www.euro.who.int/en/what-we-do/health-topics/noncommunicable-diseases/sections/news/2012/5/world-health-statistics-2012-report-increase-of-hypertension-and-diabetes. Accessed 31 July 2013.
WHO. (2013). Use of glycated haemoglobin (HbA1c) in the diagnosis of diabetes mellitus [Online]. http://www.who.int/diabetes/publications/diagnosis_diabetes2011/en/index.html. Accessed 31 July 2013.
Wickramasinghe, N., & Geisler, E. (2008). *Encyclopedia of healthcare information systems*. Hershey: IGI Global Publishers.
Wickramasinghe, N., & Goldberg, S. (2004). How $M = EC^2$ in healthcare. *International Journal of Mobile Communications, 2*, 140–156.
Wickramasinghe, N., & Schaffer, J. (2010). *Realizing value driven patient centric healthcare through technology*. Washington DC. IBM Center for The Business of Government.
Wickramasinghe, N., Troshani, I., & Goldberg, S. (2010). An investigation into the use of pervasive wireless technologies to support diabetes self-care. In A. Coronato & G. De Pietro (Eds.), *Pervasive and smart technologies for healthcare: Ubiquitous methodologies and tools* (pp. 114–129). Hershey: Medical Information Science Reference.
Wild, S., Roglic, G., Green, A., Sicree, R., & King, H. (2004). Global prevalence of diabetes: Estimates for the year 2000 and projections for 2030. *Diabetes Care, 27*, 1047–1053.
Windrum, P. (2008). *Innovation in public sector services*. New York: Edward Elgar.
Winter, A., Ammenwerth, E., Bott, O. J., Brigl, B., Buchauer, A., Gräber, S., Grant, A., Häber, A., Hasselbring, W., & Haux, R. (2001). Strategic information management plans: The basis for systematic information management in hospitals. *International Journal of Medical Informatics, 64*, 99–109.
Yin, R. (1994). *Case study research*. Thousand Oaks: Sage.
Zimmet, P. (2000). Globalization, coca-colonization and the chronic disease epidemic: Can the Doomsday scenario be averted? *Journal of Internal Medicine, 247*, 301–310.
Zuvekas, S., & Cohen, J. (2007). Prescription drugs and the changing concentration of healthcare expenditures. *Health Affairs, 26*, 249–257.

Prof. Nilmini Wickramasinghe (Ph.D.; M.B.A; Grad.Dip.Mgt.St.; B.Sc.; Amus.A, piano; Amus.A, violin) has a well-recognised research record in the field of healthcare and information technology (IT)/information science (IS). Her expertise is in the strategic application and management of technology for effecting superior healthcare solutions. She currently is the professor director of health informatics management at Epworth HealthCare and a professor at Deakin University.

Steve Goldberg started his information technology career at Systemhouse Ltd. as a trainer of minicomputer accounting applications throughout Canada and the USA. In 1998, Inet International Inc. was founded by Steve Goldberg as a Canadian technology management consulting firm. At Crowntek, he formed an executive collaboration to develop a $30 million IT services business. During his tenure at Cybermation, he transformed the organization from supporting mainframe applications to client/server applications. Prior to Inet, at Compugen, he successfully built a high-performance team to meet large government and corporate organizations' e-business needs. Today at Inet, Mr. Goldberg develops and manages an advanced worldwide network of sample providers to gain physician access for online healthcare research studies. In healthcare delivery, he built and his team utilizes the first standardised wireless technology infrastructure to deliver innovative chronic disease management solutions.

Chapter 25
Using Actor Network Theory and Agency Theory to Identify Critical Factors in the Adoption and Implementation of a Chemotherapy Ordering System: A Case Study from the Australian Private Health-Care Sector

Nilmini Wickramasinghe, Peter Haddad and Stephen Vaughan

Introduction

Cancer is one of the most common diseases in today's modern society and cancer treatment regimens are complex, have high risks associated with them, and often have unwanted variances. One area within cancer treatment today that exemplifies these issues is in the prescription and administration of complex chemotherapy protocols. Although part of drug prescribing generally, chemotherapy is much more complex than most other drug prescribing in terms of the intrinsic toxicity of the drugs, the complexity of the schedules of administration, and the necessity for close monitoring. Additional differences from other prescribing are the role of specially trained chemotherapy nurses who actually administer most of the drugs and a very high level of pharmacy engagement.

In the Australian private hospital setting, private physicians usually order the drugs in their consulting rooms, a privately contracted pharmacy manufactures the drugs, and chemotherapy nurses employed by the hospital administer the drugs in hospital facilities. These multifaceted employment arrangements in the private sector and the intrinsic complexity of the prescription process combine to create a heterogeneous network of operations that exhibits a unique set of problems and agency dilemmas due to misaligned and/or divergent goals. From a rational economic perspective, this means there are multiple or nested principal–agent relationships in a heterogeneous

N. Wickramasinghe (✉)
Deakin University and Epworth HealthCare, 60 Baker Ave, Kew East 3102, Australia
e-mail: n.wickramasinghe@deakin.edu.au

P. Haddad
185-187 Hoddle st., Richmond, VIC 3121, Australia
e-mail: peter.haddad@epworth.org.au

S. Vaughan
89 Bridge Road, Richmond, VIC 3121, Australia
e-mail: Stephen.Vaughan@epworth.org.au

N. Wickramasinghe et al. (eds.), *Contemporary Consumer Health Informatics*,
Healthcare Delivery in the Information Age, DOI 10.1007/978-3-319-25973-4_25

network in contrast to the Australian public hospital setting where the physician, nurse, and pharmacist are all employed by the public hospital so the principal/agency arrangements are more straightforward. However, a chemotherapy ordering system (COS) for the ordering, make-up, and administration of cytotoxic drugs is likely to improve the quality, safety, and efficiency of this process. A major consideration is the effectiveness of the implementation of such a system; the facilitators and barriers to this process as well as how to address them form the central focus of this paper. Hence, the objectives of this study are to answer the research questions:

> How can a group of non-employee clinicians' goals be aligned to use a single information system? What are the barriers, facilitators, and critical success factors that must be addressed?

This is reviewed in the context of the Australian private health-care sector at one of the private hospitals, referred to as the ABC Hospital throughout the chapter, located in Victoria, Australia. The ABC Hospital is Victoria's largest not-for-profit private health-care group, renowned for excellence in diagnosis, treatment, care, and rehabilitation. The ABC Hospital considers itself to be an innovator in Australia's health system, embracing the latest in evidence-based medicine to pioneer treatments and services for its patients.

To better understand the underlying critical dynamics in this context and thereby design and develop appropriate information communication technology (ICT) systems and solutions to facilitate the delivery of superior care, it is useful to model the scenario (Fig. 25.1) in terms of actor–network theory (ANT; Aarts and Koppel

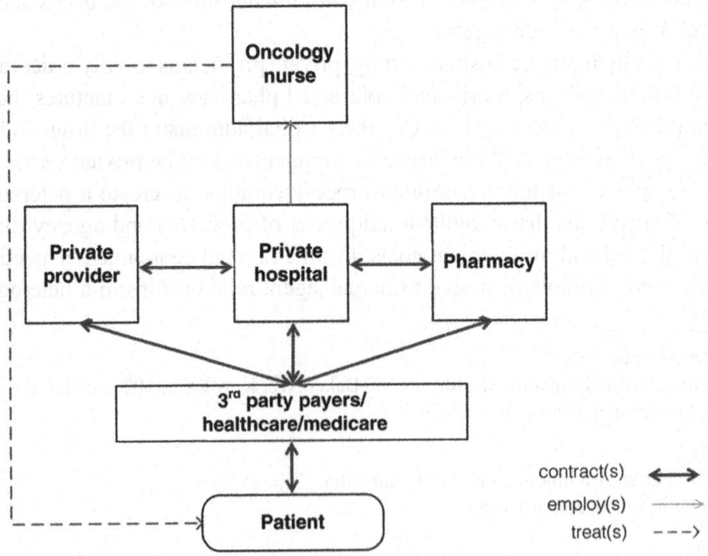

Fig. 25.1 Heterogeneous network for chemotherapy ordering

2009) and describe the relationships in terms of agency theory in the case of a knowledge worker (Aarts et al. 2007). The study involves three key phases as follows: Phase 1: an assessment of the existing technology applications at all ABC Hospital facilities and private physicians rooms with regard to the ordering of chemotherapy interventions as well as a mapping of all existing processes used in the ordering of chemotherapy interventions using the rich lens of ANT. In addition, this phase will require an in-depth analysis and synthesis of the relevant literature. Phase 2: an assessment of the specific benefits of the proposed ICT solution for this specific context as well as an assessment of the need for any process changes. Prior ICT experience of all professional staff will be assessed and their attitudes to ICT evaluated. Phase 3: recommendations and directives will be provided regarding the best way to move forward in trying to assimilate the system into the ABC Hospital context in order to realise maximum benefits and reduce any possible risks and potential barriers.

This study is assessing the benefits of a COS for the ABC Hospital context. To do this, we will focus on the following four propositions:

P1 The implementation of an organisation-wide COS to enable the ordering of chemotherapy drugs will enable higher goal-aligned behaviour according to recognised standards (Koppel 2005a; Koppel 2005b; Kotter and Schlesinger 1979) and better and safer health-care delivery.

P2 The implementation of an organisation-wide COS to enable the ordering of chemotherapy drugs will enable greater bonding activities[1] to ensue with knowledge work agents.

P3 The implementation of an organisation-wide COS to enable the ordering of chemotherapy drugs will enable better data collection and monitoring of principals and knowledge worker agents.

P4 The COS solution will enable stabilisation of the heterogeneous network.

Background

Australian health care contains two different sectors, private and public, with a different funding structure between these sectors. Recent developments have blurred this distinction a little, with private hospitals contracting to do public work and public hospitals accessing private health funds and the Medicare funding for a fee for service clinics. Nonetheless, for the purposes of analysis, the distinction is mostly valid. Private health care consists of not-for-profit and for-profit hospitals (Bloom 2002). The for-profit hospitals' primary goal is to generate profits for its shareholders. The not-for-profit hospitals, owned by religious, charity, and community organisations, are not primarily driven by profit but by committed agreements or values

[1] Bonding activities as described in agency theory pertain to non-monetary provisions given by the principle to the agent that serve to reduce frustrations and complications for agents such as a parking space or tools to make workflow and their job easier and more streamlined (Wickramasinghe 2000).

(Bloom 2002). This unique funding combination plus the mission to generate profit and achieve an acceptable return on investment determine that private hospitals must carefully plan and employ revenue as a strategic tool. Thus, they have to put their major focus on revenue that best suits their commercial and corporate objectives. This sometimes leads to less or no funding for information systems/information technology (IS/IT) investments (Leggat and Dwyer 2002).

However, research shows that using computerised systems can bring many benefits to hospitals and clinics as indicated by many researchers (Kaushal et al. 2003; Lin et al. 2014; Nolen and Rodes 2008; Redley and Botti 2013; Wickramasinghe 2013). However, new technology can contribute to system complexity and create unanticipated or new problems and opportunities for medication error (Aarts et al. 2007; Balkrishnan et al. 2009; Campbell et al. 2006; Kohn et al. 2000; Koppel 2005a; Koppel 2005b; Redley and Botti 2013), for example, human–machine interface errors and workflow problems. Further, as technology grows rapidly, system design and development at the time may have not included the new technology, features, and functions, which results in system/technology problems. The Y2K problem is a good example. System integration at the implementation is another concern to health-care organisations. Hospitals usually have many existing local/unit applications that are used for different purposes in diagnosis and treatments (Kaplan and Harris-Salamone 2009; Poon et al. 2004). Integration of the new system/solution with the existing application without affecting the workflow and creating too much extra burden to the existing operation is very important. Some system implementations went halfway and were aborted because of integration failure and workflow problems (Bloom 2002). A good system should be customised to fit the clinician's workflow and simplify and support their workflow, as recorded by Kaplan and Harris-Salamone (2009) in their research (Kaplan and Harris-Salamone 2009). Moreover, software applications may have not been fully tested and contain hidden bugs. It is reported that US Food and Drug Administration "data indicate that one in every three medical devices that makes use of software for its operation has been recalled due to failure in the software itself" (Jetley 2010). These incidences and concerns are alarms and risk factors one must consider when using an IS/IT solution such as COS.

Actor Network Theory

Actor–network theory (ANT) is a sociological theory developed by French sociologist Bruno Latour and Michel Callon and British sociologist John Law (Alchian and Demsetz 1972; Balkrishnan et al. 2009; Bloom 2002; Underwood and Richards 2013). The essence of this theory is that the world is constructed of hybrid entities (Alchian and Demsetz 1972) consisting of both human and non-human elements, for example, people, objects, and organisations known as actors or actants, and these elements cannot be studied in isolation or separately (Boyatzis 1998). ANT tries to bridge the gap between a sociotechnical divide. Emphasis is also placed on the concept of heterogeneous networks because of the non-similar nature of elements and their relationship in the network (Braithwaite et al. 2014; Campbell et al. 2006; Demsetz 1988). Using ANT, we model the context at the hospital regarding chemotherapy ordering.

Agency Theory

The primary focus of agency theory (Aarts et al. 2007; Fairbrother et al. 2014; Jensen and Meckling 1992) is the relationship between the principal and the agent as well as the achievement of goal-aligned behaviour. In health-care contexts, the agent is typically a knowledge worker agent such as a physician (Aarts et al. 2007; Jetley 2010), nurse, or pharmacist. In the private hospital sector, such as the ABC Hospital, there exist nested or multiple principal–agent relationships. Specifically, the principal requires certain specific tasks to be performed and hires knowledge worker agents (medical care professionals, who are experts with regard to these tasks) to perform them on his/her behalf. In so doing, however, the principal needs to guard against suboptimal behaviour (or low goal-aligned behaviour), that is, the divergence between the agent pursuing activities, which facilitate his/her own goals in contrast to the achievement of the principal's goals (Kaplan and Harris-Salamone 2009). ICTs in general have been shown to help reduce agency costs by enabling enhanced tacit monitoring and bonding activities as well as to enable effective and efficient operations to ensue in all areas but this is especially true in health-care contexts (Jetley 2010; Kaplan and Harris-Salamone 2009).

Overall, based on the extensive literature analysis, it is possible to identify the following key points in order to implement IS systems in health-care contexts (Table 25.1):

Conceptual Model

On combining the results from the preceding literature synthesis with an initial assessment of the data site(s), the following conceptual model was developed (Fig. 25.2). This figure serves to capture the environment and multiple actors. It is noted that COS has been defined as a computerised physician order entry COS to be consistent with the extant literature. The patient is at the centre to reflect a patient-centric view that is to be adopted at all times. Critical to an understanding of the proposed conceptual model is the defining and describing of the relevant clinical microsystems. Hospitals in many respects can be considered aggregations of clinical microsystems rather than more formal organisations in the conventional sense.

A clinical microsystem is defined as a small organised group of clinicians and staff working together with a shared clinical purpose to provide care for a defined set of patients. This conceptual model will be used to describe the delivery of chemotherapy services to cancer patients at the ABC Hospital and the impact that the introduction of a COS for chemotherapy will have on that care process. Critical processes are illustrated in Fig. 25.2 with a series of concentric hexagons which

Table 25.1 Key points in order to implement IS systems in health-care contexts

Key point	Description
Participation and involvement (Groene et al. 2014; Serapioni and Duxbury 2014; Waterson 2014)	In general, participation leads to commitment, not merely compliance (Kotter and Schlesinger 1979). Organised and scheduled resisters' participation can often forestall resistance. Participation and involvement can happen at any stage of the system development life cycle (SDLC) or project life cycle
Facilitation and support (Chaudhry et al. 2006; Waterson 2014)	It is very important that the leaders/managers are being supportive. It is most helpful when fear and anxiety lie at the heart of resistance (Bloom 2002). Support can be in many forms such as: training, giving time off, listening, providing emotional support, counselling, encouragement, etc.
Negotiation and agreement (Ludwick and Doucette 2009; Schmulson et al. 2014)	Negotiation is important in health-care IS/IT projects as it is a complex dynamic environment and it involves many players/actors, with each actor's focus on his/her own interests. Negotiation can be also used when it is clear that someone is going to lose out as a result of a change and this person/group's power to resist is significant (Bloom 2002). Negotiating written agreements can be a relatively easy way to avoid major resistance. Negotiation is particularly important with VMOs as they are not subject to the controls which an organisation has with salaried employees and there are always a number of different issues other than IT on which they must negotiate deals with hospitals which may become contemplated conflated with IT issues
Influences (Ludwick and Doucette 2009; Waterson 2014)	Give a group leader/manager or someone with respect a key role in design and implementation of the change. Consider using peer pressure before the change in plan. These actions can be an inexpensive and easy way to gain an individual's or a group's support (Bloom 2002)
Education and training (Chaudhry et al. 2006; Schmulson et al. 2014)	Educate people about the project beforehand and afterwards. An education and communication program is ideal when resistance is based on inadequate or inaccurate information and analysis, and when resister's help is needed in the implementation (Bloom 2002). Training programs must support different users and levels and should be ongoing
Communication (Carayon et al. 2014; Chaudhry et al. 2006; Kwamie et al. 2014)	This helps people see the need and logic for a change. Communication methods can be one-to-one discussions, presentations, memos, reports, briefings, focus groups, announcements, posters, emails, intranet and internet posting, etc.
Identify and mitigate risks (Chaudhry et al. 2006; Schneider et al. 2014)	Identify all the risks early, consider and analyse them deeply throughout all stages of the project. Indicate possible ways to mitigate the risks. Document in detail on risk description, category, cause, triggers, level of impact, probability, potential responses, risk owner, progress status (Schwalbe 2013)
Learn from the past and others (Ludwick and Doucette 2009; Schmulson et al. 2014)	Studying the success and failures can help prevent and avoid mistakes in conjunction with turning a bad situation around

IS/IT information systems/information technology, *VMO* visiting medical officer

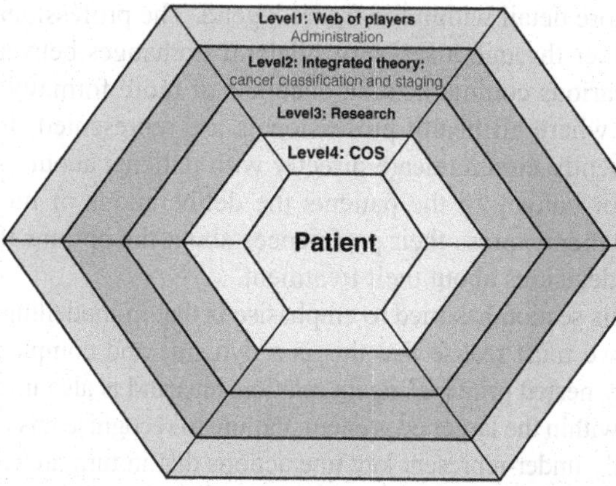

Fig. 25.2 Conceptual model. *Level 1—professional staff-web of players*: (1.1) *nursing staff*—the nurses receive a chemotherapy order from the cancer specialist, educate the patient, and deliver the chemotherapy to the patient (1.2) *pharmacy staff*—they received the chemotherapy order from the doctor and make up the chemotherapy in a form suitable for administration to the patient. They provide an educational resource to both the patient and other staff (1.3) *diagnostic services*—These include the pathology for blood tests and radiology for medical imaging. Pathology services are particularly important in the chemotherapy prescribing as it is necessary for the blood tests to be at a certain level before chemotherapy can be administered (1.4) *medical staff*—these include specialists and registrars and other staff in training. The types of specialists involved in the chemotherapy prescribing are usually either medical oncologists or haematologists but other specialists may use chemotherapy drugs for non-malignant disease which are usually then administered in the same place, that is, day stay oncology where cancer patients are treated with chemotherapy. An important distinction in this particular project is between the types of employment of specialist medical staff. All specialist medical staff at the ABC Hospital involved in cancer services are visiting medical officers (VMOs) who are not employees and over whom there is limited administrative control in most public sector organisations and medical staff who are salaried specialists and are employed by the hospital (1.5) *supportive care staff*—this includes dieticians, social workers, and psychologists (1.6) *administration*—this includes local clerical administrative staff who operate in day stay oncology as well as higher level managers throughout the organisation. *Level 2—integrated theory:* (2.1) *cancer classification and staging*—this is the process by which the cancer is classified and staged (extent) according to internationally recognised systems for this process. Oncology protocols (see below) are selected based on this classification. (2.2) *oncology protocols* (chemotherapy)—these are drug orders that specify the dose, frequency, duration, and route of drug administration with individual doses calculated for a particular patient based on patient parameters like height, body weight, renal function, or some other parameter on some patient parameter. Treatment may be multimodality, in that other treatment modalities like surgery and radiotherapy are given concurrently with or sequentially with chemotherapy. These are specified in the protocol. (2.3) *information science theories* (2.4) *design science* (2.5) *management* (2.6) *quality objectives*—the subheadings below are usually considered components of quality which is therefore made a major heading—this section requires numeric notation, and given that it is the primary objective of the system, it requires more prominence—I'm not sure how to represent this diagrammatically. *Level 3—researches (this is out of scope for the present study but noted for completeness): Level 4—COS:*—COS is the outcome of the process and is a document which is an accurate and legal drug order. Excess emphasis should not be placed on the document per se as it needs to be interpreted in the context of a complex inter-professional process, partly written, partly

are described in more detail within the figure legend. The professional processes is operationalised either through a series of bilateral exchanges between health-care professionals by various communication channels or more formally in a multidisciplinary meeting where all health professionals are represented. Individual professionals subsequently communicate directly with patients about aspects of their professional role or convey to the patients the deliberations of multidisciplinary meetings. Patients then express their preferences about the options they have been offered and make decisions about their treatment.

Overall, what this section has tried to emphasise is that in modelling the actors and their integrations, we must realise that this is a dynamic and complex environment. Further, it has many nested principal–agent relationships and is also impacted upon by exogenous factors within the larger ecosystem. Failure to recognise this complexity will serve to dramatically under-represent key interactions that in turn are relevant and impact the well-functioning of the technology solutions. Finally, while beyond the scope of the present study, it is also important to be cognizant of the wider health ecosystem which includes international and national policy, health-care systems as well as laws and regulations, since these will also have far-reaching flow-on effects to the COS, its successful implementation, adoption, and ongoing use.

Research Method

As the COS is one of the ABC Hospital-wide projects, the setting includes all hospital facilities that treat oncology patients with chemotherapy. Participants/key informants will include all individuals who will interact with the system such as private physicians, oncology nurses, pharmacy, and consumers. Participation is voluntary. Recruitment is done via email and mail to:

a. Make the relevant individuals aware of the study and
b. Request their participation.

The study adopts a primarily qualitative approach using semi-structured interviews, focus groups, and survey techniques to gather critical information and a questionnaire designed and developed in Germany specifically to assess usability and acceptance of technology in health-care contexts.

---

oral, and heavily influenced by traditional professional roles. It is a very important intermediate outcome but the ultimate outcome is the outcome for the patient as a result of the protocol administration which will not be specifically addressed in this project. *Level 5*—the patient. We note that this part of the diagram is underdeveloped. Although this is not the primary focus of this research project, we need to recognise significant developments in health generally, and particularly the concept of patient-centredness; hence, the reason for placing the patient in the middle. Integral to this is that the patient needs to be seen within a series of concentric circles with them at the centre, their immediate carers in the next circle, their community in the next circle, and their society in the outer circle

Analysis: As noted above, this is a predominantly qualitative study; thus, standard qualitative analysis techniques such as content analysis and thematic analysis are employed to analyse the collected data (Kaushal et al. 2003; Kohn et al. 2000; Koppel 2005a; Koppel 2005b). Literature, in particular ANT and agency theory, serves to inform the design of the priori themes. From the questionnaire, it is possible to run simple frequency and regression analyses that serve to confirm prevalence of themes. To help illustrate the impact of COS and the interaction between different stakeholders and the COS system, an online survey was designed to target three categories of health-care professionals and executives as follows:

1. Oncologists: 25 were targeted
2. Executives and non-users, but have access to the system: 9
3. COS users: 53 (defined as COS users comprising nursing, pharmacy, and administrative staff using COS to schedule or reference chemotherapy appointments)

Breaking the targeted respondents into these three categories helped understand the specific level to which each group deals with the system and the type and quality of this interaction, which was quite interesting. Insights generated from this survey form the basis of data analysed in this chapter.

Results

The highest response rate to the survey was 56% and resulted from the executives and non-users category, which indicates the level to which these executives were engaged with the implementation of COS at the ABC Hospital. Oncologists responded to the survey with a rate of 36%, which also indicates their level of interest in the system. The lowest rate was from the COS users categories with about 10%. This unexpected finding needs a deeper analysis of the responses to better understand COS user interaction which we plan to embark upon. It is noted that in viewing and interpreting the following, it is important to keep in mind respective user response rates to determine overall significance. Demographic and professional insights are presented in Table 25.2.

Having these demographic and professional insights as well as the way the respondents looked at computers for daily work helps to understand the following responses in three main areas of interest: user satisfaction, compatibility of the system, and expectations from this system.

- User satisfaction
  First, the survey asked the respondents how often they use the COS system for daily work. As would be expected, most of the respondents from oncologists and COS users stated they used the system several times a day, or daily, while less usage by executives was identified. Figure 25.3 provides a summary of usage by respondent groups.

Table 25.2 Demographic and professional insights

Key items	Descriptions/information
Gender	Females: 60 % of the respondents from users and executives categories
	Males: 88.9 % of the respondents from oncologists
Age	33–39: 44.4 %
	40–49: 11.1 %
	50–59: 22.2 %
	60–69: 22.2 %
Work experience	Work experience was measured by two measures; the first was the number of years at the ABC Hospital, and the second in how many organizations in the health sector people had previously worked. The answers for both measures were broadly diverse, with a tendency to long working years at the hospital and more health-care organizations previously worked at for oncologists, less years and less health-care organizations previously worked at for users, and more places previously worked at and relatively long years of work at the ABC Hospital for executives
Use of computer	All respondents from all categories felt comfortable and very comfortable with respect to using computers in general, with the majority feeling very comfortable. All respondents reported that they utilised computers during work very often, that is, more than five times per day. Answering questions indicates the advanced level of computer skills and use for all respondents, but does not reflect the significance of computers for daily work

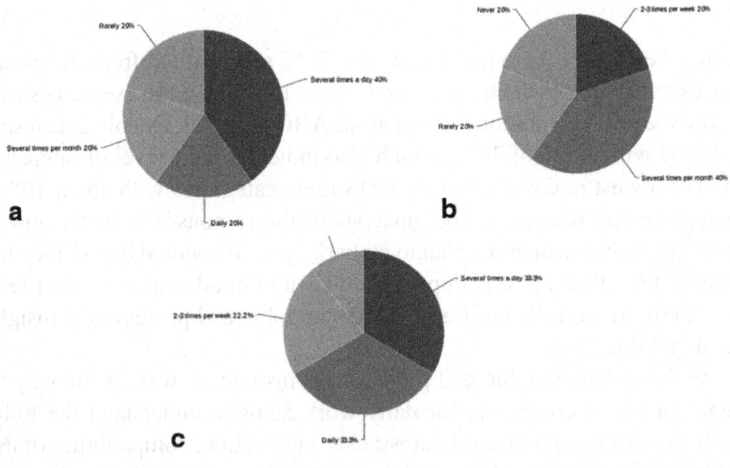

Fig. 25.3 Chemotherapy ordering system (COS) usage by: **a** COS users **b** Executives **c** Oncologists

- Compatibility of the system:
  In this section, respondents were asked about the COS system, from the perspective of core functionality. In doing so, the respondents evaluated the system in four main statements included:

1. The COS will support decision-making (reminders and warnings/alerts)
2. The COS will help preventing medication errors
3. The COS will provide an appropriate overview over the current patient situation and the daily treatment activities
4. The COS will help to improve the quality of care outcomes

The responses in general were positive across the three respondents' categories, with a few sceptical responses from the oncologists group as Table 25.3 shows. In the COS users group, all answers fell between 50/50 correct and correct, with majority tending to be correct and mostly correct. Almost the same pattern can be seen in the executives and non-users group. The responses from oncologists took a different pattern, in which the evaluations of the abovementioned statements varied from N/A to correct (Table 25.3).

- Expectations of the system
  This part of the survey forms the basis upon which better understanding of the interaction between different stakeholders and the COS could be achieved. To do so, respondents from the three groups of respondents answered questions in four main interrelated areas:

1. The role of COS
2. How COS can help do the job and its related activities
3. How to maximize the benefits of the COS system
4. How COS can enhance the job and its related activities
5. Comments

The main comments from the three groups of respondents were about the need for more bedside computers, new policies, sufficient training, more details about the system and how it works, and finally a stronger commitment from the ABC Hospital to the project as whole. Table 25.4 summarises the main themes and points for the expectations of COS by the three targeted groups (Table 25.4).

Table 25.3 The core functionality of the chemotherapy ordering system (COS) as oncologists see it

	N/A	Incorrect	Mostly incorrect	50/50	Mostly correct	Correct
1. The COS will support decision-making (reminders and warnings/alerts)	1 11.1%	0 0.0%	0 0.0%	3 33.3%	2 22.2%	3 33.3%
2. The COS will help in preventing medication errors	1 11.1%	0 0.0%	0 0.0%	1 11.1%	3 33.3%	4 44.4%
3. The COS will provide an appropriate overview over the current patient situation and the daily treatment activities	1 11.1%	1 11.1%	0 0.0%	1 11.1%	4 44.4%	2 22.2%
4. The COS will help to improve the quality of care outcomes	1 11.1%	1 11.1%	0 0.0%	2 22.2%	2 22.2%	3 33.3%

COS chemotherapy ordering system

Table 25.4 Expectations of chemotherapy operating systems (COS) as the survey revealed

Area of interest	Executives and non-users	Oncologists	Users
Concerns about the role of COS	Change management	Inflexibility	Ease of use
	Commitment of nursing and pharmacy staff to the system	Compatibility with current systems	Reliability
		Lack of control of chemotherapy ordering	Availability
How COS can help do the job and its related activities	Easy to ACCURATELY order infusions		
	Reduces errors and confusion in ordering the chemotherapy		
	Reminders for doses and treatments		
	Gives timely access to patients records		
	Increases work efficiency		
	Enables us to monitor the usage of this system	Enables improved patient care	Helps adhere to guidelines/protocols
	Enables the review of unexpected readmissions	No need to make templates for new chemotherapies for patients	Supports regimen provisions
	Helps allocate resources		Professionalises the job
	Provides important data about scheduling and other clinical outcomes data		
	Standardises the processes around medication management and nursing care delivery		
	Enables urgent clinical decision-making		
How to maximise the benefits of the COS system	The system has to be:		
	Intuitive	Compatible with current software and IS systems	Easy to use
	Support clinical workflow	Flexible	Available online for users
	Accurate	Able to generate data and send it to other database management systems	Aligned to national and international standards
	Support evidence-based medicine	Benchmarking enabler	24/7 available
	Technically supported by ITS and the vendor		

Table 25.4 (continued)

Area of interest	Executives and non-users	Oncologists	Users
	Well-taught and trained before use		
	Resourced from an oncology pharmacy perspective		
	Used by all nursing, medical specialists and practice managers at a very early stage		
How COS can enhance the job and its related activities	Enhancing clinical processes and patient safety	Being easy, fast, and simple to learn and use	Adhering to policies, protocols, and guidelines
	Reducing medication errors	Accurate	Enabling an online access to medical records
	Establishing best practice therapies	Improves communications and workflow	Enduring consistent processes
	Enabling clinicians to monitor their patients' records online	Improves reporting and recoding hospital-wide	
Comments	Painless project	Lack of details on how it works	Huge change process
	Less commitments from the ABC Hospital side		More bedside computers are required
			Policies are needed

COS chemotherapy ordering system, *IS* information systems, *ITS* information technology services

Taken together, the results from the survey as well as the invaluable lessons learned from the phase 1 implementation show the importance and need for COS at the ABC Hospital. However, it also serves to highlight critical success factors that must be considered if the full potential of the solution is to be realised at the ABC Hospital. In particular, the following must be addressed:

1. Need to examine existing processes, policies, and protocols and determine if there are possibilities to streamline and improve, standardise across all locations, and perhaps even embrace lean and six sigma principles.
2. Need to engage all clinicians and develop appropriate strategies to foster Visiting Medical Officer (VMO) sponsorship. Further, this must be addressed early to ensure optimal clinical support.
3. Need to ensure smooth assimilation of solution, appropriate level of support, training, and assistance.
4. Need to ensure correct, complete, and accurate data capture, transfer which in turn will also support future analytic potential, and seamless knowledge management.

Discussion

In this study, data analysis suggests that there are still many areas that need to be addressed before it will be possible to see germane and tangible changes to the underlying goal-aligned behaviours. This indicates that having the systems is a necessary but not sufficient requirement to enhancing the consequent goal-aligned behaviour. In order to engage users, it is important to ensure strong goal alignment between their tasks and their interactions with the system and the hospital's goals and objectives. While the answer is simple to realise, in practice, it is not. In particular, it requires engagement with user training as well as effecting appropriate change management and organisation culture/subculture modification changes. This in turn requires strong leadership and a project champion who is credible and respected by the clinical users. Key barriers, facilitators, and recommendations captured by this study are summarised in Table 25.5:

An important yet unexpected finding that emerged is that key barriers, facilitators, and recommendations captured on this study can be also used for implementing a computerised physician order entry (CPOE) system as well. CPOE systems are widely viewed as crucial for reducing prescribing errors and saving hundreds of billions in annual costs (Potts et al. 2004). These systems are expected to become more prevalent in response to resident working hour limitations and related care discontinuities and will supposedly offset causes (e.g., job dissatisfaction) and effects (e.g., ADEs) of nursing shortages (Alsweed et al. 2014; Berger and Kichak 2004).

Overall, the study served to demonstrate that the COS is of tremendous benefit to support and facilitate its delivery of excellence in care for oncology and directly aligns with the ABC Hospital's strategic priorities.

Conclusions

This study set out to answer specific research questions and address four key propositions. At this point in the assimilation of COS at the ABC Hospital, it is not possible to definitively refute or uphold these propositions; however, directional data to date suggests that all propositions are likely to be upheld. With regard to the propositions, a summary of our findings is presented in Table 25.6.

Further, in trying to answer the posed research questions, several key findings have been unearthed and significant recommendations developed. It is apparent for the study that COS holds many potential benefits to the ABC Hospital, not just in the short term but possibly more importantly in the longer term. This necessitates prudent and thoughtful assimilation so that it will be possible to realise these benefits. Furthermore, it has been noted that the full potential of COS at the hospital cannot ensue unless the six significant recommendations are embraced.

In closing, it is essential to take a holistic perspective when considering COS at the hospital. This includes adequate attention to the health ecosystem, the system structure, the delivery operations as well as the clinical structure. Further, these must be thought of simultaneously in terms of strategic, infrastructure, transitional, and

Table 25.5 Barriers, facilitators, and recommendations captured

Key barriers
Barriers should be considered in terms of people, process, and technology issues:
1. People
a. Lack of engagement
b. Poor or insufficient back fill of staff duties
c. Poor alignment of user goals with hospital goals and objectives
2. Process
a. Complex and time consuming
b. Data and information incorrect or incomplete
c. Unfamiliarity and lack of understanding of all user needs
3. Technology
a. Technical problems
b. Poor ease-of-use
c. Complex
Key facilitators
To address the aforementioned barriers, the following facilitators are suggested. However, it is noted that to be successful, strong commitment to providing these facilitators is essential:
1. Training and maintenance
2. Back fill and time provided to learn and familiarise oneself to the system
3. Introduce change management and culture/subculture change processes
4. Explore and introduce business process re-engineering (BPR), six sigma, and lean principles
5. Ensure data and information integrity and that all data is entered once but can be reused often with confidence
6. Ensure the system is user as well as organisation-centred and subscribes to a patient-centric delivery of care paradigm
Recommendations
1. Participation and engagement of all stakeholders is a critical success factor
2. Assimilation of COS should also be user-centred not just organisation-centred and subscribe to a patient-centric delivery of care paradigm
3. Ensure protocols are in place and users are trained in these protocols so that data capture is accurate and complete, that is, captured once correctly it is useful on multiple occasions with confidence
4. Perform BPR and incorporate lean and six sigma principles to ensure processes are streamlined and supportive of optimal use of the system
5. Include change management into the training
6. Recognise the dynamic nature of health care and the importance of oncology services at the ABC Hospital, build into the ongoing plans a future-oriented mindset to strategically leverage data captured, and harness the potential of business intelligence and/or business analytic capabilities to support continued best practice and state-of-the-art research

informatics perspectives. Ultimately, the potential to improve cancer care through health information technology necessitates the adoption of a learning health-care IT system (de Moor et al. 2013). It has been noted by scholars that creating such a learning cancer care system might initially be slow to evolve but its benefits are far-researching and significant (Bloom 2002). COS provides private health-care sectors with this possibility and it would behoove them to seize this opportunity.

Table 25.6 Summary of the study findings regarding the propositions

Propositions	Support from findings
P1: The implementation of an organisation-wide COS to enable the ordering of chemotherapy drugs will enable higher goal-aligned behaviour according to recognised standards (Koppel 2005a; Koppel 2005b; Kotter and Schlesinger 1979) and better and safer healthcare delivery	The implementation of the COS is not sufficient to enable higher goal-aligned behaviour to ensue. Change management and activities designed to fully engage oncologists and COS users are also required
P2: The implementation of an organisation-wide COS to enable the ordering of chemotherapy drugs will enable greater bonding activities to ensue with knowledge work agents	At this stage, it would appear that P2 is upheld. But a better assessment needs to occur after more than 1 year of using the COS
P3: The implementation of an organisation-wide COS to enable the ordering of chemotherapy drugs will enable better data collection and monitoring of principals knowledge worker agents	Indeed, the COS system does enable better data capture and monitoring
P4: The COS solution will enable stabilisation of the heterogeneous network	It is too early to state if the heterogeneous network is more stable; again, this needs to be assessed after at least 1 year of use

References

Aarts, J., & Koppel, R. (2009). Implementation of computerized physician order entry in seven countries. *Health Affairs, 28*(2), 404–414.

Aarts, J., Ash, J., & Berg, M. (2007). Extending the understanding of computerized physician order entry: Implications for professional collaboration, workflow and quality of care. *International Journal of Medical Informatics, 76,* S4–S13.

Alchian, A. A., & Demsetz, H. (1972). Production, information costs, and economic organization. *The American Economic Review,* 777–795.

Alsweed, F., Alshaikh, A., Ahmed, A., Yunus, F., & Househ, M. (2014). Impact of computerised provider order entry system on nursing workflow, patient safety, and medication errors: Perspectives from the front line. *International Journal of Electronic Healthcare, 7*(4), 287–300.

Balkrishnan, R., Foss, C. E., Pawaskar, M., Uhas, A. A., & Feldman, S. R. (2009). Monitoring for medication errors in outpatient settings. *Journal of Dermatological Treatment, 20*(4), 229–232.

Berger, R. G., & Kichak, J. (2004). Computerized physician order entry: Helpful or harmful? *Journal of the American Medical Informatics Association, 11*(2), 100–103.

Bloom, A. L. (2002). The funding of private hospitals in Australia. *Australian Health Review, 25*(1), 19–39.

Boyatzis, R. E. (1998). *Transforming qualitative information: Thematic analysis and code development.* Thousand Oaks: Sage Publications.

Braithwaite, J., Marks, D., & Taylor, N. (2014). Harnessing implementation science to improve care quality and patient safety: A systematic review of targeted literature. *International Journal for Quality in Health Care, 26,* 312–329.

Campbell, E. M., Sittig, D. F., Ash, J. S., Guappone, K. P., & Dykstra, R. H. (2006). Types of unintended consequences related to computerized provider order entry. *Journal of the American Medical Informatics Association, 13*(5), 547–556.

Carayon, P., Wetterneck, T. B., Rivera-Rodriguez, A. J., Hundt, A. S., Hoonakker, P., Holden, R., et al. (2014). Human factors systems approach to healthcare quality and patient safety. *Applied Ergonomics, 45*(1), 14–25.

Chaudhry, B., Wang, J., Wu, S., Maglione, M., Mojica, W., Roth, E., et al. (2006). Systematic review: Impact of health information technology on quality, efficiency, and costs of medical care. *Annals of Internal Medicine, 144*(10), 742–752.

de Moor, J. S., Mariotto, A. B., Parry, C., Alfano, C. M., Padgett, L., Kent, E. E., et al. (2013). Cancer survivors in the United States: Prevalence across the survivorship trajectory and implications for care. *Cancer Epidemiology Biomarkers & Prevention, 22*(4), 561–570.

Demsetz, H. (1988). The theory of the firm revisited. *Journal of Law, Economics, & Organization, 4,* 141–161.

Fairbrother, G., Trudnak, T., Christopher, R., Mansour, M., & Mandel, K. (2014). Cincinnati Beacon Community Program highlights challenges and opportunities on the path to care transformation. *Health Affairs, 33*(5), 871–877.

Groene, O., Sunol, R., Klazinga, N. S., Wang, A., Dersarkissian, M., Thompson, C. A., et al. (2014). Involvement of patients or their representatives in quality management functions in EU hospitals: Implementation and impact on patient-centred care strategies. *International Journal for Quality in Health Care, 26*(suppl 1), 81–91.

Jensen, M., & Meckling, W. (1992). Specific and general knowledge and organizational structure. http://papers.ssrn.com/abstract=6658. Accessed Dec 2014.

Jetley, R. (2010). FDA Recommends Static Analysis for Medical Devices.

Kaplan, B., & Harris-Salamone, K. D. (2009). Health IT success and failure: Recommendations from literature and an AMIA workshop. *Journal of the American Medical Informatics Association, 16*(3), 291–299.

Kaushal, R., Shojania, K. G., & Bates, D. W. (2003). Effects of computerized physician order entry and clinical decision support systems on medication safety: A systematic review. *Archives of Internal Medicine, 163*(12), 1409–1416.

Kohn, L. T., Corrigan, J. M., & Donaldson, M. S. (2000). *To err is human: Building a safer health system*. Washington, DC: National Academies Press.

Koppel, R. (2005a). Computerized physician order entry systems: The right prescription? *LDI Issue Brief, 10*(5), 1–4.

Koppel, R. (2005b). What do we know about medication errors made via a CPOE system versus those made via handwritten orders? *Critical Care-London, 9*(5), 427.

Kotter, J. P., & Schlesinger, L. A. (1979). Choosing strategies for change, *Harvard Business Review*.

Kwamie, A., van Dijk, H., & Agyepong, I. A. (2014). Advancing the application of systems thinking in health: realist evaluation of the Leadership Development Programme for district manager decision-making in Ghana. *Health Research Policy and Systems*, 12(29), 10.1186.

Leggat, S., & Dwyer, J. (2002). Innovation in Australian hospitals. *Australian Health Review, 25*(5), 19.

Lin, C. H., Yang, A. W. H., Pittayachawan, S., Vogel, D., & Wickramasinghe, N. (2014). *Investigating the possibility for IS/IT to support the delivery of Chinese medicine*. Proceedings of the first AIS-journals joint author workshop in ECIS, Tel Aviv, Israel 2014.

Ludwick, D. A., & Doucette, J. (2009). Adopting electronic medical records in primary care: Lessons learned from health information systems implementation experience in seven countries. *International Journal of Medical Informatics, 78*(1), 22–31.

Nolen, A. L., & Rodes, W. D. (2008). Bar-code medication administration system for anesthetics: Effects on documentation and billing. *American Journal of Health-System Pharmacy, 65*(7), 655–659.

Poon, E. G., Blumenthal, D., Jaggi, T., Honour, M. M., Bates, D. W., & Kaushal, R. (2004). Overcoming barriers to adopting and implementing computerized physician order entry systems in US hospitals. *Health Affairs, 23*(4), 184–190.

Potts, A. L., Barr, F. E., Gregory, D. F., Wright, L., & Patel, N. R. (2004). Computerized physician order entry and medication errors in a pediatric critical care unit. *Pediatrics, 113*(1), 59–63.

Redley, B., & Botti, M. (2013). Reported medication errors after introducing an electronic medication management system. *Journal of Clinical Nursing, 22*(3–4), 579–589.

Schmulson, M., Corazziari, E., Ghoshal, U., Myung, S. J., Gerson, C., Quigley, E., et al. (2014). A four-country comparison of healthcare systems, implementation of diagnostic criteria, and treatment availability for functional gastrointestinal disorders. *Neurogastroenterology & Motility, 26*(10), 1368–1385.

Schneider, E. C., Ridgely, M. S., Meeker, D., Hunter, L. E., Khodyakov, D., Rudin, R., et al. (2014). *Promoting patient safety through effective health information technology risk management*. Santa Monica: RAND.

Schwalbe, K. (2013). *Information technology project management*. Cengage Learning. https://cengage.com.au/product/title/information-technology-project-management/isbn/9781133526885. Accessed Dec 2014.

Serapioni, M., & Duxbury, N. (2014). Citizens' participation in the Italian health-care system: The experience of the mixed advisory committees. *Health Expectations, 17*(4), 488–499.

Underwood, A. A., & Richards, S. D. (2013). Context is everything. *Civil Engineering-ASCE, 83*(3), 68–71.

Waterson, P. (2014). Health information technology and sociotechnical systems: A progress report on recent developments within the UK National Health Service (NHS). *Applied Ergonomics, 45*(2), 150–161.

Wickramasinghe, N. (2000). IS/IT as a tool to achieve goal alignment. *International Journal of Healthcare Technology and Management, 2*(1), 163–180.

Wickramasinghe, N. (2013). Implicit and explicit knowledge assets in healthcare. In Bali et al. (Eds.), *Pervasive knowledge management* (pp. 15–26). New York: Springer.

Prof. Nilmini Wickramasinghe (Ph.D.; M.B.A.; Grad.Dip.Mgt.St.; B.Sc.; Amus.A, piano; Amus.A, violin) has a well-recognised research record in the field of health care and IT/IS. Her expertise is in the strategic application and management of technology for effecting superior health-care solutions. She currently is the professor director of Health Informatics Management at Epworth HealthCare and a professor at Deakin University.

Peter Haddad is working towards his Ph.D. from Deakin University, Australia. He is involved in different research projects that concentrate on IS/IT in health care. Mr. Haddad comes from an engineering management background and has over 12 years' experience in this area, both in academic and professional contexts.

Dr. Stephen Vaughan is the director of the Cancer Services Clinical Institute at Epworth HealthCare. He conducts a part-time practice as a locum consultant physician in haematology/medical oncology in various public and private clinics throughout Victoria and New South Wales. He has also worked as a consultant to the Health Insurance Commission on high-cost drugs and for the Department of Health and Human Services on pathology accreditation. Dr. Vaughan was previously a director of the Peter MacCallum Cancer Institute and a member of its Research Advisory and Ethics committees.

Erratum to: Satisfaction with Health Informatics System Characteristics and Their Effect on Openness to Frequent Use

Karoly Bozan and Pratim Datta

Erratum to:
Chapter 7 in: N. Wickramasinghe et al. (eds.), *Contemporary Consumer Health Informatics*, Healthcare Delivery in the Information Age,
DOI 10.1007/978-3-319-25973-4_7

The publisher regrets to inform that the name of the co-author (Pratim Datta) of Chapter 7 was missing in ToC and in the Chapter opening page of the print and online versions of the book. His affiliation and bio have been updated in the original chapter and are mentioned below:

Pratim Datta Kent State University College of Business Administration, P.O. Box 5190, Terrace Drive, Kent, OH 44242, USA

Pratim Datta (Ph.D.) is a two-time Farris Family Research Innovation Fellow and an Associate Professor of IS and Supply Chains at Kent State University. Ranked among the top 40 researchers internationally, Datta has over 55 journal articles and conference proceedings with multiple best paper awards. Datta focuses on IS and supply chain use, performance and security as well as cross-functional corporate decision-making. He has won the Paul Pfeiffer Professional and Teaching Award. He has also received the Outstanding MBA Professor Award and he is the showcased professor for the Executive MBA Program.

The online version of the original chapter can be found under
DOI 10.1007/978-3-319-25973-4_7

K. Bozan (✉)
Office: Room 540, 921 South 8th Avenue, Pocatello, ID 83209, USA
e-mail: bozakaro@isu.edu

P. Datta
Kent State University College of Business Administration, P.O. Box 5190,
Terrace Drive, Kent, OH 44242, USA
e-mail: pdatta@kent.edu

N. Wickramasinghe et al. (eds.), *Contemporary Consumer Health Informatics*,
Healthcare Delivery in the Information Age, DOI 10.1007/978-3-319-25973-4_26

Epilogue

The proceeding has served to provide an indication of the breadth of the nascent field of consumer health informatics (CHI). Clearly, it is not possible to cover all areas in one publication but we have tried to highlight key aspects including the major technologies such as mobile, social media and other Internet based solutions. We have also tried to illustrate critical considerations for success which cover people, process and technology aspects as well as highlight some domains where CHI appears to be especially relevant including nursing and oncology.

Our primary goal has been to provide the reader with a solid grounding and a basic understanding of central issues, major areas of debate and discourse as well as highlight new opportunities. The digital economy is in its infancy but as it matures so too will the opportunities for CHI. We hope this book assists our readers to be prepared and ready so they can actively participate in future research and the further defining of this domain.

The Editors
Nilmini, Indrit and Joseph

N. Wickramasinghe et al. (eds.), *Contemporary Consumer Health Informatics*, Healthcare Delivery in the Information Age, DOI 10.1007/978-3-319-25973-4

Index

N. Wickramasinghe et al. (eds.), *Contemporary Consumer Health Informatics*, Healthcare Delivery in the Information Age, DOI 10.1007/978-3-319-25973-4

Printed in the United States
By Bookmasters